Hendee's Radiation Therapy Physics

Hendee's Radiation Therapy Physics

Fourth Edition

Todd Pawlicki PhD, FAAPM

Professor and Vice-Chair
Department of Radiation Medicine and Applied Sciences
University of California, San Diego, CA

Daniel J. Scanderbeg PhD

Associate Professor
Department of Radiation Medicine and Applied Sciences
University of California, San Diego, CA

George Starkschall PhD, FACMP, FAAPM, FACR

Research Professor
Department of Radiation Physics
Division of Radiation Oncology
The University of Texas MD Anderson Cancer Center
Houston, TX

WILEY Blackwell

Published by John Wiley & Sons, Inc., Hoboken, New Jersey
Published simultaneously in Canada

For general information on our other products and services or for technical support, please contact our Customer Care Department within the United States at (800) 762-2974, outside the United States at (317) 572-3993 or fax (317) 572-4002.

Wiley also publishes its books in a variety of electronic formats. Some content that appears in print may not be available in electronic formats. For more information about Wiley products, visit our web site at www.wiley.com.

Library of Congress Cataloging-in-Publication Data

Names: Pawlicki, Todd, author. — Scanderbeg, Daniel J., author. — Starkschall, George, author. — Hendee, William R. Radiation therapy physics. Preceded by (work):

Title: Hendee's radiation therapy physics / Todd Pawlicki, Daniel J. Scanderbeg, George Starkschall.

Other titles: Radiation therapy physics

Description: Fourth edition. — Hoboken, New Jersey : John Wiley & Sons, Inc., [2016] — Preceded by Radiation therapy physics / William R. Hendee, Geoffrey S. Ibbott, Eric G. Hendee. 3rd ed. c2005. — Includes bibliographical references and index.

Identifiers: LCCN 2015039643 — ISBN 9780470376515 (cloth)

Subjects: — MESH: Radiotherapy. — Physics.

Classification: LCC RM849 — NLM WN 250 — DDC 615.8/42–dc23 LC record available at http://lccn.loc.gov/2015039643

Printed in Singapore by C.O.S. Printers Pte Ltd

10 9 8 7 6 5 4 3 2 1

CONTENTS

PREFACE TO THE FOURTH EDITION

Over ten years ago, the third edition of *Radiation Therapy Physics* was published. Since that time, the discipline of radiation therapy physics has undergone many changes. To cite just a few examples: intensity-modulated radiation therapy (IMRT) has become a routine method of radiation treatment delivery; real-time, or at least near-time, imaging has led to the frequent use of image-guided radiation therapy (IGRT); digital imaging has replaced film-screen imaging for localization and verification; protons have become a viable mode of radiation therapy in many radiation therapy centers; new approaches have been introduced to radiation therapy quality assurance, focusing more on process analysis than on specific performance testing; and the explosion in patient- and machine-related data has necessitated an increased awareness of the role of informatics in radiation therapy. The list could go on and on, resulting in the conclusion that an up-to-date edition of *Radiation Therapy Physics* is needed at this time, and should include information about all of these developments.

Another major change in medical physics has been the retirement of Bill Hendee, principal author of the first three editions of this book, from active involvement in medical physics. Consequently, new authors have been recruited to carry on the tradition of *Radiation Therapy Physics*. Recognizing Bill Hendee's tremendous influence on medical physics and this textbook, in particular, the title of the book has been changed to *Hendee's Radiation Therapy Physics*. Dr. Hendee's influence is felt throughout this textbook.

Several significant changes have been made in the book to reflect the changes in medical physics that have occurred since publication of the previous edition. Some of the existing chapters have been modified, most notably the chapter on imaging, which now reflects the diminished role of film and conventional simulation and the increased role of digital imaging and computed tomography (CT) simulation. New chapters have been added to include topics such as image-guided therapy, proton radiation therapy, radiation therapy informatics, and quality and safety improvement, all of which now play an important role in radiation therapy physics.

Furthermore, we have elected to narrow the target audience somewhat. Rather than make this textbook a source for a broad audience that includes medical physics graduate students, radiation oncology residents, and medical dosimetry students, we are focusing our attention on radiation oncology residents; our experience has shown that a single textbook cannot meet all targets. Adequate rigor in a physics text designed to be useful for medical physicist graduate students is likely to turn off most medical residents, who do not have the same quantitative background possessed by a medical physics graduate student. We have tried to make the material accessible but of a sufficient depth that the interested medical resident can pursue an understanding of the material at the fundamental level. We also hope, however, that medical physics students and medical dosimetry students may find this book a useful supplement to their studies.

Finally, the authors wish to acknowledge colleagues who have contributed greatly to this book, with both materials as well as useful discussion. GS wishes to express his thanks to colleagues at The University of Texas MD Anderson Cancer Center, in particular Dr. Peter Balter, who provided much of the material in the chapter on basics of imaging, and Dr. Narayan Sahoo, who provided much of the material in the chapter on proton radiation therapy. TP and DJS wish to thank their colleagues at The University of California, San Diego.

And lastly, we would all like to thank our families for their understanding and support during the many hours we have spent away from them working on the fourth edition of this textbook.

Todd Pawlicki, PhD
Daniel J. Scanderbeg, PhD
San Diego, CA

George Starkschall, PhD
Houston, TX

PREFACE TO THE THIRD EDITION

When Geoff Ibbott and I published the second edition of *Radiation Therapy Physics* in 1996, we anticipated that the book would be well received. However, the degree of enthusiasm over the book, although rewarding to us, caught our former publisher by surprise. The print run for the book was quickly depleted, and could not be replenished because of a merger under negotiation with a larger publishing house. Consequently, the second edition has been out of print for the past 6 years, and we have been giving permission to teachers and students to photocopy the text for their personal use.

Soon after release of the second edition, Geoff and I realized that a new edition would quickly become necessary, because the techniques of radiation therapy were evolving rapidly and dramatically. Over the past five years, treatment procedures such as conformal and intensity-modulated radiation therapy, high dose rate and vascular brachytherapy, and image-guided and intraoperative radiation therapy have become standard operating procedures in radiation therapy clinics around the world. In addition, x-ray beams from linear accelerators have replaced ^{60}Co γ rays as the standard teaching model for the parameters of external beam radiation therapy, and several new protocols have been developed for calibrating and applying radiation beams and sources for cancer treatment. These procedures, and others that represent state-of-the-art radiation therapy, are discussed at length in this new edition.

In designing the third edition, Geoff and I had an opportunity to add Eric Hendee as a third member of the writing team. Eric's broad experience in radiation therapy physics, and his ability as a clear writer, make him an excellent member of the team. In this new edition, we are presenting information in a format that reflects our understanding of the way people learn in today's culture. Throughout the book we make extensive use of self-contained segments, illustrations, highlights, sidebars, examples and problems. We hope that this approach will help students use the book as a primary source of information, rather than simply as a supplement to the classroom. We feel this approach is important because classroom time for learning is becoming a casualty of the increasing emphasis on productivity and accountability in healthcare. It is also important because increasingly each of us is forced to assimilate information in fragments rather than as a continuous process, principally as a product of the Information Age in which we live. Without judging the ultimate societal consequences of this assimilation process, we acknowledge its pervasiveness and have attempted in this text to accommodate it.

The treatment of patients with ionizing radiation is a complex undertaking that requires close collaboration among physicians, physicists, engineers, radiation therapists, dosimetrists and nurses. Together they provide a level of patient care that would be unachievable by any single group working alone. But to achieve maximum success, each member of the team must have a solid foundation in the physics of radiation therapy. It is the intent of this text to provide this foundation. We hope we have done so in a manner that makes learning enriching and enjoyable.

Many people have supported this third edition, including several investigators who have contributed data and illustrations to the text. We are grateful for their help. Luna Han, the book's editor at our new publisher, John Wiley & Sons, Inc., has encouraged and helped us to meet our deadlines without being overbearing. Our editorial assistants, Mary Beth Drapp in Milwaukee and Elizabeth Siller in Houston, have managed to keep the text and the authors organized and focused. We acknowledge that the authors were more of a challenge than the chapters. And, last but certainly not least, Geoff thanks Diane, Eric thanks Lynne, and I thank Jeannie for their forbearance during production of another edition of yet another book.

William R. Hendee

PREFACE TO THE SECOND EDITION

In 1981 the first edition of *Radiation Therapy Physics* was published as a paperback supplement to the second edition of my text *Medical Radiation Physics*. This book addressed the evolving new era of radiation therapy and covered topics such as high-energy x-rays, electron beams, consensus calibration protocols, computerized treatment planning, and the reemergence of sealed-source brachytherapy. It was received by an especially receptive audience, and the publisher's stock of books was soon depleted. The book has been out-of-print for several years, and several physics instructors have told me they have been using photocopies for their classes.

The response to the first edition has been gratifying. However, there was one recurring concern about it. Many readers complained that the book did not cover the fundamentals of radiation physics. They did not like having to buy a text on diagnostic radiologic physics to learn these principles. More recently, several teachers have called to suggest that a new edition be prepared and that it should cover fundamental physics principles as well as their applications to radiation therapy. The publisher, Mosby–Year Book, Inc. also encouraged the preparation of a new edition. This book is my response to this encouragement.

Radiation therapy has changed in many ways since the first edition was released. High-energy x-ray and electron beams have become the preferred approach to the radiation treatment of many cancers, and sealed-source implants have become more common and more complex. Imaging techniques and computers are now used routinely in treatment planning, and sophisticated methods are available for overlaying anatomical images with computer-generated multi-dimensional treatment plans. Calibration protocols have been extensively revised, and quality assurance in radiation therapy has become almost a subject in itself. A new edition of *Radiation Therapy Physics* is certainly overdue. This second edition is presented in the hope that it will satisfy the needs of radiation physicists, oncologists, and therapists for a text that explains the fundamentals of radiation physics and their applications to the radiation treatment of cancer patients.

In planning the second edition, I had to confront a dilemma. My work schedule simply did not offer enough flexibility to accommodate the efforts that would be required. I needed a coauthor. This individual had to be someone who is exceedingly knowledgeable about the physics of radiation therapy. He or she had to be a good writer. Finally, the co-author had to be a person with whom I knew I could work comfortably over the course of a couple of years. One special person came to mind, and I am pleased that Geoff Ibbott agreed to co-write the book with me. Geoff and I have worked as a team on many projects since the late 1960s, including 18 years together at the University of Colorado. If the reader learns half as much from this book as I have learned from Geoff in putting the book together, I will consider the text a success.

Many people have been supportive in the preparation of the second edition. Several investigators have contributed illustrations and data, and I am grateful for their help. Our editor at Mosby, Elizabeth Corra, has been terrific in her persistence and patience. Two individuals, Terri Komar and Claudia Johnson in our respective offices, have been invaluable in their organizational and editorial skills. Finally, Geoff thanks Diane while I remain indebted to Jeannie for their tolerance over the many nights and weekends we have spent in front of the computer. We are not quite sure why they put up with this intrusion into our respective relationships, but we know better than to question it.

William R. Hendee

PREFACE TO THE FIRST EDITION

When the First edition of *Medical Radiation Physics* was published in 1970, the study of radiology encompassed both diagnostic and therapeutic applications of radiation, and physicians and graduate student trainees in the field were required to understand both applications. Since that time, the field of radiology has bifurcated into two specialties, diagnostic imaging and radiation oncology, and the knowledge required of trainees in either field has expanded greatly. In preparing the second edition of *Medical Radiation Physics*, I confined my text to diagnostic imaging procedures.

The present text constitutes a supplement to the second edition of *Medical Radiation Physics* devoted to the physics of radiation therapy. Because it is a supplement, information presented in the second edition on the basic principles of radiologic physics is not duplicated herein. For information on topics such as atomic and nuclear structure, production and interactions of radiation, x-ray generator and tube design, and units and measurement of radiation, the reader is referred to the second edition of *Medical Radiation Physics*. Material in this text is presented with the assumption that the principles of radiologic physics are understood by the reader.

Since publication of the first edition, radiation oncology has progressed from the era of 60Co therapy to a complex clinical specialty employing megavoltage x-ray and electron beams and minicomputers dedicated to the acquisition of dosimetric data and the design of complex treatment plans for radiation therapy patients. This progression is reflected in significant expansion of many sections of the text and the addition of a number of sections related to the current practice of radiation oncology. For example, the chapter on radiation therapy units now includes a lengthy section on linear accelerators, and the chapter on absorbed dose measurements has been expanded to consider problems associated with dose measurements in high-energy x-ray beams. An entire chapter has been added on measurements associated with electron beams, and the chapter on dosimetry of radiation fields now includes sections on tissue-phantom and tissue-maximum ratios, scatter-air ratios, and computational techniques for dose estimates for mantle fields and other fields of irregular shape. Isodose distributions are discussed in part from the perspective of decrement lines, dose gradients, polar coordinates and other methods useful for computer simulation of composite dose distributions.

The use of sealed sources such as 192Ir, 125I, and 137Cs is discussed in the chapter on implant therapy, and the chapter on radiation protection has been completely rewritten for greater comprehensibility and relevance to radiation oncology. In developing this text, I have been greatly helped by Ms. Josephine Ibbott, who prepared new drawings for each chapter, and by Ms. Sarah Bemis, who typed the manuscript and kept the entire project organized. I also wish to thank Geoffrey S. Ibbott, M.S., for his helpful criticism of the entire manuscript and Russell Ritenour, Ph.D., for his assistance in verifying the solutions to problems.

William R. Hendee

1

ATOMIC STRUCTURE AND RADIOACTIVE DECAY

Objectives

After studying this chapter, the reader should be able to:
- Understand the relationship between nuclear instability and radioactive decay.
- Describe the different modes of radioactive decay and the conditions in which they occur.
- Interpret decay schemes.
- State and use the fundamental equations of radioactive decay.
- Perform elementary computations for sample activities.
- Describe the principles of transient and secular equilibrium.
- Discuss the principles of the artificial production of radionuclides.

Introduction

The composition of matter has puzzled philosophers and scientists for centuries. Even today, the mystery continues as strange new particles are detected in high-energy accelerators. Various models proposed to explain the composition and mechanics of matter are useful in certain applications, but invariably fall short in others. One of the oldest models, the atomic theory of matter devised by early Greek philosophers,[1] remains a useful approach to understanding many physical processes, including those important to the study of the physics of radiation therapy. The atomic model is used in this text, but it is important to remember that it is only a model, and that the true composition of matter remains an enigma.

Atomic and nuclear structure

The atom is the smallest unit of matter that possesses the physical and chemical properties characteristic of one of the 118 elements, 92 of which occur naturally and the others are produced artificially. The atom consists of a central positive core, termed the *nucleus*, surrounded by a cloud of electrons moving in orbits around the nucleus. The nucleus is composed of protons and neutrons, collectively termed *nucleons*, with a diameter on the

Hendee's Radiation Therapy Physics, Fourth Edition. Todd Pawlicki, Daniel J. Scanderbeg and George Starkschall.
© 2016 John Wiley & Sons, Inc. Published 2016 by John Wiley & Sons, Inc.

order of 10^{-14} meters (m). Protons are subatomic particles with a mass of 1.6734×10^{-27} kilograms (kg) and a positive charge of $+1.6 \times 10^{-19}$ Coulombs. Neutrons are subatomic particles with a mass of 1.6747×10^{-27} kg and no electrical charge. The electron cloud surrounding the nucleus has a diameter of about 10^{-10} m.

Electrons have a mass of 9.108×10^{-31} kg and a negative charge of -1.6×10^{-19} Coulombs. In the neutral atom, the number of protons in the nucleus is balanced by an equal number of electrons in the surrounding orbits. An atom with a greater or lesser number of electrons than the number of protons is termed a *negative* or *positive ion*.

An atom is characterized by the symbol $^A_Z X$, in which A is the number of nucleons in the nucleus, Z is the number of protons in the nucleus (or the number of electrons in the neutral atom), and X represents the chemical symbol for the particular element to which the atom belongs. The number of nucleons, A, is termed the *mass number* of the atom and Z is called the *atomic number* of the atom. The difference $A - Z$ is the number of neutrons in the nucleus, termed the *neutron number*, N. Each element has a characteristic atomic number but can have several mass numbers depending on the number of neutrons in the nucleus. For example, the element hydrogen has the unique atomic number of 1, signifying the solitary proton that constitutes the hydrogen nucleus, but can have zero (^1_1H), one (^2_1H), or two (^3_1H) neutrons. The atomic forms $^1H, ^2H,$ and ^3H (the subscript 1 can be omitted because it is redundant with the chemical symbol) are said to be *isotopes* of hydrogen because they contain different numbers of neutrons combined with the single proton characteristic of hydrogen. Isotopes of an element have the same Z but different values of A, reflecting a different neutron number, N. *Isotones* have the same N but different values of Z and A. $^3H, ^4He,$ and ^5Li are isotones because each nucleus contains two neutrons ($N = 2$). *Isobars* have the same A, but different values of Z and N. ^3H and ^3He are isobars ($A = 3$). *Isomers* are different energy states of the same atom and therefore have identical values of Z, N, and A. For example ^{99m}Tc and ^{99}Tc are isomers because they are two distinct energy states of the same atom. The m in ^{99m}Tc signifies a metastable energy state that exists for a finite time (6 hours half-life) before changing to ^{99}Tc. The term *nuclide* refers to an atomic nucleus in any form.

Atomic units

Units employed to describe dimensions in the macroscopic world, such as kilograms, Joules, meters, and Coulombs, are too large to use at the atomic level. Units more appropriate for the atomic scale include the atomic mass unit (amu) for mass, electron volt (eV) for energy, nanometer (nm) for distance, and electron charge (e) for electrical charge.

The *amu* is defined as 1/12 of the mass of an atom of the most common form of carbon, ^{12}C, which has 6 protons, 6 neutrons, and 6 electrons. One amu $= 1.66 \times 10^{-27}$ kg. By definition, the atomic mass of an atom of ^{12}C is 12.00000 amu. In units of amu, the masses of atomic particles are as follows:

electron $= 0.00055$ amu

proton $= 1.00727$ amu

neutron $= 1.00866$ amu

Every atom has a characteristic atomic mass, A_m. The gram-atomic mass of an isotope is an amount of the isotope in grams that is numerically equivalent to the isotope's atomic mass. For example, one gram-atomic mass of ^{12}C is exactly 12 grams. One gram-atomic mass of any isotope contains 6.0228×10^{23} atoms, which is a constant value that is known as *Avogadro's number* N_A. With these expressions, the following quantities can be computed:

$$\text{Number of atoms/g} = N_A / A_m$$
$$\text{Number of electrons/g} = (N_A Z) / A_m$$
$$\text{Number of g/atom} = A_m / N_A$$

Example 1-1

Compare the number of electrons/g for ^{12}C to the number of electrons/g for ^{40}Ar.

For ^{12}C, the atomic number is 6 and the atomic mass is 12.000. Consequently, the number of electrons/g is $6.0228 \times 10^{23} \times 6/12.000 = 3.0114 \times 10^{23}$ electrons/g.

For ^{40}Ar, the atomic number is 18 and the atomic mass is 39.948. Consequently, the number of electrons/g is $6.0228 \times 10^{23} \times 18/39.948 = 2.714 \times 10^{23}$ electrons/g.

Note that, although the atomic masses and atomic numbers of carbon and argon are widely different from one another, the electron densities are within 10% of each other. Because for most materials the mass number is approximately twice the atomic number, the electron densities will be relatively constant.

The electron volt (eV) is a unit of energy equal to the kinetic energy of a single electron accelerated through a potential difference (voltage) of 1 volt. One keV $= 10^3$ eV and 1 MeV $= 10^6$ eV. One nanometer (nm) is 10^{-9} meters. The electron unit of electrical charge $= 1.6 \times 10^{-19}$ Coulombs. One eV is equal to 1.6×10^{-19} Joules of energy.

Example 1-2

What is the kinetic energy (E_k) of an electron accelerated through a potential difference of 400,000 volts [400 kilovolts (kV)]?

$$E_k = (1 \text{ electron}) (400,000 \text{ volts})$$
$$= 400,000 \text{ eV} = 400 \text{ keV}$$

Mass defect and binding energy

The neutral ^{12}C atom contains 6 protons, 6 neutrons, and 6 electrons. The mass of the components of this atom can be computed as:

$$\text{Mass of 6 protons} = 6(1.00727\ \text{amu}) = 6.04362\ \text{amu}$$
$$\text{Mass of 6 neutrons} = 6(1.00866\ \text{amu}) = 6.05196\ \text{amu}$$
$$\underline{\text{Mass of 6 electrons} = 6(0.00055\ \text{amu}) = 0.00330\ \text{amu}}$$
$$\text{Mass of components of }^{12}\text{C} = 12.09888\ \text{amu}$$

The mass of an atom of ^{12}C, however, is 12.00000 amu by definition. That is, the sum of the masses of the components of the ^{12}C atom exceeds the actual mass of the atom. There is a *mass defect* of 0.09888 amu in the ^{12}C atom. The difference in mass must be supplied to separate the ^{12}C atom into its constituents. The mass defect can be described in terms of energy according to Einstein's expression $E = mc^2$, for the equivalence of mass and energy. In this expression, E is energy, m is mass, and c is the speed of light in a vacuum (3×10^8 m/sec). From the formula for mass-energy equivalence, 1 amu of mass is equivalent to 931 MeV of energy. For example, the energy equivalent to the mass of the electron is (0.00055 amu) (931 MeV/amu) = 0.511 MeV.

The energy associated with the mass defect of ^{12}C is (0.09888 amu)(931 MeV/amu) = 92.0 MeV. The energy equivalent to the mass defect of an atom is known as the *binding energy* of the atom and is the energy required to separate the atom into its constituent parts. Almost all of the binding energy of an atom is associated with the nucleus and reflects the influence of the strong nuclear force that binds particles together in the nucleus. For ^{12}C, the average binding energy per nucleon is 92.0 MeV/12 = 7.67 MeV/nucleon. When computing the average binding energy per nucleon as the quotient of the binding energy of the atom divided by the number of nucleons, the small contribution of electrons to the binding energy of the atom is ignored.

Example 1-3

What is the average binding energy per nucleon of ^{16}O with an atomic mass of 15.99492 amu?

$$\text{Mass of 8 protons} = 8(1.00727\ \text{amu}) = 8.05816\ \text{amu}$$
$$\text{Mass of 8 neutrons} = 8(1.00866\ \text{amu}) = 8.06928\ \text{amu}$$
$$\underline{\text{Mass of 8 electrons} = 8(0.00055\ \text{amu}) = 0.00440\ \text{amu}}$$
$$\text{Mass of components of }^{16}\text{O} = 16.13184\ \text{amu}$$
$$\text{Mass of }^{16}\text{O atom} = 15.99492\ \text{amu}$$
$$\text{Mass defect} = 16.13184\ \text{amu} - 15.99492\ \text{amu}$$
$$= 0.13692\ \text{amu}$$
$$\text{Binding energy of }^{16}\text{O} = (0.13692\ \text{amu})(931\ \text{MeV/amu})$$
$$= 127.5\ \text{MeV}$$
$$\text{Average binding energy per nucleon}$$
$$= (127.5\ \text{MeV})/16$$
$$= 7.97\ \text{MeV/nucleon}$$

The average binding energy per nucleon is plotted in Figure 1-1 as a function of the mass number of different isotopes. The greatest average binding energies per nucleon occur for isotopes with mass number in the range of 50 to 100. Heavier isotopes gain binding energy by splitting into lighter isotopes.

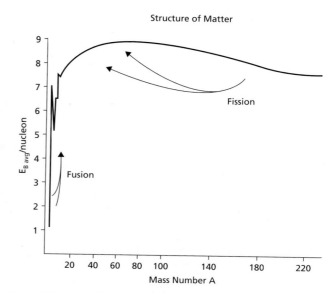

Figure 1-1 Average binding energy per nucleon versus mass number.

This is equivalent to saying that heavier isotopes release energy when they split into lighter isotopes, a process known as *nuclear fission*. The isotopes ^{233}U, ^{235}U, and ^{239}Pu fission spontaneously when a neutron is added to the nucleus. This process is the origin of the energy released during fission in nuclear reactors and fission weapons. Similarly, energy is released when light isotopes combine to form products with higher average binding energies per nucleon. This latter process is termed *nuclear fusion* and is the source of energy released during an uncontrolled fusion reaction, such as that in a "hydrogen" bomb. Uncontrolled nuclear fission is the process employed in uranium or plutonium atomic bombs. Controlled nuclear fission is the process employed in a nuclear reactor.

Electron energy levels

The model of the atom in which electrons revolve in orbits around the nucleus was developed by Niels Bohr in 1913.[2] This model represented a departure from explanations of the atom that relied on classical physics. In the Bohr model, each orbit or "shell" can hold a maximum number of electrons defined as $2n^2$, where n is the number of the electron shell. The first ($n = 1$ or K) shell can hold up to 2 electrons, the second ($n = 2$ or L) shell can contain up to 8 electrons, the third ($n = 3$ or M) shell can hold up to 18 electrons, and so on. The maximum number of electrons in a particular electron orbit is defined by the Pauli Exclusion Principle, which states that in any atom (or atomic system) no two electrons can have the same four quantum numbers. The four quantum numbers of an electron are the *principal*, *azimuthal*, *magnetic*, and *spin* quantum numbers. The outermost occupied M, N, or O electron shell, called the *valence shell*, however, can hold no more than 8 electrons. Additional electrons begin to fill the next level to create a new outermost shell before more than 8 electrons are added to an M or higher shell. The

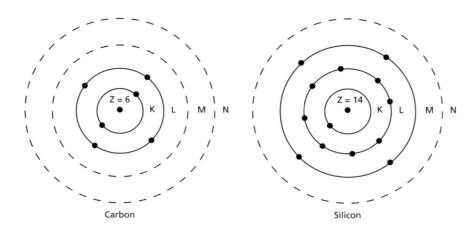

Figure 1-2 Electron "orbits" in the Bohr model of the atom for carbon ($Z = 6$) and silicon ($Z = 14$).

number of valence electrons in the outermost shell determines the chemical properties of the atom and the elemental species to which it belongs. Examples of electron orbits in representative atoms are shown in Figure 1-2.

An electron neither gains nor loses energy so long as it remains in a specific electron orbit. Energy is needed, however, to move an electron from one orbit to another farther from the nucleus because work must be done against the attractive electrostatic force of the positive nucleus for the negative electron. Similarly, energy is released when an electron moves from one orbit to another nearer the nucleus. This transition can occur only if a vacancy exists in the nearer orbit, perhaps because an electron has been ejected from that orbit by some physical process.

The energy required to remove an electron completely from an atom is defined as the *binding energy* of the electron. The positive charge of the nucleus (i.e., the Z of the atom) and the particular shell from which the electron is removed are the principal influences on the electron's binding energy. Minor influences are the particular energy subshell of the electron within the orbit and the direction of rotation as the electron spins on its own axis while it revolves in the electron orbit. The electron orbits of a particular atom can be characterized in terms of the binding energies of electrons in the orbits.

Binding energies for electron orbits in hydrogen ($Z = 1$) and tungsten ($Z = 74$) are compared in Figure 1-3. Binding energies are much greater in tungsten than in hydrogen because the higher nuclear charge exerts a stronger attractive force on the electrons. In hydrogen, an electron moving to the K shell from a level farther from the nucleus releases energy usually in the form of ultraviolet radiation. In tungsten, an electron falling into the K shell releases energy usually in the form of an x ray, a form of electromagnetic radiation much more energetic than ultraviolet radiation. The actual energy released equals the difference in binding energy between the electron orbits representing the origin and destination of the electron. For example, an electron moving from the L to the K shell in tungsten releases (69,500 − 11,280 = 58,220 eV) 58.2 keV of energy, whereas an electron falling from the M to the K shell in tungsten releases

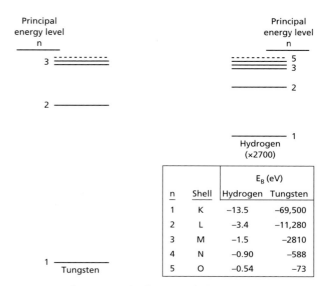

n	Shell	E_B (eV) Hydrogen	Tungsten
1	K	−13.5	−69,500
2	L	−3.4	−11,280
3	M	−1.5	−2810
4	N	−0.90	−588
5	O	−0.54	−73

Figure 1-3 Binding energies for electrons in hydrogen ($Z = 1$) and tungsten ($Z = 74$). A change in scale is required to show both energy ranges in the same diagram.

(69,500 − 2810 = 66,690 eV) 66.7 keV. X rays emitted by electron transitions between orbits are termed *characteristic x rays* because their energy is characteristic of the atomic number of the atom and the particular electron shells involved in the transition. Characteristic x rays are sometimes called *fluorescence x rays*.

When an electron falls from the L to the K shell in a heavy atom, a vacancy is created in the L shell. This vacancy is usually filled instantly by an electron from a shell farther from the nucleus, usually the M shell. The vacancy created in this shell is then filled by another electron from a more distant orbit. Hence, a vacancy in an inner shell of an atom usually results in a cascade of electrons with the emission of a range of characteristic energies, often as electromagnetic radiation. In tungsten, transitions of electrons into the K and L shell result in the release of x rays, whereas transitions into M and higher shells produce radiations too low in energy to qualify as x rays.

Energy that is liberated as an electron falls to an orbit closer to the nucleus is not always released as electromagnetic radiation. Instead, it may be transferred to another electron farther from the nucleus, resulting in the ejection of the electron from its orbit. The ejected electron is termed an *Auger electron* and has a kinetic energy equal to the energy transferred to it, decreased by the binding energy required to eject the electron from its orbit. For example, an electron falling from the L to the K shell in tungsten releases 58,220 eV of energy. If this energy is transferred to another electron in the L shell, this electron is ejected with a kinetic energy of (58,220 − 11,280 = 46,940) eV. Usually, an Auger electron is ejected from the same energy level that gave rise to the original transitioning electron. In this case, the kinetic energy of the Auger electron is $E_{bi} - 2E_{bo}$, where E_{bi} is the binding energy of the inner electron orbit that receives the transitioning electron and E_{bo} is the energy of the orbit that serves as the origin of both the transitioning and the Auger electrons.

Example 1-4

What is the kinetic energy E_k of an Auger electron released from the L shell of gold [$(E_b)_L = 13.335$ keV] as an electron falls from the L to the K shell [$(E_b)_K = 80.713$ keV]?

$$E_k = E_{bi} - 2E_{bo} = [80.713 - 2(13.335)] \text{ keV}$$
$$= 54.043 \text{ keV}$$

The emission of characteristic electromagnetic radiation and the release of Auger electrons are alternative processes that release energy from an atom during electron transitions. The *fluorescence yield*, w, defines the probability that an electron vacancy will result in the emission of characteristic radiation as it is filled by an electron from a higher orbit.

$$w = \frac{\text{Number of characteristic radiation emitted}}{\text{Number of electron shell vacancies}}$$

For low-Z nuclides, Auger electrons tend to be emitted more frequently than characteristic radiations, as shown in Figure 1-4. As Z increases, the fluorescence yield also increases, so that characteristic radiations are released more frequently than Auger electrons.[3]

Nuclear stability

The nuclei of many atoms are stable. In general, it is these atoms that constitute ordinary matter. In stable nuclei of lighter atoms, the number of neutrons is about equal to the number of protons. A high level of symmetry exists in the placement of protons and neutrons into nuclear energy levels similar to the electron shells constituting the extranuclear structure of the atom. The assignment of nucleons to energy levels in the nucleus is referred to as the *shell model* of the nucleus. For heavier stable atoms, the number of neutrons increases faster than the number of protons, suggesting that the higher energy levels are spaced more closely for neutrons than for protons. The number of neutrons (i.e., the neutron number) in the nuclei of stable atoms is plotted in Figure 1-5 as a function of the number of protons (i.e., the atomic

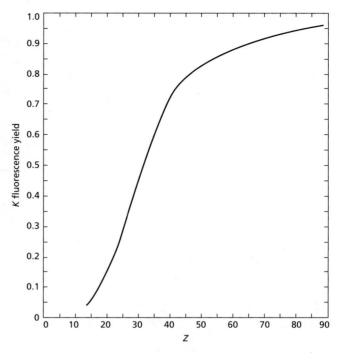

Figure 1-4 K-shell fluorescence yields as a function of atomic number.[4]

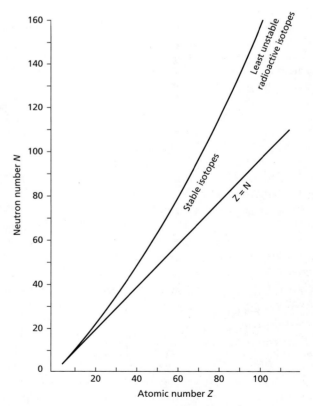

Figure 1-5 Number of neutrons (N) in stable (or least unstable) nuclei as a function of the number of protons (atomic number Z).

Table 1-1 Radioactive decay processes.

Type of Decay	New A	New Z	New N	Comments
Beta ($\beta -$)	A	$Z + 1$	$N - 1$	$E_{\beta\text{-mean}} \cong \dfrac{E_{max}}{3}$
Positron ($\beta +$)	A	$Z - 1$	$N + 1$	$E_{\beta\text{-mean}} \cong \dfrac{E_{max}}{3}$
Electron capture isomeric transition γ emission	A	$Z - 1$	$N + 1$	Characteristic + Auger electrons Metastable if $T_{1/2} > 10^{-6}$ sec
Internal conversion (IC)	A	Z	N	IC electrons: characteristic + Auger electrons
Alpha (α)	$A - 4$	$Z - 2$	$N - 2$	

number). Above $Z = 83$, no stable forms of the elements exist and the plot depicts the neutron/proton (N/Z) ratio for the least unstable forms of the elements (i.e., isotopes that exist for relatively long periods before changing).

Nuclei that have an imbalance in the N/Z ratio are positioned away from the stability curve depicted in Figure 1-5. These unstable nuclei tend to undergo changes within the nucleus to achieve more stable configurations of neutrons and protons. The changes are accompanied by the emission of particles and electromagnetic radiation (photons) from the nucleus, together with the release of substantial amounts of energy related to an increase in binding energy of the nucleons in their final nuclear configuration. These changes are referred to as the *radioactive decay* of the nucleus, and the process is described as *radioactivity*. If the number of protons is different between the initial and final nuclear configurations, Z is changed and the nucleus is transmuted from one elemental form to another. The various processes of radioactive decay are summarized in Table 1-1.

Radioactivity was discovered in 1896 by Henri Becquerel,[5] who observed the emission of radiation (later shown to be beta particles) from uranium salts. Becquerel experienced a skin burn from carrying a radioactive sample in his vest pocket. This is the first known biological effect of radiation exposure.

Radioactive decay

Radioactivity can be described mathematically without reference to the specific mode of decay of radioactive atoms. The rate of decay (the number of atoms decaying per unit time) is directly proportional to the number of radioactive atoms N present in the sample:

$$\Delta N/\Delta t = -\lambda \Delta N \tag{1-1}$$

where $\Delta N/\Delta t$ is the rate of decay. The constant λ is the *decay constant* of the particular species of atoms in the sample, and the negative sign reveals that the number of radioactive atoms

in the sample is diminishing as the sample decays. The decay constant can be expressed as:

$$\lambda = -\frac{\left(\dfrac{\Delta N}{N}\right)}{\Delta t}$$

revealing that it represents the fractional rate of decay of the atoms. The value of λ is characteristic of the type of atoms in the sample and changes from one nuclide to the next. Units of λ are $(\text{time})^{-1}$. Larger values of λ characterize more unstable nuclides that decay more rapidly.

Equation (1-1) describes the expected decay rate of a radioactive sample. At any moment the actual decay rate may differ somewhat from the expected rate because of statistical fluctuations in the decay rate. The decay constant λ is also called the *transformation constant*. The decay constant of a nuclide is truly a constant: it is not affected by external influences such as temperature and pressure, or by magnetic, electrical, or gravitational fields. The rate of decay of a sample of atoms is termed the activity A of the sample (i.e., $A = \Delta N/\Delta t$). A rate of decay of 1 atom per second is termed an activity of 1 Becquerel (Bq). That is, 1 Bq = 1 disintegration per second (dps). A common unit of activity is the megabecquerel (MBq), where 1 MBq = 10^6 dps. An earlier unit of activity, the Curie (Ci) is defined as 1 Ci = 3.7×10^{-10} dps. The Curie was defined in 1910 as the activity of 1 gram of radium. Although subsequent measures revealed that 1 gram of radium has a decay rate of 3.61×10^{10} dps, the definition of the Curie was left as 3.7×10^{10} dps.

Multiples of the Curie are the picocurie (10^{-12} Ci), nanocurie (10^{-9} Ci), microcurie (10^{-6} Ci), millicurie (10^{-3} Ci), kilocurie (10^3 Ci), and megacurie (10^6 Ci). The Becquerel and the Curie are related by 1 Bq = 1 dps = 2.7×10^{-11} Ci. The activity of a radioactive sample per unit mass (e.g., MBq/mg) is known as the *specific activity* of the sample.

Example 1-5

A. A $^{60}_{27}$C0 source has a decay constant of 0.131 y^{-1}. Find the activity in MBq of a sample containing 10^{15} atoms.

$A = \lambda N$
$\quad = 4.2 \times 10^6$ atoms/s $= 4.2 \times 10^6$ Bq
$\quad = 4.2$ MBq

B. What is the specific activity of the sample in MBq/g? The gram-atomic mass of ^{60}Co is 59.9338.

$$\text{Sample mass} = \frac{(10^{15}\ \text{atoms})\ (59.9338\ \text{g/g-atomic mass})}{6.023 \times 10^{23}\ \text{atoms/g-atomic mass}}$$
$$= 9.95 \times 10^{-8}\ \text{g}$$

$$\text{Specific activity} = (4.2\ \text{MBq})/(9.95 \times 10^{-8}\ \text{g})$$
$$= 42 \times 10^{6}\ \text{MBq/g}$$

Through the process of mathematical integration, an expression for the number N of radioactive atoms remaining in a sample after a time, t, has elapsed can be shown to equal:

$$N = N_0 e^{-\lambda t} \tag{1-2}$$

where N_0 is the number of atoms present at time $t = 0$. Equation (1-2) reveals that the number N of parent atoms decreases *exponentially* with time and can also be written as:

$$A = A_0 e^{-\lambda t} \tag{1-3}$$

where A is the activity of the sample at time t, and A_0 is the activity at time $t = 0$.

The number of radioactive atoms N^* that have decayed after time t is $N_0 - N$, or:

$$N^* = N_0(1 - e^{-\lambda t}) \tag{1-4}$$

The probability that a particular atom will not decay during time t is N/N_0 or $e^{-\lambda t}$, and the probability that the atom will decay during time t is $1 - N/N_0$ or $1 - e^{-\lambda t}$.

For small values of λt, the probability of decay $(1 - e^{-\lambda})$ can be approximated as λt or expressed as the probability of decay per unit time, p(decay per unit time) $\sim \lambda$. Radioactive decay must always be described in terms of the probability of decay; whether any particular radioactive nucleus will decay within a specific time period is never certain.

The *physical half-life*, $T_{1/2}$, of a radioactive sample is the time required for half of the atoms in the sample to decay. The half-life is logarithmically related to the decay constant of the sample.

$$T_{1/2} = (\ln 2)/\lambda = 0.693/\lambda$$

Each radioactive isotope has a unique decay constant and, therefore, a unique half-life. The average life t_{avg} of a radioactive sample, sometimes referred to as the *mean life*, is the average time for decay of atoms in the sample. The average life is $t_{avg} = 1/\lambda = 1.44(T_{1/2})$.

Example 1-6

What are the half-life and average life of the sample of $^{60}_{27}$Co described in Example 1-5?

$$T_{1/2} = 0.693/\lambda = 0.693/0.131 \text{y}^{-1}$$
$$= 5.3\text{y}$$
$$T_{avg} = 1.44(T_{1/2}) = 1.44(5.3\text{y})$$
$$= 7.63\text{y}$$

The percent of original activity remaining in a radioactive sample is depicted in Figure 1-6(a) as a function of elapsed time. This variable is replotted in Figure 1-6(b) on a semilogarithmic graph (activity on a vertical logarithmic scale and time on a horizontal linear scale) to yield a straight line. Semilogarithmic plots yield straight lines of variables, such as activities that vary according to an exponential relationship, and are useful in depicting several quantities in radiation therapy (e.g., radioactive decay, attenuation of radiation, and survival of tumor cells following irradiation).

Example 1-7

The physical half-life of ^{131}I is 8.0 days.
A sample of ^{131}I has a mass of 100 μg. How many ^{131}I atoms are present in the sample?
Number of atoms, N:

$$= \frac{(\text{Number of grams})\ (\text{Number of atoms/gram-atomic mass})}{(\text{Number of grams/gram-atomic mass})}$$
$$= \frac{(100 \times 10^{-6}\text{grams})\ (6.02 \times 10^{23}\text{atoms/gram-atomic mass})}{131\ \text{grams/gram-atomic mass}}$$
$$= 4.6 \times 10^{17}\ \text{atoms}$$

How many ^{131}I atoms remain after 20 days have elapsed?

$$N = N_0 e^{-(0.693\,t/T_{1/2})}$$
$$= (4.6 \times 10^{17}\text{atoms})e^{-(0.693/8\,\text{d})(20\,\text{d})}$$
$$= 8.1 \times 10^{16}\text{atoms}$$

What is the activity of the sample after 20 days?

$$A = \lambda N$$
$$= (0.693/8.0\,\text{d})(1/86,400\,\text{s/d})(8.1 \times 10^{16}\text{atoms})$$
$$= 8.2 \times 10^{10}\text{atoms/sec}$$
$$= 8.2 \times 10^{4}\text{MBq}$$

What is the specific activity of the ^{131}I sample?

$$SA = 8.2 \times 10^{4}\text{MBq}/0.1\text{mg}$$
$$= 8.2 \times 10^{5}\text{MBq/mg}$$

What activity should be ordered at 8 AM Monday to provide an activity of 8.2×10^{4} MBq at 8 AM on the following Friday?

$$\text{Elapsed time} = 4\ \text{days}$$
$$N = N_0 e^{-\lambda t}$$
$$8.2 \times 10^{4}\ \text{MBq} = N_0 e^{-(0.693/8\text{d})(4\text{d})}$$
$$8.2 \times 10^{4}\ \text{MBq} = N_0(0.7072)$$
$$N_0 = 11.6 \times 10^{4}\ \text{MBq must be ordered}$$

Types of radioactive decay

The process of radioactive decay often is described by a decay scheme in which energy is depicted on the vertical (y) axis

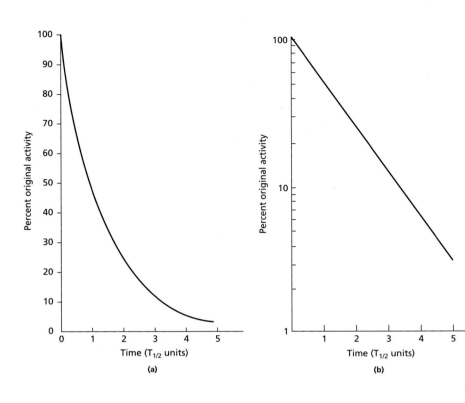

Figure 1-6 Percentage of original activity of a radioactive sample as a function of time in units of half-life. (a) Linear plot. (b) Semilogarithmic plot.

and the atomic number is shown on the horizontal (x) axis. A generic decay scheme is illustrated in Figure 1-7. The original nuclide (or *parent*) is depicted as $_Z^A X$, and the product nuclide (or "progeny") is denoted as element *P*, *Q*, *R*, or *S* depending on the decay path. Parent and progeny nuclei are also referred to as *mother* and *daughter*. In the path from *X* to *P*, the nuclide gains stability by emitting an alpha (α) particle, two neutrons, and two protons ejected from the nucleus as a single particle. In this case, the progeny nucleus has an atomic number of $Z - 2$ and a mass number of $A - 4$ and is positioned at reduced elevation in

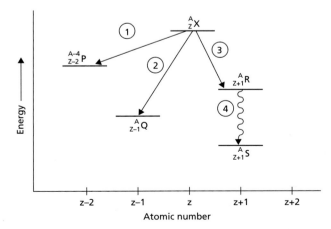

Figure 1-7 Symbolic radioactive decay scheme. A decay scheme is a useful way to assimilate and depict the decay characteristics of a radioactive nuclide.

the decay scheme to demonstrate that energy is released as the nucleus gains stability through radioactive decay. The released energy is referred to as the *transition energy*. The transition *energy* released during radioactive decay is also referred to as the *disintegration energy* and the *energy of decay*. In the path from *X* to *Q*, the nucleus gains stability through the process in which a proton in the nucleus changes to a neutron. This process can be either positron decay or electron capture and yields an atomic number of $Z - 1$ and an unchanged mass number *A*. The path from *X* to *R* represents negatron decay in which a neutron is transformed into a proton, leaving the progeny with an atomic number of $Z + 1$ and an unchanged mass number *A*. In the path from *R* to *S*, the constant *Z* and constant *A* signify that no change occurs in nuclear composition. This pathway is termed an *isomeric transition between nuclear isomers* and results only in the release of energy from the nucleus through the processes of γ emission and internal conversion.

Alpha decay

Alpha decay is a decay process in which greater nuclear stability is achieved by emission of 2 protons and 2 neutrons as a single alpha (α) particle (a nucleus of helium) from the nucleus. Alpha emission is confined to relatively heavy nuclei. The sum of mass numbers and the sum of atomic numbers after the transition equal the mass and atomic numbers of the parent before the transition. In α decay, energy is released as kinetic energy of the α particle, and is sometimes followed by energy

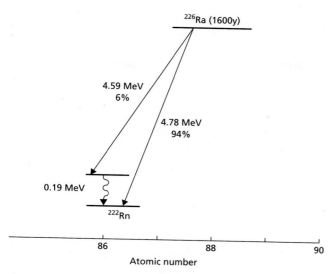

Figure 1-8 Radioactive decay scheme: α decay of ^{226}Ra.

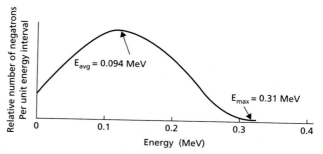

Figure 1-9 Energy spectrum of electrons from $^{60}_{27}Co$.

released during an isomeric transition resulting in emission of a γ ray or conversion electron. Alpha particles are always ejected with energy characteristic of the particular nuclear transition.

An example of alpha decay is the decay of ^{226}Ra:

$$^{226}_{88}Ra \rightarrow\, ^{222}_{86}Rn +\, ^{4}_{2}He$$

An alpha transition is depicted in Figure 1-8, in which the parent ^{226}Ra decays directly to the final energy state (ground state) of the progeny ^{222}Rn in 94% of all transitions. In 6% of the transitions, ^{226}Ra decays to an intermediate higher energy state of ^{222}Rn, which then decays to the ground state by isomeric transition. For each of the transition pathways, the transition energy between parent and ground state of the progeny is constant. In the example of ^{226}Ra, the transition energy is 4.78 MeV.

Beta decay

Nuclei with an N/Z ratio that is above the line of stability tend to decay by a form of beta (β) decay that is sometimes referred to as *negatron emission*. In this mode of decay, a neutron is transformed into a proton, and the Z of the nucleus is increased by 1 with no change in A. In this manner, the N/Z ratio is reduced, and the product nucleus is nearer the line of stability. Simultaneously an electron is ejected from the nucleus together with a neutral massless particle, an antineutrino, that carries away the remainder of the released energy that is not accounted for by the negatron. Neutrinos and antineutrinos seldom interact with matter and are not important to applications of radioactivity in medicine.

The process of beta decay may be written:

$$^{1}_{0}n \rightarrow\, ^{1}_{1}p +\, ^{0}_{-1}e + \bar{\nu}$$
$$\rightarrow\, ^{1}_{1}p +\, ^{0}_{-1}\beta + \bar{\nu}$$

where $^{0}_{-1}e$ depicts the ejected beta particle and $^{0}_{-1}\beta$ reflects the nuclear origin of the electron. The symbol ν represents the antineutrino. An example of beta decay is the beta decay of ^{60}Co:

$$^{60}_{27}Co \rightarrow\, ^{60}_{28}Ni +\, ^{0}_{-1}\beta + \bar{\nu} + \text{isomeric transition}$$

with the isomeric transition often accomplished by the release of cascading γ rays of 1.17 and 1.33 MeV. A decay scheme for ^{60}Co is shown in Figure 1-10 below. The transition energy for decay of ^{60}Co is 2.81 MeV.

A discrete amount of energy is released when an electron is emitted from the nucleus. This energy is depicted as the maximum energy E_{max} of the electron. Electrons, however, usually are emitted with some fraction of this energy and the remainder is carried from the nucleus by the antineutrino. The mean energy of the electron is $E_{max}/3$. An energy spectrum of 0.31 MeV E_{max} electrons emitted from ^{60}Co is shown in Figure 1-9. Electron energy spectra are specific for each electron transition in every nuclide by this mode of nuclear transformation.

Example 1-8

Determine the transition energy and the E_{max} of electrons released during the decay of $^{60}_{27}Co$ (atomic mass 59.933814 amu) $^{60}_{28}Ni$ (atomic mass 59.930787 amu).

$$\text{Transition}: {}^{60}_{27}Co\left[+{}^{60}_{27}e\right]. \rightarrow\, ^{60}_{28}Ni. +\, ^{0}_{-1}\beta + \bar{\nu}$$
$$+\text{isomeric transmission}$$

where the $^{0}_{-1}e$ on the left side of the transition must be added from outside the atom to balance the additional positive nuclear charge of ^{60}Ni compared with ^{60}Co.

$$\text{Mass difference} = \text{mass}(^{60}_{27}Co +\, ^{0}_{-1}e) - \text{mass}\left(^{60}_{28}Ni +\, ^{0}_{-1}\beta\right)$$
$$= (59.933814 + 0.00055)\text{amu}$$
$$-(59.930787 + 0.00055)\text{amu}$$
$$= 0.003027\text{amu}$$
$$\text{Transition energy} = (0.003027\text{ amu})(931\text{ MeV/amu})$$
$$= 2.81\text{ MeV}$$

The isomeric transition in ^{60}Co accounts for $(1.17 + 1.33) = 2.50$ MeV (Figure 1-10). Hence the electron E_{max} is $2.81 - 2.50 = 0.31$ MeV.

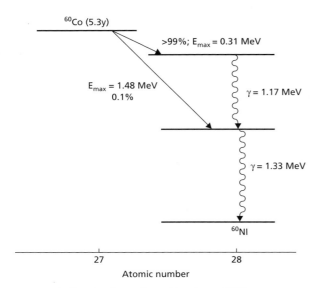

Figure 1-10 Radioactive decay scheme: Beta decay of ^{60}Co.

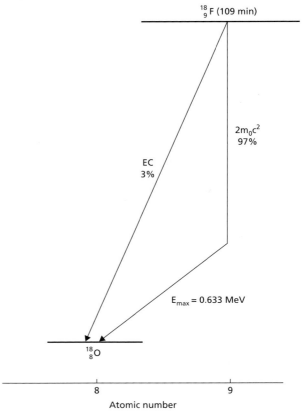

Figure 1-11 Radioactive decay scheme: $^{0}_{+1}\beta$: e capture decay of $^{18}_{8}F$.

Nuclei below the line of stability are unstable because they have too few neutrons for the number of protons in the nucleus. These nuclei tend to gain stability by a decay process in which a proton is transformed into a neutron, resulting in a unit decrease in Z with no change in A. One possibility for this transformation is positron decay:

$$^{1}_{1}p \rightarrow\, ^{1}_{0}n +\, ^{0}_{+1}e + v$$
$$\rightarrow\, ^{1}_{0}n +\, ^{0}_{+1}\beta + v$$

where $^{0}_{+1}\beta$ represents the nuclear origin of the emitted positive electron (positron). A representative positron transition is:

$$^{18}_{9}F \rightarrow\, ^{18}_{8}O +\, ^{0}_{+1}\beta + v$$

where v represents the release of a neutrino, a noninteractive particle similar to an antineutrino except with opposite axial spin. In positron decay, the atomic mass of the decay products exceeds the atomic mass of the atom before decay. This difference in mass must be supplied by energy released during decay according to the relationship $E = mc^2$. The energy requirement is 1.02 MeV. Hence, nuclei with a transition energy less than 1.02 MeV cannot undergo positron decay. For nuclei with transition energy greater than 1.02 MeV, the energy in excess of 1.02 MeV is shared among the kinetic energy of the positron, the energy of the neutrino, and the energy released during isomeric transitions. Decay of ^{18}F is depicted in Figure 1-11 below, in which the vertical component of the positron decay pathway represents the 1.02 MeV of energy that is expressed as increased mass of the products of the decay process.

The emission of positrons from radioactive nuclei was discovered in 1934 by Irène Curie (daughter of Marie Curie) and her husband Frédéric Joliot.[6] In bombardments of aluminum by α particles, they documented the following transmutation:

$$^{4}_{2}He +\, ^{27}_{13}Al \rightarrow\, ^{4}_{2}P +\, ^{1}_{0}n$$
$$^{30}_{15}P \rightarrow\, ^{30}_{14}Si +\, ^{0}_{+1}\beta + v$$

An alternate pathway to positron decay is electron capture, in which an electron from an extranuclear shell, usually the K shell, is captured by the nucleus and combined with a proton to transform it into a neutron. Electron capture of K-shell electrons is known as *K-capture*; electron capture of L-shell electrons is known as *L-capture*; and so on.

The process is represented as:

$$^{1}_{1}P +\, ^{0}_{1}e \rightarrow\, ^{0}_{1}n + v$$

Electron capture does not yield a mass imbalance before and after the transformation. Hence, there is no transition energy prerequisite for electron capture. Low N/Z nuclei with transition energy less than 1.02 MeV can decay only by electron capture. Low N/Z nuclei with transition energy greater than 1.02 MeV can decay by both positron decay and electron capture. For these nuclei, the electron capture branching ratio describes the probability of electron capture, and (1 – branching ratio) depicts the probability of positron decay. Usually, positron decay occurs more frequently than electron capture for nuclei that decay by either process. In Figure 1-11, illustrating electron capture and positron decay, the branching ratio for electron capture of ^{18}F is 3%.

Example 1-9

Determine the transition energy and E_{max} of positrons released during the transformation of $^{18}_{9}F$ (atomic mass = 18.000937 amu) to $^{18}_{8}O$ (atomic mass = 17.999160 amu). There are no isomeric transitions in this decay process.

Transition: $^{18}_{9}F \rightarrow {}^{18}_{8}O + {}^{0}_{1}\beta + \nu + {}^{0}_{1}\theta$

where the $^{0}_{1}e$ on the right side of the transition must be released from the atom to balance the reduced positive nuclear charge of ^{18}O compared with ^{18}F.

$$\text{Mass difference} = \text{mass}\left({}^{18}_{9}F\right) - \text{mass}^{18}_{8}O + {}^{0}_{+1}\beta + \nu + {}^{0}_{+1}e$$
$$= (18.000937)\ \text{amu}$$
$$-(17.999160 + 2(0.00055)\ \text{amu}$$
$$= 0.000677\ \text{amu}$$

$$\text{Energy available as } E_{max} = (0.000677\ \text{amu})(931\ \text{MeV/amu})$$
$$= 0.630\ \text{MeV}$$

The energy equivalent to the mass of the $^{0}_{+1}\beta$ and $^{0}_{1}e$ is $2(0.00055\ \text{amu})(931\ \text{MeV/amu}) = 1.02\ \text{MeV}$. Hence the total transition energy is $(0.63 + 1.02)\ \text{MeV} = 1.65\ \text{MeV}$.

A few unstable nuclei can decay by negatron decay, positron emission, or electron capture. For example, the decay scheme for ^{74}As reveals that electron decay occurs 32% of the time, positron emission occurs with a frequency of 30%, and the nuclide decays by electron capture 38% of the time.

Gamma emission and internal conversion

Frequently during radioactive decay, a product nucleus is formed in an "excited" energy state above the ground energy level. Usually the excited state decays instantly to a lower energy state, often the ground energy level. Occasionally, however, the excited state persists with a finite half-life. An excited energy state that exists for a finite time before decaying is termed a *metastable energy state* and denoted by an "m" following the mass number (e.g., ^{99m}Tc, which has a half-life of 6 hours). The transition from an excited energy state to one nearer the ground state, or to the ground state itself, is termed an *isomeric transition* because the transition occurs between isomers with no change in Z, N, or A. An isomeric transition can occur by either of two processes: γ emission or internal conversion.

Gamma rays are a form of high-energy electromagnetic radiation and differ from x rays only in their origin. Gamma rays are emitted during transitions between isomeric energy states of the nucleus, whereas x rays are emitted during electron transitions outside the nucleus. Gamma rays and other electromagnetic radiation are described by their energy E and frequency ν, two properties that are related by the expression $E = h\nu$, where

h = Planck's constant ($h = 6.62 \times 10^{-34}$ J-sec). The frequency, ν, and wavelength, λ, of electromagnetic radiation are related by the expression $\nu = c/\lambda$, where c is the speed of light in a vacuum.

No radioactive nuclide decays solely by γ emission; an isomeric transition is always preceded by a radioactive decay process, such as electron capture or emission of an alpha particle, negatron, or positron. Isomeric transitions for ^{60}Co (as depicted in an earlier marginal figure) yield γ rays of 1.17 and 1.33 MeV with a frequency of more than 99%. Gamma rays are frequently used in medicine for the detection and diagnosis of a variety of ailments, as well as for the treatment of cancer.

Internal conversion is a competing process to γ emission for an isomeric transition between energy states of a nucleus. In a nuclear transition by internal conversion, the released energy is transferred from the nucleus to an inner electron, which is ejected with a kinetic energy equal to the transferred energy reduced by the binding energy of the electron. Internal conversion is accompanied by the emission of x rays and Auger electrons as the electron structure of the atom resumes a stable configuration following ejection of the conversion electron. The *internal conversion coefficient* is the fraction of conversion electrons divided by the number of γ rays emitted during a particular isomeric transition. The conversion coefficient can be expressed in terms of specific electron shells denoting the origin of the conversion electron. The probability of internal conversion increases with Z and the lifetime of the excited state of the nucleus.

Radioactive equilibrium

Some progeny nuclides produced during radioactive decay are themselves unstable and undergo radioactive decay in a continuing quest for stability. When a radioactive nuclide is produced by the radioactive decay of a parent, a condition can be reached in which the rate of production of the progeny equals the parent's rate of decay. In this condition, the number of progeny atoms and therefore the progeny activity reach their highest level and are constant for a moment in time. This constancy reflects an equilibrium condition known as *transient equilibrium* because it exists only momentarily. In some texts, transient equilibrium is defined as the extended period over which the progeny decays with an apparent half-life equal to the half-life of the parent. This definition is not appropriate because no equilibrium exists beyond the moment when the rate of production of the progeny equals its rate of decay. In cases in which a shorter-lived radioactive progeny is produced by decay of a longer-lived parent, the activity curves for parent and progeny intersect at the moment of transient equilibrium. This intersection reflects the occurrence of equal activities of parent and daughter at that particular moment. After the moment of transient equilibrium has passed, the progeny activity decays with an apparent half-life equal to that of the longer-lived parent. The apparent half-life of the progeny reflects the simultaneous production and decay of the progeny.

If no progeny atoms are present at time $t = 0$, the number N_2 of progeny atoms at any later time t is:

$$N_2 = [\lambda_1/(\lambda_2 - \lambda_1)]N_0 e^{-\lambda_1 t} \qquad (1\text{-}5)$$

In this expression, N_0 is the number of parent atoms present at time $t = 0$, λ_1 is the decay constant of the parent, and λ_2 is the decay constant of the progeny. If progeny atoms are present at time $t = 0$, the expression for N_2 is written:

$$N_2 = (N_2)_0 e^{-\lambda_2 t} + [\lambda_1/(\lambda_2 - \lambda_1)]N_0(e^{-\lambda_1 t} - e^{-\lambda_2 t})$$

Transient equilibrium for a hypothetical nuclide Y formed by decay of the parent X is illustrated in Figure 1-12. The activity of Y is greatest at the moment of transient equilibrium and exceeds the activity of X at all times after transient equilibrium is achieved, provided that no amount of Y is removed from the sample. After transient equilibrium, the activity of progeny Y decays with an apparent half-life equal to that of the parent X. The ratio of activities A_1 and A_2 for X and Y, respectively, is:

$$A_1/A_2 = (\lambda_2 - \lambda_1)/\lambda_2$$

In the hypothetical transient equilibrium between parent X and progeny Y, equilibrium occurs:

- at only one instant of time
- when Y reaches its maximum activity
- when the activity of Y is neither increasing or decreasing
- when the activities of X and Y are equal.

The principle of transient equilibrium is employed in the production of short-lived nuclides useful in nuclear medicine. The nuclide ^{99m}Tc ($T_{1/2} = 6$ hours), used in more than 85% of all nuclear medicine examinations, is produced in a radionuclide generator in which the progeny ^{99m}Tc is produced by decay of

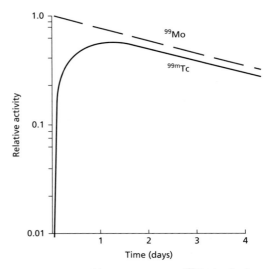

Figure 1-13 Transient equilibrium. Formation of ^{99m}Tc by the decay of ^{99}Mo.

the parent ^{99}Mo ($T_{1/2} = 67$ hours). This process is illustrated in Figure 1-13, in which the moment of transient equilibrium is illustrated as the point of greatest activity in the curve for ^{99m}Tc. In this case, the ^{99m}Tc activity never reaches that of the parent ^{99}Mo because not all of the ^{99}Mo atoms decay through the isomeric energy state ^{99m}Tc. In a ^{99m}Tc generator, the progeny atoms are removed periodically by "milking the cow" (i.e., removing activity from the generator) by using saline solution to flush an ion exchange column to which the parent is firmly attached. This process gives rise to abrupt decreases in ^{99m}Tc activity, as depicted in Figure 1-14.

When the half-life of the parent greatly exceeds that of the progeny (e.g., by a factor of 10^4 or more), equilibrium of the progeny activity is achieved only after a long period of time has

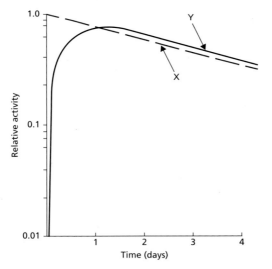

Figure 1-12 Transient equilibrium. Hypothetical radionuclide Y formed by the decay of parent X.

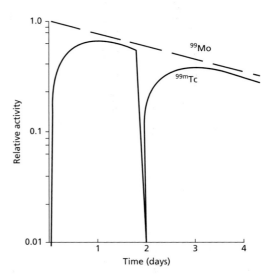

Figure 1-14 Transient equilibrium. Reestablishment of equilibrium after "milking" a ^{99m}Tc generator.

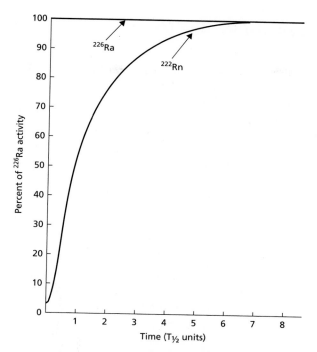

Figure 1-15 Growth of activity and secular equilibrium of ^{222}Rn formed by the decay of ^{226}Ra.

elapsed. The activity of the progeny becomes relatively constant, however, as the progeny activity approaches that of the parent, a condition depicted in Figure 1-15. This condition is known as *secular equilibrium* and is a useful approach for the production of the nuclide ^{222}Rn, which was used at one time in radiation therapy. For radionuclides approaching secular equilibrium, the activities of parent (A_1) and progeny (A_2) are equal, and the number of atoms of parent N_1 (which is essentially N_0 because few atoms have decayed since time $t = 0$) and progeny (N_2) are related by the expression:

$$A_1 = A_2$$
$$\lambda_1 N_1 = \lambda_2 N_2$$
$$N_0/(T_{1/2})_1 = N_2/(T_{1/2})_2$$

An intraophthalmic irradiator containing ^{90}Sr sometimes is used to treat various conditions of the eye. The low-energy beta particles from ^{90}Sr are not useful clinically, but the higher-energy beta particles from the progeny ^{90}Y are useful. The relatively short-lived Y ($T_{1/2} = 64$ hours) is contained in the irradiator in secular equilibrium with the longer-lived parent ^{90}Sr ($T_{1/2} = 28$ years) so that the irradiator can be used over many years without replacement. Radium needles and capsules that were formerly used widely in radiation oncology contained many decay products in secular equilibrium with the long-lived ($T_{1/2} = 1600$ years) parent ^{226}Ra.

Natural radioactivity and decay series

Most radionuclides in nature are members of one of three naturally occurring radioactive decay series. Each series consists of a sequence of radioactive transformations that begins with a long-lived radioactive parent and ends with a stable nuclide. In a closed environment such as the earth, intermediate radioactive progeny exist in secular equilibrium with the long-lived parent, and decay with an apparent half-life equal to that of the parent. All naturally occurring radioactive nuclides decay by emitting either alpha or negative beta particles. Hence, each transformation in a radioactive series changes the mass number by either 4 or 0 and changes the atomic number by −2 or +1.

The uranium series depicted in Figure 1-16 begins with the isotope ^{238}U and ends with the stable nuclide ^{206}Pb. The parent and each product in this series have a mass number that is divisible by 4 with remainder of 2; the uranium series is also known as the *4n + 2 series*. The naturally occurring isotopes ^{226}Ra and ^{222}Rn are members of the uranium series. The actinium (4n + 3) series begins with ^{235}U and ends with ^{207}Pb, and the thorium (4n) series begins with ^{232}Th and ends with ^{208}Pb. Members of the hypothetical neptunium (4n + 1) series do not occur in nature because no long-lived parent is available. Fourteen naturally occurring radioactive nuclides are not members of a decay series. These nuclides, all with relatively long half-lives, are ^{3}H, ^{14}C, ^{40}K, ^{50}V, ^{87}Rb, ^{115}In, ^{130}Te, ^{138}La, ^{142}Ce, ^{144}Nd, ^{147}Sm, ^{176}Lu, ^{187}Re, and ^{192}Pt.

Artificial production of radionuclides

Radioactive isotopes with properties useful in biomedical research and clinical medicine may be produced by bombarding selected nuclei with neutrons or high-energy charged particles. Nuclides with excess neutrons that subsequently decay by

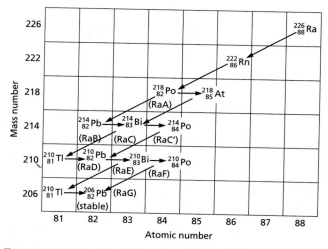

Figure 1-16 Uranium (4n + 2) decay series. Note that ^{238}U (with mass number 238 and atomic number 92) is not shown on this graph.

negatron emission are created by bombarding nuclei with neutrons in a nuclear reactor or from a neutron generator. Typical reactions are:

$$^{13}_{6}C + ^{1}_{0}n \rightarrow ^{14}_{6}C + \text{isomeric transition}$$

$$^{13}_{15}P + ^{1}_{0}n \rightarrow ^{32}_{15}P + \text{isomeric transition}$$

Useful isotopes produced by neutron bombardment include ^{3}H, ^{35}S, ^{51}Cr, ^{60}Co, ^{99}Mo, ^{133}Xe, and ^{198}Au. Because the isomeric transition frequently results in the prompt emission of a γ ray, neutron bombardment often is referred to as an (n, γ) reaction. The reaction yields a product nuclide with an increase in A of 1 and no increase in Z. The complete transformation, including radioactive decay that results from neutron bombardment, is demonstrated by the example of ^{60}Co:

$$^{59}_{27}Co + ^{1}n \rightarrow ^{60}_{27}Co + \text{isomeric transitions}$$

$$^{60}_{27}Co \rightarrow ^{60}_{28}Ni + ^{0}_{-1}\beta + v + \text{isomeric transitions}$$

The transition can be represented as ^{59}Co$(n, \gamma)^{60}$Co. The decay of ^{60}Co occurs with a half-life of 5.27 years. The isomeric transitions accompanying this decay process almost always result in the emission of cascading γ rays of 1.17 and 1.33 MeV.

Radionuclides with excess protons are produced when nuclei are bombarded with high-energy positively charged particles from a particle accelerator. These radionuclides then decay by electron capture and, if the transition energy is adequate, positron decay. A typical reaction is:

$$^{11}_{5}B + ^{1}_{1}P \rightarrow ^{11}_{6}C + ^{1}_{0}n$$

where $^{1}_{0}n$ denotes that a neutron is ejected from the nucleus during bombardment so that the parent and progeny nuclei are isobars. This reaction can be represented as ^{11}B$(p, n)^{11}$C and is termed a (p, n) reaction. Other representative charged-particle interactions include:

$$^{14}_{7}N + ^{4}_{2}He \rightarrow ^{17}_{8}O + ^{1}_{1}p \quad [(\alpha, p) \text{ reaction}]$$

$$^{68}_{30}Zn + ^{1}_{1}p \rightarrow ^{67}_{31}Ga + 2^{1}_{1}n \quad [(p, 2n) \text{ reaction}]$$

$$^{27}_{13}Al + ^{4}_{2}He \rightarrow ^{30}_{15}P + ^{1}_{0}n \quad [(\alpha, n) \text{ reaction}]$$

$$^{12}_{6}C + ^{1}_{1}p \rightarrow ^{13}_{7}N + y \quad [(p, \gamma) \text{ reaction}]$$

$$^{3}_{1}H + ^{2}_{1}d \rightarrow ^{4}_{2}He + ^{1}_{0}n \quad [(p, n) \text{ reaction}]$$

where d stands for deuteron, a particle composed of a proton and neutron (i.e., a nucleus of deuterium).

Radioactive nuclides are also produced as a result of nuclear fission. These nuclides can be recovered as fission byproducts from the fuel elements used in nuclear reactors. Isotopes such as ^{90}Sr, ^{99}Mo, ^{131}I, and ^{137}Cs can be recovered in this manner.

Fission-produced nuclides (fission byproducts) are often mixed with other stable and radioactive isotopes of the same element, and cannot be separated chemically as a solitary radionuclide.[7] As a consequence, fission byproducts are less useful in research and clinical medicine than are radionuclides that are produced by neutron or charged-particle bombardment.

Summary

- Radioactive decay is the consequence of nuclear instability.
- Negatron decay occurs in nuclei with a high N/Z ratio.
- Positron decay and electron capture occur in nuclei with a low N/Z ratio.
- Alpha decay occurs with heavy unstable nuclei.
- Isomeric transitions occur between different energy states of nuclei and result in the emission of γ rays and conversion electrons.
- The activity A of a sample is:

$$A = A_o e^{-\lambda t}$$

where λ is the decay constant (fractional rate of decay).
- The half-life $T_{1/2}$ is the time required for half of a radioactive sample to decay.
- The half-life and the decay constant are related by:

$$T_{1/2} = 0.693/\lambda$$

- The common unit of activity is the Becquerel (Bq), with 1 Bq = 1 disintegration/second.
- Transient equilibrium may exist when the progeny nuclide decays with a $T_{1/2} < T_{1/2}$ parent.
- Secular equilibrium may exist when the progeny nuclide decays with a $T_{1/2} \ll T_{1/2}$ parent.
- Most radioactive nuclides found in nature are members of naturally occurring decay series.

Problems

1-1 What are the atomic and mass numbers of the oxygen isotope with 17 nucleons? Calculate the mass defect, binding *energy*, and binding *energy* per nucleon for this nuclide, with the assumption that the mass defect is associated with the nucleus. The mass of the atom is 16.999133 amu.

1-2 Natural oxygen contains three isotopes with atomic masses in amu of 15.9949, 16.9991, and 17.9992 and relative abundances of 2500:1:5. Determine to three decimal places the average atomic mass of oxygen.

1-3 Determine the *energy* required to move an electron from the K to the L shell in tungsten and in hydrogen, and explain the difference.

1-4 What is the *energy* equivalent to the mass of an electron? A proton?

1-5 The *energy* released during the nuclear explosion at Hiroshima has been estimated as equivalent to that released by 20,000 tons of TNT. Assume that 200 MeV is released when a ^{235}U nucleus absorbs a neutron and fissions and that 3.8×10^{9}J is released during detonation of 1 ton of TNT. How many nuclear fissions occurred at Hiroshima, and what was the total decrease in mass?

1-6 Group the following nuclides as isotopes, isotones, and isobars:

$$^{14}_{6}C, \, ^{14}_{7}N, \, ^{15}_{7}N, \, ^{15}_{6}C, \, ^{16}_{7}N, \, ^{16}_{8}O, \, ^{17}_{8}O$$

1-7 The half-life of ^{32}P is 14.3 days. What interval of time is required for 100 mCi of ^{32}P to decay to 25 mCi? What time is required for the decay of 7/8 of the ^{32}P atoms?

1-8 A radioactive needle contains $^{222}_{86}Rn$ ($T_{1/2} = 3.83$ days) in secular equilibrium with $^{222}_{88}Ra$ ($T_{1/2} = 1600$ years). How long is required for the $^{222}_{86}Rn$ to decay to half of its original activity?

1-9 In nature, $^{222}_{88}Ra$ ($T_{1/2} = 1600$ years) exists in secular equilibrium with $^{238}_{92}U$ ($T_{1/2} = 4.5 \times 10^9$ years). What fraction of the world's supply of radium will be left after 1600 years?

1-10 What is the mass in grams of 100 MBq of pure ^{32}P? How many ^{32}P atoms constitute 100 MBq? What is the mass in grams of 100 MBq of Na_3PO_4 if all the phosphorus in the compound is radioactive?

1-11 If a radionuclide decays for an interval of time equal to its average life, what percentage of the original activity remains?

1-12 What are the wavelength and frequency of a 1 MeV photon? A 15 MeV photon?

1-13 ^{126}I nuclei decay by negatron emission, positron emission, and electron capture. Write the decay equation for each mode of decay and identify the daughter nuclide.

1-14 How many atoms and grams of ^{90}Y are in secular equilibrium with 50 mCi of ^{90}Sr?

1-15 How many MBq of ^{132}I ($T_{1/2} = 2.3$ hours) should be ordered so that the sample activity will be 500 MBq when it arrives 24 hours later?

1-16 $^{127}_{53}I$ is the only stable isotope of iodine. What mode(s) of decay would be expected for ^{131}I? ^{125}I?

1-17 For a nuclide X with the decay scheme how many γ rays are emitted per 100 disintegrations of X if the coefficient for interval conversion is 0.25?

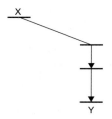

1-18 ^3H (3.016050 amu) decays to ^3_2He (3.016030 amu) by negatron emission. What is the transition *energy* and negatron E_{max} if no isomeric transitions occur?

1-19 $^{11}_{6}C$ (11.011432 amu) decays to $^{11}_{5}B$ (11.009305 amu) by positron emission and electron capture. What is the transition *energy* and positron E_{max} if no isomeric transitions occur?

References

1 Bailey, C. *The Greek Atomists and Epicurus*. New York, Oxford University Press, 1928.

2 Bohr, N. On the constitution of atoms and molecules. *Philos. Mag.* 1913; **26**:476, 875.

3 Bohr, N. Neutron capture and nuclear constitution. *Nature* 1936; **137**:344.

4 Broyles, C. D., Thomas, D. A., and Haynes, S. K. K-shell fluorescence yields as a function of atomic number. *Phys. Rev.* 1953; **89**:715.

5 Becquerel, H. Sur les radiations émises par phosphorescence. *Compt. Rend.* 1896; **122**:420.

6 Curie, I., and Joliot, F. Physique nucléaire: Un nouvean type de radioactivité. *Compt. Rend.* 1934; **198**:254.

7 Hendee, W. R., and Ritenour, E. R., *Medical Imaging Physics*, 4th edition. New York, John Wiley & Sons, Inc., 2001.

CHAPTER

2

INTERACTIONS OF X RAYS AND GAMMA RAYS

Objectives

After studying this chapter, the reader should be able to:
- Perform simple computations related to x- and γ-ray attenuation and transmission.
- Distinguish among various attenuation and absorption coefficients and convert one to another.
- Explain exponential attenuation and broad- and narrow-beam geometry.
- Outline the principles and the variables that influence:
  ○ Photoelectric interactions
  ○ Compton interactions
  ○ Pair production.
- Compute the energy of Compton-scattered photons.
- Define the concepts of:
  ○ Half-value layer and tenth-value layers
  ○ Mean free path
  ○ Linear attenuation coefficient
  ○ Compton wavelength.

Introduction

An x or γ ray impinging on a material leads to one of three possible outcomes. The photon may be (1) transmitted through the material without interaction, (2) scattered in a different direction during one or more interactions, or (3) absorbed by the transfer of its energy to the material through one or more interactions. Photons that traverse a material without interaction are referred to as primary photons or *primary radiation*, whereas photons that are scattered are considered *secondary radiation*. If the photon is absorbed or scattered, it is said to have undergone *attenuation*. Attenuation processes can involve single or multiple interactions and can result in the transfer of all or only part of the photon's energy to the material. Scattering usually removes photons from an x- or γ-ray beam but does not always do so, especially if the beam is broad or the scattering occurs

Hendee's Radiation Therapy Physics, Fourth Edition. Todd Pawlicki, Daniel J. Scanderbeg and George Starkschall.
© 2016 John Wiley & Sons, Inc. Published 2016 by John Wiley & Sons, Inc.

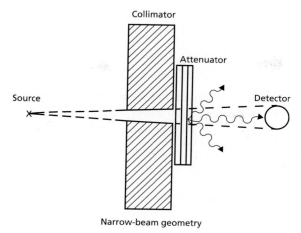

Figure 2-1 Narrow-beam (good) geometry.
Source: Hendee and Ritenour 2001.[1] Reproduced with permission from John Wiley and Sons, Ltd.

through small angles. As the distance increases on the far side of a scattering material, the number of scattered photons decreases in an x- or γ-ray beam, because the scattered photons have a greater likelihood of escaping from the beam. A measurement of x- or γ-ray intensity for a narrow beam of photons at a location far from a scatterer is said to be taken under conditions of narrow-beam geometry. A similar measurement obtained near a scatterer or for a broad beam of photons is considered to have been acquired under conditions of broad-beam geometry. These concepts are illustrated in Figure 2-1 and Figure 2-2 and summarized in Table 2-1.[1]

Attenuation of x rays and gamma rays

The fractional number of photons $\Delta I/I$ attenuated in an infinitesimally thin slab of material of thickness Δx is $\Delta I/I =$

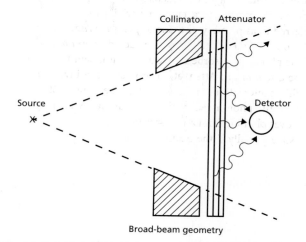

Figure 2-2 Broad-beam (poor) geometry for attenuation measurements.
Source: Hendee and Ritenour 2001.[1] Reproduced with permission from John Wiley and Sons, Ltd.

Table 2-1 Narrow beam versus broad beam geometry.

Narrow-beam geometry	Broad-beam geometry
Very small beam (highly collimated)	Wide beam (large collimation)
Attenuator far from detector	Attenuator near detector
Very little scatter reaches detector	Large amount of scatter reaches detector

$-\mu\Delta x$, where μ is referred to as the *linear attenuation coefficient*.[1] This can be rewritten as $\mu = -\left(\Delta I/I\right)/\Delta x$. In this form, we can interpret the equation to mean that the linear attenuation coefficient is the fractional decrease in the number of photons per unit thickness of absorber. This is often a more useful way of understanding the linear attenuation coefficient. For example, a linear attenuation coefficient of 0.001 cm^{-1} means that 0.1% (0.001) of the photons in the beam are attenuated per cm of absorber. We will see why this interpretation is useful later in the chapter. Under conditions of narrow-beam geometry, the number of photons, I, transmitted through a material of finite thickness, x, is:

$$I = I_o e^{-\mu x}$$

There is no exact analytical expression for the transmission of photons under broad-beam conditions. The expression usually encountered is:

$$I = BI_0 e^{-\mu x}$$

where B is a *build-up factor* that varies with the area and energy of the photon beam and the nature of the attenuating material.

The fractional transmission is $I/I_0 = e^{-\mu x}$, where I_0 is the number of photons reaching the same point on the far side of the attenuating material in the absence of the material. The expression $e^{-\mu x}$ represents the exponential quantity, e, raised to the power $-\mu x$, where $e = 2.7183$. The number of x or γ rays attenuated (absorbed or scattered) in the material is I^*, where:

$$I^* = I_0 - I = I_0 - I_0 e^{-\mu x}$$
$$= I_0(I - e^{-\mu x})$$

The fractional attenuation is $I^*/I_0 = I - e^{-\mu x}$.

The exponent of e must carry no units. Hence, if the thickness x has units of cm, μ must have units of 1/cm (or m and 1/m, mm and 1/mm, and so on). The value of the linear attenuation coefficient depends on the energy of the x or γ rays and the composition (atomic number and physical density) of the material.

At times, the dependence of μ on the physical density (g/cm^3) of the attenuating material is troublesome, and a coefficient that is independent of density is desirable. The *mass attenuation coefficient*, μ_m, has this advantage and is defined as the linear attenuation coefficient divided by the density of the material. Sometimes the relationship is explicitly written as μ/ρ. Mass attenuation coefficients have units of area/mass, such as cm^2/g or m^2/kg. Thicknesses are often expressed in units of mass/area (e.g., g/cm^2 or kg/m^2) when they are used in combination with mass attenuating coefficients. A thickness expressed in units of

Table 2-2 Relationships among attenuation coefficients.

Coefficient	Symbol	Unit
Linear	μ	m^{-1}
Mass	μ_m	m^2/kg
Atomic	μ_a	$m^2/atom$
Electronic	μ_e	$m^2/electron$

mass per unit area is termed *areal density* and is computed as the product of the linear thickness (cm or m) times the physical (mass) density (g/cm³ or kg/m³).

Attenuation coefficients may also have other units. For example, the *atomic attenuation coefficient*, μ_a, has units of area/atom (e.g., cm²/atom or m²/atom), and corresponding thicknesses have units of atoms/area. The atomic attenuation coefficient, μ_a, is related to the linear attenuation coefficient, μ, by $\mu_a = \mu M/\rho N_a$, where M is the gram-atomic mass and N_a is Avogadro's number.

Another coefficient encountered occasionally is the *electronic attenuation coefficient*, μ_e, with units of area/electron. Corresponding attenuator thicknesses have units of electrons/area. The electronic attenuation coefficient is related to the linear attenuation coefficient μ by $\mu_e = \mu_a/Z = \mu M/\rho N_a Z$. Note that, for most materials, M/Z lies between 2.0 and 2.5. Since N_a is a constant ($= 6.02 \times 10^{23}$ atoms/g-atomic mass), the electronic attenuation coefficient will be approximately a constant times the mass attenuation coefficient.

The relationships among the various attenuation coefficients are illustrated in Table 2-2.

Conversion among attenuation coefficients and computations with different coefficients is illustrated in Example 2-1.

Example 2-1

A A narrow beam of 5000 monoenergetic photons is reduced to 1000 photons by a copper absorber 2 cm thick. What is the linear attenuation coefficient of the copper absorber for these photons?

$$I = I_0 e^{-\mu x}$$
$$I/I_0 = e^{-\mu x}$$
$$I_0/I = e^{\mu x}$$
$$\ln I_0/I = \mu x$$
$$\ln\left[\frac{5000}{1000}\right] = \mu[2 \text{ cm}]$$
$$\mu = \ln(5)/2 \text{ cm} = 1.61/2 \text{ cm}$$
$$\mu = 0.81 \text{ cm}^{-1}$$

B What are the mass (μ_m), atomic (μ_a), and electronic (μ_e) attenuation coefficients? Copper has a density of ρ of 8.9 g/cm³, a gram-atomic mass M of 63.6, and an atomic number Z of 29.

The mass attenuation coefficient is the linear attenuation coefficient divided by the mass density, or:

$$\mu_m = \mu/\rho = 0.81 \text{ cm}^{-1}/8.9 \text{ g/cm}^3$$
$$= 0.091 \text{ cm}^2/\text{g}$$

The atomic attenuation coefficient is the mass attenuation coefficient divided by the number of atoms per unit mass, or:

$$\mu_a = \frac{\mu M}{\rho N_A} = \frac{(0.81 \text{ cm}^{-1})(63.6 \text{ g/g-atomic mass})}{(8.9 \text{ g/cm}^3)(6.02 \times 10^{23} \text{ atoms/g-atomic mass})}$$
$$= 9.6 \times 10^{-24} \text{ cm}^2/\text{atom}$$

The electronic attenuation coefficient is the mass attenuation coefficient divided by the number of electrons per unit mass, or:

$$\mu_e = \mu_a/Z = (9.6 \times 10^{-24} \text{ cm}^2/\text{atom})/29 \text{ electrons/atom}$$
$$= 3.3 \times 10^{-25} \text{ cm}^2/\text{electron}$$

C An additional 2 cm of copper is added to the copper absorber in part A. How many photons remain in the beam?

$$I = I_0 e^{-\mu x} = 5000 e^{-(0.81 \text{ cm}^{-1})(4 \text{ cm})}$$
$$= 5000 e^{-3.24}$$
$$= 5000(0.0392)$$
$$= 200 \text{ photons}$$

The first 2 cm of copper absorbed 4000 photons (80%), leaving 1000 photons in the beam. An additional 800 photons (80%) are absorbed by the second 2 cm of Cu, leaving 200 photons in the beam.

D What is the thickness x_e in electrons per square centimeter for the 4 cm absorber?

$$x_e = x_a Z = \frac{x N_a \rho Z}{M}$$
$$\frac{(4 \text{ cm})(6 \times 10^{23} \text{ atom/g-atomicmass})(8.9 \text{ g/cm}^3)(29 \text{ electron/atom})}{(63.6 \text{ g/g-atomicmass})}$$
$$= 9.77 \times 10^{24} \text{ electrons/cm}^2$$

E Repeat the calculation in part C using the electronic attenuation coefficient.

$$I = I_0 e^{-\mu x}$$
$$= 5000 e - (3.3 \times 10^{-25} \text{ cm}^2 \text{ electron})$$
$$\times (9.77 \times 10^{24} \text{ electrons/cm}^2)$$
$$= 5000(0.0392)$$
$$= 200 \text{ photons}$$

The *mean path length*, also called the *mean free path* or *relaxation length*, is the average distance traveled by x or γ rays before they interact with a particular material. The mean path length is $1/\mu$, where μ is the linear attenuation coefficient of the material for particular photons.

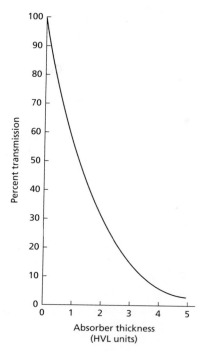

Figure 2-3 Linear plot of percent transmission of a narrow beam of monoenergetic photons as a function of the thickness of an attenuator in units of HVL.

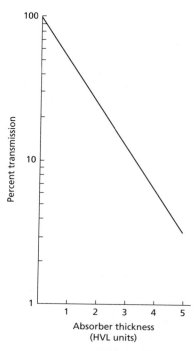

Figure 2-4 Semilogarithmic plot of percent transmission of a narrow beam of monoenergetic photons as a function of the thickness of an attenuator in units of HVL.

The thickness of a material required to reduce the intensity of an x- or γ-ray beam to half its initial value under conditions of narrow-beam geometry is called the *half-value layer* (*HVL*), or *half-value thickness* (*HVT*). The HVL is related to the attenuation coefficient by the expression HVL = 0.693/μ, where 0.693 is the natural logarithm of 2. In Example 2-1, the HVL is 0.693/0.81 cm^{-1} = 0.85 cm of Cu. Half-value layers can be expressed in other units, such as g/cm^2, atoms/cm^2, or electrons/cm^2.

The expression I = $I_0 e^{-\mu x}$ is termed an *exponential equation*. A narrow beam of monoenergetic x or γ rays passing through a material of constant composition is said to be attenuated exponentially. Figure 2-3 illustrates a graph of exponential behavior.

Rewriting the exponential equation in logarithmic form yields:

$$\ln(I/I_0) = -\mu x$$

This expression reveals that ln (I/I_0) decreases linearly with increasing thickness of the attenuator. The ratio I/I_0, expressed as percent transmission, can be plotted on both a linear and a logarithmic axis as a function of thickness x of the attenuator on a linear axis. A graph of I/I_0 on a logarithmic axis and x on a linear axis is termed a *semilogarithmic plot*. Figure 2-4 illustrates such a graph on a semilogarithmic plot.

For an x- or γ-ray beam to be attenuated exponentially, it must be monoenergetic and measured under conditions of narrow-beam geometry. A polyenergetic beam such as an x-ray beam from a linear accelerator is not attenuated exponentially because the absorber selectively removes lower-energy x rays from the beam. As a consequence, the beam's average energy, and therefore its attenuation coefficient, changes as the beam proceeds through the material. These changes result in a gradual increase in the penetrating ability of the x-ray beam as it moves through the attenuator and lower-energy x rays are selectively removed.

From measurements of the HVL of a polyenergetic beam, an effective attenuation coefficient, μ_{eff}, can be estimated as μ_{eff} = 0.693/HVL. The effective energy can then be determined as the energy of monoenergetic photons that have an attenuation coefficient identical to μ_{eff}.

The *homogeneity coefficient* is the ratio of the first HVL (the thickness of attenuator required to reduce the beam's intensity to half) divided by the second HVL (the thickness required to reduce the intensity from half to one-quarter). For a narrow, monoenergetic beam, the homogeneity coefficient is unity; for polyenergetic beams, it is less than unity.

In general, the attenuation coefficient of a material decreases with increasing energy of incident photons. Consequently, lower-energy photons are attenuated more readily than those of higher energy. A polyenergetic beam becomes more penetrating (it is said to become "harder") after it has traversed an attenuating material because lower-energy photons have been selectively removed from the beam.

Example 2-2

1.2 mm of copper is required to reduce the intensity of an x-ray beam to half, and an additional 1.4 mm is needed to reduce the intensity from half to one-quarter. What are the first HVL, homogeneity coefficient, effective linear and mass attenuation coefficients, and effective energy of the x-ray beam?

$$HVL = 1.2 \text{ cm Cu}$$

$$\text{Homogeneity coefficient} = \frac{(HVL)_1}{(HVL)_2} = \frac{1.2 \text{ mm Cu}}{1.4 \text{ mm Cu}}$$

$$= 0.86$$

$$\mu_{eff} = 0.693/HVL = 0.693/1.2 \text{ mm Cu}$$

$$= 0.58 \text{ mm}^{-1} = 5.8 \text{ cm}^{-1}$$

$$(\mu_{eff})_m = \mu_{eff}/\rho = 5.8 \text{ cm}^{-1}/8.9 \text{ g/cm}^3$$

$$= 0.652 \text{ cm}^2/\text{g}$$

Monoenergetic photons of 88 keV have a total mass attenuation coefficient of 0.65 cm^2/g in copper. Consequently, the effective energy of the x-ray beam is 88 keV.

The linear attenuation coefficient and mass attenuation coefficients give us a measure of the fractional decrease in number of photons per unit absorber thickness. Often, however, we are more interested in how energy is transferred from the radiation beam to charged particles in the absorber as a result of an interaction process. As we shall see later in this chapter, not all of the energy of the incident photon is transferred to charged particles. If $\bar{E}_{tr}$ is the mean energy transferred from the incident radiation beam to charged particles in the absorber, then $\bar{E}_{tr}/h\nu$ is the fraction of energy transferred from the radiation beam. The *energy transfer coefficient*, $\mu_{tr} = \mu \left[\bar{E}_{tr}/h\nu\right]$, is a measure of the fraction of energy of the beam that is transferred from the beam per unit absorber thickness. In addition to an energy transfer coefficient, we could also have a *mass energy transfer coefficient*, an *atomic energy transfer coefficient*, and an *electronic energy transfer coefficient*.

Example 2-3a

An incident photon beam of energy 100 keV transfers a mean energy of 60 keV to charged particles in the absorber. If the linear attenuation coefficient is 0.500 mm^{-1}, what is the energy transfer coefficient?

$$\mu_{tr} = \mu \left[\bar{E}_{tr}/h\nu\right]$$

$$= 0.500 \text{ mm}^{-1}(60 \text{ keV})/(100 \text{ keV})$$

$$= 0.300 \text{ mm}^{-1}$$

The energy transferred to the charged particles in the absorber can be converted back into photons through the production of Bremsstrahlung or characteristic radiation, or it can be absorbed locally by the charged particles. Of particular interest in dosime-

try is the energy that is absorbed locally. If we let g be the fraction of energy that is re-radiated in the form of Bremsstrahlung or characteristic radiation, then the *energy absorption coefficient*, μ_{en}, given by $\mu_{en} = \mu_{tr}[1 - g]$, is a measure of the energy absorbed in the attenuator per unit absorber thickness.

Example 2-3b

If in Example 2-3a 1% of the incident energy were re-radiated as Bremsstrahlung or characteristic radiation, what would be the energy absorption coefficient?

$$\mu_{en} = \mu_{tr}\left[1 - g\right]$$

$$= 0.300 \text{ mm}^{-1}(0.99)$$

$$= 0.297 \text{ mm}^{-1}$$

The *mass energy absorption coefficient*, $[\mu_{en}]_m = \mu_{en}/\rho$, is particularly important in radiation therapy because it provides us with the connection between the number of photons in a beam and the energy absorbed per unit mass in the absorber, or the radiation dose. Attenuation and energy absorption coefficients for water (a medium that closely simulates muscle) are plotted in Figure 2-5 as a function of photon energy.

Example 2-4

The linear attenuation coefficient is 0.071 cm^{-1} for 1 MeV photons in water. If the energy absorption coefficient for 1 MeV photons in water is 0.031 cm^{-1}, find the average energy absorbed in

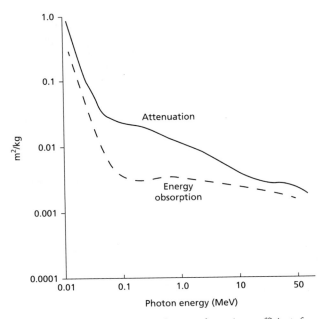

Figure 2-5 Total mass attenuation and energy absorption coefficients for water as a function of photon energy.

water per photon interaction.

$$\mu_{en} = \mu \frac{E_a}{h\nu}$$

$$\begin{aligned}
E_a &= \frac{\mu_{en}}{\mu}(h\nu) \\
&= \frac{0.031 \text{ cm}^{-1}}{0.071 \text{ cm}^{-1}}(1 \text{ } MeV) \\
&= 0.44 \text{ MeV} \\
&= 440 \text{ keV}
\end{aligned}$$

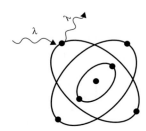

Figure 2-6 Coherent scattering in which the photon is absorbed and reradiated in a different direction with no significant loss of energy.

X-ray and gamma-ray interactions

X rays and γ rays can interact by several different mechanisms, including coherent scattering, photoelectric absorption, Compton scattering, pair production, and photodisintegration. These possibilities can be depicted as:

$$e^{-\mu x} = (e^{-\omega x}) \cdot (e^{-\tau x}) \cdot (e^{-\sigma x}) \cdot (e^{-\kappa x}) \cdot (e^{-\pi x}) = e^{-(\omega+\tau+\sigma+\kappa+\pi)x}$$

where $e^{-\mu x}$ is the probability that a photon traverses a medium of thickness x without interacting, and $e^{-\omega x} \dots e^{-\pi x}$ represent the probabilities that the photon does not interact by specific interaction mechanisms. The total linear attenuation coefficient can be partitioned into separate coefficients for coherent scattering (ω), photoelectric absorption (τ), Compton scattering (σ), pair production (κ), and photodisintegration (π). At times, this expression can be simplified to fewer coefficients because certain mechanisms of interaction are negligible. A diagnostic x-ray beam cannot interact by pair production or photodisintegration, because the energy of the x rays is too low. Hence, the expression for μ simplifies to $\mu = \omega + \tau + \sigma$ for a diagnostic x-ray beam. Similarly, a therapeutic x-ray beam may not interact by coherent scattering or photodisintegration, permitting simplification of the expression for μ to $\mu = \tau + \sigma + \kappa$. The individual coefficients for various interactions have equivalent expressions for mass, atomic, and electronic coefficients. For example:

$$\mu_m = \frac{\mu}{\rho}; \ \omega_m = \frac{\omega}{\rho}; \ \tau_m = \frac{\tau}{\rho}; \ \sigma_m = \frac{\sigma}{\rho}; \ \kappa_m = \frac{k}{\rho}; \ \pi_m = \frac{\pi}{\rho}$$

Coherent scattering

Low-energy photons can be deflected or scattered by the process of *coherent (Rayleigh) scattering*, sometimes referred to as *classical scattering*.[2] In this interaction, the energy of a photon is transferred completely to an atom, which then radiates the energy of the photon in a different direction (Figure 2-6). Hence the incoming photon appears to have shifted in direction (i.e., to have been scattered) with no change in energy.

Coherent scattering is negligible for high-energy photons interacting in relatively low-Z tissues, such as those in the body. Hence, it can be ignored in essentially all applications of radiation therapy.

Photoelectric interactions

A *photoelectric interaction* results in a transfer of the total energy of a photon to an inner-shell electron of an atom of the absorbing medium (Figure 2-7). The electron, termed a *photoelectron*, is ejected from the atom with kinetic energy $E_k = h\nu - E_b$, where $h\nu$ is the energy of the photon and E_b is the binding energy of the ejected electron. Vacancies created by ejected electrons are filled by cascading electrons, resulting in the emission of characteristic photons and Auger electrons. When photons interact in tissue via the photoelectric effect, the characteristic photons and Auger electrons have energies less than 0.5 keV, and are readily absorbed in tissue in the immediate vicinity of the site of interaction.

Photoelectric interactions occur primarily for x and γ rays of relatively low energy, and the probability of this type of interaction decreases rapidly with increasing photon energy. In general, the mass attenuation coefficient for photoelectric absorption decreases as $(1/h\nu)^3$, where $h\nu$ is the photon energy. Shown in Figure 2-8 are the mass attenuation coefficients for photoelectric interaction in muscle and lead, plotted as a function of photon energy. Discontinuities in the plot of photoelectric absorption coefficients for lead, termed *absorption edges*, occur at photon energies equal to the binding energy of electrons in the inner electron shells. Photons with energy less than the binding energy of K-shell electrons cannot eject K electrons from the atom. These photons can interact via the photoelectric effect

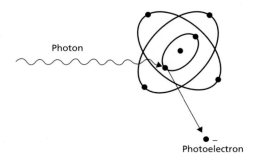

Figure 2-7 Photoelectric interaction in which the photon disappears and is replaced by an electron ejected from the atom with kinetic energy $E_k = h\nu - E_b$, where E_b is the electron binding energy. Characteristic radiation and Auger electrons are emitted as cascading electrons replace the ejected photoelectron.

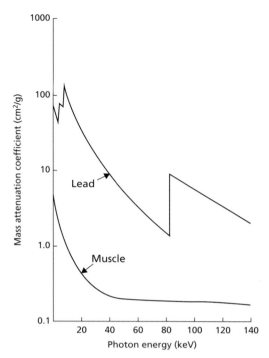

Figure 2-8 Mass attenuation coefficient for photons in muscle and lead as a function of photon energy. K- and L-absorption edges are depicted in lead.

only with more loosely bound electrons in the L, M, and other shells. Photons with energy greater than the K-shell binding energy selectively interact with K-shell electrons through the photoelectric process. Exceeding the threshold energy for photoelectric interactions with K-shell electrons causes an abrupt increase in the photoelectric attenuation coefficient at the K-shell binding energy. In soft tissue, the binding energy of K-shell electrons is too low to be depicted in Figure 2-8. The elements iodine and barium have binding energies of 33 and 36 keV, respectively, and are considered almost ideal absorbers of x rays in the diagnostic energy range. For this reason, they are widely employed as contrast agents in diagnostic radiology.[3]

The probability of a photoelectric interaction depends on the atomic number of the absorbing material as well as on the energy of the x or γ rays. In general, the photoelectric mass attenuation coefficient varies directly with Z^3. The likelihood of photoelectric interaction of low-energy photons is almost four times greater in bone ($Z_{eff} = 11.6$) than in an equal mass of soft tissue ($Z_{eff} = 7.4$) because $(11.6/7.4)^3 = 3.8$. The expression Z_{eff} represents the effective atomic number of a multielement absorber, defined as the Z of an imaginary single element that attenuates x and γ rays in the same manner as the absorber. The effective atomic number is discussed further in Chapter 5.

The incident photon beam can be looked on as a transverse electromagnetic wave in which the electric field is perpendicular to the direction of propagation of the photon beam. The photoelectrons can be viewed as moving with the electric field; consequently, when ejected from the atom, they will be preferentially ejected perpendicular to the direction of the incident photons. As the energy of the photon beam increases, the photon beam will carry more momentum in a forward direction. In order to conserve momentum, the photoelectrons will be ejected in a more forward direction.

Example 2-5

What is the kinetic energy of a photoelectron ejected from the K shell of lead ($E_b = 88$ keV) by photoelectric absorption of a 200 keV photon?

$$E_k = hv = E_b$$
$$= 200 \text{ keV} - 88 \text{ keV}$$
$$= 112 \text{ keV}$$

Selective attenuation of photons by photoelectric interactions in materials with different atomic numbers and different physical densities is one of the principal reasons why low-energy x rays are useful for producing images in diagnostic radiology. Prior to the introduction of megavoltage radiation therapy, the presence of photoelectric interactions resulted in an enhanced dose to bone over soft tissue. Photoelectric interactions rarely occur at the higher photon energies currently employed in radiation therapy. Hence, differences in atomic number among different media are relatively unimportant in determining the likelihood of photon interactions in radiation therapy. This property is advantageous in therapy because it permits delivery of relatively large doses of soft tissue tumors without excessive doses to higher-Z structures such as bone.

To summarize, photoelectric interactions:
- involve only bound electrons
- increase in likelihood with Z^3
- decrease in likelihood with $(hv)^3$
- in tissue involve K electrons more than 80% of the time.

Compton interactions

X and γ rays with energies between 30 keV and 30 MeV interact in soft tissue principally by Compton scattering. In this type of photon interaction, part of the energy of the photon is transferred to a loosely bound or "free" electron in the medium (Figure 2-9). The electron, termed a *Compton electron*, is set into motion with a kinetic energy equal to the energy transferred by

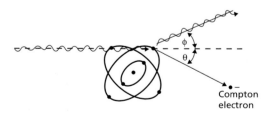

Figure 2-9 Compton scattering of an incident photon, with the photon scattered at an angle φ and the Compton electron ejected at an angle θ with respect to the direction of the incident photon.

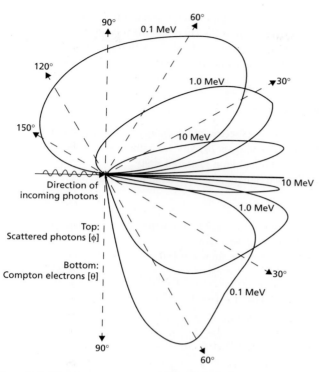

Figure 2-10 Electron scattering angle θ as a function of the energy of incident photons. Both θ and φ decrease as the energy of incident photons increases.[1]

the incident photon, less any binding energy (almost always negligible) that must be overcome in ejecting the electron from its atom. Because of the need to conserve momentum, the direction of the Compton electron, defined as the electron scattering angle, θ, is confined to the forward hemisphere (i.e., $\pm 90°$) with respect to the direction of the incident photon. In the interaction process, the incident photon is scattered with reduced energy at the photon scattering angle, φ, with respect to its original direction. This angle may be any value (i.e., up to $\pm 180°$) with respect to the original photon direction. Both θ and φ tend to narrow with increasing energy of the incident photon (Figure 2-10).

If the energy of an incident photon undergoing Compton scattering is $h\nu$, then the energies $h\nu'$ and E_k of the scattered photon and electron, respectively are:

$$h\nu' = h\nu \left[\frac{1}{1 + \alpha(1 - \cos\varphi)} \right]$$

$$E_k = h\nu - h\nu' = h\nu \left[\frac{\alpha(1 - \cos\varphi)}{1 + \alpha(1 - \cos\varphi)} \right]$$

where $\alpha = h\nu/m_0 c^2$ and $m_0 c^2$ is the rest mass energy of the electron (0.511 MeV). During a Compton interaction, the change in wavelength ($\Delta\lambda$) in nanometers of the x or γ ray is $\Delta\lambda = 0.00243 (1 - \cos\varphi)$, where φ is the scattering angle of the photon. The wavelength λ' of the scattered photon is $\lambda = \lambda + \Delta\lambda$, where λ is the wavelength of the incident photon.

Example 2-6

A 250 keV photon is scattered at an angle of 60° during a Compton interaction. What are the energies of the scattered photon and the Compton electron?

Because the formula for change in wavelength in Compton scatter is fairly simple, we are best working in terms of wavelengths. The wavelength λ of the incident photon is:

$$\lambda = \frac{1.24}{h\nu} = \frac{1.24}{250\ keV}$$
$$= 0.005 \text{ nm}$$

The change in wavelength $\Delta\lambda$ during the scattering process is:

$$\Delta\lambda = 0.00243(1 - \cos\phi)$$
$$= 0.00243(1 - \cos(60°))$$
$$= 0.00243(1 - 0.5)$$
$$= 0.00122 \text{ nm}$$

The wavelength λ' of the scattered photon is:

$$\lambda' = \lambda + \Delta\lambda$$
$$= (0.0050 + 0.0012) \text{ nm} = 0.0062 \text{ nm}$$

The energy of the scattered photon is:

$$h\nu' = \frac{1.24}{\lambda'} = \frac{1.24}{0.0062 \text{ nm}}$$
$$= 200 \text{ keV}$$

The energy of the Compton electron is:

$$E_k = h\nu - h\nu' = (250 - 200) \text{ keV}$$
$$= 50 \text{ keV}$$

The energy of the scattered photon and Compton electron can also be determined with the expressions:

$$h\nu' = h\nu \left[\frac{1}{1 + \alpha(1 - \cos\varphi)} \right]$$
$$= 250 \text{ keV} \left[\frac{1}{1 + (250/511)(1 - \cos(60°))} \right]$$
$$= 250 \text{ keV} \left[\frac{1}{1 + (0.489)(1 - 0.5)} \right]$$
$$= 250 \text{ keV}[0.8]$$
$$= 200 \text{ keV}$$

$$E_k = h\nu - h\nu' = h\nu \left[\frac{\alpha(1 - \cos\varphi)}{1 + \alpha(1 - \cos\varphi)} \right]$$
$$= 250 \text{ keV} \left[\frac{0.489(0.5)}{1 + 0.489(1 - 0.5)} \right]$$
$$= 250 \text{ keV}[0.2]$$
$$= 50 \text{ keV}$$

Example 2-7

A 50 keV photon is scattered by a Compton interaction. What is the maximum energy transferred to the Compton electron?

The energy transferred to the electron is greatest when the change in wavelength is maximum; the change in wavelength is maximum when $\varphi = 180°$.

$$\Delta\lambda_{max} = 0.00243[1 - \cos(180°)] \text{ nm}$$
$$= 0.00243[1 - (-1)] \text{ nm}$$
$$= 0.00486 \text{ nm}$$
$$\cong 0.005 \text{ nm}$$

The wavelength of a 50 keV photon is:

$$\lambda = \frac{1.24}{50 \text{ keV}} = 0.025 \text{ nm}$$

The wavelength λ' of the photon scattered at 180° is:

$$\lambda' = \lambda + \Delta\lambda$$
$$= (0.025 + 0.005) \text{ nm} = 0.03 \text{ nm}$$

The energy $h\nu'$ of the scattered photon is:

$$h\nu' = \frac{1.24}{\lambda'} = \frac{1.24}{0.03}$$
$$= 41.3 \text{ keV}$$

The energy of the Compton electron is:

$$E_k = h\nu - h\nu'$$
$$= (50 - 41.3) \text{ keV} = 8.7 \text{ keV}$$

When a relatively low-energy photon undergoes a Compton interaction, most of the energy of the incident photon is retained by the scattered photon, and only a small portion of the energy is transferred to the electron.

Example 2-8

A 5 MeV photon is scattered by a Compton interaction. What is the maximum energy transferred to the recoil electron?

The wavelength $\Delta\lambda$ of a 5 MeV photon is:

$$\lambda = \frac{1.24}{5000 \text{ keV}} = 0.00025 \text{ nm}$$

The change in wavelength of a photon scattered at 180° is 0.005 nm (see Example 2-6). The wavelength λ of the photon scattered at 180° is:

$$\lambda = \lambda + \Delta\lambda$$
$$= (0.00025 + 0.005) \text{ nm}$$
$$= 0.00525 \text{ nm}$$

The energy of the scattered photon is:

$$h\nu' = \frac{1.24}{\lambda} \frac{1.24}{0.0052} = 240 \text{ keV}$$

The energy E_k of the Compton electron is:

$$E_k = h\nu - h\nu'$$
$$= (5000 - 236) \text{ keV}$$
$$= 4760 \text{ keV}$$

When a relatively high-energy photon undergoes a Compton interaction, most of the energy of the incident photon is transferred to the electron and only a small fraction of the energy is retained by the scattered photon.

Example 2-9

Show that, irrespective of the energy of the incident photon, the maximum energy is 255 keV for a photon scattered at 180° and 511 keV for a photon scattered at 90°.

The wavelength λ of a scattered photon is:

$$\lambda' = \lambda + \Delta\lambda$$

For photons at very high energy, λ is very small and may be neglected relative to $\Delta\lambda$.

For a photon scattered at 180°:

$$\lambda' \cong \Delta\lambda = 0.00243(1 - \cos(180°))$$
$$= 0.00243(1 - (-1))$$
$$= 0.00486 \text{ nm}$$
$$h\nu' = \frac{1.24}{\lambda} = \frac{1.24}{0.00486 \text{ nm}}$$
$$= 255 \text{ keV}$$

For photons scattered at 90°:

$$\lambda' \cong \Delta\lambda = 0.00243(1 - \cos(90°))$$
$$= 0.00243(1 - 0)$$
$$= 0.00243 \text{ nm}$$
$$h\nu' = \frac{1.24}{\lambda} = \frac{1.24}{0.00243 \text{ nm}}$$
$$= 511 \text{ keV}$$

The likelihood of Compton interaction decreases gradually with increasing photon energy, as depicted in Figure 2-11. Note that an increase in energy of a factor of 1000 results in a decrease in the attenuation coefficient by a factor of about 6.

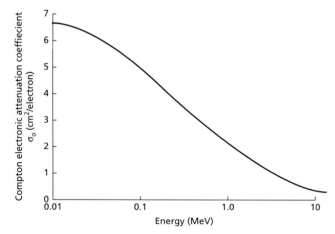

Figure 2-11 Compton electronic attenuation coefficient as a function of photon energy.

Table 2-3 Variables that influence principal modes of interaction of x and γ rays.

Dependence of Linear Attenuation Coefficient on			
Mode of Interaction	Photon Energy hν	Atomic Number Z	Electron Density ρ_e or Physical Density ρ
Photoelectric	$\dfrac{1}{(h\nu)^3}$	Z^3	ρ
Compton	$\dfrac{1}{h\nu}$	—	ρ_e
Pair production	$h\nu$ (>1.02 MeV)	Z	ρ

Compton interactions occur principally with loosely bound ("free") electrons, thus the mass attenuation coefficient varies directly with the electron density (number of electrons per gram) of the attenuating material, because a material with a higher electron density provides a higher concentration of electrons with which incident photons can interact. Recall that the number of electrons per gram is given by ZN_a/M, where Z is the atomic number (number of electrons per atom), N_a is Avogadro's number (number of atoms per gram-atomic mass), and M is the atomic mass (grams per gram-atomic mass). N_a is a constant, and Z/M is approximately the same for all materials, ranging from 0.4 to 0.5 for all materials except ordinary hydrogen, for which Z/M is approximately equal to 1. Hence, photons interact by Compton interaction more readily in materials with high concentrations of hydrogen. Compared with other tissue constituents, fat has a greater concentration of hydrogen. For this reason, a gram of fat absorbs more energy by Compton interaction than does, for example, a gram of bone. However, the physical density (g/cm^3) is greater for bone than for fat. Therefore, a greater number of electrons are present in a given volume of bone than in the same volume of fat, even though the electron density (electrons/g) is greater in fat. Hence a volume of bone attenuates more photons by Compton interaction than does an equal volume of fat or muscle, even though less energy is deposited in each gram of bone compared with the other tissue constituents.

In an image acquired with x rays in the diagnostic energy range (i.e., a radiographic or fluoroscopic image), various tissues can be distinguished because of differences in optical density in the image. These differences are referred to collectively as *contrast* in the image. Image contrast is a reflection of differences in the transmission of x rays through various regions of the patient. In radiation therapy, a localization (*portal*) image that is created using the high-energy x rays from the treatment machine, and used to verify alignment of the treatment beam, yields an image with greatly subdued contrast compared with that of a diagnostic image. The difference in the two images is due principally to the difference in the dominant photon interactions contributing to the images. The diagnostic x-ray beam interacts in part by photoelectric interactions that yield a major distinction in x-ray transmission through constituents of different Z within the patient. The higher energy therapeutic x-ray beam interacts only rarely by photoelectric interaction and almost exclusively by Compton interaction. The transmitted therapy beam used to form the portal image differs in intensity as a reflection only of variations in the physical and electron densities of various tissues. These properties vary only slightly among muscle, bone, and fat (see Table 2-3 below). In addition, the scattered x rays produced as a result of the Compton interaction reach the detector without providing useful information as to where the interactions took place, thus adding to noise on the detector and further degrading the portal image. In the diagnostic x-ray energy regime, the majority of interactions arise from the photoelectric effect, which does not produce any scattered photons. Hence the localization portal image yields much less contrast compared with the diagnostic x-ray image. This difference is depicted in Figure 2-12 for a lateral image of a patient's head using low-energy x-ray beams (in kilovoltage energy range typically used in diagnostic radiology) and with high-energy x-ray beams typically used in radiation therapy.

To summarize, Compton interactions:
- occur with loosely bound electrons

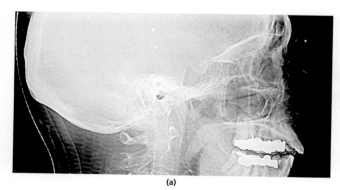

(a)

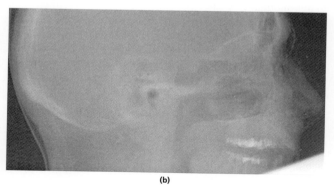

(b)

Figure 2-12 (a) Image obtained with a kilo-voltage x-ray beam, and (b) image obtained with a 6 MV x-ray beam.

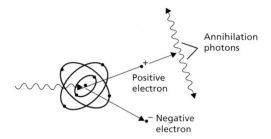

Figure 2-13 Pair production interaction of a high-energy photon near a nucleus. Annihilation photons are produced when the positron and an electron annihilate each other.

- have a likelihood of occurrence that is independent of Z
- have a likelihood of occurrence that decreases slowly with increasing (hv)
- increase the fraction of incident photon energy transferred to the Compton electron with increasing (hv)
- dominate photon interaction in soft tissue between 30 keV and 30 MeV.

Pair production

For an x or γ ray above a threshold energy of 1.02 MeV, *pair production* is an additional type of interaction available to the photon. This type of interaction occurs near the nucleus of an atom in the absorbing medium and results in the complete disappearance of the photon. In its place appears a positron-electron pair (Figure 2-13). Pair production exhibits a threshold energy because the photon must possess enough energy to create the mass of the positron and electron (2×0.51 MeV = 1.02 MeV). Energy in excess of 1.02 MeV is distributed as kinetic energy of the two particles. Although the nucleus recoils slightly when pair production occurs in its vicinity, the energy transferred to the nucleus during the interaction usually can be neglected. As the positron and the electron travel, they deposit energy along their tracks. When the positron has deposited all of its energy, it combines with an electron. Both particles are said to be annihilated, and two γ rays, each with energy 0.511 MeV, are ejected at 180° to one another.

Example 2-10

A 6 MeV photon interacts by pair production. Residual energy is shared equally between the negative and positive electrons. What are the kinetic energies of the particles?

$$hv(MeV) = 1.02 + (E_k)_{e-} + (E_k)_{e+}$$
$$(E_k)_{e-} = (E_k)_{e+} = \frac{(hv - 1.02)MeV}{2}$$
$$= 2.49 \text{ MeV}$$

Occasionally, pair production occurs near an electron, rather than a nucleus of an atom in the absorbing medium. For 10 MeV

photons in soft tissue, for example, about 10% of all pair production interactions occur in the vicinity of an electron. This type of photon interaction is referred to as *triplet production* because the existing electron receives energy from the photon and is ejected from its atom simultaneously with the creation of negative and positive electrons. Hence three ionizing particles, two electrons and one positron, are set into motion during triplet production. The threshold energy for triplet production is twice (2.04 MeV) that for pair production. The ratio of triplet to pair production increases with the energy of the incident photons and decreases with increasing atomic number of the medium. Pair and triplet production must occur in the presence of a charged particle (a nucleus or an electron) so that momentum is conserved in the interaction.

The mass attenuation coefficient κ_m for pair production varies almost linearly with the atomic number of the attenuating material. It also increases slowly with the energy of incident photons above the threshold energy of 1.02 MeV. Consequently, at energies in which pair production predominates, the penetrating ability of the radiation decreases with increasing energy. Thus, there is an effective upper limit of 25–35 MeV for the photon energies used in radiation therapy. In diagnostic radiology, pair production does not occur because the x rays do not possess enough energy to undergo this type of interaction. Pair production can be a significant interaction for x rays used in high-energy radiation therapy.

To summarize, the pair-production interaction:
- cannot occur with photons below 1.02 MeV
- initially increases rapidly for photons above 1.02 MeV
- increases in likelihood with Z
- transfers ($hv - 1.02$ MeV) to the electron–positron pair
- yields a positron that ultimately interacts with an electron to produce two annihilation photons of 0.51 MeV each.

Photodisintegration

Except for pair production, interactions of x and γ rays with nuclei are significant only if the photons have very high energy. *Photodisintegration* interactions occur when photons have sufficient energy to eject a nuclear particle when they are absorbed by a nucleus. Most photodisintegration interactions are either (γ, n) or (γ, p) interactions in which a photon is absorbed and either a neutron or a proton is ejected. Photodisintegration rarely occurs in tissue, but can take place in shielding materials around high-energy accelerators. Neutron production as a result of photodisintegration becomes an issue when designing shielding for linear accelerators producing photons of energies greater than 10 MeV. Photodisintegration interactions also can be used to measure the energy of photons in a high-energy x-ray beam. An example of this procedure is the use of a beryllium foil in combination with elemental silver to calibrate the energy of an x-ray beam. A beryllium foil exposed to high-energy x rays can experience the reaction with a threshold energy of 1.65 MeV. A

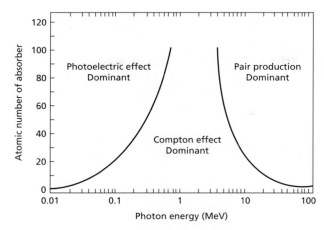

Figure 2-14 Relative importance of the three principal interactions of x and γ rays.

silver foil adjacent to the beryllium is activated by the ejected neutrons and emits γ rays in a (γ, n) reaction. One can detect γ rays by an external detector only if neutrons are released by the beryllium, signifying that x rays of at least 1.65 MeV are present in the high-energy x-ray beam. By substituting other foils with different threshold energies for the beryllium, the range of energies in the x-ray beam can be determined.

Likelihood of interactions

The relative importance of photoelectric, Compton, and pair production interactions in different media is depicted in Figure 2-14. In muscle or water (Z_{eff} = 7.4), the probabilities of photoelectric and Compton interactions are equal at a photon energy of 35 keV. However, equal energies are not deposited in tissue at this energy because a photoelectric interaction deposits the total energy of the photon, whereas only part of the photon energy is transferred during a Compton interaction. The energy depositions from photoelectric and Compton interactions are equal at about 60 keV in muscle or water, where more Compton interactions compensate for less energy transferred per interaction.

A summary of the variables that influence the linear attenuation coefficient for photoelectric, Compton, and pair production interactions is provided in Table 2-3.

Summary

- Equations important to photon transmission and attenuation include:

$$\mu = \frac{(dI/I)}{dx} = \text{fractional rate of attenuation}$$
$$I = I_0 e^{-\mu x} = \text{number of photons transmitted}$$
$$I^* = I_0(1 - e^{-\mu x}) = \text{number of photons attenuated}$$

- Useful attenuation and absorption coefficients include μ (linear attenuation), μ_m (mass attenuation), μ_a (atomic attenuation), μ_e (electronic attenuation), and μ_{en} (mass energy absorption).
- Half-value layer measurements should be acquired under conditions of narrow-beam (good) geometry.
- The total attenuation coefficient is the sum of ω (coherent scattering), τ (photoelectric absorption), σ (Compton scattering), κ (pair production), and π (photodisintegration).
- The likelihood of photoelectric effect varies with Z^3 and $(1/h\nu)^3$.
- The likelihood of Compton scattering varies with the electron density and decreases slowly with increasing energy, but is independent of Z.
- The maximum energy of a photon scattered at 90° is 511 keV, and at 180° it is 255 keV.
- Pair production does not occur for photons below 1.02 MeV in energy.

Problems

2-1 The tenth-value layer (TVL) is the thickness of a material necessary to reduce the intensity of x or γ rays to 1/10 the intensity with no material present. For conditions of good geometry and monoenergetic photons, show that the TVL equals $2.30/\mu$, where μ is the total linear attenuation coefficient.

2-2 Assume that the exponent μx in the equation $I = I_0 e^{-\mu x}$ is equal to or less than 0.1. Show that, with an error of less than 1%, the number of photons transmitted is $I_0(1 - \mu x)$ and the number attenuated is $I_0 \mu x$. (*Hint*: Expand the term $e^{-\mu x}$ into a series.)

2-3 The mass attenuation coefficient of copper is 0.0589 cm²/g for 1.0 MeV photons. The number of 1.0 MeV photons in a narrow beam is reduced to what fraction by a copper absorber 1 cm thick? The density of copper is 8.9 g/cm³.

2-4 Copper has a density of 8.9 g/cm³ and a gram-atomic mass of 63.56. The total atomic attenuation coefficient of copper is 3.3×10^{-24} cm²/atom for 5 MeV photons. What thickness (cm) of copper is required to attenuate 5 MeV photons to half the original number?

2-5 K- and L-shell binding energies for cesium are 28 keV and 5 keV, respectively. What are the kinetic energies of photoelectrons released from the K and L shells as 30 keV photons interact with cesium?

2-6 Compute the energy of a photon scattered at 45° during a Compton interaction, if the energy of the incident photon is 150 keV. What is the kinetic energy of the Compton electron? Is the energy of the scattered photon increased or decreased if the photon scattering angle is increased to more than 45°?

2-7 A γ ray of 2.75 MeV from ^{24}Na undergoes pair production in a lead shield. The negative and positive electrons possess equal kinetic energy. What is their kinetic energy?

2-8 Prove that, regardless of the energy of the incident photon, a photon scattered at an angle greater than 60° during a Compton interaction cannot undergo pair production.

2-9 What thickness (cm) of lead is required to reduce the intensity of 2 MeV photons to 0.1% if $\mu_m = 0.046$ cm^2/g and $\rho = 11.3$ g/cm^3 for lead?

2-10 5 mm of aluminum ($\rho = 2.7$ g/cm^3) transmits 30% of a beam of 30 keV photons. What is the mass attenuation coefficient of aluminum for these photons?

2-11 A linear attenuation coefficient of 0.001 cm^{-1} means that 0.1% of the photons in the beam are attenuated per cm of absorber. Does this mean that 1000 cm of absorber will attenuate all the photons in the beam? How do you justify your answer?

2-12 What would have to occur for the homogeneity coefficient to be greater than unity? Under what circumstances might this be possible?

2-13 As the energy of an incident photon increases, the scattered photon is more likely to be scattered in a forward direction. Compare the effect of field size on scattered dose for 6 MV vs 18 MV photons.

References

1 Hendee, W. R., and Ritenour, E. R. *Medical Imaging Physics*, 4th edition. New York, John Wiley & Sons, Ltd., 2001.

2 Lord Rayleigh. *Philos. Mag.* **41**:274, 1871; **47**:375–284, 1899, reprinted in *Scientific Papers* **1**:87; **4**:397.

3 Grodstein, G. W. *X-Ray Attenuation Coefficients from 10 keV to 100 MeV*. Washington, DC, U.S. National Bureau of Standards, Pub. No. 583, 1957.

CHAPTER

3

INTERACTIONS OF PARTICULATE RADIATION WITH MATTER

Objectives

After studying this chapter, the reader should be able to:
- Recognize the differences in interactions between charged and uncharged particles, and between light and heavy charged particles.
- Describe the interactions of charged particles with electrons, including the concept of ionization, excitation, work function, specific ionization, and linear energy transfer.
- Describe the interactions of charged particles with nuclei, including the concepts of cross section and Bremsstrahlung radiation.
- Identify the ratio of radiative energy loss to collisional energy loss for both electrons and heavy charged particles.

Introduction

Interactions of charged particles with matter are important to understand, especially in radiation oncology. Radiation treatments have been delivered for many years with charged particles (electrons), and many new facilities are being built to treat patients with charged particles (protons). Neutrons and heavy charged particles, such as carbon ions, have also played a role in radiation therapy. Charged particles exhibit some similarities in the nature of their interactions with matter, but also exhibit some

differences. Another reason for studying interactions of charged particles with matter is that after a photon has initially interacted with a target atom secondary electrons are produced. These secondary electrons generally cause many more ionizations than the primary photon. In many respects, the consequences of an interaction of a photon with matter are those of the interactions of the secondary electrons with matter.

Differences between charged particles and photons

The major differences between the manner in which charged particles interact with matter and the manner in which photons interact with matter lie in the nature of their collisions. The interaction of electrons with other electrons and the nuclei of a medium are termed *Coulombic interactions* because they occur between charged particles in which each particle exerts a Coulombic force of attraction or repulsion upon the other. Most charged particle interactions with matter are interactions with the electrons that surround the nucleus, although interactions with the nuclei can also occur. As a result of these interactions, the charged particles impart a small portion of their kinetic energy to secondary electrons. An approximation that is

Hendee's Radiation Therapy Physics, Fourth Edition. Todd Pawlicki, Daniel J. Scanderbeg and George Starkschall.
© 2016 John Wiley & Sons, Inc. Published 2016 by John Wiley & Sons, Inc.

frequently used to derive properties of charged particles passing through matter is the continuous slowing-down approximation (CSDA). For example, as we shall see later in this chapter, an electron passing through tissue will lose 30–35 electron volts in each interaction in which it is involved. Thus, a 3 MeV electron will undergo approximately 100,000 interactions before it loses all of its kinetic energy and comes to rest. Assuming the energy loss to be continuous is a very good approximation.

As a beam of charged particles interacts with the target material, the beam loses energy, but the intensity, related to the number of charged particles in the beam, does not change. Energy is lost in a continuous manner until the charged particles lose all their kinetic energy, at which point they stop and do not continue to pass through the absorber. Consequently, the radiation dose, the energy deposited by a charged particle beam, is, to a first approximation, constant from the patient's skin surface to a maximum depth of penetration, called the *range*, beyond which it is essentially zero.

A photon interaction, on the other hand, is referred to as a *catastrophic interaction*, in which the photon is completely absorbed in the absorbing material and an electron is ejected. Alternatively, the photon may eject an electron along with a photon of lower energy (i.e., a scattered photon). Because the energy is the only way we have to identify a photon, we say that in such an interaction the initial photon is absorbed and a new, scattered photon is ejected. Consequently, the photon entering an interaction is attenuated (removed from the beam) and a secondary electron, and possibly a secondary photon, is produced. The photon beam intensity decreases with depth of penetration, whereas the photon beam energy, at least for a monochromatic beam, does not change.

Table 3-1 summarizes the differences between photon and particle interactions.

Classification of particles

Particulate radiation is classified into three categories: (1) electrons/positrons, (2) heavy charged particles, and (3) neutrons. The classification is based on the differences in interactions between the particulate radiation and matter. Electrons, for example, can undergo collisional interactions with other electrons and radiative interactions with nuclei. These interactions will be examined in more detail later in this chapter. Heavy

Table 3-1 Differences between photon and particle interactions.

	Photons	Particles
Beam intensity (number)	Decreases with depth, never reaches zero	Uniform until max range is reached, then zero
Beam energy	Uniform with depth*	Decreases with depth until max range is reached

*This is strictly true only for a monoenergetic photon beam.

Table 3-2 Classification of neutron energies.

Thermal	0–0.5 keV
Epithermal	0.5–10 keV
Intermediate	10–500 keV
Fast	> 500 keV

charged particles are similar to electrons in that they undergo collisional interactions with electrons. However, because of their masses, radiative interactions involving heavy charged particles are far less probable. Moreover, when electrons cause ionization and eject other electrons, there exists some ambiguity as to which is the incident electron and which is the ejected electron. By convention, the electron with the greater energy is designated as the incident electron. Such ambiguity does not exist when the incident particle is a heavy charged particle and the ejected particle is an electron.

Neutrons are different from charged particles in that they cannot interact with nuclei or electrons through the long-range electrostatic force, but rather interact with nuclei through a short-range interaction. The specific interactions by which neutrons transfer energy to charged particles (remembering that it is the secondary charged particles that cause the ionizations) depend on the energy of the incident neutrons. Table 3-2 shows the classification of neutron energies. It is important to recognize, however, that the boundaries between energy classes are somewhat fuzzy.

Low-energy (thermal and epithermal) neutrons interact primarily via neutron capture reactions. For example, neutron capture by carbon results in the ejection of a proton, which can induce ionization, and neutron capture by hydrogen results in the ejection of a γ ray, which can also induce ionization. At higher energies, elastic scatter, and, at even higher energies, inelastic scatter, are more prevalent. Elastic scatter results in the transfer of some kinetic energy from the neutron to the target nucleus, which then can dissipate energy through ionization. Inelastic scatter causes the target nucleus to become excited, overcoming nuclear binding energy, and ejecting a charged particle from the nucleus.

Collisional interactions

As a beam of energetic charged particles moves through a medium, the charged particles can interact by transferring part of their energy to an electron in the medium. In this transfer, the impinging charged particle loses energy and is deflected (scattered) at some angle with respect to its original direction. Charged particles are scattered by electrons in the medium imparting small amounts of energy to the electrons in the medium as they ionize the atoms of the medium. The *collisional stopping power* is a measure of this energy loss, and is defined to be the energy loss per unit length along the track of the charged particle traversing the medium. More commonly used is the

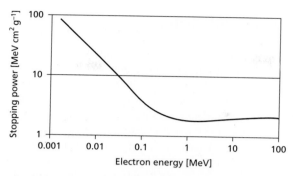

Figure 3-1 Mass collisional stopping power of an electron beam in water as a function of electron energy.

mass collisional stopping power, which is the collisional stopping power divided by the density of the medium. The mass collisional stopping power of a charged particle beam is proportional to the square of the atomic number of the target material and inversely proportional to $(v/c)^2$, where v is the velocity of the charged particle and c is the speed of light in vacuum (3.00 $\times 10^8$ m sec^{-1}). Note that for lower energy charged particles, the mass collisional stopping power decreases with increasing energy, because the velocity increases, but for relativistic particles, such as electrons at therapeutic energies (several MeV), the velocity is constant (approximately equal to c) so that the mass collisional stopping power is approximately constant, and equal to approximately 2 MeV cm^2 g^{-1}. This means that in water, with density 1 g cm^{-3}, an electron beam will lose approximately 2 MeV for every cm it traverses the medium. Figure 3-1 illustrates the mass collisional stopping power of an electron beam as a function of its energy.

In an electron–electron interaction the electron receiving the energy may be raised to a shell farther from the nucleus of the atom to which it belongs, or it may be ejected completely from the atom.

When an electron is raised to a shell farther from the nucleus, the atom is unstable and said to be *excited*. Usually the atom remains in this state only momentarily and quickly regains stability through one or more electron transitions, emitting characteristic x rays, until all vacancies in the lower energy levels are filled.

If an electron is ejected during an electron–electron interaction, its kinetic energy, E_k, is given by:

$$E_k = E - E_b$$

where E is the energy transferred to the ejected electron and E_b is the binding energy of the ejected electron. If the binding energy is negligible, the sum of the kinetic energy of the scattered and ejected electrons is equal to the kinetic energy of the original electron before the interaction. When kinetic energy is *conserved* in an interaction, the interaction is said to be *elastic*. Elastic scattering interactions of electrons are sometimes referred to as *billiard-ball collisions*. If the binding energy cannot be

ignored, kinetic energy is not conserved, and the interaction is said to be *inelastic*.

When an electron is ejected from an atom through a process such as an interaction with an incident electron, the atom is said to be *ionized*. The ejected electron and residual positive ion constitute a primary *ion pair* (IP). In air, an average energy of 33.97 eV is expended in producing an ion pair.[1] The average value is represented by the symbol $\bar{W}/e$ where:

$$\frac{\bar{W}}{e} = 33.97 \text{ eV/IP}$$

The energy needed to overcome the binding energy of the most loosely bound electrons in air is considerably less than $\bar{W}/e$. The quantity $\bar{W}/e$ includes not only the electron's binding energy but also the average kinetic energy of the ejected electron and the average energy lost in the processes of exciting atoms, interacting with nuclei, and increasing the rotational and vibrational energy states of molecules in the medium. On average, 2.2 atoms are excited for each atom ionized in air by incident electrons.

An electron ejected from an atom may possess enough kinetic energy to ionize nearby atoms. Ion pairs produced by this process are termed *secondary ion pairs*. The number of primary and secondary ion pairs produced per unit path-length of an incident electron is termed the *specific ionization* (SI) of the electron, usually expressed in units of ion pairs per centimeter (IP/cm). In air, at *standard temperature and pressure* (STP), the SI of an electron with a kinetic energy less than 10 MeV can be estimated as:

$$SI = 45 \, (v/c)^2 \text{ IP/cm}$$

where v and c were defined earlier.

The specific ionization is related to $\bar{W}/e$ and the *linear energy transfer* (LET)* by the relation:

$$SI = LET/(\bar{W}/e)$$
$$= LET/33.7 \text{ (eV/IP)}$$

so that the LET can be determined by multiplying the SI by $(\bar{W}/e)$.

Example 3-1

Determine the SI and LET of 0.1 MeV electrons in air ($v/c = 0.548$)

$$SI = \frac{45}{(v/c)^2}$$
$$= 45/(0.548)^2$$
$$= 160 \text{ IP/cm}$$
$$LET = (SI)(\bar{W}/e)$$
$$= (160 \text{ IP/cm})(33.97 \text{ eV/IP})(10^{-3} \text{keV/eV})$$
$$= 5.4 \text{ keV/cm}$$

*The LET is the same as the collisional stopping power.

A positron traversing a medium interacts in a manner similar to that of an electron, with one exception. As the positron transfers energy to surrounding atoms, it loses kinetic energy and finally combines with an electron. The two particles momentarily revolve around each other and then annihilate with the release of electromagnetic radiation with a total energy equivalent to the mass of the two particles. Usually, the energy is released as two 0.511 MeV photons moving in opposite directions (180° apart). This interaction is termed *pair annihilation* and the radiation that is produced is referred to as *annihilation radiation*. Annihilation radiation is detected in *positron emission tomography* (PET) imaging following administration of a positron-emitting radionuclide to a patient.

Generally, a charged particle loses energy continuously as it penetrates absorbing medium. Consequently, if the charged particle enters the absorber with specified energy, it will lose energy in collisional interactions until it runs out of energy, and then stop; hence the origin of the term *stopping power*. A charged particle beam, then, has a finite range in medium equal to the initial energy divided by the collisional stopping power. The collisional stopping power of an electron beam in water is approximately 2 MeV/cm. A useful rule of thumb is that the range of an electron beam in cm is approximately the initial energy of the beam in MeV divided by 2. For example, a 12 MeV electron beam will have a range of approximately 6 cm in water.

We noted before that as the energy of a charged particle decreases the energy loss per unit track length increases. Hence the particle will lose a great deal of energy toward the end of its range, depositing an increased dose at the end of its range. This increase in dose is called a *Bragg peak* and is illustrated in Figure 3-2.

This enhancement in dose is used advantageously in particle-beam radiation therapy (e.g., proton-beam therapy), in which the energy of the beam is selected to deliver the enhanced dose to the depth of the tumor. After radiative interactions are discussed later in the chapter, it will be clear why electron beams do not exhibit a Bragg peak.

Radiative interactions

An electron traveling through a medium may be scattered at reduced energy during interaction with a nucleus in the medium. In some interactions, kinetic energy is conserved because the sum of the kinetic energy of the scattered electron and the "recoil" nucleus equals that of the incident electron.

The probability of the elastic scattering of impinging electrons is about equal for electrons and nuclei in hydrogen. In absorbers of higher Z, elastic scattering by nuclei is more likely because its probability increases with Z^2, whereas the likelihood of elastic scattering by electrons increases with Z. The probability of interaction often is referred to as the *cross section* for the interaction, sometimes expressed in units of *barns*, where 1 barn = 10^{-24} cm^2.

Most scattering interactions of electrons with nuclei are inelastic rather than elastic because the kinetic energy of the interacting particles is not conserved in the interaction. The loss of kinetic energy is pressed as energy released as electromagnetic radiation during the interaction. Energy radiated as an electron (or any charged particle) slows by interacting with a nucleus of an absorbing medium is termed *Bremsstrahlung*, or *braking radiation*. A Bremsstrahlung photon may possess energy up to the entire kinetic energy of the incident electron. For low-energy electrons, Bremsstrahlung is released predominantly at right angles to the direction of the electrons. The angle narrows for electrons of higher energy (Figure 3-3).

Similar to the elastic scattering of electrons by nuclei, the probability of Bremsstrahlung production varies with Z^2 of the medium. Consequently, media of high Z are much more effective in producing Bremsstrahlung than are absorbers of low Z. A typical Bremsstrahlung spectrum is shown in Figure 3-4. The area under the spectrum (i.e., the amount of

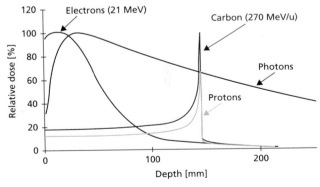

Figure 3-2 Ionization of carbon and proton beams as a function of depth in water illustrating the enhanced ionization that takes place at the end of the particle beam range. For a color version of this figure, see the color plate section.

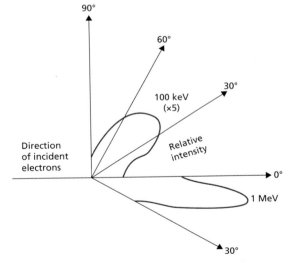

Figure 3-3 Relative intensity of Bremsstrahlung radiated at different angles for electrons with kinetic energies of 100 keV and 1 MeV.
Source: Data from O. Scherzer[2] and H. Andrews[3].

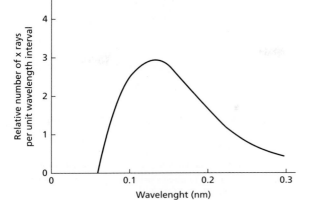

Figure 3-4 Bremsstrahlung spectrum for a molybdenum ($Z = 42$) target bombarded by electrons accelerated through 20 kV.
Source: Data from M. Wehr and J. Richard,[5] with permission.

Bremsstrahlung produced) increases dramatically with the Z of the medium, but the relative shape of the spectrum along the energy axis remains constant. The ratio of energy lost by electrons due to inelastic interactions with nuclei [radiative energy loss (Bremsstrahlung)], to that lost by excitation and ionization during interactions with electrons (collisional energy loss) is approximately:

$$\frac{\text{Radiative energy loss}}{\text{Collisional energy loss}} = \frac{E_k Z}{820}$$

where E_k is the kinetic energy of the incident electrons in MeV and Z is the atomic number of the medium. For example, Bremsstrahlung and ionization-excitation contribute about equally to the energy lost by 10 MeV electrons traversing lead ($Z = 82$). This ratio is important in the design of x-ray tubes used for medical diagnosis and radiation therapy. Table 3-3 shows relative collisional and radiative energy losses of electrons in water and lead.

Example 3-2

What is the approximate ratio of radiation to collisional energy loss of 20 MeV electrons in a gold transmission x-ray target ($Z = 79$) used for radiation therapy? Compare this value with the ratio of 0.1 MeV electrons striking a tungsten target ($Z = 74$) in a diagnostic x-ray tube.

$$\frac{\text{Radiative energy loss}}{\text{Collisional energy loss}} = \frac{E_k Z}{820}$$

For 20 MeV electrons in gold:

$$\frac{E_k Z}{820} = \frac{(20)(79)}{820} = 1.9$$

That is, energy released as radiation energy loss (Bremsstrahlung) is almost twice that expended in collisional energy losses.

For 0.1 MeV electrons in tungsten:

$$\frac{E_k Z}{820} = \frac{(0.1)(74)}{820} = 0.0090$$

In a diagnostic x-ray tube, almost all (> 99%) of the electron energy is expended through collisional energy mechanisms, producing low-energy electrons, leading to heat production in the target. Less than 1% of the electron energy is released as radiation energy loss. In radiation therapy, x rays are generated at much higher voltages, and the ratio of x rays to heat is much greater. At a few megavolts, for example, x-ray production may account for 50% or more of the energy delivered by electrons to the x-ray target.

Radiative stopping power is inversely proportional to the square of the mass of the charged particle. A proton has a mass of about 2000 times the mass of an electron, so the amount of Bremsstrahlung production in an electron beam is over 10^6 times that in a proton beam. Because electron beams interact with nuclei with a greater probability, especially at higher energies, electrons will undergo considerably more scatter than heavy charged particles. For a heavy charged particle beam, which does not undergo a great deal of scatter, the penetration depth and the path length will be quite similar, and such beams exhibit a Bragg peak. However, for an electron beam, the end of the particle track can occur at a range of depths, resulting in an unobservable Bragg peak.

Summary

- Charged particle interactions are of importance in radiation oncology because charged particles are used in radiation treatment and because most of the ionizations that result from photon interactions are actually the result of the interactions of secondary electrons.
- When a beam of charged particles interacts with target material, the energy of the beam decreases while the intensity of the beam is unchanged. This is different from the interactions of a photon beam, in which the intensity of the beam decreases but the energy of the beam is unchanged.

Table 3-3 Relative (percent) collisional and radiative energy losses of electrons in water (tissue) and lead.

	100 keV	1 MeV	10 MeV	25 MeV
Water				
Collision	99.9	99	92	80
Radiative	0.1	1	8	20
Lead				
Collision	97	86	49	25
Radiative	3	14	51	75

Source: Jayaraman and Lanzl 1996.[4]

- Charged particles can interact with matter either by collisional interactions, in which orbital electrons are ejected, or by radiative interactions, in which the charged particles are deflected emitting Bremsstrahlung x rays.

Problems

3-1 What is the ratio of the number of interactions that a 20 MeV electron undergoes in coming to rest compared to a 6 MeV electron?

3-2 Electrons with a kinetic energy of 1.0 MeV have an SI in air of about 60 IP/cm. Estimate the stopping power of these electrons in air.

3-3 Alpha particles of 2.0 MeV have an LET in air of 0.175 keV/μm. What is the SI of these particles in air if W/e is assumed to be 33.97 eV/IP?

3-4 Approximately how far does a 6 MeV electron travel in water? A 20 MeV electron?

3-5 What is the ratio of radiative energy loss to collisional energy loss for a 6 MeV electron in water? A 20 MeV electron? Note, the effective atomic number of water is approximately 7.4.

3-6 Describe the process of charged particle interactions that play a role in collision stopping power.

References

1 Boutillon, M., and Perroche-Roux, A. M. Re-evaluation of the W value for electrons in dry air. *Phys. Med. Biol.* **32**(2):213–220.

2 Scherzer, O. Radiation emitted on the stopping of protons and fast electrons. *Ann. Physik.* 1932; **13**:137.

3 Andrews, H. *Radiation Physics*. Englewood Cliffs, NJ, Prentice-Hall International, 1961.

4 Jayaraman, S., and Lanzl, L., *Clinical Radiotherapy Physics. Vol 1: Basic Physics and Dosimetry*, Boca Raton, FL, CRC Press, 1996.

5 Wehr, M., and Richard, J. *Physics of the Atom*. Reading, MA, Addison-Wesley, 1960:150.

Objectives

After studying this chapter, the reader should be able to:
- Describe the components and characteristics of conventional x-ray tubes, including the filament, cathode assembly, tube voltage, modes of rectification, three-phase and high-frequency generators, x-ray target, target materials, anode, focal spot, and line focus principle.
- Depict x-ray spectra and how spectra are influenced by x-ray tube current and voltage and by beam filtration.

- Discuss the historical developments leading to the design of modern treatment equipment.
- Describe the characteristics of radiation beams produced by treatment equipment found in clinical use.
- Identify the major components of a modern linear accelerator and explain their purpose and function.
- Compare the operation and clinical utility of linear accelerators with several other megavoltage treatment machines.

Hendee's Radiation Therapy Physics, Fourth Edition. Todd Pawlicki, Daniel J. Scanderbeg and George Starkschall.
© 2016 John Wiley & Sons, Inc. Published 2016 by John Wiley & Sons, Inc.

History of x rays

X rays were discovered on November 8, 1895, by Wilhelm Röntgen, a physicist at the University of Wurzburg in Germany.[1] Röntgen was studying the properties of "cathode rays" produced by applying a high voltage across a partially evacuated glass tube. During his experiments, Röntgen noticed that barium platinocyanide crystals in his laboratory glowed when voltage was applied to the tube. He then determined that the glow diminished, but did not disappear, when dense objects were placed between the cathode-ray tube and the crystals. The glow could not be caused directly by the cathode rays because it was known that cathode rays could travel no more than a few centimeters in air. Röntgen concluded that the glow was produced by a new type of penetrating radiation released from the cathode-ray tube. He named the new radiation *x rays*.

Over the next few weeks, Röntgen documented several properties of x rays.[2,3] He noted that x rays travel in straight paths, are not affected by magnetic fields, and are attenuated by a material according to its physical density and elemental composition (now characterized as the material's atomic number). He also determined that x rays darken photographic film and used this property to measure the amount of x-ray radiation reaching the film under different experimental conditions. He used photographic film to produce images of objects that are opaque to visible light. His observations are now understood to have resulted from x rays that were released as residual gas molecules in the cathode-ray tube that were ionized by electrons that were emitted as cathode rays when they interacted with various components of the cathode-ray tube.

Cathode-ray tubes were unreliable sources of x rays and produced radiation at low intensity. In 1913, Coolidge developed the "hot cathode" x-ray tube, in which a wire filament was heated with electrical current to release electrons by the process of thermionic emission (sometimes called the *Edison effect*).[4] The released electrons were repelled by a negative charge on the filament and accelerated toward a positively charged metal target. X rays were released as the high-speed electrons interacted in the target. The Coolidge tube was the prototype for x-ray tubes in use today.

Conventional x-ray tubes

The basic principle of x-ray production was identified in Chapter 3. High-energy electrons, interacting with a target, can be deflected by the nuclei in the target, producing Bremsstrahlung x rays. Consequently, the basic necessities to produce a useful x-ray beam are as follows: (a) electron source, (b) high voltage supply, (c) target for x-ray production, (d) vacuum, and (e) collimator. The components of a stationary anode x-ray tube are depicted in Figure 4-1. A filament heated by an electrical current serves as a source of electrons. The electrons are accelerated

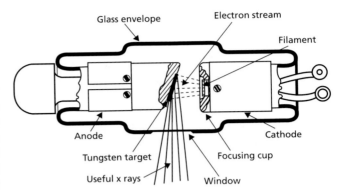

Figure 4-1 Simplified x-ray tube with a stationary anode and a heated filament.
Source: Bloom et al. 1965.[5]

toward a tungsten target by application of a high potential difference (voltage) between the filament housing (the cathode) and the target (the anode). X rays are produced as the electrons interact with nuclei of the target atoms. The x rays emerge from the target in all directions and are collimated to produce a useful x-ray beam of defined cross-sectional area. The glass envelope surrounding the components of the x-ray tube is evacuated to prevent the electrons from interacting with gas molecules before they reach the x-ray target.

Electron source

The filament of the x-ray tube is a metal wire that conducts electricity and has a high melting point. Tungsten (melting point 3370°C) filaments are used in most x-ray tubes. The filament is housed within a negatively charged focusing cup, which, together with the filament, serves as the *cathode assembly* for the x-ray tube. A current of a few amperes (the filament current) is used to heat the filament to a temperature at which thermionic emission occurs. If the released electrons are attracted to the target as soon as they are emitted from the filament, no pile-up of electrons occurs around the filament, and the rate of flow of electrons across the x-ray tube (the tube current) is said to be *filament-emission limited*. In this condition, the tube current can be increased only by heating the filament to a higher temperature, through use of a greater filament current. X-ray tubes operating at high voltage, or relatively low tube current, function in the filament-emission limited condition.

At relatively low voltages across the x-ray tube, electrons released by thermionic emission tend to accumulate around the filament because they are not pulled immediately to the target. This accumulation of electrons is referred to as a *space charge*. The negative cloud of electrons prevents additional electrons from leaving the filament and thereby limits the tube current. Under this condition, the tube current is said to be *space-charge limited*. Space-charge-limited operation is encountered primarily in x-ray tubes operated at relatively low voltages, such as those employed for mammography. X-ray tubes can operate in one of these two modes: (1) filament-emission limited or (2) space-charge limited.

The focal spot of an x-ray tube is the volume of x-ray target in which electrons are absorbed and x rays are produced. For the most sharply defined x-ray beams, a small focal spot is needed. A small focal spot requires a small or "fine" filament as an electron source. If the filament is too small, however, thermionic emission is limited, and the rate of production of x rays is restricted. In this case, longer exposures are required and patient motion during an exposure can become troublesome. In any x-ray exposure, a compromise must be reached between (a) use of a small focal spot to provide a sharp x-ray beam and consequently a high-resolution image and (b) use of a larger focal spot to furnish an x-ray beam of higher intensity.[6-8] This compromise is reflected in the presence of two filaments in most x-ray tubes. The small filament is used when low tube currents can be tolerated and a small focal spot is desired to yield a sharply defined x-ray beam. When patient motion is a problem and higher x-ray intensities are needed to limit exposure times, the large filament is used to provide higher tube currents. An x-ray tube with two focal spots is called a *dual-focus x-ray tube*.

X-ray tube voltage

The potential difference (voltage) between the filament (cathode) and target (anode) of an x-ray tube influences the intensity and spectral distribution of x rays furnished by the tube. A positive electrode is termed an *anode* because negative ions (anions) are attracted to it. A negative electrode is referred to as a *cathode* because positive ions (cations) are attracted to it. Alternating voltage and current (AC) are used as the source of electrical power for most x-ray tubes because it is the type of electrical power supplied by electrical utilities in most countries. In the United States, alternating current is supplied at a frequency of 60 hertz (Hz), with 1 Hz = 1 cycle per second. With 60 Hz AC, the voltage changes polarity and the current changes direction 120 times each second, with two changes in polarity or direction constituting one cycle. X-ray tubes, however, are designed to operate only when the x-ray target is positive and the filament is negative. Hence, x-ray units must convert the AC furnished by the utility to direct current (DC) for use in the x-ray tube. This conversion is accomplished by the process of *rectification*. A rectifier is any device that converts alternating current to direct current.

One of the simplest ways to operate an x-ray tube is to use AC and rely on the x-ray tube itself to control the flow of electrons in only one direction, from filament to target. The composition and configuration of the filament is ideal for producing the elevated temperatures necessary to release electrons by thermionic emission. When the filament is negative and the target is positive, these electrons flow to the x-ray target and produce x rays. Under normal circumstances, the x-ray target is not an efficient source of electrons. When the polarity of the alternating voltage is reversed and the target is negative and the filament is positive, electrons are not available from the target, and therefore no electrons flow from target to filament. In this condition, known as *self-rectification*, the x-ray tube itself is rectifying the AC power. Self-rectification is a satisfactory method of controlling electron flow in an x-ray tube, provided that the target does not reach an elevated temperature at which electrons are released from the target by thermionic emission. This provision is satisfied by circumstances in which the tube current is relatively low and the target remains relatively cool. At high tube currents, however, greatly elevated temperatures are achieved by the target. Under these conditions, thermionic emission, and therefore reverse electron flow, can occur. High-energy electrons bombarding the filament can destroy it; hence, self-rectification is employed only in circumstances in which the tube current is intrinsically limited, such as in some low-current generators used for mobile radiography and radiation therapy.[9]

With two rectifiers in the high-voltage circuit, one pulse of x rays is produced per cycle of the supplied alternating electrical power. This method, termed *half-wave rectification*, is a relatively inefficient use of the supplied power because the reverse half-cycle of the electrical power is discarded. This reverse half-cycle can be captured and used by the process of *full-wave rectification*, which employs a more complex rectification circuit.

With full-wave rectification, current from both the positive and the negative phases of the voltage waveform emerges from the rectification circuit in a single direction and is always presented to the x-ray tube with the filament at negative potential and the anode at positive potential. In full-wave rectification, the negative pulses in the voltage waveform are essentially "flipped over" so that they also can be used to produce x rays. In this manner, a full-wave rectification circuit converts an AC waveform into a DC waveform with two pulses per cycle or 120 pulses per second.

The efficiency of x-ray production can be further increased by maintaining the voltage wave-form at high potential, rather than allowing it to decrease to zero twice during each voltage cycle. Three-phase (3φ) power permits this goal to be approached. Three-phase power is supplied through three separate cables connected to the x-ray tube. The voltage waveform in each cable varies slightly out of phase with that in the other two cables. These voltage waveforms are presented to the x-ray tube so that the voltage across the tube is always at or near maximum. The voltage waveforms are full-wave rectified to provide six voltage pulses to the x-ray tube during each power cycle. The circuit that supplies the rectified waveforms is known as a *3φ, 6-pulse circuit*. A refinement of 3φ circuitry yields a slight phase delay for the waveform presented to the anode compared with that to the cathode. This refinement, known as a *3φ, 12-pulse circuit*, provides a smaller ripple (about 3%) in the voltage applied to the x-ray tube compared with a 3φ, 6-pulse circuit, for which the ripple may be as great as 12%.

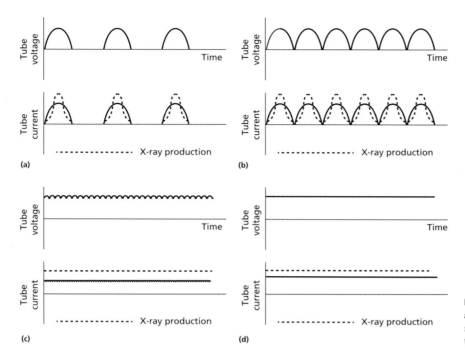

Figure 4-2 Voltage and current waveforms across the x-ray tube for (a) half-wave rectification, (b) full-wave rectification, (c) three-phase, and (d) constant potential.

Voltage waveforms across the x-ray tube are depicted in Figure 4-2 for half-wave and full-wave rectification and for 3φ and constant potential operation. This latter condition is approached in *high-frequency x-ray generators*, in which the voltage pulses are supplied to the x-ray tube at frequencies from 1 to 100 kHz. High-frequency x-ray generators provide the greatest efficiency achievable for x-ray production.

X-ray spectra

Several factors influence the distribution of photon energies in an x-ray beam. The energy of electrons impinging on the target varies with the voltage applied across the x-ray tube. For electrons of a specific energy Bremsstrahlung photons are produced with energies up to a maximum keV equal numerically to the kVp across the x-ray tube. The kVp designation depicts the maximum (p = peak) voltage in kilovolts (kV). Characteristic x rays are also generated, and these x rays have energies independent of the impinging electrons so long as the threshold energy for characteristic x-ray emission is exceeded.

Every x-ray beam is filtered by materials naturally present in the x-ray beam, including the target, glass envelope of the x-ray tube, insulating oil surrounding the tube, and exit window in the tube housing. These materials are collectively referred to as the *inherent* or *intrinsic filtration of the x-ray beam*, usually expressed as millimeters aluminum equivalent (mm Al eq). The inherent filtration in most diagnostic x-ray tubes is about 1 mm Al eq. Additional filtration is always inserted to "harden" the x-ray beam by selectively removing x rays of lower energy. If these x rays were not removed by filtration, they would be absorbed in the patient and increase the patient's radiation dose. An x-ray beam with higher average energy is said to be "harder"

because it is able to penetrate more dense (i.e., harder) substances such as bone. An x-ray beam of lower average energy is said to be "softer" because it can penetrate only less dense (i.e., softer) substances such as fat and muscle. In x-ray beams used for diagnosis, the added filtration is usually a few millimeters of aluminum. For the higher-energy *orthovoltage* (a few hundred kVp) x-ray beams employed in radiation therapy, a filter of aluminum, copper, and tin often is used. A filter of aluminum, copper, and tin is termed a *Thoraeus filter* after its developer, R. Thoraeus, who first described it in 1932.

Emission spectra for a tungsten-target diagnostic x-ray tube are shown in Figure 4-3 for the three thicknesses of added

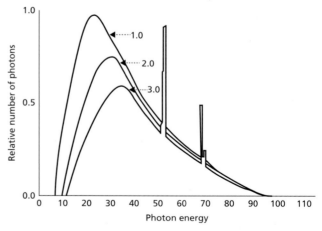

Figure 4-3 X-ray spectra for a 100 kVp tungsten target x-ray tube with total filtration values of 1.0, 2.0, and 3.0 mm Al. KVp and mAs are the same for the three spectra.

Source: Computer simulation courtesy of Todd Steinberg, St. Louis, MO.

aluminum filtration. The added filtration decreases the total number of x rays but increases the average energy of the x rays in the beam. These changes are reflected in a decrease in the overall height of the x-ray spectrum and a shift of the spectral peak toward higher energy.

The material used as the target of an x-ray tube affects the x-ray spectrum by influencing the efficiency of x-ray production and determining the energies of the characteristic x rays. The efficiency of x-ray production is the ratio of the energy emitted as x-ray radiation divided by the energy deposited in the target by electrons accelerated from the filament. The rate of energy deposition in the target is the power deposition, P_d, in watts, where $P_d = VI$ (V is the tube voltage in volts and I is the tube current in amperes). The rate at which energy is released as radiation is the emitted power, P_r, in watts:

$$P_r = 0.9 \times 10^{-9} (Z)(V^2)(I)$$

where Z is the atomic number of the target. The ratio of these quantities is the x-ray production efficiency:

$$\text{Efficiency} = P_r/P_d = 0.9 \times 10^{-9} (Z)(V)$$

As shown in this equation, the efficiency of x-ray production increases with the atomic number of the target and the voltage across the x-ray tube. At voltages in the range of 100 kVp used in diagnostic radiology, x-ray production is an inefficient process, with less than 1% of the energy that is delivered to the target being released as radiation. Almost all of the electron energy deposited in the target is degraded to heat, causing an elevated temperature of the target. To prevent the target from overheating, mechanisms are employed to limit the target temperature. These mechanisms include use of large-diameter rotating anodes, beveled targets to spread the deposited energy over a larger target volume, and water or oil recirculating systems as well as radiating fins for lower-power x-ray tubes.

Example 4-1

In 0.5 sec, 1.25×10^{18} electrons (400 mA) are accelerated across a constant potential difference of 100 kV. At what rate is energy deposited in the x-ray target?

$$P = VI$$
$$= (105\,V)(0.4\,A)$$
$$= 4 \times 10^4 \text{ watts}$$

Example 4-2

If the x-ray tube in Example 4-1 has a tungsten target ($Z = 74$), determine the power (P_r) emitted as x radiation and the efficiency of x-ray production.

$$P_r = 0.9 \times 10^{-9}(Z)(V^2)(I)$$
$$= 0.9 \times 10^{-9}(74)(10^5)^2(0.4)$$
$$= 2.7 \times 10^2 \text{ watts}$$

$$\text{Efficiency} = 0.9 \times 10^{-9}(Z)(V)$$
$$= 0.9 \times 10^{-9}(74)(10^5)$$
$$= 0.67 \times 10^{-2} \cong 0.7\%$$

At tube voltages employed in diagnostic radiology, x rays are emitted approximately at right angles to the incident electrons, and a reflectance target is used to produce an x-ray beam at a 90° angle to the axis of the x-ray tube. In radiation therapy, the increased efficiency of x-ray production also permits use of stationary, rather than rotating, x-ray targets.

The energies of characteristic x rays from an x-ray target reflect the binding energies of electrons in the target, particularly those in the K, L, and M shells. In a typical x-ray spectrum, the principal peak of characteristic x rays reflects electron transitions from the L to the K shell, and a second peak depicts transitions from the M to the K shell. In either case, the x rays have energies slightly below the K binding energies of electrons in the target material. As described in Chapter 2 x rays with energies slightly below the binding energy of K electrons of a material are transmitted through the material with little attenuation. Therefore, a filter of the same material as an x-ray target transmits characteristic x rays from the target with little attenuation. This property is employed in mammographic x-ray tubes, in which a molybdenum target is used to provide characteristic x rays (17–20 keV) of a desirable energy for imaging soft tissue. A molybdenum filter placed in the x-ray beam transmits the characteristic x rays with little attenuation, but absorbs many of the Bremsstrahlung photons of lower energies. In all but the heaviest elements, transitions of electrons into the L and higher shells result in the release of electromagnetic radiations that are too low in energy to be classified as x rays, or so low in energy that they are readily absorbed by the inherent and added filtration in the x-ray beam.

As mentioned earlier, interaction of a high-energy electron with a target nucleus can produce a Bremsstrahlung photon with any energy up to the total kinetic energy of the electron. Such a photon would possess the maximum energy (and therefore minimum wavelength) of the photons in an x-ray beam generated at a particular tube voltage. Hence the minimum wavelength photons in an x-ray beam are related to the peak kilovoltage applied across the x-ray tube. With λ_{min} expressed in nanometers, the relationship is:

$$\text{Maximum photon energy (keV)} = h\nu_{max}$$
$$= \text{maximum tube voltage (kVp)}$$

But $\nu_{max} = c/\lambda_{min}$, where c is the speed of light in a vacuum, so:

$$\frac{hc}{\lambda_{min}} = V\,(kVp)$$
$$\lambda_{min} = hc/V\,(kVp)$$
$$\lambda_{min}(nm) = 1.24/V\,(kvp)$$

with the minimum wavelength λ_{min} expressed in nm.

Example 4-3

0.00025 nm (0.00025×10^{-3} μm) is the λ_{min} of x rays in a therapeutic x-ray beam. What is the maximum energy x ray that corresponds to λ_{min}, and what voltage characterizes the x-ray beam?

$$\lambda_{min} (nm) = 1.24/E\,(keV)$$
$$E\,(keV) = 1.24/\lambda_{min} = 1.24/0.00025\ nm$$
$$= 4.96\ MeV$$

Since $E(keV) = V(kVp)$, the x-ray beam voltage is said to be "4.96 MV."

Note: At energies above the orthovoltage range, x-ray beams are generated by mechanisms that accelerate electrons uniformly, so the *p* to designate *peak* kilovoltage is not used.

The voltage across the x-ray tube determines the maximum x-ray energy and the efficiency of x-ray production. The number of electrons impinging on the target also influences the quantity of x rays during an exposure. The number of electrons is a function of the tube current (milliamperes) and the exposure time (seconds), often expressed as the mAs of the exposure. That is, the kVp influences both the "quality" (energy or penetrating ability) and the quantity of x rays present in the x-ray beam, whereas the mAs influences only the quantity.

Example 4-4

Compute the total number of electrons impinging on the target of an x-ray tube operated at 400 mA for 0.05 sec.

The Ampere (*A*), the unit of electrical current, equals one Coulomb per second, and the product of current and time equals the total charge in Coulombs.

$$400\,mA = 0.4\,A,\ and\ one\ electron$$
$$= 1.6 \times 10^{-19}\ Coulombs\{Q[Coulombs]$$
$$= [I(Amperes)] \times [t(sec)]\}$$

$$Number\ of\ electrons = \frac{(0.4\,A)(Coulombs/sec - A)(0.05\ sec)}{1.6 \times 10^{-19} Coulombs/electron}$$
$$= 1.25 \times 10^{17} electrons$$

To produce x-ray images of the highest quality, the x rays should emerge from a small volume of reflectance target to provide a sharply defined x-ray beam. This volume of target is referred to as the *focal spot* of the x-ray tube. To reduce the focal spot, the target usually is beveled at a steep angle with respect to the direction of the incident electrons. With the target at a steep angle, the x rays appear to originate from an "apparent focal spot" that appears much smaller than the "true focal spot" (Figure 4-4). This approach to focal spot reduction is termed the *line focus principle* and is widely employed in diagnostic x-ray tubes in which target angles between 6° and 17° are used. The line focus principle is important in x-ray tubes employed in x-ray and computed tomography simulators used for treatment planning and patient monitoring in radiation therapy.

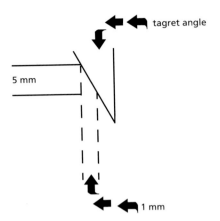

Figure 4-4 Line focus principle in which the apparent focal spot is much smaller than the true focal spot.

At the megavoltage energies employed in radiation therapy, x-ray production is much more efficient, and stationary anodes of reduced mass can be used. At these electron energies, x rays are produced in the forward direction (in the direction of the impinging electrons). Thin *transmission targets* are used that transmit the x rays with little attenuation on their way from the target to the patient. The efficiency of x-ray production is sufficiently high that anodes of large mass are not required for purposes of heat dissipation. Hence the x rays can be transmitted in a forward direction through the target without substantial attenuation. Transmission targets frequently employ a cooling mechanism, such as circulating water, to control the target temperature. The line focus principle is not applicable to most x-ray sources used in radiation therapy because transmission rather than reflectance targets are employed.

Low-energy therapy x-ray units

The practice of radiation therapy began almost immediately following Röntgen's discovery of x rays. Emil Grubbe of Chicago may have been one of the first practicing radiation therapists. He used an early Crookes x-ray tube and reported treating numerous patients with cancer with this device, beginning in January 1896. Until the advent of ^{60}Co units in the 1950s, however, most radiation therapy was conducted with x rays generated at potentials below about 300 kV. Since then, many low-energy treatment units have been replaced by megavoltage units. Many radiation oncology departments have retained a low-energy x-ray unit and make use of it, particularly for the treatment of skin lesions.

Grenz–ray units

Grenz rays are defined as radiation produced at potentials of less than 20 kV. They are nonpenetrating and consequently have little value in radiation therapy.

Contact therapy units

Contact therapy units operate at potentials of 40–50 kV and produce x rays with half-value layers of 1 or 2 mm Al. The x-ray tube is designed so that the surface to be irradiated is placed in contact with the housing, and approximately 2 cm from the target. The combination of low energy and short treatment distance causes an extremely rapid decrease in the depth dose. These x-ray beams are suitable only for treatment of surface lesions.

An advantage of contact therapy units is that their design facilitates use in operating rooms. Contact therapy machines have been used for intraoperative therapy because exposed tissues can be irradiated to high doses, while deeper tissues are spared. Their use fell out of popularity because they have been replaced by electron-beam units. Contact therapy, however, is making a comeback with modern devices specifically designed to produce ≤ 50 keV x-ray beams for brachytherapy applications.[10]

Superficial therapy units

X-ray machines operating in the kilovoltage range are primarily suited to treatment of superficial tissues. To distinguish them from *deep* therapy units, machines operating in the range of 50–150 kV are described as *superficial* therapy machines. Aluminum filters of up to 5 or 6 mm are added to increase the penetrating quality of the beam. The resulting half-value layers are generally in the range of 1–8 mm Al.

Glass or stainless-steel cones are used to collimate the beam, and the surface to be treated is placed in contact with the end of the cone. Dose rates as high as several hundred cGy per minute are available. A typical superficial unit is shown in Figure 4-5.

Orthovoltage therapy units

As higher-voltage equipment became available, x-ray machines operating in the range of 200–350 kV were developed. For

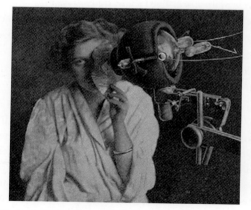

Figure 4-5 A representative superficial x-ray unit.
Source: Courtesy of Nucletron Corporation of America.

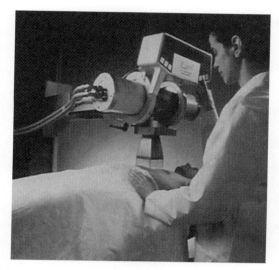

Figure 4-6 A representative orthovoltage x-ray unit.
Source: Courtesy of Nucletron Corporation of America.

many years, these units provided the most penetrating x-ray beams available to radiation therapists, and consequently they were called *deep therapy machines*. Because their energies fall between those provided by superficial units and so-called supervoltage units, they are also called *orthovoltage units*. A number of orthovoltage units are still in place, particularly outside the United States. However, they have largely been replaced by linear accelerators with electron beams, which provide more uniform irradiation of tissues than do orthovoltage x rays.

Orthovoltage units are typically equipped with adjustable collimators and a *light localizer*, which aids in the placement of the patient for treatment. Relatively short treatment distances, such as 50 cm, are routinely used. At least one modern orthovoltage unit is provided with an internal dose-monitoring system and state-of-the-art digital controls. A representative orthovoltage unit is shown in Figure 4-6.

Supervoltage therapy units

A class of treatment units operating in the 500–1000 kV range appeared in the late 1940s and 1950s. The use of conventional transformers limited the operation of x-ray machines to about 350 kV. Supervoltage machines relied on devices such as *resonant transformers* to generate higher potentials. Due to the development of alternative high-energy electrical systems and isotope treatment units, supervoltage x-ray generators were promoted for only a few years.

Megavoltage x-ray units

Several types of x-ray machines operating at more than 1000 kV have been developed, including Van de Graaff generators, betatrons, and linear accelerators. Of the three, only linear accelerators are now in widespread use. These units combine the advantages of high dose rates, compact design, and high reliability. Linear accelerators are discussed in detail in later sections of this chapter.

Isotope teletherapy units

Cobalt units

Before 1951, the only teletherapy units were *teleradium units*, which contained a few grams of radium in a sealed capsule. Teleradium units were expensive, furnished a radiation beam of low intensity, and were considered impractical for routine clinical therapy. After World War II, nuclear reactors were constructed to furnish radioactive nuclides for public use. The first high-activity ^{60}Co source for medical use was produced in Canada in 1951. In 1952, Johns and co-workers described the first ^{60}Co teletherapy unit.[11–13] As of the late 1990s, only a few ^{60}Co units are being built, primarily for sale in countries outside the United States and Western Europe.

Source capsule

A standard container for encapsulating ^{60}Co sources has been accepted by manufacturers of teletherapy units. The ^{60}Co source is retained within two stainless-steel canisters that are welded to prevent escape of the radioactive material. To attenuate γ rays emitted in undesired directions, shields of tungsten, uranium, or lead surround the source. Gamma rays emitted in the desired direction traverse a thin steel plate and are attenuated only slightly.

Source exposure mechanism

Various methods have been devised for exposing and shielding the ^{60}Co source. Some manufacturers mount the source on a metal wheel. The wheel is rotated 180 degrees to expose the source. A motor holds the source in the "on" position. A spring attached to the wheel returns the source to the "off" position when power to the motor is interrupted. An alternative method to expose the source uses air pressure generated by a small compressor to hold the source in the "on" position. The source is drawn to the shielded position by a spring when the compressed air is allowed to escape. Both of these designs are considered fail-safe in that the source returns to the shielded position if power to the unit is interrupted.

Collimators

With the source in the "on" position, γ rays from the source capsule enter a diverging channel in the lead or depleted uranium source head. A collimator mounted below the diverging channel is used to vary the size of the radiation beam leaving the source

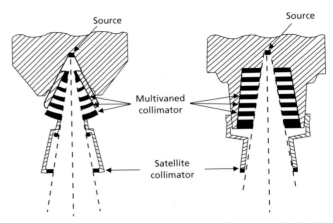

Figure 4-7 Two type of interleaved, multivaned collimators equipped with satellite collimators. *Source:* Hendee 1970.[14]

head. Modern ^{60}Co teletherapy units have an interleaved, multivaned collimator with vanes of lead or tungsten, as shown in Figure 4-7.

Often a satellite collimator (also referred to as a *penumbra trimmer*) is attached to the end of the collimator nearest the patient. The satellite collimator sharpens the edge of the radiation beam. To reduce contamination of the γ-ray beam with electrons that were produced from photon interactions, the end of the collimator should be at least 15 cm above the patient's skin.[15] At shorter distances, a significant number of electrons may reach the skin and produce severe skin reactions.

To indicate the location of the γ-ray beam and assist in the positioning of patients for treatment, a light localizer is provided. A mirror positioned inside the collimator reflects light from a bulb to provide a light field, which is coincident with the radiation beam emerging from the collimator.

Beam edge unsharpness

The finite size of a teletherapy source creates an indistinct border for the radiation field. This indistinct border is termed the *geometric penumbra*. The lack of sharpness at the skin surface and at a depth, d, within the patient is illustrated in Figure 4-8.

The width, W, of the geometric penumbra at the skin surface is:

$$W = c\frac{SSD - SCD}{SCD}$$

where c represents the diameter of the source, SSD is the source-to-skin distance, and SCD is the source-to-collimator distance. The geometric penumbra is independent of the size of the radiation field. The geometric penumbra at the patient's surface could be eliminated by placing the end of the collimator on the skin. Then $SSD = SCD$ and the penumbra $W = 0$. However, this practice must be avoided with high-energy x and γ beams because electrons from the collimator would contaminate the radiation

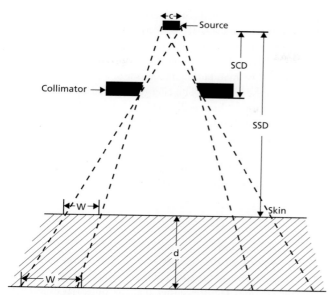

Figure 4-8 Diagram of the lack of sharpness of the beam edge caused by the finite size of a teletherapy source.
Source: Hendee 1970.[14]

beam at the skin surface. To minimize the size of the geometric penumbra, sources with high specific activity are constructed with the smallest possible diameter. Such sources can supply a radiation beam of reasonable intensity and relatively small penumbra.

The width, W', of the geometric penumbra at the depth, d, within a patient is:

$$W' = c\frac{SSD + d - SCD}{SCD}$$

The geometric penumbra is larger at any depth within the patient than it is on the skin surface.

Example 4-5

Determine the width of the geometric penumbra of a ^{60}Co beam at 10 cm depth in a patient undergoing treatment at 80 cm SSD. The source diameter is 2 cm, and the patient's surface is 35 cm from the distal end of the collimator.

The SCD is $80 - 35 = 45$ cm. From Equation (4-1), the penumbra width at depth is:

$$W' = c\frac{SSD + d - SCD}{SCD}$$
$$W' = 2\frac{80 + 10 - 45}{45}$$
$$W' = 2\text{ cm}$$

The total penumbra at the surface or at some depth below the surface sometimes is defined as the distance between the 90% and 10% *decrement lines* along the beam edge.[16] Decrement lines are lines through points at which the absorbed dose is a certain percent (e.g., 90%, 80%, 70%, and so forth) of the energy

absorbed at the same depth along the central axis of the radiation beam. The total penumbra at the skin surface and at depths below the surface should be considered during treatment planning, particularly when adjacent (abutting) radiation fields are used.

Isocentric units

Both stand-mounted and isocentrically mounted ^{60}Co teletherapy units have been available and may still be found in radiation therapy departments.

The primary advantage of isocentric treatment units is in setting up patients for treatment. With an isocentric unit, the patient needs only to be positioned once, in preparation for treatment of a single target volume with beams directed from two or more angles. In contrast, a stand-mounted unit often requires that the patient position be changed (i.e., the patient be moved from the supine to the prone position) or that the treatment couch be moved to permit repositioning of the source head.

An additional advantage of an isocentric unit is that it permits rotation or *arc therapy*. With arc therapy, the gantry rotates during treatment to move the source head around the isocenter. The patient is positioned so that the center of the target volume is located at the isocenter and the beam irradiates the target volume during its arc.

Most isocentric teletherapy installations include wall and ceiling lights or lasers that produce narrow light beams that interact at the isocenter. Superposition of the laser beams on marks on the patient's skin permits rapid alignment of the patient for treatment. With most teletherapy units, a counterweight balances the weight of the source head during rotation. Often the counterweight serves as a primary barrier to absorb radiation transmitted by the patient and reduces the shielding required for walls of the treatment room.

^{137}Cs teletherapy units

A teletherapy unit with a ^{137}Cs source was described by Brucer in 1956.[17] A few cesium units were used until the early 1990s to treat lesions at relatively shallow depths, such as head-and-neck tumors. Collimators and source-exposure mechanisms for most ^{137}Cs units were similar to those for ^{60}Co units, although some ^{137}Cs equipment was supplied with cones rather than collimators. Compared with a ^{60}Co source of equal physical size, the radiation intensity from a source of ^{137}Cs is relatively low because the maximum specific activity is only 3.2×10^{12} Bq/g (87 Ci/g) for ^{137}Cs (Example 4-6) and because γ rays are emitted during only 83% of all nuclear transitions of ^{137}Cs. Sources of sufficient activity to provide a radiation beam of reasonable intensity at a long treatment distance also furnish a large, unsharp beam edge. A smaller source increases the sharpness, but provides a beam of reasonable intensity only if the treatment distance is short. Consequently, most ^{137}Cs units were used at treatment distances of less than 35 cm. The rapid divergence of the beam resulting from the use of short treatment distances caused the distribution of a radiation dose within a patient treated with ^{137}Cs photons to resemble that from x rays generated at about 400 kVp.

Example 4-6

What is the maximum specific activity for ^{137}Cs?

Activity is calculated from the number of atoms and the decay constant:

$$A = \lambda N$$

If N is the number of atoms of ^{137}Cs per gram, the activity is the specific activity. For a source of pure ^{137}Cs ($T_{1/2} = 30$ years):

$$\text{Number of atoms/gram } N = \frac{6.02 \times 10^{23} \text{ atoms/g-atomic mass}}{137 \text{ g/g-atomic mass}}$$

$$= 4.4 \times 10^{21} \text{ atom/g}$$

$$\text{Decay constant, } \lambda, \text{ for}^{137}\text{Cs} = \frac{\ln 2}{(T_{1/2})}$$

$$= \frac{0.693}{30y}$$

$$= 2.3 \times 10^{-2} \text{ y}^{-1}$$

$$= 7.3 \times 10^{-10} \text{ sec}^{-1}$$

$$\text{Specific activity} = \lambda N$$

$$= (7.3 \times 10 - 10 \text{ sec}^{-1})(4.4 \times 10^{21} \text{ atoms/g})$$

$$= 3.2 \times 10^{12} \text{ Bq/g}$$

Linear accelerators

Modern linear accelerators (*linacs*) are now found in virtually all radiation therapy departments, having replaced most other therapy units. They are used to treat patients with beams of electrons or Bremsstrahlung x rays following interactions of electrons in a suitable target. Intense electron beam currents are achievable with an accelerator to provide high dose rates for both x-ray and electron treatments. Hence, treatment times are short even at relatively long target-to-patient distances. Many modern linacs provide multiple electron and photon beam energies in the megavoltage energy range. The term *MV* is typically used to describe photon beams (e.g., 6 MV) whereas the term *MeV* is typically used to describe an electron beam (e.g., 6 MeV).

Historical development

The earliest linear accelerators were so-called direct accelerators, in which charged particles were accelerated by an electric field created by placing a high potential difference over an insulated column.

In the simplest form of linear accelerator, such as the simple x-ray tube shown in Figure 4-1, electrons are boiled off the cathode surface (which is heated by a filament) and accelerated toward the anode. The accelerating force is provided by a static electric field produced by maintaining the anode at a positive potential V relative to the cathode. The energy acquired by an electron accelerated in this fashion is determined by the voltage, V; electrons accelerated through a potential difference of 1 V gain an energy of 1 electron volt (eV). This corresponds to 1.6×10^{-19} Joules, although the unit eV (or MeV) is most commonly used.

The velocity of the accelerated electron can be determined from the classic equation for kinetic energy:

$$T = \frac{1}{2}m_e v^2 \tag{4-1}$$

where m_e is the electron's mass and v is its velocity. It is straightforward to calculate the velocity of a 1 eV electron as 1.87×10^7 m/sec, or 6.25% of the speed of light. To accelerate electrons to higher energies requires either that the potential difference be increased (impractical at voltages above a few hundred thousand volts) or that the accelerating force be repeated numerous times. Note that Equation (4-1) cannot be used once the electron becomes *relativistic* (i.e., when its velocity exceeds approximately 20% of the speed of light), because the change in electron mass must be considered.

The first linear accelerator was developed by Wideröe in 1928 to accelerate heavy ions.[18] Wideröe's accelerator consisted of a series of metal cylinders, termed *drift tubes*, with alternate cylinders connected to opposite terminals of an oscillating radio frequency voltage (Figure 4-9).

Because adjacent drift tubes are connected to opposite terminals of the power supply, an electric field develops between the ends of the tubes. Ions are accelerated across the gaps between adjacent drift tubes.

While inside the drift tubes, the ions are shielded from the electric fields produced by the radiofrequency voltage. The length of each tube is sufficient to allow ions to drift undisturbed through the tube each time the radiofrequency voltage changes polarity. In this manner, ions are accelerated from one drift tube to the next only after the correct polarity has been established across the gap between tubes. As the energy, and therefore the velocity, of the particles increases, the drift tubes must increase in length. Although useful for accelerating heavy ions, the Wideröe accelerator was not suitable for accelerating electrons, because the high speed of the electrons would have required inordinately long drift tubes.

Development of the electron linac was made possible by the invention in the late 1930s and early 1940s of the microwave cavity and by the development of klystron and magnetron tubes as sources of microwave power.

Between 1948 and 1955, the first electron linacs were designed and built by groups working independently in England and in the United States. Fry and associates at the Telecommunications Research Group, Great Malvern, England (later to become

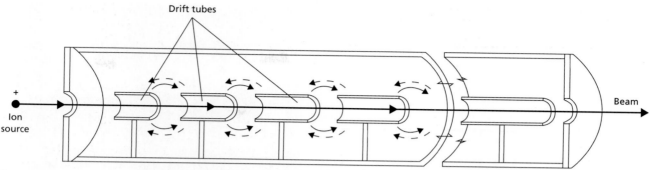

Drift tubes

+
Ion
source

Beam

Figure 4-9 An early linear accelerator, in which drift tubes were suspended in an evacuated accelerator waveguide and connected to opposite terminals of a power supply.

part of the Atomic Energy Research Establishment at Harwell) designed a 0.5 MeV linac in 1946 and accelerated electrons later that same year.[19] Independently, Ginzton and associates in Palo Alto, California, USA, developed a 1.7 MeV accelerator, which became operational in early 1947.[20] By late 1947, both groups had achieved energies of 3.5 to 6 MeV. Also during this period, Chodorow, Ginzton, and Hansen constructed multimegawatt klystrons, having many orders of magnitude greater power than those developed for wartime radar applications.[21] These microwave sources made possible the development of traveling-wave linacs with high beam currents and energies of up to 1000 MeV.

In a microwave accelerator, microwaves are guided into a cylindrical metal tube known as an *accelerator waveguide*. Simultaneously, electrons or other charged particles are introduced into one end of the accelerator waveguide. The presence of the electromagnetic field induces an electric current within the walls of the accelerator waveguide. The current generates an electric field, which exerts a force on the particles, accelerating them to high velocities.

The microwave power, P, required to establish the electric field within the accelerator depends on several characteristics of the waveguide:

$$P = \frac{V^2}{ZL}$$

where V is the potential difference developed within the guide through which particles are accelerated, Z is the *shunt impedance* of the accelerator waveguide, and L is the length of the waveguide. The shunt impedance is a measure of the efficiency of the guide. To develop the potential to accelerate particles to an energy of 10 MeV in a structure with a shunt impedance of 100 MΩ/m and a length of 1 m, 1 MW of electromagnetic power is consumed. (*Note*: MΩ represents the quantity "mega ohms," where "ohm" is a unit of impedance.) Additional power is consumed by the accelerated particles themselves, as well as by other components of the linac. Consequently, a source of 2 MW or more of microwave power is required. A 2 MW magnetron is often used in low-energy linacs, whereas klystrons

with power ratings of up to 10 MW are used in higher-energy units.

To regulate the phase velocity of the microwave (the velocity at which a peak of the microwave appears to travel), barriers such as metal discs may be placed in the waveguide at regular intervals (Figure 4-10). The term *phase velocity* refers to the velocity of a peak or valley of an electromagnetic wave. A linear accelerator designed by use of this principle allows the crest of the electromagnetic wave to travel at less than the speed of light, permitting the charged particle to keep up. The energy carried by the electromagnetic wave always moves at the speed of light.

The electric field established by the microwaves develops between the discs. In some accelerator structures, a *forward*-directed field develops between one pair of discs, while a *backward*-directed field develops between the adjacent pair of discs. Consequently, a wavelength spans two adjacent cavities (Figure 4-11). Particles in the space between the first pair of discs are accelerated in the forward direction, while particles in the second space (between the second and third discs) are accelerated in the backward direction. Naturally, particles would arrive

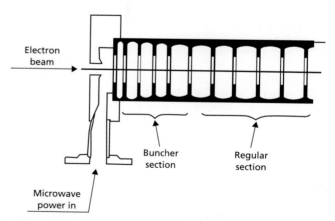

Electron beam

Buncher section

Regular section

Microwave power in

Figure 4-10 A disc-loaded waveguide for electron acceleration. The spacing between discs in the *buncher section* is less than that in the *regular section*. The buncher section accelerates electrons to relativistic energies and forms them into bunches for efficient acceleration by the regular section.

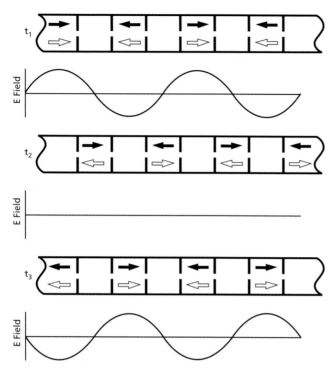

Figure 4-11 A schematic of an accelerator waveguide showing separate forward and backward waves and their superposition. In each diagram, the *solid arrows* indicate the positive and negative peaks of a microwave electric field moving from left to right, whereas the *open arrows* indicate a field reflected from the right moving to the left. At t_1 and t_3, the forward and reflected waves superimpose constructively. At t_2, they interfere destructively, and the electric field intensity is zero everywhere. *Source:* Adapted from Karzmark et al. 1993.[23]

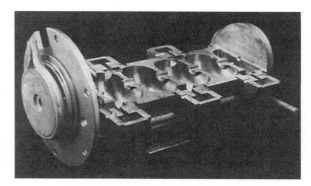

Figure 4-12 An example of a side-coupled standing-wave linear accelerator waveguide. *Source:* Karzmark et al. 1993.[23]

at the second space only if they were accelerated in the forward direction while in the first space. The distance between the discs is determined by the velocity of the particles:

$$L_n = \frac{V_n}{2v}$$

where L_n is the distance between adjacent discs, V_n, is the velocity of the particles, and v is the frequency of the microwaves. In medical electron linacs, the electrons quickly approach the speed of light as they are accelerated down the waveguide. Consequently, the spacing between discs quickly reaches a maximum distance. In the more common $\pi/2$ mode, one wavelength spans four cavities, and particles are accelerated only in alternate cavities. The microwave field has zero intensity in the remaining cavities (Figure 4-11). The benefits of this design are described later in this chapter.

Early medical linacs were of the *traveling wave* design. Microwaves were injected into one end of the accelerator and traveled to the other end, where they were extracted. As they traveled, they carried the electrons along with them. The extracted microwaves could be conducted back to the proximal end of the accelerator and re-injected. The disc-loaded design

limited the shunt impedance to maximum values less than 60 MΩ/m, which restricted the *accelerator gradient*, or attainable electron energy in MeV/m, to fairly low values.

In 1968, Knapp et al. invented the *side-coupled standing wave accelerator*, in which the microwaves were reflected from the ends of the accelerator waveguide.[22] The backward traveling wave interferes with the forward traveling wave, alternately constructively and destructively. The resulting *standing wave* has a magnitude of approximately double that of the traveling wave, and the peak intensity travels along the waveguide at the phase velocity of the traveling wave. In alternate spaces between discs, the magnitude of the wave is always at or near zero (Figure 4-11).

In standing wave structures, the spaces between discs are optimized by changing the shape of the discs. The resulting *cavities* permit the microwaves to resonate, improving the efficiency with which their energy is transferred to the accelerated electrons. An additional improvement is that the microwave electric field intensity is at or near zero in alternate cavities. Although necessary to conduct the microwave energy, these cavities play no role in accelerating particles. By moving them to the side (Figure 4-12), off the waveguide axis, the accelerating cavities can be placed closer together. The overall length of the structure becomes shorter, facilitating the placement of the guide in the treatment unit and improving its efficiency.

Major components of medical electron accelerators

Modern linear accelerators consist of several major subsystems. These components produce the electrical power required to generate microwaves, conduct the microwave power to the accelerator waveguide, and transport the accelerated beam ultimately to the patient.

Modulator and pulse-forming network

Linear accelerators require fairly large amounts of electrical power. The power must be provided in large pulses because

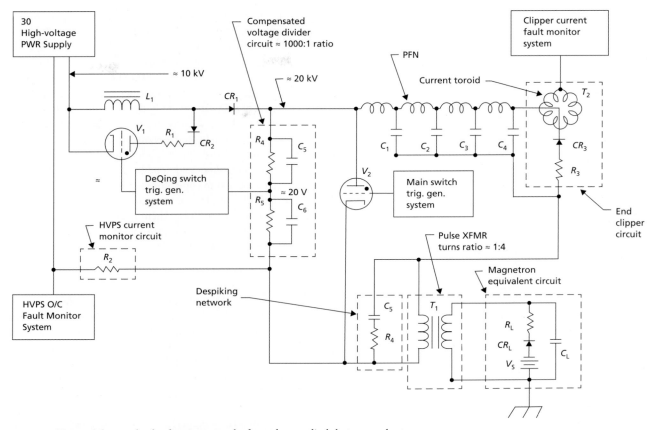

Figure 4-13 The modulator and pulse-forming network of a modern medical electron accelerator. *Source:* Karzmark et al. 1993.[23]

linacs accelerate particles in bursts. The *modulator* consists of a power supply that converts the incoming alternating current into direct current, along with a *pulse-forming network* that modulates the current into pulses.

A diagram of a modulator appears in Figure 4-13. The direct current charges a bank of capacitors, which store the charge until a pulse is required. The charging cycle lasts about a millisecond. On receiving a signal from a timing circuit, a switching tube closes, completing a circuit from the capacitor bank, through a transformer, to ground. The capacitors discharge rapidly, but because of the inductor connecting them, they discharge in sequence. The resulting pulse is nearly square.

The switching tube, or *thyratron*, is a gas-filled triode (Figure 4-13). When the grid is charged positively, electrons flow from the cathode to the anode. The gas within the tube ionizes and conducts larger currents than do other switching devices. At the end of the pulse, the grid voltage is removed, preventing further current flow while the pulse-forming network recharges. This cycle is repeated between 50 and 500 times each second.

The output of the pulse transformer is conducted to the microwave-producing tube, either a magnetron or a klystron. The resulting microwave pulse, similar in shape to the electrical pulse, is about 6 μsec long and consists of several megawatts of power.

Magnetrons

The cavity-type magnetron was invented in 1940 by Boot and Randall and made high-definition radar (radio detection and ranging) possible in World War II.[23] Magnetrons are commonly used in low-power linear accelerators. A magnetron of this type consists of a cylindrical diode containing a central cathode, which is heated by internal filaments. The coaxial anode is constructed of solid copper with coupled resonant cavities formed in the wall (Figure 4-14).

An axial magnetic field is supplied by a large permanent magnet. When a DC pulse is applied to the diode, electrons from the cathode are accelerated toward the anode and assume a spiral path because of the magnetic field. The individual electrons follow complex cycloidal paths around the cathode. As the electrons swirl along their spiral pathway, they induce intense local variations in the axial magnetic field. The radiofrequency energy induced in the magnetic field by this process is trapped in the resonant cavities. Oscillation of this trapped energy forms varying electrical fields across the lips of each cavity. These varying electrical fields channel electrons to the more positive regions of the anode, and the spiraling electron cloud appears to sweep around the cathode as it tracks the more positive regions. The sweeping electron cloud induces additional intense variations

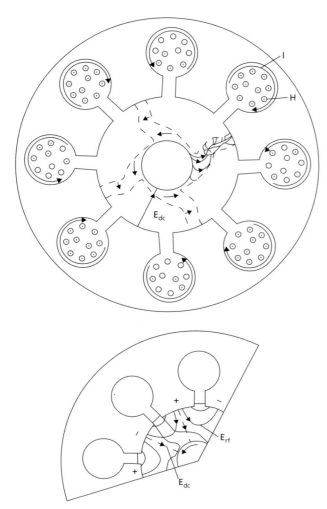

Figure 4-14 A cutaway view of a magnetron microwave power tube. *Source:* Karzmark et al. 1993.[23]

in the magnetic field, which are in resonance and coupled with the cavities of the coaxial anode. A loop antenna inserted in one of the cavities taps the radiofrequency energy in the cavities and transfers it to a waveguide for transmission to the accelerator waveguide. Magnetrons transform DC power to radiofrequency power with efficiencies as high as 60%. Typically, such magnetrons provide 2 MW peak power.

The microwave wavelength must be of an appropriate length so that the accelerator components are reasonably easy to design and manufacture. Most modern medical linacs operate with microwaves of about 3000 MHz, in what is known as the *S-band*. The wavelength in a vacuum may be determined from the frequency v and speed of light c as:

$$\lambda = \frac{c}{v}$$

For microwaves of 3000 MHz, the wavelength in a vacuum is on the order of 10 cm. In a waveguide, the wavelength is reduced somewhat because the phase velocity of the radiation is reduced.

During operation of a linac, the temperature of various components tends to increase. Changes in temperature may adversely affect the operation of the accelerator and must be avoided. In particular, a temperature rise of the accelerator guide of as little as 1°C may cause sufficient expansion to change the resonant frequency by 60 kHz. A change in resonant frequency of as little as 20 kHz can seriously degrade the performance of the accelerator. This sensitivity means that the frequency of the microwaves must be adjusted to compensate. Consequently, the magnetron must be *tunable*, to permit continuous matching of the frequency. Early linacs equipped with fixed-frequency magnetrons required that the operator manually adjusted the flow of water around the accelerator waveguide, to regulate the size of the resonant cavities and keep them matched to the microwave frequency. Modern magnetrons are equipped with motor-driven tuners that are controlled by a circuit that senses the microwave frequency.

Klystrons

The principle of the klystron microwave power tube is illustrated in Figure 4-15. The tube requires a low-power radiofrequency oscillator to supply RF power to the first cavity, termed the *buncher*. The low-power RF source used with a klystron is known as the *RF driver* and typically delivers a power level of a few hundred watts. By application of an accelerating voltage supplied as a DC pulse from the DC power supply (the pulse forming network described earlier), electrons with energies of several keV are injected into the cavity. In the buncher cavity, the velocity of the electrons is modulated by the electric field component of the microwave field. This modulation of velocity causes the electrons to group together into closely spaced electron bunches. As the electron bunches arrive at the second cavity, termed the *catcher cavity*, they are decelerated, and their energy is transformed into a pulse of microwave power. High-power klystrons containing additional cavities have achieved direct current-to-microwave conversion efficiencies of up to 55%, with peak powers as high as 24 MW.

Microwave power-handling equipment

Microwaves from the magnetron or klystron are conducted to the accelerator waveguide by rectangular sections of waveguide (Figure 4-16). The microwaves are confined by the metal walls of the waveguide and propagate through a dielectric gas such as Freon or sulfur hexafluoride. The dimensions of such waveguides are typically 0.6 λ in width by (0.2–0.5) λ in height. The circular accelerator waveguide is normally energized in the TM01 mode, meaning that the magnetic field is transverse to the longitudinal axis of the guide. Consequently, the electric field is axial, and the force exerted by the electric field on the particles accelerates them along the longitudinal axis of the guide.

In single-modality accelerators (those capable of producing only an x-ray beam of selected energy), the waveguide and other microwave power-handling equipment are straightforward.

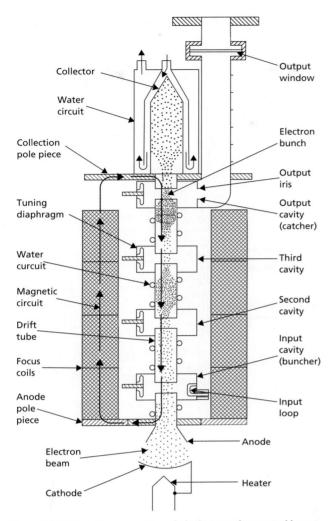

Figure 4-15 Schematic cross-section of a high-power four-cavity klystron power tube.

Multimodality accelerators, capable of producing beams of electrons as well as x-ray beams of one or more energies, require alteration of the microwave power delivered to the accelerator structure, so that particles can be accelerated to different energies. Because magnetrons and klystrons are generally adjustable over only small ranges, other means are required to vary the power. One available device is called a *power splitter*. A variable fraction of the power directed to this device is returned to the accelerator waveguide. The remainder is absorbed in a water-filled *load*. Of the power directed to the accelerator waveguide, a portion may be reflected from the guide. A *circulator* or *directional coupler* directs this reflected power away from the magnetron or klystron, to avoid interfering with its operation.

So-called *dual-energy* or *multi-energy* linacs have the capability of producing x-ray beams of two or more energies. They incorporate accelerator waveguides of sufficient length to accelerate electrons to the energy required for the highest-energy photon beam desired, but must be able also to accelerate

electrons to lesser energies. This capability requires radiofrequency power-handling equipment of greater complexity, to ensure that the electron bunches remain focused and that the variation in energy of the electrons remains small. An *energy switch* employed by one manufacturer is shown in Figure 4-17. It provides control over the amount of radiofrequency power passing from the left-hand cavity into the remainder of the guide.

Vacuum pump

The accelerator guide of a linac requires a high vacuum (on the order of 10^{-8} mm Hg) to prevent power loss and electrical arcing caused by interactions of electrons with gas molecules. Although older models used mechanical fore-pumps and oil diffusion vacuum pumps, all newer models use *sputter-ion (Vac-Ion)* pumps to maintain good vacuum.

A sputter-ion pump typically consists of multiple cylindrical anodes positioned between two cathodes. The cathodes are sandwiched between the poles of a magnet. The cathodes are composed of a reactive sputtering material such as titanium. Electrons ejected spontaneously from the cathode are attracted toward the anode and assume a spiral path in the magnetic field. As a consequence, they oscillate between the cathodes and collide with gas molecules to produce considerable ionization. The resulting positive ions bombard the cathodes, causing ejection (*sputtering*) of neutral atoms of titanium, which are deposited chiefly on the anodes. By this mechanism, gas molecules are continuously removed from the electron accelerator section.

Bending magnet

Low-energy linacs require short accelerating structures that can be mounted directly in line with the path from the x-ray target to the patient. Higher-energy linacs require longer structures that are often mounted horizontally (or nearly so) within the linac gantry. A *bending magnet* is used to change the direction of the accelerated electron beam from horizontal to vertical. The angle of bend may be 90°, but many accelerators use a 270° *achromatic* magnet. As described below, a magnet with multiple 90° bends provides greater stability of the resulting photon beam.

The electrons accelerated in a linac do not all reach the bending magnet with exactly the same velocity. By equating the force on a particle in an electromagnetic field with the centripetal force, we can show that an electron in a magnetic field follows a curved path with a radius given:

$$r = \frac{mv}{qB}$$

Example 4-7

What is the radius of the path of a 10 MeV electron passing through a magnetic field of strength = 7000 Gauss (0.7 Tesla or 0.7 Weber/m²)?

$$r = \frac{mv}{qB}$$

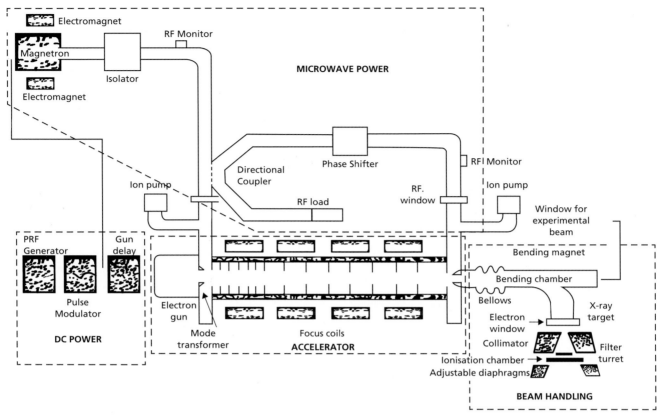

Figure 4-16 RF power-handling equipment for a linear accelerator.

where v is the velocity of the 10 MeV electron (99.88% of the speed of light) and m is the mass of the electron; m is related to m_0, the rest mass of the electron (9.11×10^{-31} kg) by:

$$m = \frac{m_0}{\sqrt{1 - \dfrac{v^2}{c^2}}}$$

Therefore, $m = 1.86 \times 10^{-29}$ kg. The intensity of the magnetic field $B = 0.7$ Weber/m^2 and the charge of an electron

$q = 1.6 \times 10^{-19}$ C. Therefore:

$$r = \frac{(1.86 \times 10^{-29} \text{ kg})(3 \times 10^8 \text{ m/s})}{(1.6 \times 10^{-19} \text{ C})(0.7 \text{ weber/m}^2)}$$

$$r = 0.05 \text{ m or 5 cm}$$

The Weber is a unit of magnetic flux and describes the integral of the magnetic field strength over a surface. Magnetic field

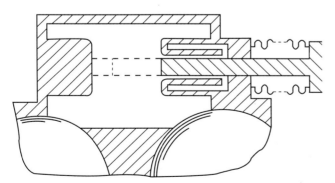

Figure 4-17 A noncontact-type microwave energy switch for a standing-wave accelerator guide.
Source: Karzmark et al. 1993.[23]

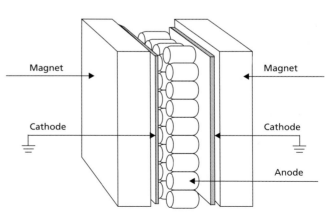

Figure 4-18 A representative sputter-ion pump.

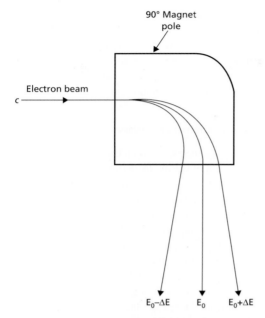

Figure 4-19 A simple 90° bending magnet, showing the paths of electrons of three energies.

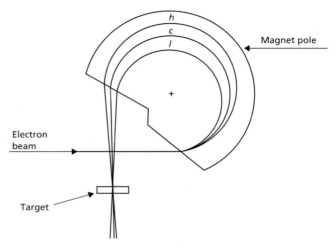

Figure 4-20 A modern 270° *achromatic* bending magnet, showing the paths of electrons of three energies.

strength is defined by the force exerted by the field on a charged particle:

$$F = qv \times B$$

B therefore is expressed in units of $\frac{\text{newton}}{\text{coulomb (m/s)}}$, which has been given the special name Weber/meter^2: 1 Weber/meter^2 = 1 Tesla = 10^4 Gauss. The Earth's magnetic field is about 0.000025–0.000065 Tesla or 0.25–0.65 Gauss.

For a chosen magnetic field strength, electrons with higher energy (higher values of mv) are bent through a larger radius than are lower-energy electrons. As shown in Figure 4-19 of a 90° bending magnet, lower-energy electrons strike the target at a different point than the higher-energy component of the beam. However, in a 270° achromatic bending magnet, as shown in Figure 4-20, the low-energy and high-energy components of the beam converge at a point called the *triple focus*. A target positioned at this point intercepts all electrons emerging from the bending magnet. Many bending magnets are equipped with an energy-defining slit consisting of barriers that intercept electrons whose energies vary from the desired energy by more than a selected amount.

The energy-defining slit of a modern linear accelerator consists of a mechanical barrier placed near the midpoint of the bending magnet. A window in the barrier allows electrons of the selected energy range (correct radius of bend) to pass through. Electrons outside the range are stopped. The choice of barrier material is important to minimize the production of x rays. Nevertheless, the bending magnet is a major source of leakage radiation. If an accelerator is not tuned properly, it can steer a large

fraction of the electron beam into the energy slits. The resulting leakage radiation may exceed regulatory limits.

X-ray target

When an x-ray beam is desired, a *target* of an appropriate material is moved into the path of the electrons. The material usually has a high atomic number (e.g., tungsten) in low-energy linacs, but may be of intermediate atomic number (e.g., copper) in high-energy units. In contrast to conventional x-ray tubes, an accelerator target is generally a *transmission* target, meaning that the generated x rays are transmitted through the target material to reach the patient. The thickness of the target is a compromise between one that ensures every electron interacts and one that absorbs the fewest x rays. The ideal thickness is related to the *radiation length*, the thickness in which $1/e$ of the electron beam is absorbed. Bremsstrahlung x rays leave the location of production at an angle relative to the direction of incident electrons. At low electron energies, the mean angle of emission (ϕ) is large. As the energy, E, of the incident electrons increases, ϕ decreases so that at megavoltage energies the x rays are emitted predominantly in the forward direction. Consequently, a reflection target of the type used in lower-energy x-ray tubes is not used in a linear accelerator. Instead, a thin transmission target is used.

Flattening filter and scattering foil

The x-ray beam from a linac is frequently strongly *forward peaked*. The mean scattering angle subtended by the beam is related to the electron energy by the *Rossi–Griesan equation*:

$$\langle\phi\rangle = \frac{15}{E_0} \sqrt{\frac{X}{X_0}}$$

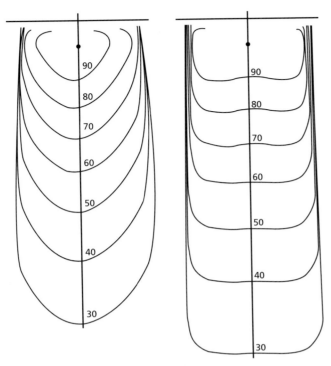

Figure 4-21 Isodose distributions for a 10 MV x-ray beam without (left) and with (right) the beam-flattening filter in place. Lateral horns of the distribution are apparent near the surface for the distribution obtained with the beam-flattening filter.

where ϕ is the mean scattering angle in steradians, E_0 is the energy in MeV of the incident electrons, X is the target thickness, and X_0 is the radiation length (a characteristic of a material, related to the energy loss of the electrons with the material). For example, a 15 MeV electron beam incident on a target whose thickness is equal to the radiation length generates a photon beam whose mean scattering angle is only 1 steradian.

A *flattening filter* is used to create a beam of sufficient area and uniformity for clinical use. The effect of a flattening filter on the *raw lobe* of a 10 MV beam is shown in Figure 4-21. Today's medical linac uses a flattening filter so that the x-ray beam reaching the patient is as uniform as possible. Treatment techniques recently introduced, such as intensity-modulated radiation therapy (IMRT), do not require a uniform beam and may allow the production of machines without flattening filters and the *flattening filter free* (FFF) mode is now used clinically. The raw lobe beams are starting to be used for very high output treatments, which is one of the main benefits of FFF mode. However, one should always use FFF beam in conjunction with CT-based treatment planning as the non-flat beams will produce significantly different dose distributions than conventional flat beams. A summary of the strengths and weaknesses of FFF beams is provided by Georg et al.[24]

The electron beam exiting from the accelerator waveguide or bending magnet is often no more than 1 or 2 mm in diameter.

When the electron beam is to be used for treatment, a *scattering foil* is employed to provide a uniform beam of dimensions suitable for treatment. Modern scattering foils are of complex design, to scatter the beam without generating an unacceptable quantity of Bremsstrahlung radiation or degrading the beam energy by too great an amount.

Monitor ionization chamber

In contrast to ^{60}Co units, in which the source decays predictably to furnish a beam of slowly decreasing intensity, the dose rate of an accelerator beam may vary unpredictably or by design. Consequently, it is not possible to rely on the elapsed time to control the dose delivered to a patient. Instead the radiation leaving the target or scattering foil passes through a *monitor ionization chamber* (Figure 4-22), where it produces an ionization current that is proportional to the beam intensity. The ionization current is conducted to the control panel, where it is converted to a digital display of *monitor units* (MUs). The dose delivered to the patient is controlled by programming the accelerator to deliver a prescribed number of MUs.

Collimator

The final control over the beam, before it is delivered to the patient, is exerted by the collimator. In contrast to ^{60}Co sources, which are often several centimeters in diameter, the source of x rays in a linac is only 1 or 2 mm in diameter. As a result, the collimator can be of simpler design because the geometric penumbra is smaller. For x-ray beams, the collimator consists of jaws made of a high atomic number material, such as lead or tungsten. In most cases, the jaws are adjusted under motor control to create rectangular beams of almost any size. Most modern accelerators can deliver beams of up to 40×40 cm^2. A modern linear accelerator is shown in Figure 4-23.

Because electrons can be scattered easily by the intervening air between the scattering foil and the patient, the final stage of collimation of an electron beam must be close to the skin surface. An *electron applicator* or *cone*, such as those shown in Figure 4-24, is used to shape electron beams. Although the cone is rectangular, a slot is often provided to place a shaped insert to customize the field shape to the patient's target volume.

Treatment couch

To support the patient during treatment, a treatment couch is provided as part of a linear accelerator. The couch is usually mounted so that it pivots about an axis that passes through the gantry isocenter. Sometimes an eccentric axis of rotation is provided to provide greater convenience for patients or to permit extended lateral movement of the couch. Typical weight limits for a treatment couch are about 400 lb but can be greater for new robotic-style couches. One should always confirm with the vendor before loading a couch with more than 300 lb.

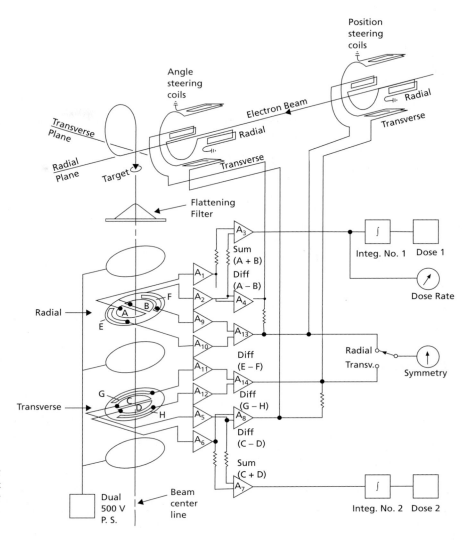

Figure 4-22 A modern multisegment monitor ion chamber showing the role of each segment in measuring the beam flatness and symmetry as well as the dose rate.
Source: Karzmark et al. 1993.[23]

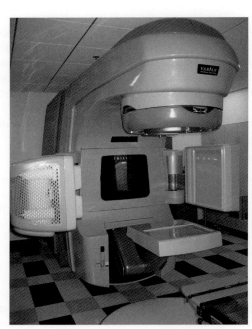

Figure 4-23 A modern dual-energy linear accelerator for radiation therapy.

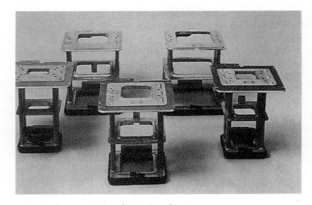

Figure 4-24 Representative electron applicators.
Source: Courtesy of Varian Associates, Inc.

Other medical accelerators

The first particle accelerator developed by Van de Graaff was described in 1931.[25] Van de Graaff generators used in research provide beams of positively charged particles with energies of 20 MeV and higher. In radiation therapy, Van de Graaff generators have been used to accelerate electrons to energies of up to 3 MeV but are no longer used.

Betatrons have largely been replaced in the clinic by linear accelerators, but for several decades after their introduction they enjoyed considerable popularity. However, presently, there are not any in clinical operation in the United States. The first betatron, constructed by Kerst in 1941, accelerated electrons to an energy of 2 MeV.[26] In later years, electrons and x rays with energies of up to 45 MeV were available from betatrons, but, primarily because of their relatively low dose rates, betatrons are no longer routinely used for patient treatments.

Cyclotrons

The first cyclotron, developed by Lawrence and Livingston in 1932, provided the background for modern orbital accelerators.[27] Electrons are not accelerated in cyclotrons, but, proton facilities almost exclusively use cyclotrons for accelerating protons. Cyclotrons are also used extensively to produce radioactive nuclides, including positron emitters that are useful in nuclear imaging and medical research.

The operation of a cyclotron is outlined in Figure 4-25. Two hollow, semicircular electrodes, or *dees*, are mounted between the poles of an electromagnet and separated from each other by a gap of 2–5 cm. The electromagnet is energized by direct current and furnishes a magnetic field of constant intensity across the dees. An alternating voltage applied to the dees oscillates with a frequency that is chosen with consideration for the intensity of the magnetic field and the type of particle being accelerated. For most cyclotrons available commercially, the frequency is between 10 and 40 MHz.

Positive ions (e.g., ^{1}H+, ^{2}H+, ^{3}He^2+, or ^{4}He^2+) are released by a cathode-arc source in the gap between the dees and are accelerated in bunches toward the negative dee. After the ions enter the dee, they are shielded from the electric field. The magnetic field forces the particles into a circular path, which the particles follow with constant speed. Just as the polarity reverses across the dees, the ions emerge from the first dee and accelerate across the gap toward the second dee. The ions follow a circular orbit in the second dee and emerge as the polarity reverses again. In this manner, the particles are accelerated each time they cross the dee aperture until they attain the desired energy.

The radius of the orbit followed by ions within a dee is described by:

$$r = \frac{mv}{Bq}$$

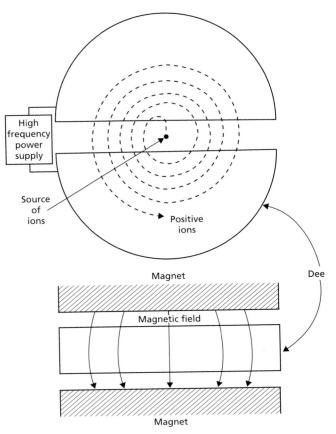

Figure 4-25 Conventional two-dee cyclotron. The path of positively charged particles is denoted by the *dashed curve*. The particles are accelerated each time they cross the gap between the dees.

where r is the radius, m is the mass of the accelerated particles, v is the velocity of the particles, B is the magnetic field intensity, and q is the charge of the particles. This equation is identical to the equation that describes the equilibrium orbit of electrons in a betatron and in a bending magnet. If the magnetic field intensity, B, and the mass, m, are constant, the radius of the orbit increases linearly with the velocity of the accelerated particles.

The time, T, for a half-revolution of the particles in a dee is:

$$T = \frac{\pi m}{Bq}$$

If the mass of the particles remains constant, the time for a half-revolution is also constant, and the emergence of the particles from the dees is synchronized easily with changes in the dee polarity. However, the relativistic mass, m, of a particle moving with velocity, v, is:

$$m = \frac{m_0}{\sqrt{1 - \frac{v^2}{c^2}}}$$

When the velocity of particles in a cyclotron reaches about $0.2c$, the increased mass of the particles disturbs the synchronization between the emergence of particles from the dees and the changing polarity across the dees. For example, deuterons may be accelerated in a cyclotron to a maximum energy of about 35 MeV. A deuteron is a combination of a proton and a neutron. Above 35 MeV, the relativistic increase in mass causes the deuterons to emerge from the dees out of phase with the changing polarity of the dees. Electrons reach the limiting velocity of $0.2c$ when their kinetic energy is only about 10 keV. Consequently, electrons are not accelerated in cyclotrons.

To maintain the synchronization between particle emergence from the dees and changing polarity of the dees, the frequency of the alternating voltage applied to the dees may be reduced as the particles gain energy. This approach is used in the synchrocyclotron, and deuterons have been accelerated to energies of up to 200 MeV in these machines.

For experimental studies, a beam of heavy particles may be extracted from a cyclotron. Additionally, radioactive nuclides may be produced in a cyclotron by directing accelerated particles onto a target. An increasing number of medical institutions are using a cyclotron to produce short-lived, positron-emitting radioactive nuclides (^{11}C, ^{13}N, ^{15}O, ^{18}F) useful in nuclear medicine. These nuclides are used in combination with *positron emission tomography* (PET).

Microtrons

With the availability of microwave accelerator cavities came the development of another device for accelerating electrons in circular or elliptical orbits. This device, called the *microtron*, combines the static magnetic field of the cyclotron with the accelerating cavity of the linear accelerator.[28] In contrast to the linear accelerator, electrons pass through the accelerating cavity multiple times, gaining energy each time. The path of the electron bunch is bent by the static magnetic field in a circular or racetrack shape, bringing the electrons back to the cavity.

As electrons reach velocities close to the speed of light, they can be considered to be traveling at constant velocity during the entire acceleration process. As their energy increases, however, their momentum increases proportionately, and their bending radius increases as well.

In a circular microtron, the electron's energy increases in equal increments, and therefore the circumference of the path increases by corresponding increments. Consequently, the electron bunch arrives at the accelerating cavity at the correct moment to be accelerated again.

The maximum energy of electrons in a microtron is essentially limited only by the dimensions and strength of the static magnetic field. In practice, microtrons can accelerate electrons to energies of up to 50 MeV.[28] Difficulties with the stability of operation have made microtrons unreliable in the clinic, and pursuit of their clinical application has been discontinued.

Summary

- An x-ray tube may be operated under either space-charge-limited or filament-emission-limited conditions.
- X-ray production efficiency may be increased by the use of rectification (self-, half-wave, full-wave) and special x-ray circuits (three-phase and high frequency).
- X-ray spectra are influenced by tube current, tube voltage, x-ray circuitry (three-phase, high frequency), and beam filtration.
- The line-focus principle is employed to reduce the size of the apparent focal spot.
- Radiation treatment unit design has evolved significantly since the first x-ray tubes became available in 1896.
- The use of x rays for radiation therapy began within months of their discovery.
- Low-energy x-ray units are in use in many clinics for the treatment of superficial disease.
- The introduction of the ^{60}Co teletherapy unit made "megavoltage" radiation therapy affordable and practical.
- The development of the side-coupled standing-wave electron linear accelerator allowed the construction of a 4 MV linac that is physically no larger than a ^{60}Co unit.
- Refinements have made dual-photon energy linacs practical and affordable for many radiation therapy departments.
- ^{60}Co units remain a practical and economic alternative in countries where accelerator service capabilities are limited.

Problems

4-1 How many electrons flow from the filament to the target each second in an x-ray tube with a tube current of 200 mA? If the tube voltage is a constant 100 kV, what is the power (energy/second) delivered to the target?

4-2 An apparent focal spot of 1 mm is projected from an x-ray target with a "true" focal spot of 5 mm (see diagram below). What is the target angle?

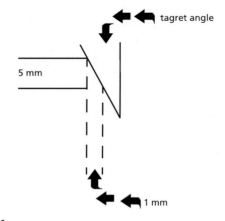

tagret angle

5 mm

1 mm

Figure 4-26

4-3 What is the kinetic energy of electrons accelerated through a potential difference of 250 kV? What fraction of the energy is expended as radiation energy loss as the electrons interact in a tungsten target? What is the λ_{min} of the x rays?

4-4 The source-to-collimator distance is 62 cm for a particular ^{60}Co unit. The ^{60}Co source has a diameter of 2 cm. What are the widths of the geometric penumbra at the skin and at 15 cm below the skin when the source-skin distance is 80 cm?

4-5 (A) The beam penumbra of a linac is measured at the surface of a phantom at 100 cm source-to-surface and found to be 8 mm. The source-to-collimator distance is 55 cm. If the measured penumbra equals the geometric penumbra, what must the effective source diameter be? (B) How much smaller would the penumbra be if tapered blocks were positioned in the beam at 65 cm from the source?

4-6 What is the maximum specific activity for ^{60}Co?

4-7 What is the wavelength for a 6 MV linear accelerator photon beam?

4-8 What is the fractional increase in mass of a particle moving with a velocity of 0.1c? 0.5c? 0.99c?

4-9 Electrons of 15 MeV enter a bending magnet with a magnetic field strength of 0.7 Tesla. What is the radius of the path of the electrons? What range of energies could electrons have and still be confined to orbits with radii within 5% of the 15 MeV electrons?

4-10 Distinguish between the operation of magnetron and klystron microwave tubes.

4-11 Distinguish between a standing wave and a traveling wave linear accelerator.

References

1 Röntgen, W. C. Über eine Art von Strahlen (vorläufige Mitteilung), *Sitzungs- Berichte der Physikalisch-medicinischen Gesellschaft zu Wurzurg*, 1895; **9**:132.

2 Donizetti, P. *Shadow and Substance: The Story of Medical Radiography*. Oxford, Pergamon Press, 1967.

3 Glasser, O. *Dr. W. C. Roentgen*, 2nd edition. Springfield, IL, Charles C. Thomas, 1958.

4 Coolidge, W. A powerful roentgen ray tube with a pure electron discharge. *Phys. Rev.* 1913; **2**:409.

5 Bloom, W., Hollenbach, J., and Morgan, J. (eds.) *Medical Radiographic Technic*, 3rd edition. Springfield, IL, Charles C. Thomas, 1965.

6 Chaney, E., and Hendee, W. Effects of x-ray tube current and voltage on effective focal-spot size. *Med. Phys.* 1974; **1**:141.

7 Dance, D. R. Diagnostic radiology with x rays. In *The Physics of Medical Imaging*, S. Webb (ed.). Philadelphia, Institute of Physics, 1988, pp. 20–73.

8 Hendee, W., and Chaney, E. X-ray focal spots: Practical considerations. *Appl. Radiol.* 1974; **3**:25.

9 Curry, T. S., Dowdey, J. E., and Murray, R. C. *Christensen's Physics of Diagnostic Radiology*, 4th edition. Malvern, PA, Lea & Febiger, 1990.

10 Park, C. C., Yom, S. S., Podgorsak, M. B., Harris, E., Price, R. A. Jr, et al. Electronic Brachytherapy Working Group. American Society for Therapeutic Radiology and Oncology (ASTRO) Emerging Technology Committee report on electronic brachytherapy. *Int. J. Radiat. Oncol. Biol. Phys.* 2010; **76**(4):963–972.

11 Johns, H., Bates, L., and Watson, T. 1000 curie cobalt units for radiation therapy: I. The Saskatchewan cobalt-60 unit. *Br. J. Radiol.* 1952; **25**:296–302.

12 Johns, H. E., Epp, E. R., Cormack, D. V., and Fedoruk, S. O. Depth dose data and diaphragm design for the Saskatchewan 1000 curie cobalt unit. *Br. J. Radiol.* 1952; **25**:302–308.

13 Johns, H., et al. Physical characteristics of the radiation in cobalt-60 beam therapy. *J. Can. Assoc. Radiol.* 1952; **3**:2.

14 Hendee, W. R. *Medical Radiation Physics*, 1st edition, Chicago, Mosby–Year, 1970.

15 Ibbott, G., and Hendee, W. Beam-shaping platforms and the skin-sparing advantage of ^{60}Co radiation. *AJR* 1970; **108**:193–196.

16 Debois, J. The determination of the penumbra at different depths. *J. Belg. Radiol.* 1966; **49**:200–205.

17 Brucer, M. An automatic controlled pattern cesium-137 teletherapy machine. *AJR* 1956; **75**:49–55.

18 Wideröe, R. Uber ein neues prinzip zur Herstellung hohen Spannungen, *Arch. Elektrotech.* 1928; **21**:387.

19 Fry, D. W., Harvie, S.-R., Mullet, L. B., and Walkinshaw, W. Traveling-wave linear accelerator for electrons. *Nature* 1947; **160**:351–352.

20 Ginzton, E. L., Hansen, W. W., and Kennedy, W. R. A linear electron accelerator. *Rev. Sci. Instr.* 1948; **19**:89–108.

21 Chodorow, M., Ginzton, E. L., and Hansen, W. W. Design and performance of a high-power pulsed klystron. *Proc. IRE*, 1953; **41**:1584.

22 Knapp, E. A., Knapp, B. C., and Potter, I. M. Standing wave high energy linear accelerator structures. *Rev. Sci. Instr.* 1968; **39**:979–991.

23 Karzmark, C. J., Nunan, C. S., and Tanabe, E. *Medical Electron Accelerators*. New York, McGraw-Hill, 1993.

24 Georg, D., Knöös, T., and McClean, B. Current status and future perspective of flattening filter free photon beams. *Med. Phys.* 2011; **38**:1280.

25 Van de Graaff, R. A 1,500,000 volt electrostatic generator. *Phys. Rev.* 1931; **348**:1919–1920.

26 Kerst, D. Acceleration of electrons by magnetic induction. *Phys. Rev.* 1941; **60**:47–53.

27 Lawrence, E., and Livingston, M. The production of high speed light ions without the use of high voltages. *Phys. Rev.* 1932; **40**:19–35.

28 Brahme, A., and Svensson, H. Radiation beam characteristics of a 22 MeV microtron. *Acta Radiol. Oncol.* 1979; **18**:244–272.

CHAPTER

5

MEASUREMENT OF IONIZING RADIATION

Objectives

After studying this chapter, the reader should be able to:
- Define the following concepts used to describe radiation quantity: photon fluence, photon fluence rate, energy fluence, energy fluence rate, exposure, kerma, dose, and dose equivalent.
- Describe the purpose and operation of the free-air ionization chamber.
- Explain the concepts of electron equilibrium, effective atomic number, mass stopping power, and the Bragg–Gray principle.
- Identify the correction factors necessary for measurements of exposure and dose with an ionization chamber.
- Delineate the principles of radiation dose measurements by calorimetry, photographic film, chemical dosimetry, scintillation dosimetry, and thermoluminescent dosimetry.
- Describe radiation quality and factors that influence it.

Introduction

The term *radiation* refers to energy that can be transferred in space from one location to another. The term *ionizing radiation* refers to radiation with sufficient energy to remove electrons from atoms. Ionizing radiation encompasses directly ionizing charged particles, indirectly ionizing uncharged particles (e.g., neutrons), and electromagnetic energy (x- and γ-ray photons). A *radiation quantity* describes an amount of energy measured in some fashion at a specific position in space over a prescribed period of time. The method of measurement defines the unit employed to describe radiation quantity. Common units of radiation quantity are described in this chapter. The term *radiation intensity* is used generically in the literature to describe

Hendee's Radiation Therapy Physics, Fourth Edition. Todd Pawlicki, Daniel J. Scanderbeg and George Starkschall.
© 2016 John Wiley & Sons, Inc. Published 2016 by John Wiley & Sons, Inc.

radiation quantity. In this text, radiation intensity is given a specific definition.

Radiation intensity

The number, N, of x or γ rays (electromagnetic photons, hereafter referred to simply as *photons*), crossing a unit area, A, at a location in a beam of radiation is known as the *photon fluence* Φ ($\Phi = N/A$) at the specific location. The rate at which the photons cross the area is termed the *photon fluence rate*, $\dot{\Phi}$, ($\dot{\Phi} = \Phi/t = N/At$, where t represents time). If the fluence varies with time, the fluence rate must be specified at a particular moment or expressed as an average over time.

If all the photons in a beam of radiation possess the same energy, the *energy fluence*, Ψ, is simply the product of the photon fluence and the energy per photon ($\Psi = \Phi E = NE/A$). The *energy fluence rate*, $\dot{\Psi}$, (often termed the *radiation intensity*) is the photon fluence rate multiplied by the energy per photon ($\dot{\Psi} = \dot{\Phi}E = NE/At$). If the radiation beam contains photons of different energies ($E_1, E_2, \ldots, E_m$), the intensity or energy fluence rate is expressed as:

$$\Psi = \sum_{i-1}^{m} f_i \dot{\Phi}_i E_i$$

where f_i represents the fraction of photons with energy E_i and the symbol $\sum_{i=1}^{m}$ indicates that the intensity is determined by summing the components of the beam at each of the m energies.

Example 5-1

A 6 MV x-ray portal image requires 10^{16} x rays over an exposure time of 2 seconds with an area of 1500 cm^2. With the assumption that the average photon energy is 2 MeV, determine the photon fluence rate, photon fluence, energy fluence rate, and energy fluence.

Photon fluence $\Phi = \dfrac{N}{A} = \dfrac{10^{16} \text{ photons}}{1.5 \times 10^{-1} \text{ m}^2}$
$$= 6.7 \times 10^{16} \text{ photons/m}^2$$

Photon fluence rate $\dot{\Phi} = \dfrac{N}{At} = \dfrac{\Phi}{t} = \dfrac{6.7 \times 10^{16} \text{ photons/m}^2}{2 \text{ sec}}$
$$= 3.4 \times 10^{16} \text{ photons/m}^2\text{-sec}$$

Energy fluence $\psi = \dfrac{NE}{A} = \Phi E$
$$= (6.7 \times 10^{16} \text{ photons/m}^2)(2 \text{ MeV/photon})$$
$$= 1.3 \times 10^{17} \text{ MeV/m}^2$$

Energy fluence rate $\dot{\psi} = \dfrac{NE}{At} = \dfrac{\psi}{t} = \dfrac{1.3 \times 10^{17} \text{ MeV/m}^2}{2 \text{ sec}}$
$$= 6.7 \times 10^{16} \text{ MeV/m}^2\text{-sec}$$

An x-ray beam actually contains a spectrum of energies. A more exact computation of energy fluence and energy fluence rate would involve a weighted sum of the contributions of the various photon energies. This procedure is illustrated in Example 5-2.

Example 5-2

Gamma rays of 1.17 and 1.33 MeV are released each time a ^{60}Co atom decays. What are the photon fluence and energy fluence at 1 m from a ^{60}Co source in which 10^6 atoms decay?

The surface area of a sphere of radius r is $4\pi r^2$. The surface area of a sphere of 1 m radius is $4\pi(1 \text{ m})^2$. Because γ rays are emitted isotropically (equal numbers in all directions) from a radioactive source, the photon fluence is equal at all locations on the sphere surface if the source is positioned at the center of the sphere. The fraction of the photons intercepted by a 1 m^2 area on the sphere surface is:

$$\text{Fraction of total emissions} = \frac{1 \text{ m}^2}{4\pi(1 \text{ m})^2} = 7.96 \times 10^{-2}$$

Because 2 photons are released per decay, 2×10^6 photons are released during 10^6 decays:

Photon fluence $= \Phi = (2 \times 10^6 \text{ photons})(7.96 \times 10^{-2})$
$$\cong 16 \times 10^4 \text{ photons/m}^2$$

The energy fluence is:

$$\psi = \sum_{i=1}^{2} f_i \Phi E_i = (0.5)(16 \times 10^4)(1.17 \text{ MeV})$$
$$+ (0.5)(16 \times 10^4)(1.33 \text{ MeV})$$

where the photon fluence of 16×10^4 photons/m^2 is composed of equal numbers of photons (8×10^4 photons/m^2) of 1.17 and 1.33 MeV:

$$\Psi = (9.36 \text{ MeV/m}^2 + 10.64 \text{ MeV/m}^2) \times 10^4 = 20 \times 10^4 \text{ MeV/m}^2$$

Although photon and energy fluences and fluence rates are important in many computations, these quantities are not easily measured. Usually, radiation quantity is expressed in units that are related directly to common methods of radiation measurement. Several units of radiation quantity have been used over the years including the Röntgen (R), the radiation absorbed dose (rad), and the Röntgen equivalent man (rem). Today the preferred units of radiation are part of the Système International definition of units (SI units) and are the Gray (Gy), replacing the rad, and the Sievert (Sv), replacing the rem. Conversions from traditional to SI units are shown in Table 5-1.

Radiation exposure

Primary ion pairs (electrons and positive ions) are produced as ionizing radiation interacts in a medium. These ion pairs (IP) produce additional ionizations (secondary IP) as they dissipate

Table 5-1 Traditional (T) and Système International (SI) units.

Unit Quantity	To Convert from T to SI		
	T	SI	Multiply by
Exposure	Röntgen (R)	Coulombs/kg	2.58×10^{-4}
Absorbed dose (kerma)	Rad	Gray (Gy)	0.01
Dose equivalent	Rem	Sievert (Sv)	0.01

Table 5-2 Mass energy-absorption coefficient $(\mu_{en})_m$, m_2/kg $\times 10^3$.

Photon Energy (MeV)	Water	Air	Compact Bone	Muscle
0.010	489	466	1900	496
0.020	52.3	51.6	251	54.4
0.040	6.47	6.40	30.5	6.77
0.060	3.04	2.92	9.79	3.12
0.080	2.53	2.36	5.20	2.55
0.10	2.52	2.31	3.86	2.52
0.20	3.00	2.68	3.02	2.97
0.40	3.29	2.96	3.16	3.25
0.60	3.29	2.96	3.15	3.26
0.80	3.21	2.89	3.06	3.18
1.0	3.11	2.80	2.97	3.08
2.0	2.60	2.34	2.48	2.57
4.0	2.05	1.86	1.99	2.03
6.0	1.80	1.63	1.78	1.78
8.0	1.65	1.50	1.65	1.63
10.0	1.55	1.44	1.59	1.54

Source: International Commission on Radiation Units and Measurements: Physical Aspects of Irradiation, *National Bureau of Standards Handbook*.

their energy by interacting with nearby atoms. The total number of IP produced is proportional to the energy absorbed as the radiation interacts in the medium. If the medium is air, the total charge Q (negative or positive) of the ionization produced as the radiation interacts with a unit mass, m, of air is known as the *radiation exposure X* ($X = Q/m$). The charge, Q, includes both primary and secondary IP, with the secondary IP produced both inside and outside of the volume of air of mass m. The SI unit of radiation exposure is Coulombs/kg. The earlier unit of exposure is the Röntgen (R), defined as 1 R = 2.58×10^{-4} Coulombs/kg of air. This definition is numerically equivalent to an older description of the Röntgen that states that 1 R equals 1 electrostatic unit of charge (esu) released per cubic centimeter (cm^3) of air at standard temperature and pressure (STP), where STP = 0 °C temperature and 1 atmosphere (760 mm Hg) pressure. Under these conditions, 1 m^3 of air has a mass of 1.293 kg. The unit Röntgen has virtually disappeared from use as the SI unit of Coulombs/kg has become accepted.

Measurement of radiation exposure is applicable only to x and γ radiation. The concept of exposure cannot be used for beams of particles or high-energy photons. For reasons that will become clear in the section "Free air ionization chamber", the measurement of exposure is limited to x- or γ-ray energies below about 3 MeV.

Energy and photon fluence per unit exposure

The energy, E_a, absorbed per unit mass of air during an exposure of X Coulombs/kg is:

$$E_a = \frac{(X \text{ Coulombs/kg})(33.97 \text{ eV/IP})(1.6 \times 10^{-19} \text{ J/eV})}{(1.6 \times 10^{-19} \text{ Coulombs/IP})}$$
$$= 33.97 \cdot X [(J/kg)]$$

where 33.97 eV/IP is known as the *work function* and is defined as the average energy expended per IP produced by ionizing radiation in air. The absorbed energy, E_a, is also the product of the energy fluence and the total mass energy absorption coefficient $(\mu_{en})_m$ for the x or γ rays that contribute to the energy fluence.

$$E_a = \psi (J/m^2) \cdot (\mu_{en})_m [(m^2/kg)]$$
$$= \psi (\mu_{en})_m [(J/kg)]$$

The coefficient $(\mu_{en})_m$ is $\mu_m (E_a/h\nu)$, where μ_m is the total mass attenuation coefficient of air for photons of energy, $h\nu$, and E_a represents the average energy transformed into kinetic energy

of electrons and positive ions per photon absorbed or scattered from the x- or γ-ray beam, corrected for energy released as characteristic radiation and Bremsstrahlung as electrons interact with electrons and nuclei in the medium. Mass energy absorption coefficients for a few selected media, including air, are listed in Table 5-2.

By combining the equations for $E_a = (\mu_{en})_m \psi = 33.97 (X)$, the energy fluence per unit exposure (ψ/X) is:

$$\psi/X = 33.97/(\mu_{en})_m$$

where $(\mu_{en})_m$ is expressed in units of m^2 per kg, ψ in J/m^2, and X in Coulombs/kg. For monoenergetic photons, the photon fluence per unit exposure Φ/X is the quotient of the energy fluence per unit exposure divided by the energy per photon:

$$\Phi/X = \psi X[1/(h\nu \cdot 1.6 \times 10^{-13} \text{ J/MeV})]$$

with $h\nu$ expressed in MeV and in Φ units of photons per m^2.

The photon fluence and energy fluence per unit exposure are plotted in Figure 5-1 as a function of photon energy. At lower energies, the large influence of photon energy on the energy absorption coefficient of air is reflected in the rapid change in the energy and photon fluence per unit exposure. Above 100 keV, the energy absorption coefficient is relatively constant, and the energy fluence per unit exposure does not vary greatly. However, the photon fluence per unit exposure decreases steadily as the energy per photon increases.

Example 5-3

Determine the energy and photon fluence per unit exposure in C/kg for ^{60}Co γ rays. The average energy of the γ rays is 1.25 MeV, and the total energy absorption coefficient is

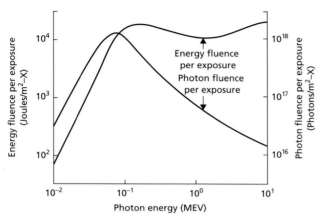

Figure 5-1 Photon and energy fluence per unit exposure, plotted as a function of the photon energy in MeV. To convert the vertical axis to exposure in Röntgens, multiply the vertical scale by 2.58×10^{-4}.

2.67×10^{-3} m²/kg (Table 5-2).

$$\psi/X = 33.97/(\mu_{en})_m = 33.97/2.67 \times 10^{-3} \text{ m}^2/\text{kg}$$
$$\cong 12,600 \text{ J/m}^2$$

$$\Phi/X = 12,600 \frac{\text{J}}{\text{m}^2}[1/(1.6 \times 10^{-13} \text{ J/MeV})(1.25 \text{ MeV})]$$
$$= 6.4 \times 10^{16} \text{ photons/m}^2$$

Measurement of radiation exposure

By rearranging one of the previous equations, the energy fluence can be expressed as $\psi = E_a/(\mu_{en})_m$. However, $E_a = E/\rho$, where E is the energy absorbed per unit volume and ρ is the density of air (1.29 kg/m³ at STP). If J_g is the number of primary and secondary IP produced by this energy deposition, then $E = J_g \overline{W}/e$, where $\overline{W}/e = 33.97$ eV/IP. The energy fluence is:

$$\psi = J_e \frac{W/e}{\rho}\bigg/(\mu_{en})_m$$

Example 5-4

A 1 cm³ volume of air is exposed to a photon fluence of 10^{15} photons/m². Each photon has energy of 1 MeV, and the total mass energy absorption coefficient of air is 2.80×10^{-3} m²/kg for photons of this energy. How many IP are produced inside the 1 cm³ volume? How much charge of either sign is measured if all of the IP are collected?

$$\Psi = \Phi h\nu$$
$$= (10^{15} \text{ photons/m}^2)(1 \text{ MeV/photon})(1.6 \times 10^{-13} \text{ J/MeV})$$
$$= 1.6 \times 10^2 \text{ J/m}^2$$

But:

$$\psi = J_g \frac{\overline{W}/e}{\rho}\bigg/(\mu_{en})_m \quad \text{and} \quad J_g = \frac{\psi\rho(\mu_{en})_m}{\overline{W}/e}$$

$$J_g = \frac{\begin{array}{c}(1.6 \times 10^2 \text{ J/m}^2)(1.29 \text{ kg/m}^3)(2.8 \times 10^{-3} \text{ m}^2/\text{kg}) \\ \times (10^{-6} \text{ m}^3/\text{cm}^3)(1 \text{ cm}^3)\end{array}}{(33.97 \text{ eV/IP})(1.6 \times 10^{-19} \text{ J/eV})}$$
$$= 10.7 \times 10^{10} \text{ IP}$$

The charge, Q, collected is:

$$Q = (10.7 \times 10^{10} \text{ IP})(1.6 \times 10^{-19} \text{ Coulombs/IP})$$
$$\cong 17 \times 10^{-9} \text{ Coulombs}$$

When energy is deposited in a small collecting volume of air, some secondary electrons are produced outside the collecting volume by primary IPs (particularly electrons) that escape the collecting volume. It is not possible to collect and measure all of these secondary electrons. However, the collecting volume may be chosen so that ionization created outside the volume by IP originating inside the volume is balanced by ionization created inside the volume by IP originating outside the volume. This condition, known as *electron equilibrium*, results in the collection of a number of IP inside the volume equal to the total ionization J_g. The principle of electron equilibrium is fundamental to the measurements of radiation exposure and is employed in the free-air ionization chamber.

Free-air ionization chamber

Fundamental measurements of radiation exposure can be achieved in standards laboratories with an instrument known as the *free-air ionization chamber*. These measurements can be used to form the standard against which measurements obtained with more clinically useful instruments are compared to yield calibration factors for the simpler instruments. The clinical instruments can then be used in the clinical setting to measure radiation exposures from sources of x and γ rays employed clinically.

X or γ rays incident on a free-air chamber are collimated into a beam with a cross-sectional area, A, at the center of the chamber (Figure 5-2). Inside the chamber, the beam traverses an electrical field between parallel electrodes A and B, with electrode A at ground potential and the potential of electrode B highly negative. The collecting volume of air inside the chamber has an area A and a length L. The charge Q (positive or negative) collected by the chamber is $Q = N$ (1.6 × 10⁻¹⁹ Coulombs/IP), where N is the total number of IPs collected. For an accurate measurement of N, the range of electrons liberated by the incident radiation must be less than the distance between each electrode and the collecting volume. Also the photon fluence rate must remain constant across the chamber, and the distance from the collimator to the border of the collecting volume must exceed

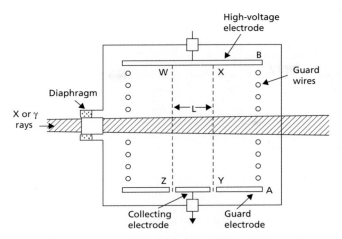

Figure 5-2 A free-air ionization chamber. The collecting volume of length *L* is enclosed within the region WXYZ. The air volume exposed directly to the x-ray and γ-ray beam is depicted by the hatched area.

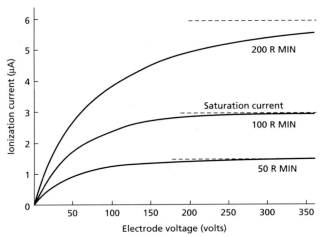

Figure 5-3 Current in a free-air ionization chamber as a function of the potential difference across the electrodes of the chamber. Saturation currents are shown for different exposure rates. Data were obtained from a chamber with electrodes 1 cm apart.
Source: Johns and Cunningham 1969.[1]

the electron range. If these requirements are satisfied, electronic equilibrium is achieved in the collecting volume, and the number of ion pairs liberated by the incident photons per unit volume of air is N/AL.

Electronic equilibrium exists in a volume when the energy deposited outside the volume by ionization created within equals the energy deposited in the volume by ionization created outside. In the free-air chamber, the voltage between electrodes A and B must be large enough to collect all of the ionization without significant recombination, yet not so large that the ions are accelerated to an energy where they create additional ionization on their way to the electrodes. The length *L* of the collecting volume is defined by guard electrodes positioned adjacent to the collecting electrodes.

Because 1 R = 2.58×10^{-4} Coulombs/kg, the number of Röntgens, *X*, corresponding to a charge *Q* in Coulombs collected in a free-air ionization chamber is:

$$X = Q/[AL\rho(2.58 \times 10^{-4} \text{ Coulombs/kg-R})]$$

where ρ is the density of air in kg/m³ and *AL* is expressed in m³. As mentioned earlier, the preferred unit of radiation exposure is Coulombs/kg rather than Röntgen, so the conversion factor of 2.58×10^{-4} Coulombs/(kg-R) is no longer needed in exposure measurements with a free-air chamber.

To prevent IP from recombining before expending all their energy by producing secondary ionization, the potential difference between the electrodes in a free-air chamber must be sufficient to attract all ion pairs to the electrodes. This potential difference is referred to as a *saturation voltage*. As shown in Figure 5-3, the saturation voltage increases with exposure rate. A potential difference between the electrodes below the saturation voltage permits IP to recombine before they are collected. Measurements obtained at a potential difference below the saturation voltage underestimate the true exposure. Errors caused

by IP recombination can be especially severe during measurements of x-ray beams in which the x rays are furnished in short pulses of high intensity. Such beams are commonly furnished by linear accelerators employed in radiation therapy. Recombination errors must be guarded against when measurements are obtained with conventional ionization chambers used in the clinical setting. When recombination cannot be prevented in a pulsed x-ray beam, a correction factor must be applied to correct the chamber response for a decrease in collection efficiency caused by IP recombination.

The range of released electrons in air increases rapidly with the energy of incident x or γ rays (Table 5-3). Electrodes in a free-air chamber used to measure 1 MV x rays would have to be separated by about 4 m. A chamber this large is impractical, particularly since a uniform electrical field would be difficult to maintain over such a distance. Other problems, such as reduced efficiency of IP collection, would also be encountered. In general, it is difficult to determine how many secondary IP are produced outside the measurement volume by ionization originating inside the volume (and vice versa). This problem restricts the exposure measurements to x- and γ-ray beams of relatively low energy. However, free-air chambers operated at elevated air pressures permit extension of their use to photon energies as high as 3 MeV. This energy is an upper limit to the use of free-air chambers as well as to the definition of the Röntgen. At lower energies, free-air ionization chambers can achieve accuracies to within ± 0.5% for measurements of x- and γ-ray beams under carefully controlled conditions. Free-air chambers are too fragile and bulky to be used routinely in the clinical setting. Hence, their application is limited to use as a standard against which the response of more rugged and useful chambers can be compared.

Table 5-3 Range and percent of total ionization produced by photoelectrons and Compton electrons for x rays generated at 100, 200, and 1000 kVp.

X-ray Tube Voltage (kVp)	Photoelectrons Range in Air (cm)	Photoelectrons % of Total Ionization	Compton Electrons Range in Air (cm)	Compton Electrons % of Total Ionization	Electrode Separation in Free-Air Ionization Chamber at STP[a]
100	12	10	0.5	90	12 cm
200	37	0.4	4.6	99.6	
1000	290	0	220	100	4 m

[a]STP, standard temperature and pressure; defined as 273°K (0°C) and 760 mm Hg.
Source: W. Meredith and J. Massey.[2]

All ionization chambers, including free-air chambers, operate at or near the saturation voltage. Factors applied to free-air ionization measurements usually include corrections for air attenuation, ion pair recombination, temperature, pressure, humidity, and ionization produced by scattered photons.

Thimble chambers

The amount of ionization collected in a small volume of air is not influenced by the physical density of the medium surrounding the collecting volume of air, provided that the medium has an atomic number equal to the effective atomic number of air. Consequently, the large volume of air surrounding the collecting volume in a free-air chamber may be replaced by a lesser thickness of a more dense material with an effective atomic number equal to that of air. That is, the large distances in air required for electron equilibrium in a free-air chamber may be replaced by smaller thicknesses of a denser *air-equivalent* material with an effective atomic number close to 7.64, the effective atomic number of air.

The *effective atomic number*, $\overline{Z}$, of a material is the atomic number of a hypothetical single element that attenuates photons at the same rate as the material. When photoelectric and Compton interactions are the dominant processes of photon attenuation, the $\overline{Z}$ of a mixture of element is:

$$\overline{Z} = (a_1 Z_1^{2.94} + a_2 Z_2^{2.94} + \cdots + a_n Z_n^{2.94})^{1/2.94}$$

where $Z_1, Z_2, \ldots, Z_n$ are the atomic numbers of elements in the mixture and $a_1, a_2, \ldots, a_n$ are the fractional contributions of each element to the total number of electrons in the mixture. A reasonable approximation for $\overline{Z}$ may be obtained by rounding 2.94 to 3. The $\overline{Z}$ of air is 7.64, as computed in Example 5-5. Chambers with air-equivalent walls are known as *thimble chambers* because they resemble a sewing thimble.

Example 5-5

Calculate $\overline{Z}$ for air. Air contains 75.5% nitrogen, 23.2% oxygen, and 1.3% argon. Gram-atomic masses are nitrogen, 14.007; oxygen, 15.999; and argon, 39.948.

The number of electrons contributed to 1 g of air is as follows:

For nitrogen:
$$\frac{(1\text{ g})(0.755)(6.02 \times 10^{23}\text{ atoms/g-atomic mass}) \times (7\text{ electrons/atom})}{(14.007\text{ g/g-atomic mass})}$$
$$= 2.27 \times 10^{23}\text{ electrons}$$

For oxygen:
$$\frac{(1\text{ g})(0.232)(6.02 \times 10^{23}\text{ atoms/g-atomic mass}) \times (8\text{ electrons/atom})}{(15.999\text{ g/g-atomic mass})}$$
$$= 0.70 \times 10^{23}\text{ electrons}$$

For argon:
$$\frac{(1\text{ g})(0.013)(6.02 \times 10^{23}\text{ atoms/g-atomic mass}) \times (18\text{ electrons/atom})}{(39.948\text{ g/g-atomic mass})}$$
$$= 0.04 \times 10^{23}\text{ electrons}$$

Total electrons = $(2.27 + 0.70 + 0.04) \times 10^{23} = 3.01 \times 10^{23}$ electrons.

The fractional contributions of electrons are:

$$\alpha_N = \frac{2.27 \times 10^{23}}{3.01 \times 10^{23}} = 0.753$$

$$\alpha_O = \frac{0.70 \times 10^{23}}{3.01 \times 10^{23}} = 0.233$$

$$\alpha_A = \frac{0.04 \times 10^{23}}{3.01 \times 10^{23}} = 0.013$$

$$\overline{Z}_{air} = \left[\alpha_N Z_N^{2.04} + \alpha_O Z_O^{2.94} + \alpha_A Z_A^{2.94} \right]^{1/2.94}$$
$$= [(0.753)(7)^{2.94} + (0.233)(8)^{2.94} + (0.013)(18)^{2.94}]^{1/2.94}$$
$$= 7.64$$

In a thimble chamber, most of the ionization collected in the air volume originates during interactions of photons in the air-equivalent wall of the chamber. The ionization in an air-filled cavity is shown in Figure 5-4 as a function of the thickness of the wall surrounding the cavity. The ionization increases with wall thickness until the thickness equals the range of electrons liberated by the incident photons. At this thickness, electrons from

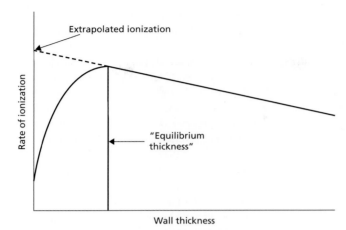

Figure 5-4 Ionization in an air-filled cavity exposed to x or γ radiation is expressed as a function of the thickness of the air-equivalent wall surrounding the cavity.

the outer portion of the wall just reach the cavity, and the ionization inside the cavity is at a maximum. A thinner wall would not provide electron equilibrium, and a thicker wall would attenuate the photons unnecessarily, as reflected in the slow decline in ionization beyond the equilibrium thickness. The wall thickness required for electron equilibrium increases with photon energy. Extrapolation of the curve in Figure 5-4 to zero wall thickness denotes the ionization that would occur in the cavity if photons were not attenuated at all in the surrounding wall.

A thimble chamber is diagrammed in Figure 5-5. The inside of the chamber is coated with a conducting material (e.g., carbon), and the central positive electrode is a conductor such as aluminum. The chamber response may be varied by changing the size of the collecting volume of air, the thickness of the chamber coating, or the length of the central electrode. The response of the chamber can be calibrated at several photon energies to provide accurate measurements of radiation exposure over a range of photon energies.

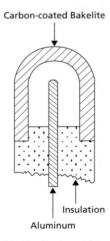

Carbon-coated Bakelite

Insulation

Aluminum

Figure 5-5 Diagram of a thimble chamber with an air-equivalent wall.

Condenser ("ionization") chambers

The ratio of the charge, Q, collected by an ionization chamber to the voltage reduction, ΔV, across the chamber caused by the collected charge is known as the *chamber capacitance C*, typically expressed in units of Farads. That is, $C = Q/\Delta V$. If a chamber of volume, v, is exposed to X Coulombs/kg, the charge, Q, collected is $Q = X(C/kg) \cdot \rho(kg/m^3) \cdot v(m^3) = X\rho v$. For an air density of 1.29 kg/m^3 at STP, $Q = 1.29\ Xv$. The reduction in voltage ΔV is $Q/C = (1.29\ Xv)/C$, and the voltage reduction per unit exposure $\Delta V/X = 1.29\ v/C$, where v is the volume of the chamber in m^3 and C is the capacitance of the chamber in Farads. The voltage reduction per unit exposure, termed the *sensitivity* of the chamber, can be decreased by reducing the volume or increasing the capacitance of the chamber.

Most ionization chambers used for radiation measurements consist of a thimble chamber connected to a capacitor (sometimes called a *condenser*) to reduce the sensitivity to a value appropriate for routine clinical use. The total capacitance, C, of the resulting *condenser chamber* is $C = C_t + C_s$, where C_t and C_s are the capacitance of the thimble and condenser stem and cable. Usually, $C_s \gg C_t$. The sensitivity $\Delta V/X$ of a condenser chamber is $\Delta V/X = 1.29\ V/(C_t + C_s)$.

Various instruments are available commercially for measuring radiation exposure with a condenser chamber. In most of these devices, the chamber is connected during exposure to an electrometer used to measure the small electrical charge or current generated during the exposure. While in the x- or γ-ray beam, the chamber is made sensitive to radiation for a selected interval of time, and the exposure rate or cumulative exposure is determined. A typical exposure-measuring device is shown in Figure 5-6. If the electrometer has a capacitance of C_e, the sensitivity $\Delta V/X$ of the entire device is $\Delta V/X = 1.29\ V/(C_t + C_s + C_e)$.

A thin-wall thimble chamber designed for measurement of low-energy photons can be used at higher energies by placing a cap around the chamber to produce a wall of adequate thickness. Such a cap is called a *buildup cap*.

Example 5-6

The capacitance ($C_t + C_s$) of a condenser chamber is 100 picofarads (1 picofarad = 10^{-12} Farads), and the capacitance of the charger-reader is 15 picofarads. The air volume of the chamber is 0.46 cm^3. What is the sensitivity of the chamber? What voltage reduction occurs across the chamber following an exposure of 0.015 Coulombs/kg?

$$\text{Sensitivity} = \frac{\Delta V}{X} = 1.29V/(C_t + C_s)$$

$$= \frac{1.29(0.46\,\text{cm}^3)(10^{-6}\,\text{m}^3/\text{cm}^3)}{(100 + 15) \times 10^{-12}\,\text{Farads}}$$

$$= 5.2 \times 10^3\ \text{volts/Coulomb/kg}$$

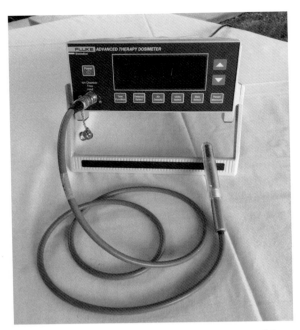

Figure 5-6 Integrated ionization chamber and electrometer used for radiation measurements irradiation therapy.

The reduction in voltage following an exposure of 0.015 Coulombs/kg is $\Delta V = (5.2 \times 10^3 \text{ volts/Coulombs/kg}) \cdot (0.015 \text{ Coulombs/kg}) = 78.0$ volts.

Chambers with different air volumes are available to yield different sensitivities, and chambers with different wall thicknesses are provided so that the device can be used to measure exposures for beams of different energies. The chamber shown in Figure 5-6 is often referred to as a *Farmer chamber*, because it was originally designed by the physicists Aird and Farmer.

Correction factors

When a condenser chamber is exposed to a radiation beam, all of the thimble must be irradiated to yield an accurate measurement of radiation exposure. Usually, all or part of the stem is also exposed and additional ionization may be produced in the stem itself. This extraneous ionization can produce slight differences in the measured exposure depending on how much of the stem is irradiated. These differences must be accounted for with a *stem correction factor*. This correction factor is obtained by measuring the response of the chamber with different amounts of stem exposed, and comparing this response with that measured under conditions (usually full stem irradiation) employed when the calibration factor for the chamber is determined. The stem correction factor can be obtained by making several measurements with the chamber positioned at one end of a rectangular field, with the chamber oriented differently for each measurement so that different amounts of stem are exposed.[3] In modern chambers, the stem effect is very small due to chamber design.

In some applications of condenser chambers, the efficiency of IP collection differs slightly, depending on whether the chamber wall is negative and the central electrode positive, or vice versa. This *polarity effect*, noticed most often when electron or high-energy photon beams are measured with an ionization chamber, is usually caused by slight differences in the collection efficiency of ionization originating outside the collecting volume of air.[4] It can be minimized by averaging measurements obtained with normal and reversed polarities across the chamber. Measurements obtained with opposite polarities should not differ by more than 0.5% to ensure that the averaging procedure yields a reasonable correction for the polarity effect. The polarity effect is a result of several processes, including the *Compton current*, an electric created by high-energy Compton electrons ejected during interactions of energetic photons, and ionization collected outside the collecting volume ("extra-cameral current"). The polarity effect is typically more significant for electron beams than for photon beams.

Most condenser chambers are not sealed and therefore are open to the atmosphere. In these chambers, the number of air molecules in the collecting volume varies with the air density, which, in turn, is affected by the ambient temperature and atmospheric pressure. The response of an unsealed chamber must be normalized to the atmospheric conditions existing when the chamber calibration factor was determined. In the United States, these conditions are 1 atmosphere (760 mm Hg) of barometric pressure and 22 °C (295 K) temperature. The *temperature-pressure correction factor*, $C_{T,P}$, for a chamber is:

$$C_{T,P} = [760/P(\text{mm Hg})] \cdot [(273 + T(^\circ\text{C}))/295]$$

where P is the atmospheric pressure in mm Hg, and the value of 273 corrects the ambient temperature, T, in degrees Celsius to absolute degrees (Kelvin). An all-too-common error in exposure measurements is use of an ambient pressure obtained from a weather station in which a correction has been applied to convert the pressure to an equivalent pressure at sea level. At an elevation of 1 mile above sea level, the use of ambient pressure "corrected to sea level" can produce an error of more than 20% in exposure measurements. When ambient pressure is obtained from a local weather station, it is advisable to request the uncorrected *station pressure* and to be aware of differences in elevation between the location of the station and the site of exposure measurements.

Example 5-7

Determine $C_{T,P}$ for an ambient temperature of 25 °C and an atmospheric pressure of 630 mm Hg at 1 mile (1609 m) elevation above sea level:

$$
\begin{aligned}
C_{T,P} &= (760/P) \cdot [(273 + T)/295] \\
&= (760/630) \cdot [(273 + 25)/295] \\
&= (1.21)(1.01) = 1.22
\end{aligned}
$$

In measurements of radiation exposure with a condenser chamber, the readings M should be corrected by the following expression to obtain true measurements of exposure X:

$$X = M \cdot N_C \cdot C_{P,T} \cdot C_i \cdot C_s$$

where N_c is the chamber calibration factor, $C_{T,P}$ is the temperature-pressure correction factor, C_i is the correction for collection efficiency loss caused by recombination, and C_s is the stem correction factor. The exposure, X, obtained by this procedure represents the true exposure at the location of measurement in the absence of the chamber because any perturbation of the radiation caused by the presence of the chamber, including attenuation of photons in the chamber wall, is included in the chamber calibration factor, N_c.

Example 5-8

A reading of 68 Coulombs/kg (uncorrected) is obtained in air with a condenser chamber with a calibration factor of 1.03 at full-stem irradiation for the average energy of x rays in the x-ray beam. The pressure-temperature correction is 1.22; the ionization collection efficiency is 100% when the entire stem of the chamber is exposed. What is the corrected exposure?

$$X = M \cdot N_C \cdot C_{P,T} \cdot C_i \cdot C_s$$
$$= (68) \cdot (1.03) \cdot (1.22) \cdot (1.0) \cdot (1.0)$$
$$= 85.4 \, \text{Coulombs/kg}$$

In the United States, chamber calibration factors are acquired by sending the chamber and associated electrometer to an accredited dosimetry calibration laboratory (ADCL).

Extrapolation and parallel-plate chambers

At times, a measurement of exposure is desired at the surface of a medium. This measurement can be obtained with an extrapolation chamber such as that illustrated in Figure 5-7a. The radiation beam enters the chamber through a thin foil that serves as the upper electrode. The lower electrode is backed by the backscattering material in the chamber. The thickness of the electrode spacing (and therefore the collecting volume) can be varied by micrometer screws that cause the upper electrode to descend toward the lower electrode. The ionization per unit collection volume is plotted against electrode spacing and extrapolated to zero spacing to yield a measure of the exposure at the surface of the medium (Figure 5-7b).

The parallel-plate ionization chamber is similar to an extrapolation chamber except that the electrodes are immobile. Ionization between the closely spaced electrodes is measured as the thickness of the medium above the upper electrode is increased. In this manner, the exposure can be measured as a function of depth at shallow depths where a cylindrical thimble chamber would perturb the radiation field.

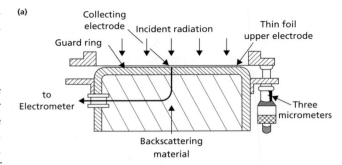

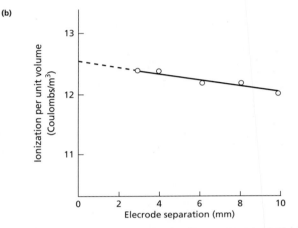

Figure 5-7 (a) Failla extrapolation chamber. (*Source:* From F. M. Khan. *The Physics of Radiation Therapy*. Baltimore, Williams & Wilkins, 1984. As redrawn from J. W. Boag, used with permission.)[4] (b) Ionization current per unit chamber volume as a function of electrode spacing in an extrapolation chamber. (*Source:* Stanton 1968.)[5]

Radiation dose

Chemical and biological changes in tissue exposed to ionizing radiation are caused by the deposition of energy from the radiation into the tissue. This deposition is described by two closely related quantities: kerma and absorbed dose. The SI unit for kerma and absorbed dose is the Gray (Gy), defined as 1 Joule/kg of irradiated medium. The centigray (cGy) is 0.01 Gy.

Favorable characteristics of ion chambers used for routine clinical measurements include minimum variation in sensitivity with photon energy, minimum variation in response with the direction of incident radiation, linear response over the expected range of exposures, minimum stem correction, and minimum ion pair recombination.

The *kerma* (the acronym for kinetic energy released in matter) is the sum of the initial kinetic energies of all IP liberated in a volume element of matter, divided by the mass of matter in the volume element. The *absorbed dose* is the energy actually absorbed per unit mass in the volume element. If ion pairs escape the volume element without depositing all of their energy, and if they are not compensated by ion pairs originating outside the volume element but depositing energy within it (electron equilibrium), the kerma exceeds the absorbed dose. The kerma also is greater than the absorbed dose when energy is radiated from the volume element as Bremsstrahlung or characteristic radiation. Under conditions in which electron equilibrium is achieved and the radiative energy loss is negligible, the kerma and absorbed dose are identical. The output of x-ray tubes is sometimes described in terms of *air kerma* expressed as the energy released per unit mass of air.

Example 5-9

A dose of 2 Gy (200 cGy) is delivered to a 1000 g tumor during a single radiation therapy session. How much energy is delivered to each gram of tumor and to the entire tumor?

$$\frac{\text{Energy absorbed}}{\text{per gram}} = 2\,\text{Gy}\left(1\frac{\text{J}}{\text{kg-Gy}}\right)\left(10^{-3}\frac{\text{kg}}{\text{g}}\right)$$
$$= 2 \times 10^{-3}\,\text{J/g}$$

$$\frac{\text{Energy absorbed}}{\text{in 1000 gram}} = 2 \times 10^{-3}\frac{\text{J}}{\text{G}}(1000\,\text{g})$$
$$= 2\,\text{J}$$

The difference between kerma and absorbed dose is useful in explaining the skin-sparing effect of high-energy photons such as multi-MV x rays used in radiation therapy. As shown in Figure 5-8, the kerma is greatest at the surface of irradiated tissue because the photon intensity is highest at the surface and causes the greatest number of interactions with the medium. The photon intensity diminishes gradually as the photons interact on their way through the medium. The electrons set into motion during the photon interactions at the surface travel several millimeters in depth before their energy is completely dissipated (Figure 5-9). The actual distance that the liberated elec-

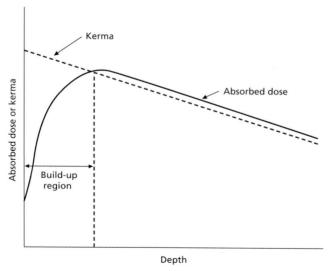

Figure 5-8 Kerma and absorbed dose as a function of depth in an irradiated medium.

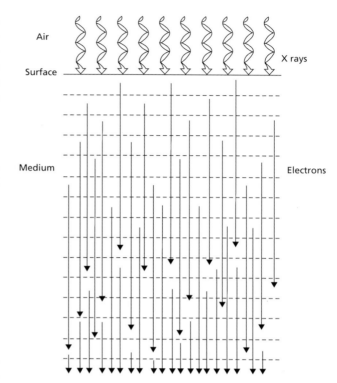

Figure 5-9 Dose buildup below the surface of a medium irradiated with high-energy photons as liberated electrons travel several millimeters before dissipating their energy.

trons travel depends on the energy of the incident photon beam. These electrons add to the ionization produced by photon interactions occurring at greater depths. Hence, the absorbed dose increases below the surface to reach the greatest dose at the depth of maximum dose (d_{max}) several millimeters to several centimeters below the surface. This buildup of absorbed dose below the skin is responsible for the clinically important skin-sparing effect of high-energy x and γ rays. Beyond d_{max}, the absorbed dose also decreases gradually as the photons are attenuated. At depths greater than d_{max}, the kerma curve falls below that for the absorbed dose because the kerma reflects the photon intensity at each depth, whereas the absorbed dose reflects in part the photon intensity at shallower depths that sets electrons into motion that penetrate to the depth.

The absorbed dose is a measure of the energy absorbed per unit mass of irradiated material. The total energy absorbed is termed the *integral dose* in the irradiated material.

Kerma, k, may be defined as:

$$k = \frac{\Delta E_{tr}}{\Delta m}$$

and absorbed dose, D, may be defined as:

$$D = \frac{\Delta E_{\text{ab}}}{\Delta m}$$

where E_{tr} is the energy transferred, E_{ab} is the energy absorbed, m is the mass of the irradiated material, and Δ represents an infinitesimal quantity.

The absorbed dose, D, in Gy delivered to a small mass, m, in kg is $D\,(Gy) = E/m \cdot (1\ J/kg\text{-}Gy)$, where E is the energy in Joules absorbed in the small mass. The energy, E, is the total energy deposited in the small volume, corrected for energy removed from the volume in any way (loss of ionization and radiative energy loss caused by Bremsstrahlung and characteristic radiation) that is not compensated by energy entering the volume from outside. During an exposure of 1 Coulomb per kilogram, the energy absorbed in air is 33.97 J/kg (or 33.97 Gy), as demonstrated earlier. An exposure of 1 R corresponds to an absorbed dose of (1 R) $(33.97\ J/kg/C/kg)\,(1\ Gy/J/kg) \cdot 2.58 \times 10^{-4}$ C/kg-R $= 87.6 \times 10^{-4}$ Gy (or 0.876 rad) in air.

Measurement of radiation dose

A radiation dosimeter provides a measurable response to the energy absorbed in a medium from incident radiation. To be most useful, the dosimeter should absorb an amount of energy equal to that which would be absorbed in the medium displaced by the dosimeter. A dosimeter used to measure absorbed dose in soft tissue should absorb an amount of energy equal to that absorbed by the same mass of soft tissue. Such a dosimeter is said to be *tissue-equivalent*. Few dosimeters are exactly tissue-equivalent, and corrections usually are required to determine the soft-tissue dose when a radiation dosimeter is used.

Calorimetric dosimetry

Almost all of the energy absorbed from radiation is eventually degraded to heat. If an absorbing medium is insulated from its environment, the rise in temperature of the medium is proportional to the absorbed energy. The temperature rise, ΔT, may be measured with a temperature-measuring device such as a thermocouple or thermistor. In a calorimeter insulated from its environment, the absorbed dose, D, in Gy is:

$$D(Gy) = E/m = [4.186\ (J/calorie) \cdot s \cdot \Delta T](1/1\ J/kg\text{-}Gy)$$

where E is the energy absorbed in Joules, m is the mass in kg, s is the specific heat of the absorber in calories per kg-°C, and is the ΔT temperature rise in °C. For a calorimetric measurement of dose to mimic the absorbed dose in soft tissue, the absorbing medium must resemble soft tissue. Graphite is often used as the absorbing medium in a *tissue dose* calorimeter, although water has been used with some success.

If the medium in a calorimeter is thick and dense enough to absorb all of the incident radiation, the increase in temperature reflects the total energy in the radiation beam. A measurement of this type, referred to as *absolute calorimetry*, usually employs a massive lead block as the absorbing medium.

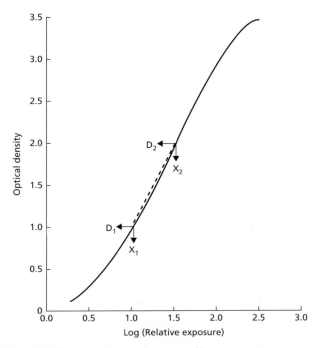

Figure 5-10 Characteristic curve for an x-ray film.

Radiographic film dosimetry

The emulsion of a photographic film contains crystals of a silver halide (e.g., AgBr) embedded in a gelatin matrix. When the film is developed, metallic silver is deposited in regions that have been exposed to radiation. Unaffected crystals of silver halide are removed during fixation of the film. The transmission of light through a region of the processed film varies with the amount of deposited silver and therefore with the energy absorbed from the radiation incident on the region of film. The transmittance, T, is usually expressed as the optical density, OD, of the film, where $OD = \log (1/T) = \log (I_0/I)$ and I and I_0 are the light intensity measured with and without the film in place. In Figure 5-10 the curve of OD versus log (exposure) is called the H–D *curve* of a film after the inventors Hurter and Driffield, who in 1890 developed this approach to describing the characteristics of photographic film. An H–D curve is sometimes referred to as a *characteristic* or *sensitometric curve*.

Radiographic film dosimetry is subject to severe errors for several reasons. The optical density of a film depends not only on the radiation exposure to the emulsion but also on variables such as the type and energy of the radiation and the conditions under which the film is developed. Photographic film consists of several high-Z elements and thus interacts with photons in ways different from soft tissue, especially when the photons are relatively low in energy. Photoelectric interactions dominate in high-Z materials for lower-energy photon beams. Photographic dosimetry is said to be *energy-dependent* because photographic film responds to x rays and γ rays differently from the response of air or soft tissue. The OD measured for an exposed film must be interpreted by comparison with a calibration H–D curve obtained under identical conditions of exposure. This requirement is often difficult to satisfy, especially when films are exposed in a medium in which a large amount of scattered radiation is present. Other problems of photographic dosimetry include the rapid attenuation of photons in a dense, high-Z film emulsion and variations in the thickness and composition of the photographic emulsion from one film or film batch to the next. Developing the film is also a source of uncertainty as it depends on the temperature and chemical consistency of the developing solution.

Radiochromic film dosimetry

Radiochromic film dosimetry is based on media that change color after irradiation. One feature that distinguishes radiochromic film dosimetry from radiographic film dosimetry is the mechanism of coloration. Whereas radiographic film needs to be developed, radiochromic film is self-developing.

Radiochromic film was introduced as a dosimetry tool in the early 1990s.[6] While the exact construction depends on the vendor, it generally consists of 1–2 sheets of polyester layers that contain 1–2 active layers (emulsion) sometimes with an adhesive. The thickness of the different layers is about 10–90 μm. The dominant elements of the film materials are hydrogen, carbon, nitrogen, and oxygen. Physical densities are about 1–1.2 g/cm^3 with effective atomic number (Z_{eff}) of 6–9, which means that radiochromic film is more tissue-like than radiographic film. Furthermore, radiochromic film is not sensitive to visual light, as is radiographic film, so handling radiochromic film is easier than handling radiographic film. However, care must still be taken when using radiochromic film because oils on the skin/hands can affect the measurement of absorbance. Therefore, tweezers or gloves should be used.

Film and reader systems should be calibrated together by exposing a series of films to different dose levels that cover the range of clinical use. Off-the-shelf document scanning systems can be used for absorbance measurements.[7] Each film sheet may be cut into smaller pieces but radiochromic film has an orientation dependence of the film response so this needs to be remembered so that the orientation of each film piece on the scanning system is the same.[8] Details of the handling and calibration process are provided by Soares.[9] Radiochromic film has minimal dose rate and energy dependence, and the AAPM TG55 report provides additional details of using radiochromic film for dosimetry.[10] There are some temperature and time-to-readout dependencies. To minimize these effects, it is recommended that the films should be stored in a temperature-controlled environment for at least 24 hours post-irradiation before performance an absorbance measurement.[11]

The process of radiochromic film colorization after irradiation is based on polymerization of diacetylene molecules, causing dye polymers to be formed. The polymers are blue in color and hence cause the film to absorb light in the red part of the spectrum. The signal formation is similar to that of radiographic film in terms of light transmission and optical density. For off-the-shelf flatbed scanners that use broadband visible light sources, the optical density depends on multiple factors. This means that the sensitivity curve will be unique to the flatbed scanner, film model, and dosimetry protocol. However, the emulsion has chromophores that are like needles, which are aligned in parallel with the emulsion coating direction. This results in the dependence of radiochromic film on the scanning direction. Nonetheless, radiochromic film dosimetry has been used successfully for an array of applications, including skin dose measurements,[12] brachytherapy,[13-15] total-body irradiation,[16] total-skin electron therapy,[17] and across photon, electron, and proton external beam treatment modalities.[18]

Typically, radiochromic film requires radiation doses of 2 Gy to 100 Gy in order to produce an image of sufficient optical density. One benefit of the range of radiochromic film is that it can be used to check dose distributions of high-dose modalities such as hypofractionated treatments.

Chemical dosimetry

Oxidation and reduction reactions may be initiated when chemical solutions are exposed to ionizing radiation. The number of molecules affected in a solution depends on the energy absorbed in the solution. Measuring the extent of oxidation or reduction is the technical basis of *chemistry dosimetry*.

The solution used most often to measure radiation dose is ferrous sulfate ($FeSO_4$), sometimes referred to as a *Fricke dosimeter*.[19] For high-energy photons that interact primarily by Compton scattering, the ratio of the energy absorbed in $FeSO_4$ to that absorbed in soft tissue is 1:1.024, the ratio of the electron densities (electrons/m^3) in the two media. Although the Fricke dosimeter is reasonably accurate ($\pm 3\%$), it is relatively insensitive, and doses of 50–500 Gy are required before the oxidation of Fe^{2+} to Fe^{3+} is measurable. The Fricke dosimeter is sometimes used to measure absorbed doses from beams of electrons and other charged particles.[20]

The yield of a chemical dosimeter such as $FeSO_4$ is described by its G value, defined as the number of molecules affected per 100 eV of energy absorbed. The G value for the Fricke dosimeter varies from 15.3 to 15.7 molecules/100 eV over a range of photon energies from ^{137}Cs (662 keV) to 30 MV x rays. For electrons from 1 to 30 MeV, the G value for $FeSO_4$ is often taken as 15.4 molecules/100 eV. After exposure, the amount of Fe^{3+} in the solution is determined by measuring the transmission of ultraviolet light of 305 nm wavelength through the solution. Once the number of affected molecules is known, the absorbed dose can be computed by dividing the number of affected molecules per unit mass of solution by the G value and converting energy units appropriately. The G value for chemical dosimetry is similar in concept to the work function $\bar{W}/e$ for ionization dosimetry.

Example 5-10

A solution of ferrous sulfate is exposed to 6 MV x rays. Measurement of the ultraviolet light (305 nm) transmitted through the solution reveals the presence of Fe^{3+} at a concentration of 0.00008 g-molecular weight/L. What was the absorbed dose in the solution, and what would the equivalent dose have been to soft tissue?

$$\text{Number of } Fe^{3+} \text{ ions/kg} = \frac{\begin{array}{c}(0.00008 \text{ g-mol wt/L}) \\ \times (6.02 \times 10^{23} \text{ molecules/g-mol wt})\end{array}}{(1 \text{ kg/L})}$$
$$= 4.82 \times 10^{19} \text{ molecules/kg}$$

For a G value of 15.6 molecules per 100 eV for $FeSO_4$, the absorbed dose in the solution is:

$$D(Gy) = \frac{(4.82 \times 10^{19} \text{ molecules/kg})(1.6 \times 10^{-19} \text{ J/eV})}{(15.6 \text{ molecules/100 eV})(1 \text{ J/kg-Gy})}$$
$$= 49.4 \text{ Gy}$$

The equivalent dose to soft tissue is:

$$D(Gy) = (49.4 \text{ Gy})(1.024)$$
$$= 50.6 \text{ Gy}$$

where 1.024 is the ratio of electron densities in tissue compared with $FeSO_4$.

Scintillation and semiconductor dosimetry

Certain materials fluoresce, or *scintillate*, during exposure to ionizing radiation. The intensity of emitted light depends on the rate of absorption of energy in the scintillator. With a solid scintillation detector such as thallium-activated sodium iodide, NaI(Tl), a light guide directs the emitted light onto a photomultiplier tube. The photomultiplier tube releases electrons in proportion to the intensity of the received light. The number of electrons is multiplied at each of several dynodes in the photomultiplier tube to yield an electrical signal at the final electrode (the anode) that is proportional to the energy deposited in the scintillator by the incident radiation.

Scintillation detectors furnish a measurable response at low dose rates and respond linearly over a wide range of radiation intensities. However, most scintillators contain high-Z atoms, and their response is strongly energy dependent compared with air or soft tissue. The energy dependence of scintillators such as NaI(T1) is the major limitation in using these detectors for the measurement of absorbed dose in soft tissue.

Semiconductors are materials with properties for electrical conduction that are intermediate between those of conductors and insulators. Semiconductor materials can be intentionally modified with impurities to yield an excess of electrons (n-type) or electron "holes" (p-type). When a voltage is applied with *reverse bias* across a junction between n-type and p-type semiconductors, a depletion zone devoid of excess electrons or holes is created. Radiation interacting in the depletion zone of the semiconductor diode can induce a current proportional to the dose delivered by incident radiation. Measurement of this current constitutes use of the semiconductor diode as a radiation dosimeter.

Luminescent dosimetry

Luminescence is the process of emission of optical radiation from a material. Thermoluminescence is the thermally accelerated return of an electron from an excited state via a metastable state. Both thermoluminescent dosimeters (TLD) and optically stimulated luminescent dosimeters (OSLD) contain materials that are used to measure ionizing radiation by measuring the amount of visible light emitted from the material after exposure to ionizing radiation.

LiF is frequently used for measurement of absorbed dose in patients and soft tissue-equivalent media (phantoms). Dosimetric LiF may be purchased as loose crystals, solid extruded rods, pressed pellets, or crystals embedded in a Teflon matrix. Dosimetric LiF contains selected impurities to provide the electron traps required for the thermoluminescent process. Pure LiF is useless as a radiation dosimeter.

A TLD is a device that releases light when it is heated following exposure to ionizing radiation. Shown in Figure 5-11 are electron energy levels in crystals of a thermoluminescent material such as LiF or $Li_2B_4O_7$. When energy is absorbed from incident radiation, electrons are raised from the valence energy to the conduction energy band. Some of the electrons return instantly to the valence band, but others are "trapped" in intermediate energy levels supplied by impurities in the crystals. The number of trapped electrons is proportional to the energy absorbed from the radiation. Unless energy is supplied to the crystals, most of the trapped electrons remain in the intermediate energy levels for an indefinite period. If the crystals are heated, however, the trapped electrons are released and return to the conduction

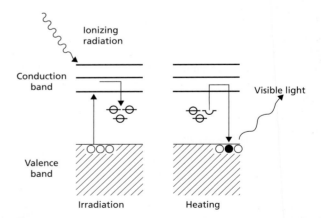

Figure 5-11 Electron transitions occurring when a thermoluminescent material is irradiated and then subsequently heated.

band. These electrons then fall to the valence band, releasing light in the process. The light is directed onto a photomultiplier tube to generate an electrical signal proportional to the energy originally deposited in the crystals by the radiation. Detection of this signal yields a measure of the absorbed dose in the crystals. Because the $\bar{Z}$ of LiF (8.18) and $Li_2B_4O_7$ (7.4) are close to that of air (7.64) and soft tissue (7.4), the energy absorbed by these materials is close to that absorbed by an equal mass of air or soft tissue. Small differences in the energy absorption are reflected in the *energy-dependence* curves for LiF and $Li_2B_4O_7$ shown in Figure 5-11. CaF_2:Mn is an especially sensitive thermoluminescent material and is often used in personnel monitors. The presence of high-Z components makes this material more energy dependent than LiF or $Li_2B_4O_7$ (Figure 5-11).

The amount of light released when TLD crystals are heated depends on several factors in addition to the energy absorbed in the TLDs from the radiation. The factors include the temperature to which the crystals are heated, the reflectivity of the heating pan, and the time over which the crystals are heated. Hence, TLD measurements must be calibrated against the light from crystals receiving a known dose of radiation.

Light from thermoluminescent dosimeters is measured under carefully controlled conditions, including exacting requirements for the temperature of the heating pan for the crystals, heating cycle, position of the photomultiplier tube, and amplification in the photomultiplier tube itself.

OSLDs are similar to TLDs in terms of the dosimetry physics. However, for OSLDs, trapped energy is released using light, which is faster and more precise than heating. Similar to TLDs, the amount of light released in reading out the OSLDs is proportional to the amount of absorbed radiation.

An OSLD is a plastic disk infused with carbon-doped aluminum oxide. Each OSLD can be used for many exposures and readouts. The dosimeters are small (e.g., 1 mm × 1 mm × 2 mm). OSLDs have a linear response of up to about 3 Gy. OSLDs are highly stable over time and do not have an angular, energy, dose rate, or temperature dependence. They have a build-up of about 3 mm. A calibration curve is required and must be measured prior to use.[21] A nonlinear curve should be created if it is expected that doses will be measured in excess of 3 Gy. OSLDs have been used successfully for an array of applications including brachytherapy,[22,23] kV x rays,[24] and across photon, electron, and proton external beam treatment modalities.[25]

Absorbed dose measurements with an ionization chamber

Determining estimates of absorbed dose in soft tissue or any other medium can be obtained by measurements of ionization in a small gas-filled cavity in the medium. The conversion of ionization in the gas-filled cavity to absorbed dose in the medium is accomplished by application of the *Bragg–Gray cavity theory*. This theory underlies many of the dosimetric measurements made in routine clinical dosimetry important to radiation oncology.

Bragg–Gray cavity theory

Suppose that a small gas-filled cavity is suspended in a homogeneous medium exposed to a beam of x or γ rays. As the photons interact in the medium, high-energy electrons are released that penetrate the gas-filled cavity and produce ionization in it. If the cavity is small, its presence does not influence the number or energy of primary and secondary electrons that traverse the medium at the location of the cavity. The energy, E_g, absorbed in eV per unit mass (kg) of gas in the cavity is $E_g = J_g \cdot \overline{W}/e$, where J_g is the ionization in IP/kg in the gas, and $\overline{W}/e$ is the average energy expended per ion pair produced in the gas (33.97 eV/IP if the gas is air). E_g is the absorbed dose to the gas in units of eV/kg.

If the cavity described in the paragraph above were replaced by an equal amount of medium, the energy E_m that would be absorbed per unit mass of medium would be $E_m = \bar{s}_m E_g$, where $\bar{s}_m$ is the ratio of the average mass stopping powers of the medium and the gas for the electrons traversing the cavity. The dose, D_m, in Grays to the medium at the location of the cavity is:

$$D_m = E_m (1.6 \times 10^{-19} \text{ J/eV})/[(1 \text{ J/kg-Gy})$$
$$\times (1.6 \times 10^{-19} \text{ Coulombs/IP})] = (\bar{s}_m \cdot J_g \cdot \overline{W}/e)$$

where $\overline{W}/e$ is expressed in units of eV/IP and J_g is described in units of C/kg. These expressions are known as the *Bragg–Gray relationship*.

The *mass stopping power*, s_m, of a medium describes the rate of energy loss of electrons traversing the medium, divided by the density of the medium. The *mass stopping power ratio*, $\bar{s}_m$, describes the rate of energy loss of electrons in one medium compared with another. Stopping power ratios are computed with the *Bethe–Bloch formula* and corrected for the density (polarization) effect.[26,27] The density effect accounts for a reduction in the influence of a charged particle on a distant atom caused by polarization of the atoms between the particle and the distant atom. Listed in Table 5-4 are average mass stopping power ratios relative to air in a few materials for electrons set into motion by high-energy x rays and ^{60}Co γ rays ($E_{avg} = 1.25$ MeV). Tables of mass stopping power ratios are available in the literature.[28,29]

For measurement of absorbed dose in a medium according to the Bragg–Gray relationship, the gas-filled cavity should be so small (< 1 cm in diameter) that its presence does not affect the electrons set into motion as photons interact in the surrounding medium. For high-energy photon beams, this is less than 1 cm in diameter. That is, none of the high-energy electrons traversing the cavity should originate or terminate in the cavity. In actual practice, the gas-filled cavity is part of a thimble chamber with a wall that separates the cavity from the surrounding medium.

Table 5-4 Average mass stopping power $\bar{s}_m$ relative to air for photon beams in selected materials.

Nominal Accelerating Potential (MV)	Water	Polyethylene	Acrylic	Graphite	Bakelite	Nylon
^{60}Co	1.134	1.113	1.103	1.012	1.081	1.142
2	1.135	1.114	1.104	1.015	1.084	1.146
5	1.129	1.106	1.096	1.005	1.073	1.130
10	1.117	1.094	1.085	0.992	1.060	1.114
15	1.106	1.083	1.074	0.982	1.051	1.097
20	1.096	1.074	1.065	0.977	1.042	1.087

Source: Radiation Therapy Committee 1983.[30] Reproduced with permission from American Association of Physicists in Medicine.

The chamber wall should be infinitesimally thin so that all electrons traversing the cavity originate in the medium and none is released from the wall.

A gas-filled cavity in a medium can be considered a Bragg–Gray cavity if it is so small that (a) the direct interaction of photons with the cavity gas is negligible, (b) the ionization in the cavity is attributable entirely to particles that originate in the medium and cross the cavity, and (c) the range of the particles is much greater than the cavity dimensions.

Alternatively, the chamber wall may have a finite thickness, provided that the wall composition is identical to the surrounding medium. Often, these conditions are not satisfied, and the ionization chamber slightly disturbs the distribution of absorbed dose in the medium. This disturbing influence is accounted for by introducing a *perturbation correction p* into the Bragg–Gray relationship:

$$D_m = (p \cdot \bar{s}_m \cdot J_g \cdot \overline{W}/e)$$

The Bragg–Gray relationship is essential to the calibration of radiation beams from high-energy accelerators employed for radiation therapy in clinical radiation oncology. In practice, there are many corrections that need to be used to apply the Bragg-Gray relationship to radiotherapy dosimetry using an ion chamber. Documents such as the AAPM TG51 report[31] and IAEA 398 report[32] provide guidance on the basis and techniques for applying these correction factors to commercially available ionization chambers for the purpose of dose measurements.

Dose equivalent

Most chemical and biological effects of radiation depend not only on the amount but also on the distribution of energy absorbed in an irradiated medium. That is, various types and energies of radiation may elicit different chemical and biological responses even though the absorbed doses delivered by the radiations are identical. The *relative biological effectiveness* (RBE) of a particular type or energy of radiation describes the efficiency with which the radiation evokes a particular response. The RBE

is determined by comparing chemical or biological results produced by a particular radiation with those obtained with a reference radiation:

$$RBE = \frac{\text{Dose of reference radiation required to produce a particular response}}{\text{Dose of radiation in question required to produce the same response}}$$

By convention, the relative biological effectiveness of 200 kV x rays is taken as 1. For a particular type of radiation, the RBE may vary from one chemical or biological response to another, as well as from one biological system or organism to another. Shown in Table 5-5 are the results of investigations into the RBE of ^{60}Co for eliciting a variety of biological effects. For these data, the reference radiation is medium-energy x rays.

Often the effectiveness with which different types of radiation produce a particular chemical or biological effect varies with the linear energy transfer (LET) of the radiation. The dose equivalent, H, in Sv is the product of the absorbed dose in Gy and a quality factor, Q, that varies with the LET of the radiation. That is, $H(\text{Sv}) = D(\text{Gy}) \cdot Q$. In traditional units of dose equivalent H is in rem, where H (rem) = D (rad) $\cdot Q$. Quality factors are listed in Table 5-6 for different types of radiation. The quality factor $Q = 1$ is reserved for radiations of average linear energy

Table 5-5 Relative biological effectiveness of ^{60}Co gammas, with different biological effects used as a criterion for measurement.

Effects	RBE of ^{60}Co Gammas	Source
30-day lethality and testicular atrophy in mice	0.77	Storer et al.[33]
Splenic and thymic atrophy in mice	1.00	Storer et al.[33]
Inhibition of growth in *Vicia faba*	0.84	Hall[34]
LD^{50} in mice, rat, chick embryo, and yeast	0.82–0.93	Sinclair[35]
Hatchability of chicken eggs	0.81	Loken et al.[36]
HeLa cell survival	0.90	Krohmer[37]
Lens opacity in mice	0.80	Upton et al.[38]
Cataract induction in rats	1.00	Focht et al.[39]
L cell survival	0.76	Till and Cunningham[40]

Table 5-6 Quality factors for different radiations.

Type of Radiation	Quality Factor
X rays, γ rays, and beta particles	1.0
Thermal neutrons	5
Neutrons and protons	20
Particles from natural radionuclides	20
Heavy recoil nuclei	20

Source: National Council on Radiation Protection and Measurements 1991.[42]
Note: These data should be used only for purposes of radiation protection.

transfer in water $(\overline{LET}) \leq 2.5$ keV/μm; $Q = 1$ to 2 for radiations of $\overline{LET} = 2.5$ to 7.0 keV/μm; $Q = 2$ to 5 for radiations of $\overline{LET} = 7.0$ to 23 keV/μm; $Q = 5$ to 10 for radiations of $\overline{LET} = 23$ to 53 keV/μm; and $Q = 10$ to 20 for $\overline{LET} = 53$ to 175 keV/μm.[41] The dose equivalent reflects differences in the effectiveness of different radiations to elicit a biological response from a small region of irradiated tissue as a reflection of the LET of the radiation.

Example 5-11

A person received an average whole-body x-ray dose of 0.8 mGy and 0.6 mGy from 10 MeV neutrons. What is the whole-body dose equivalent in mSv?

$$H(\text{mSv}) = \sum_{i=1}^{2} D_i(\text{mGy}) \cdot Q_i$$
$$= (0.8\,\text{mGy})(1) + (0.6\,\text{mGy})(20)$$
$$= 12.8\,\text{mSv}$$

For a particular response in a specific biological system, the RBE may vary with several factors, including dose rate, fractionation schedule, temperature, degree of oxygenation, spatial distribution of dose, and sample volume. The quality factor, Q, however, varies with a physical property of the radiation (LET) rather than with the response of a biological system. Consequently, it has a fixed value for a particular radiation. Although Q is not related to any particular biological result, its use in radiation protection is directed primarily to the carcinogenic and mutagenic effects of radiation.

Example 5-12

A person accidentally ingests a small amount of ^{32}P (β particle $E_{\text{max}} = 1.7$ MeV). The average dose to the gastrointestinal tract is estimated to be 10 mGy. What is the dose equivalent to the gastrointestinal tract in mSv?

$$H(\text{mSv}) = D(\text{mGy}) \cdot Q$$
$$= (10\,\text{mGy}) \cdot (1.0)$$
$$= 10\,\text{mSv}$$

Factors other than the LET may influence the biological effectiveness of radiations. For example, a distribution factor, DF, may be included to account for changes in the radiation response caused by the nonuniform distribution of radioactivity in a region of tissue. In this case, the expression for H is written as $H\,(\text{Sv}) = D\,(\text{Gy}) \cdot Q \cdot DF$.

Often the region of tissue of interest is sufficiently large that the absorbed dose and LET vary across the region. The mean dose equivalent (sometimes called the *equivalent dose*) $\bar{H}$ is defined as the average absorbed dose in a region of tissue multiplied by an effective quality factor $\overline{Q}$ (more commonly referred to as a *radiation weighting factor*, w_r) that depends on the LET of the radiation averaged over the region of exposed tissue. Also, different organs in the body vary in terms of their radiation sensitivity and relative importance to the overall well-being of the individual. These variations are reflected in the effective dose equivalent H_e, in which doses of different tissues are adjusted by a tissue weighting factor, w_t.

Radiation quality

An x-ray beam is not described completely by stating the exposure or dose it delivers to a region within an irradiated medium. The penetrating ability of the radiation, termed the *quality* of the radiation, must also be known before estimates can be made of the exposure or dose at other locations in the medium, the differences in energy absorption between regions of different composition, and the biological effectiveness or quality factor of the radiation.

Spectral distributions

The spectral distribution of an x-ray beam depicts the relative number of photons of different energies in the beam. The quality of an x-ray beam is described explicitly by the spectral distribution. The spectral distribution of an x-ray beam may be computed from an attenuation curve for the beam measured under conditions in which the area of the beam is small and the measurements are obtained at a considerable distance from the location where attenuating materials are placed in the beam. A variety of curve-fitting techniques may be applied to the attenuation curve to obtain equations used to compute the spectral distribution.[43,44]

Most measurements of x-ray spectra are obtained with a scintillation or semiconductor detector. The pulse-height distribution must be corrected for statistical fluctuations in the energy distribution, incomplete absorption of photons in the detector, and selective absorption of lower-energy photons in the detector (i.e., the detector's energy dependence). A measured x-ray spectrum with appropriate corrections applied is shown in Figure 5-12 together with the results from Monte Carlo calculations.

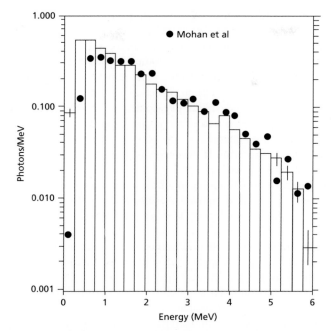

Figure 5-12 Energy distribution of x-ray photons in a beam generated at 6 MV.
Source: Chaney and Cullip 1994.[45] Reproduced with permission from American Association of Physicists in Medicine.

The *half-value layer* (HVL), sometimes called the *half-value thickness*, of an x-ray beam is the thickness of a material that reduces the exposure rate of the beam to half. The units of HVL are usually expressed in mm, such as mm Al, mm Cu, or mm Pb. Although the HVL alone furnishes a description of radiation quality that is adequate for most clinical situations, a second parameter, such as the kVp or the homogeneity coefficient, is sometimes stated with the HVL. The homogeneity coefficient is the quotient of the thickness of attenuator required to reduce the exposure to half, divided by the thickness of attenuator required to reduce the exposure further from one-half to a fourth. The homogeneity coefficient is the ratio of the first and second HVLs.

Example 5-13

The following attenuation data are measured for a therapy x-ray beam. What are the first and second HVLs and the homogeneity coefficient?

From the curve the Figure 13-example, the first HVL is approximately 1.9 mm Cu, and the second HVL is approximately 2.1 mm Cu. The homogeneity coefficient is:

$$\text{Homogeneity coefficient} = \frac{(\text{HVL})_1}{(\text{HVL})_2} = \frac{1.9\,\text{mm Cu}}{2.1\,\text{mm Cu}}$$
$$= 0.90$$

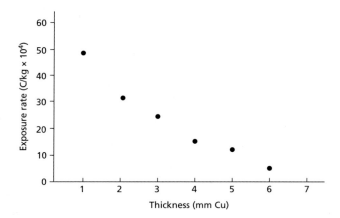

HVLs are measured with solid attenuators, such as thin sheets of aluminum, copper, or lead of uniform thickness. The attenuators are placed between the x-ray source and an ionization chamber, and measurements of exposure are obtained as the total thickness of attenuator is increased. Measurements of HVL should always be made under conditions of narrow-beam ("good") geometry so that only primary and not scattered photons enter the chamber. Narrow-beam geometry requires that the measuring chamber be positioned far from the attenuators and that an x-ray beam of small cross-sectional area be used. Conditions of narrow-beam ("good") and broad-beam ("poor") geometry are depicted in Figure 5-13 and Figure 5-14, respectively.

Measurements of HVL under these conditions are compared in Figure 5-15. With broad-beam geometry, increasing numbers of photons are scattered into the detector as additional attenuators are added to the beam. Consequently, broad-beam conditions yield inappropriately high values of the HVL. Such values, however, are useful in the computation of shielding requirements for walls surrounding sources of radiation.

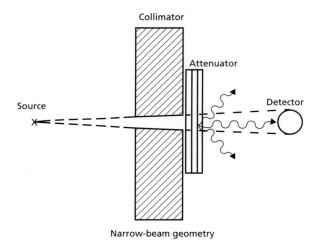

Narrow-beam geometry

Figure 5-13 Narrow-beam (good) geometry.
Source: Hendee and Ritenour 2001.[46] Reproduced with permission from John Wiley and Sons.

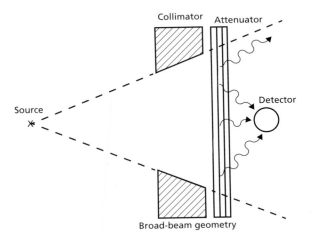

Figure 5-14 Broad-beam (poor) geometry.
Source: Hendee and Ritenour 2001.[46] Reproduced with permission from John Wiley and Sons.

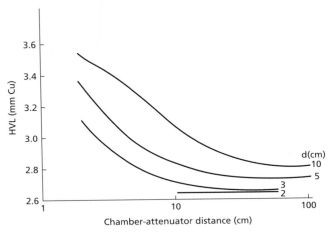

Figure 5-15 Variation of the HVL with the diameter, *d*, of an x-ray beam at the attenuator for various distances between the attenuator and the radiation detector.
Source: NCRP Report 85.[47]

Summary

- Radiation quantity may be described explicitly by the concepts of photon and energy fluence and fluence rate. The energy fluence rate is often referred to as *radiation intensity*.
- Radiation exposure [in units of Coulombs/kilogram or, formerly, Röntgen (R)] is defined in terms of the ionization that radiation produces in air.
- Measurements of radiation exposure with a free-air, thimble, or condenser chamber require that electronic equilibrium be established in the collecting volume of air.
- The effective atomic number of a material is the atomic number of a hypothetical element that attenuates x and γ rays at the same rate as the material.
- The sensitivity of air ionization chambers is the voltage reduction across the chamber per unit exposure to radiation.
- Ionization chamber readings may need correction for several influences, including a calibration factor, temperature and pressure (if the chamber is open to the atmosphere), stem irradiation, polarity effect, and collection efficiency.
- Extrapolation and parallel-plate ionization chambers are used for exposure measurements at or slightly below the surface of an irradiated material.
- Kerma is a measure of the energy deposited per unit mass of irradiated material.
- Absorbed dose is a measure of the energy absorbed per unit mass of irradiated material. Absorbed dose is the kerma corrected for energy lost by Bremsstrahlung and characteristic radiation.
- Absorbed dose can be determined from ionization measurements through the application of the Bragg–Gray principle.
- Methods for the measurement of absorbed dose include calorimetry and ionization, film, chemical, scintillation, and thermoluminescent dosimetry.
- The dose equivalent (in Sieverts) is a product of the absorbed dose (in Grays) multiplied by a quality factor (also called the *radiation weighting factor*) that varies with the LET of the radiation.
- The effective dose equivalent, also known as the *effective dose*, is the absorbed dose to a tissue multiplied by radiation and tissue weighting factors.
- Radiation quality is a measure of the penetrating ability of an x-ray beam.
- Radiation quality is often described in terms of the half-value layer (HVL), defined as the thickness of attenuation required to reduce the radiation exposure to half.

Problems

5-1 For an exposure of 43 R, what are the number of ion pairs and the charge in Coulombs liberated per kilogram of air? How much energy is absorbed per cubic meter and per kilogram of air? What is the absorbed dose in air?

5-2 For a ^{60}Co beam, a deflection of 57 scale divisions/min is recorded with a 100 R condenser chamber (full-scale deflection = 100 divisions). The chamber has a calibration factor of 0.95 for ^{60}Co γ rays determined at 22 °C. The temperature and pressure are 24 °C and 645 mm Hg. For 100% collection efficiency and a stem correction factor of 1.02, what is the exposure rate in R/min?

5-3 The photon flux is 10^{11} photons/m^2/sec for a beam of photons. Two-thirds of the photons have an energy of 600 keV, and one-third have an energy of 1.15 MeV. What is the energy flux of the beam? If the photon flux is constant over time, what is the energy fluence over a 20-second interval?

5-4 The total energy absorption coefficient of air is 2.8×10^{-3} m²/kg for photons of 1.0 MeV. What are the energy and photon fluence required for an exposure of 0.03 Coulombs/kg?

5-5 Water is 89% oxygen (gram-atomic mass 15.999) and 11% hydrogen (gram-atomic mass 1.008) by weight. Compute the effective atomic number of water.

5-6 A thimble chamber with an air-equivalent wall receives an exposure of 0.025 Coulombs/kg in 1 minute. The volume of the chamber is 0.52 cm³. What is the ionization current from the chamber?

5-7 A condenser chamber has a sensitivity of 1.43×10^4 volts/Coulombs/kg and a volume of 0.52 cm³. The capacitance of the chamber is five times that of the electrometer. What is the capacitance of the chamber?

5-8 A miniature ionization chamber has a sensitivity of 1 V/R. The chamber is discharged by 300 V during an exposure to x rays. What exposure in Röntgen did the chamber receive?

5-9 An 800 g organ receives a uniform absorbed dose of 10 Gy. How much energy is absorbed per gram, and what is the total energy absorbed in the organ?

5-10 A particular type of lesion recedes satisfactorily after receiving a dose of 55 Gy from ^{60}Co γ rays. When the lesion is treated with 10 MV x rays, a dose of 65 Gy is required to obtain the same response. Relative to ^{60}Co γ rays, what is the RBE of 10 MV x rays for treating this lesion?

5-11 A patient undergoing a nuclear medicine procedure receives a dose of 2.5 cGy to the thyroid. A total of 2.1 cGy is delivered by beta particles and 0.4 cGy is contributed by γ rays. What is the dose equivalent in cSv to the thyroid?

5-12 The specific heat of graphite is 170 cal/(kg °C). A uniform dose of 10 Gy is delivered to a graphite block that is insulated from its environment. What is the temperature rise of the block?

5-13 With $G = 15.4$ molecules/100 eV, how many Fe^{2+} ions are oxidized to Fe^{3+} when a dose of 100 Gy is delivered to a 10 mL solution of $FeSO_4$? (Assume that the density of $FeSO_4$ is 1 kg/L.)

5-14 Attenuation measures for a diagnostic x-ray beam yield the following results:

Added Filtration (mm Al)	Percent Transmission
1.0	60.2
2.0	41.4
3.0	30.0
4.0	22.4
5.0	16.9

Plot the data on semi-logarithmic graph paper, and determine the first and second HVL and the homogeneity coefficient.

References

1 Johns, H., and Cunningham, J. *The Physics of Radiology*, 3rd edition. Springfield, IL, Charles C. Thomas, 1969.

2 Meredith, W., and Massey, J. *Fundamental Physics of Radiology*. Baltimore, MD, Williams & Wilkins, 1968.

3 Ibbott, G. S., Barne, J. E., Hall, G. R., and Hendee, W. R. Stem correction for ion chambers. *Med. Phys.* 1975; **2**:328–330.

4 Boag, J. W. Ionization chambers. In *Radiation Dosimetry*, vol. II, 2nd edition, F. H. Attix and W. C. Roesch (eds.). New York, Academic Press, 1969.

5 Stanton, L. *Basic Medical Radiation Physics*. New York, Appleton-Century-Crofts, 1968.

6 McLaughlin, W. L., Yun-Gong, C., Soares, C. G., Miller, A., Van Dyke, G. and Lewis, D. F. Sensitometry of the response of a new radiochromic film dosimeter to gamma radiation and electron beams. *Nucl. Instrum. Meth. Phys. Res. A.* 1991; **302**:165–176.

7 Devic, S., Seuntjens, J., Sham, E., Podgorsak, E. B., Schmidtlein C. R., et al. Precise radiochromic film dosimetry using a flat-bed document scanner. *Med. Phys.* 2005; **32**:2245–2253.

8 Buston, M. J., Cheung T., Yu, P. K. N. Scanning orientation effects of Gafchromic EBT film dosimetry. *Australas. Phys. Eng. Sci. Med.* 2006; **29**(3):281–284.

9 Soares, C. G. Radiochromic film dosimetry. *Radiat. Meas.* 2006; **41**:S100–S116.

10 Niroomand-Rad, A., Blackwell, C. R., Coursey, B. M., Gall, K. P., McLaughlin, W. L., et al. Radiochromic dosimetry: Recommendations of the AAPM Radiation Therapy Committee Task Group 55. *Med. Phys.* 1998; **25**:2093–2115.

11 Ali, I., Costescu, C., Vicic, M., Dempsey, J. F., and Williamson, J. F. Dependence of radiochromic film optical density post-exposure kinetics on dose and dose fractionation *Med. Phys.* 2006; **30**:1957–1967.

12 Devic, S., Seuntjens, J., Abdel-Rahman, W., Evans, M., Olivares, M., et al. Accurate skin dose measurements using radiochromic film in clinical applications. *Med. Phys.* 2006; **33**:1116–1124.

13 Evans, M. D., Devic, S., and Podgorsak, E. B. High dose-rate brachytherapy source position quality assurance using radiochromic film. *Med. Dosim.* 2007; **32**:13–15.

14 Steidley, K. D. Use of radiochromic dosimetry film for HDR brachytherapy quality assurance. *Med. Dosim.* 1998; **23**:37–38.

15 Taccini, G., Cavagnetto, F., Coscia, G., Garelli, S., and Pilot, A. The determination of dose characteristics of ruthenium ophthalmic applicators using radiochromic film. *Med. Phys.* 1997; **24**:2034–2037.

16 Su, F. C., Shi, C. Y., and Papanikolaou, N. Clinical application of GAFCHROMIC (R) EBT film for in vivo dose measurements of total body irradiation radiotherapy. *Appl. Radiat. Isot.* 2008; **66**:389–394.

17 Bufacchi, A., Carosi, A., Adorante, N., Delle Canne, S., Malatesta, T., et al. In vivo EBT radiochromic film dosimetry of electron beam for Total Skin Electron Therapy (TSET). *Phys. Med.* 2007; **23**:67–72.

18 Sorriaux, J., Kacperek, A., Rossomme, S., Lee, J. A., Bertrand, D., et al. Evaluation of Gafchromic EBT3 film characteristics in therapy photon, electron, and proton beams. *Physica. Medica.* 2013; **29**:599–606.

19 Fricke, H., and Morse, S. The action of x rays on ferrous sulfate solutions. *Philos. Mag.* 1929; **7**:129–141.

20 ICRU Report 21. *Radiation Dosimetry: Electrons with Initial Energies between 1 and 50 MeV.* Washington, DC, International Commission on Radiological Units and Measurements, 1972.

21 Jursinc, P. A. Characterization of optically stimulated luminescent dosimeters, OSLDs for clinical dosimetry measurements. *Med. Phys.* 2007; **24**:4594–4603.

22 Tien, C. J., Ebeling, R., Hiatt, J. R., Curran, B., Sternick, E. Optically stimulated luminescent dosimetry for high dose rate brachytherapy. *Front. Oncol.* 2012; **2**:91.

23 Sharma, R., and Jursinic, P. A. In vivo measurements for high dose rate brachytherapy with optically stimulated luminescent dosimeters. *Med. Phys.* 2013; **40**(7).

24 Al-Senan, R. M., and Hatab, M. R. Characteristics of an OSLD in the diagnostic energy range. *Med. Phys.* 2011; **38**(7):4396–4405.

25 Reft, C. S. The energy dependence and dose response of a commercial optically stimulated luminescent detector for kilovoltage photon, megavoltage photon, and electron, proton, and carbon beams. *Med. Phys.* 2009; **36**(5):1609.

26 Bethe, H. Quantenmechanik der ein- and zwei-elektronen problems. In *Hanbuchder Physik*, vol. 24, part 1, 2nd edition, G. Geiger and K. Scheel (eds.). Berlin, Julius Springer, 1933, pp. 273–551.

27 Sternheimer, R. The density effect for the ionization loss in various materials. *Phys. Rev.* 1957; **88**:851–859.

28 Berger, M. J., and Seltzern, S. M. *Stopping Powers and Ranges of Electrons and Positrons*, 2nd edition. Washington, DC, National Bureau of Standards, 1983.

29 Burlin, T. Cavity chamber theory. In *Radiation Dosimetry*, vol. 1, 2nd edition, F. H. Attix and W. C. Roesch (eds.). New York, Academic Press, 1968.

30 Task Group 21. Radiation Therapy Committee, American Association of Physicists in Medicine: A protocol for the determination of absorbed dose from high energy photons and electron beams. *Med. Phys.* 1983; **10**:741.

31 Almond, P. R., Biggs, P. J., Coursey, B. M., Hanson, W. F., Huq, M. S., et al. AAPM's TG-51 protocol for clinical reference dosimetry of high-energy photon and electron beams. *Med. Phys.* 1999; **26**:1847–1870.

32 International Atomic Energy Agency. Absorbed dose determination in external beam radiotherapy: An international code of practice for dosimetry based on standards of absorbed dose to water. IAEA Technical Report Series No. 398. Vienna: IAEA, 2000.

33 Storer, J. B., Harris, P. S., Furchner, J. E., and Langham, W. H. Relative biological effectiveness of various ionizing radiations in mammalian systems. *Radiat. Res.* 1957; **6**:188.

34 Hall, E. Relative biological efficiency of x rays generated at 200 kVp and gamma radiation from cobalt 50 therapy unit. *Br. J. Radiol.* 1961; **34**:313.

35 Sinclair, W. Relative biological effectiveness of 22-MeVp x-rays, cobalt 60 gamma rays and 200 kVp rays: 1. General introduction and physical aspects. *Radiat. Res.* 1962; **16**:336.

36 Loken, M. K., Beisang, A. A., Johnson, E. A., and Mosser, D. G. Relative biological effectiveness of ^{60}Co gamma rays and 220 kVp x-rays on viability of chicken eggs. *Radiat. Res.* 1960; **12**:202.

37 Krohmer, J. RBE and quality of electromagnetic radiation at depths in water phantom. *Radiat. Res.* 1965; **24**:547.

38 Upton, A. C., and Odell, T. T. Jr. Relative biological effectiveness of neutrons, x-rays, and gamma rays for production of lens opacities: Observations on mice, rats, guinea pigs and rabbits. *Radiology* 1956; **67**:686.

39 Focht, E. F., Merriam, G. R. Jr., Schwartz, M. S., and Parsons, R. W. The relative biological effectiveness of cobalt 60 gamma and 200 kV x radiation for cataract induction. *Am. J. Roentgenol.* 1968; **102**:71.

40 Till, J., and Cunningham J. Unpublished data. In *The Physics of Radiology*, 3rd edition, H. Johns and J. Cunningham (eds.). Springfield, IL, Charles C. Thomas, 1969, p. 720.

41 International Commission on Radiological Protection. Recommendations of the ICRP. *Br. J. Radiol.* 1955; **28**(Suppl. 6).

42 National Council on Radiation Protection and Measurements. *Recommendations on Limits for Exposure to Ionizing Radiation*, Report 91. Washington, DC, NCRP, 1991.

43 Kramers, H. A. On the theory of x-ray absorption and the continuous x-ray spectrum. *Philos. Mag.* 1923; **46**(Series 6): 836–871.

44 Schiff, L. I. Energy-angle distribution of thin target bremsstrahlung. *Phys. Rev.* 1951; **83**:252–253.

45 Chaney, E. L., and Cullip, T. J. A Monte Carlo study of accelerator head scatter. *Med. Phys.* 1994; **21**:1383–1390.

46 Hendee, W. R., and Ritenour, E. R. *Medical Imaging Physics*, 4th edition. New York, John Wiley & Sons, Ltd., 2001.

47 NCRP Report 85. *Physical Aspects of Irradiation*. Washington, DC, National Bureau of Standards Handbook 85, 1964.

CHAPTER

6

CALIBRATION OF MEGAVOLTAGE BEAMS OF X RAYS AND ELECTRONS

Objectives

By studying this chapter, the reader should be able to:
- Describe the procedures for calibrating beams of x and γ rays and electrons.
- Discuss the pathways by which exposure, air kerma, and dose calibration standards are promulgated in the United States.
- Explain the similarities and differences among past and current U.S. calibration protocols and among international protocols.
- Describe the influences on the response of an ionization chamber and the procedures for correcting for these influences.

Introduction

The term *calibration* is often used interchangeably with output measurement. In order to calibrate a radiation producing machine, the dose delivered (output) at a reference point must be measured. The act of adjusting the response of the machine (linear accelerator monitor chamber) so that the dose output is 1 cGy per monitor unit (MU) is termed *calibration*. Calibration must be performed before a radiation beam can be used for the treatment of patients and is repeated on a regular basis to

Hendee's Radiation Therapy Physics, Fourth Edition. Todd Pawlicki, Daniel J. Scanderbeg and George Starkschall.
© 2016 John Wiley & Sons, Inc. Published 2016 by John Wiley & Sons, Inc.

ensure constancy and safety in dose delivery. Most often, calibration involves a measurement of ionization, followed by calculations to estimate the dose at the location of measurement. Alternate methods of measuring dose have been described (e.g., calorimetry), but are not practical for routine use. Methods for measuring exposure are described in Chapter 5 and the relationship between exposure and dose is also discussed there. The procedures that must be used to calibrate radiation beams in standard practice are described in this chapter. In order to discuss these procedures, first the role of calibration standards and laboratories must be discussed and several other terms need to be defined.

Calibration standards and laboratories

Many of the ionization measurement procedures described in Chapter 5 require knowledge of the mass of air inside an ionization chamber. Determination of the exact mass of air inside the collecting volume of a thimble chamber is beyond the capabilities of a practicing physicist. Instead, the instrument is submitted to a calibration laboratory where its response is determined in relation to one or more radiation quantities. This relationship is called a *calibration coefficient*. In the United States, instruments are calibrated by accredited dosimetry calibration laboratories (ADCLs).[1] The American Association of Physicists in Medicine (AAPM) supervises the promulgation of dosimetry standards in the United States. The ADCLs calibrate radiation dosimetry instruments primarily for medical physicists working in the United States. Elsewhere in the world, a network of secondary standard dosimetry laboratories (SSDLs) provides a similar function. The SSDLs are supervised by the International Atomic Energy Agency (IAEA), headquartered in Vienna, Austria.

An ADCL provides the practicing physicist with the ratio of the known exposure, air kerma, or dose at the location of the chamber (with the chamber removed from the beam) to the response of the chamber in Coulombs. The *air-kerma calibration coefficient*, N_k, is the ratio of the air kerma at the location of the chamber to the chamber signal. Likewise, the ratio of exposure at the location of the chamber to the chamber signal is termed the *exposure calibration coefficient*, N_X. When the instrument is placed in the customer's beam, the product of chamber signal, in Coulombs, and the coefficient N_X, yields the exposure at the location of measurement. However, the user must specify the energy or quality of the beam in which the calibration is to be performed. ADCLs generally provide chamber calibrations in x-ray beams with half-value layers (HVLs) from about 0.1 mm Al to 3 mm Cu, as well as in ^{60}Co γ-ray beams. Calibrations are not provided in accelerator-produced x-ray or electron beams because of the expense and impracticality of maintaining modern linear accelerators at the National Institute of Standards and Technology (NIST), formerly the National Bureau of Standards, and at the ADCLs. Instead, calibration

protocols provide mathematical corrections to account for the change in ionization chamber response with energy. The ADCLs possess ionization chambers that are periodically submitted for calibration by the NIST. The NIST maintains the U.S. dosimetry standards and is therefore the U.S. primary standard dosimetry laboratory (PSDL). Most developed countries have a PSDL, and these trace their dosimetry standards to the Bureau International des Poids et Mesures (BIPM), located in Paris, France. Accredited dosimetry calibration laboratories must also participate in periodic *measurement quality assurance* (MQA) tests to verify constancy of calibrations. The NIST-calibrated instruments are used to calibrate x- and γ-ray beams at the ADCL under carefully controlled conditions. The instruments submitted by clinical medical physicists are placed in the same beams and calibration coefficients are thus derived. The customers' instruments are said to be *directly traceable* to NIST because they are no more than one step removed from a NIST calibration. Again, *directly traceable* means that an instrument has been calibrated at NIST or an ADCL and then it follows that *indirectly traceable* means that an instrument has been calibrated by comparison with an instrument having a directly traceable calibration coefficient.

NIST has adopted terminology in general use throughout the world.[2] The term *calibration coefficient* is used for parameters with dimensions such as Gy/C, whereas a *calibration factor* is dimensionless. A calibration factor would be used to correct an instrument reading that is already in desired units, such as cGy.

Example 6-1

An ion chamber has an exposure calibration coefficient N_X of 4.0×10^9 R/C determined by an ADCL in a ^{60}Co beam. During exposure in air in the user's ^{60}Co beam, an electrometer connected to the chamber records a signal of 1.5×10^{-8} C. What is the exposure in the beam at the location of the chamber?

Exposure $= 4.0 \times 10^9$ R/C $\cdot$ 1.5×10^{-8} C

Exposure $= 60.0$ R

ADCLs offer the choice of calibrating an ionization chamber by itself or together with an electrometer as a system. If only the chamber is to be calibrated, the calibration laboratory substitutes the customer's chamber for its own and uses the ADCL electrometer to obtain the reading. In this way, the calibration coefficient of the customer's chamber is determined by direct comparison with the ADCL instrument. If a chamber is submitted with an electrometer with which it is to be calibrated as a system, the ADCL may use the customer's electrometer to determine the chamber response. Alternatively, the ADCL may determine a calibration coefficient for the customer's electrometer independently. The *system calibration coefficient* may be reported in terms of exposure per unit electrometer reading, which often is described in *Röntgens*. Consequently, the calibration coefficient is dimensionless (and is called the *calibration factor*) or has the units R/reading. Obtaining a system calibration factor for an ion chamber and electrometer that are used together is convenient because only one factor needs to be obtained and documented. However, it also means that if either component fails or is damaged the system is not suitable for use as a system for calibration. By obtaining a calibration coefficient for each component, any calibrated chamber can be used with any calibrated electrometer.

The quality of calibrations at NIST and at the ADCLs is very high. Estimates of the calibration uncertainty introduced by these facilities indicate that a customer's instrument, such as a cable-connected ionization chamber of good quality, can be calibrated with an *overall uncertainty* of 1.5% (expressed at the 2 standard deviation level, or 95% confidence level).[3,4] The world's PSDLs work hard to ensure that their dosimetry standards are accurate and in good agreement. An international comparison, conducted by circulating a set of ionization chambers, revealed that each PSDL assigned calibration coefficients to the instruments that were within 0.5% of the mean value, and that most were within 0.2% of the mean.[5]

Calibration coefficient as a function of energy

As mentioned previously, the value of N_X or N_K for an ionization chamber generally varies with photon-beam energy and N_X for the user's beam might be determined by interpolation between the N_X values assigned by the ADCL. The N_X values for a representative ionization chamber are shown in Figure 6-1 as a function of HVL. In general, the calibration coefficient increases as the beam energy decreases, reflecting an increased attenuation of lower-energy radiation in the wall of the chamber. The *dose-to-water calibration coefficient*, $N_{D,w}$, is the ratio of the dose to water at the chamber location in a water phantom to the chamber

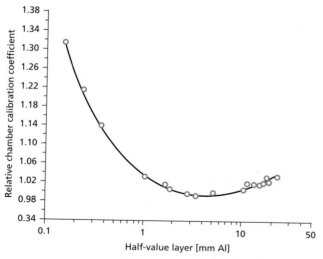

Figure 6-1 A graph of N_X as a function of photon-beam HVL. The data are for an Exradin A-2 chamber.

signal. However, $N_{D,w}$ is not determined at energies other than ^{60}Co at NIST or the ADCLs.

Estimation of dose to a medium from a calibration in air

Once the exposure calibration coefficient, N_X, for an ionization chamber is known for the beam energy to be measured, a measurement of exposure is straightforward, as described previously and also in Chapter 5. Calculation of dose from exposure at the location of measurement requires several additional steps. If, as is often the case, the chamber wall is made from an air-equivalent material such as graphite or air-equivalent plastic, the dose to the air in the chamber, or to the chamber wall material, is computed by multiplying the exposure in C/kg by the *work function*, the energy absorbed by air per unit ionization.

Work function

The determination of dose from a measurement of ionization is accomplished through knowledge of the energy absorbed by the air to produce the ionization. It is generally accepted that the *work function* (alternately known as the *W-quantity*), the average energy required to ionize dry air, has the value 33.97 eV/ion pair.[6,7] This does not mean that the binding energy for an electron in a typical air atom is 33.97 eV. Instead, it means that, on average, 33.97 eV are expended for every atom ionized. For each ion pair produced, several atoms are excited but not ionized.

For convenience, the work function can be described in SI units as 33.97 Joules (J)/Coulomb and the symbol $\overline{W}/e$ is used. When the total charge (in Coulombs) produced by ionization (of either sign) per unit mass of dry air is known, multiplying the value by $\overline{W}/e$ yields the energy absorbed by the medium in Joules. A small correction must be applied for laboratory air with about 50% humidity.[6] In this case, $\overline{W}/e = 33.77$ J/C. A humidity correction to N_X is applied by the ADCLs, so $\overline{W}/e = 33.97$ J/Coulomb should be used in calculations of the type described here. Of note, when exposures are expressed in units of Röntgens, the definition of the Röntgen, $k = 2.58 \times 10^{-4}$ C/kg · R, is needed. The product of $\overline{W}/e \cdot k$ is 0.876×10^{-2} J/kg · R.

Example 6-2

An ionization chamber filled with dry air records a charge of 1.5×10^{-8} Coulombs during irradiation with a 4 MV x-ray beam. How much energy was deposited in the air by the beam?

$$1.5 \times 10^{-8}\,\text{C} \cdot 33.97\,\text{J/C} = 5.10 \times 10^{-7}\,\text{J}$$

Dose to air

The special unit of absorbed dose is the Gray (Gy). A dose of 1 Gy corresponds to 1 J of energy absorbed per kilogram of medium.

The dose (in J/kg or Gy) absorbed by air is therefore determined as:

$$D_{air} = M \cdot N_X \cdot 0.876 \times 10^{-2} \, [\text{J/kg}]$$

where the product of the chamber reading, M, and the exposure calibration coefficient, N_X, yields the exposure, X, in air. When X is expressed in Röntgens, the dose to air is:

$$D_{air} = X \cdot 0.876 \times 10^{-2} \left[\frac{Gy}{R}\right] \tag{6-1}$$

ADCLs provide the calibration coefficient for an ionization chamber in terms of the air kerma, as well as the exposure. As discussed in Chapter 5, the term *air kerma* describes the energy transferred from the beam to the medium, without correction for energy reradiated from the local area of absorption.

Air kerma, K_{air}, is related to exposure, X, by:

$$K_{air} = \frac{x \cdot \overline{W}/e \cdot k}{(1-g)} \tag{6-2}$$

where g is a correction for energy dissipated as Bremsstrahlung outside the volume of interest. For ^{60}Co γ rays, the value of g is 0.003.[6] The air-kerma calibration coefficient, N_K, is the ratio of the air-kerma to the chamber signal. The air-kerma and exposure calibration coefficients are related by:

$$N_K = \frac{N_X \cdot \overline{W}/e \cdot k}{(1-g)}$$

Comparing the above formula with Equation (6-1) reveals that air kerma is closely related, but not equal, to the dose to air. The air-kerma calibration coefficient may not be substituted directly for the exposure calibration coefficient, and caution must be exercised when values of air kerma are available. ADCLs routinely provide the air-kerma calibration coefficient N_k for thimble and parallel-plate ionization chambers. However, N_k is not used in all calibration protocols recommended for use in the United States and a significant error would result if N_k were to be used inappropriately.

Example 6-3

An ionization chamber/electrometer system has a system calibration factor $N_X = 0.94$, determined in a beam of HVL = 0.5 mm Cu (effective energy = 55 keV). Following a 1-minute exposure in a beam of x rays of the same quality, the electrometer reads 213 R. What is the dose to air at the location of the chamber (when the chamber is removed)?

$$D_{air} = M \cdot N_X \cdot 0.876 \times 10^{-2} \, [\text{J/kg}]$$
$$D_{air} = 213 \, R \cdot 0.94 \cdot 2.58 \times 10^{-4} \, \text{C/kg-R}$$
$$\cdot 33.97 \, \text{J/C} \cdot 1 \, \text{Gy/J/kg}$$
$$D_{air} = 1.75 \, \text{Gy}$$

Dose to another medium

The dose to air is rarely of great interest. Instead, we usually wish to know the dose to tissue or tissue-equivalent material. As described in Chapter 5, the mass energy absorption coefficient $(\mu_{en})_m$ [also written (μ_{en}/ρ)] describes the rate at which energy is absorbed in an irradiated medium.[8] To determine the energy-absorption characteristics of a medium such as tissue, the ratio of its mass energy absorption coefficient to that of air may be determined at the energy of interest:

$$D_{tissue} = D_{air} \cdot \frac{(\mu_{en}/\rho) \, \text{tissue}}{(\mu_{en}/\rho) \, \text{air}} \tag{6-3}$$

This calculation yields the dose to an infinitesimal mass of tissue suspended in air at the location of the ionization chamber with the chamber removed. The mass of tissue must be only large enough to provide electron equilibrium. For convenience, the ratio in Equation (6-3) is often written $(\mu_{en}/\rho)_{air}^{tissue}$. A correction, A_{eq}, must be included to correct for attenuation of photons in the equilibrium thickness of the chamber wall. Values of A_{eq} vary from unity for photons less than 400 keV to 0.985 for ^{60}Co γ rays.

Combining equations (6-1) and (6-3) yields:

$$D_{tissue} = X \cdot 0.876 \times 10^{-2} \frac{Gy}{R} \cdot (\mu_{en}/\rho)_{air}^{tissue} \cdot A_{eq} \tag{6-4}$$

The product of 2.58×10^{-4} C/kg-R $\cdot$ 33.97 J/C $\cdot (\mu_{en}/\rho)_{air}^{tissue} \cdot$ 100 has been named the *f-factor*; therefore, Equation (6-4) reduces to:

$$D_{tissue} = X \cdot f_{tissue} \cdot A_{eq} \tag{6-5}$$

When the *f-factor* is used, and exposure is expressed in R, the dose to tissue is expressed in cGy (rads). Values of absorption coefficients and *f-factors* are found in Table 6-1 and Table 6-2. However, use of Equation (6-5) is not recommended; instead, a calibration protocol such as one described later in this chapter should be used for the calibration of x- and γ-ray beams. Although the use of the *f*-factor for the calibration of therapeutic x- and γ-ray beams is not recommended, the principles described up to this point are important to establish the foundation for modern calibration procedures.

Example 6-4

Referring to Example 6-3, determine the dose to a small mass of muscle tissue in air at the location of the chamber.

The dose to muscle is determined from Equation (6-4) or (6-5):

$$D_{muscle} = X[R] \cdot 0.876 \times 10^{-2} \frac{Gy}{R} \cdot (\mu_{en}/\rho)_{air}^{muscle} \cdot A_{eq}$$
$$D_{muscle} = 213 \, R \cdot 0.94 \cdot 0.876 \times 10^{-2} \frac{Gy}{R} \cdot 1.068 \cdot 1.00$$
$$D_{muscle} = 1.87 \, \text{Gy}$$

Table 6-1 Photon mass attenuation coefficients, μ/ρ, and mass energy-absorption coefficients, μ_{en}/ρ, in m²/kg for energies 1 keV to 20 MeV.[a]

Photon Energy (eV)	Air, Dry Z = 7.78 ρ = 1.205 kg/m³(20°C) 3.006 × 10²⁶ e/kg		Water Z = 7.51 ρ = 1000 kg/m³ 3.343 × 10²⁶ e/kg		Muscle Z = 7.64 ρ = 1040 kg/m³ 3.312 × 10²⁶ e/kg	
	μ/ρ	μ_{en}/ρ	μ/ρ	μ_{en}/ρ	μ/ρ	μ_{en}/ρ
1.0 + 03	3.617 + 02	3.616 + 02	4.091 + 02	4.089 + 02	3.774 + 02	3.772 + 02
1.5 + 03	1.202 + 02	1.201 + 02	1.390 + 02	1.388 + 02	1.275 + 02	1.273 + 02
2.0 + 03	5.303 + 01	5.291 + 01	6.187 + 01	6.175 + 01	5.663 + 01	5.651 + 01
3.0 + 03	1.617 + 01	1.608 + 01	1.913 + 01	1.903 + 01	1.828 + 01	1.813 + 01
4.0 + 03	7.751 + 00	7.597 + 00	8.174 + 00	8.094 + 00	8.085 + 00	7.963 + 00
5.0 + 03	3.994 + 00	3.896 + 00	4.196 + 00	4.129 + 00	4.174 + 00	4.090 + 00
6.0 + 03	2.312 + 00	2.242 + 00	2.421 + 00	2.363 + 00	2.421 + 00	2.354 + 00
8.0 + 03	9.721 − 01	9.246 − 01	1.018 + 00	9.726 − 01	1.024 + 00	9.770 − 01
1.0 + 04	5.016 − 01	4.640 − 01	5.223 − 01	4.840 − 01	5.284 − 01	4.895 − 01
1.5 + 04	1.581 − 01	1.300 − 01	1.639 − 01	1.340 − 01	1.668 − 01	1.371 − 01
2.0 + 04	7.643 − 02	5.255 − 02	7.958 − 02	5.367 − 02	8.099 − 02	5.531 − 02
3.0 + 04	3.501 − 02	1.501 − 02	3.718 − 02	1.520 − 02	3.754 − 02	1.579 − 02
4.0 + 04	2.471 − 02	6.691 − 03	2.668 − 02	6.803 − 03	2.674 − 02	7.067 − 03
5.0 + 04	2.073 − 02	4.031 − 03	2.262 − 02	4.155 − 03	2.257 − 02	4.288 − 03
6.0 + 04	1.871 − 02	3.004 − 03	2.055 − 02	3.152 − 03	2.045 − 02	3.224 − 03
8.0 + 04	1.661 − 02	2.393 − 03	1.835 − 02	2.583 − 03	1.822 − 02	2.601 − 03
1.0 + 05	1.541 − 02	2.318 − 03	1.707 − 02	2.539 − 03	1.693 − 02	2.538 − 03
1.5 + 05	1.356 − 02	2.494 − 03	1.504 − 02	2.762 − 03	1.491 − 02	2.743 − 03
2.0 + 05	1.234 − 02	2.672 − 03	1.370 − 02	2.966 − 03	1.358 − 02	2.942 − 03
3.0 + 05	1.068 − 02	2.872 − 03	1.187 − 02	3.192 − 03	1.176 − 02	3.164 − 03
4.0 + 05	9.548 − 03	2.949 − 03	1.061 − 02	3.279 − 03	1.052 − 02	3.250 − 03
5.0 + 05	8.712 − 03	2.966 − 03	9.687 − 03	3.299 − 03	9.599 − 03	3.269 − 03
6.0 + 05	8.056 − 03	2.953 − 03	8.957 − 03	3.284 − 03	8.876 − 03	3.254 − 03
8.0 + 05	7.075 − 03	2.882 − 03	7.866 − 03	3.205 − 03	7.795 − 03	3.176 − 03
1.0 + 06	6.359 − 03	2.787 − 03	7.070 − 03	3.100 − 03	7.006 − 03	3.072 − 03
1.5 + 06	5.176 − 03	2.545 − 03	5.755 − 03	2.831 − 03	5.702 − 03	2.805 − 03
2.0 + 06	4.447 − 03	2.342 − 03	4.940 − 03	2.604 − 03	4.895 − 03	2.580 − 03
3.0 + 06	3.581 − 03	2.054 − 03	3.969 − 03	2.278 − 03	3.932 − 03	2.257 − 03
4.0 + 06	3.079 − 03	1.866 − 03	3.403 − 03	2.063 − 03	3.370 − 03	2.043 − 03
5.0 + 06	2.751 − 03	1.737 − 03	3.031 − 03	1.913 − 03	3.001 − 03	1.894 − 03
6.0 + 06	2.523 − 03	1.644 − 03	2.771 − 03	1.804 − 03	2.743 − 03	1.785 − 03
8.0 + 06	2.225 − 03	1.521 − 03	2.429 − 03	1.657 − 03	2.403 − 03	1.639 − 03
1.0 + 07	2.045 − 03	1.446 − 03	2.219 − 03	1.566 − 03	2.195 − 03	1.548 − 03
1.5 + 07	1.810 − 03	1.349 − 03	1.941 − 03	1.442 − 03	1.918 − 03	1.424 − 03
2.0 + 07	1.705 − 03	1.308 − 03	1.813 − 03	1.386 − 03	1.790 − 03	1.367 − 03

Photon Energy (eV)	Fat Z = 6.46 ρ = 920 kg/m³ 3.192 × 10²⁶ e/kg		Bone Z = 12.31 ρ = 1850 kg/m³ 3.192 × 10²⁶ e/kg		Polystyrene Z = 5.74 ρ = 1046 kg/m³ 3.238 × 10²⁶ e/kg	
	μ/ρ	μ_{en}/ρ	μ/ρ	μ_{en}/ρ	μ/ρ	μ_{en}/ρ
1.0 + 03	2.517 + 02	2.516 + 02	3.394 + 02	3.392 + 02	2.047 + 02	2.046 + 02
1.5 + 03	8.066 + 01	8.055 + 01	1.148 + 02	1.146 + 02	6.227 + 01	6.219 + 01
2.0 + 03	3.535 + 01	3.526 + 01	5.148 + 01	5.133 + 01	2.692 + 01	2.683 + 01
3.0 + 03	1.100 + 01	1.090 + 01	2.347 + 01	2.303 + 01	8.041 + 00	7.976 + 00
4.0 + 03	4.691 + 00	4.621 + 00	1.045 + 01	1.025 + 01	3.364 + 00	3.312 + 00
5.0 + 03	2.401 + 00	2.345 + 00	1.335 + 01	1.227 + 01	1.704 + 00	1.659 + 00
6.0 + 03	1.386 + 00	1.338 + 00	8.129 + 00	7.531 + 00	9.783 − 01	9.375 − 01
8.0 + 03	5.853 − 01	5.474 − 01	3.676 + 00	3.435 + 00	4.110 − 01	3.773 − 01
1.0 + 04	3.048 − 01	2.716 − 01	1.966 + 00	1.841 + 00	2.150 − 01	1.849 − 01
1.5 + 04	1.022 − 01	7.499 − 02	6.243 − 01	5.726 − 01	7.551 − 02	5.014 − 02
2.0 + 04	5.437 − 02	3.014 − 02	2.797 − 01	2.450 − 01	4.290 − 02	2.002 − 02
3.0 + 04	3.004 − 02	8.881 − 03	9.724 − 02	7.290 − 02	2.621 − 02	6.059 − 03
4.0 + 04	2.377 − 02	4.344 − 03	5.168 − 02	3.088 − 02	2.177 − 02	3.191 − 03
5.0 ± 04	2.118 − 02	2.980 − 03	3.504 − 02	1.625 − 02	1.982 − 02	2.387 − 03

(continued)

Table 6-1 (*Continued*)

Photon Energy (eV)	Fat Z = 6.46 ρ = 920 kg/m³ 3.192 × 10²⁶ e/kg		Bone Z = 12.31 ρ = 1850 kg/m³ 3.192 × 10²⁶ e/kg		Polystyrene Z = 5.74 ρ = 1046 kg/m³ 3.238 × 10²⁶ e/kg	
	μ/ρ	μ_{en}/ρ	μ/ρ	μ_{en}/ρ	μ/ρ	μ_{en}/ρ
6.0 + 04	1.974 − 02	2.514 − 03	2.741 − 02	9.988 − 03	1.868 − 02	2.153 − 03
8.0 + 04	1.805 − 02	2.344 − 03	2.083 − 02	5.309 − 03	1.724 − 02	2.152 − 03
1.0 + 05	1.694 − 02	2.434 − 03	1.800 − 02	3.838 − 03	1.624 − 02	2.293 − 03
1.5 ± 05	1.506 − 02	2.747 − 03	1.490 − 02	3.032 − 03	1.448 − 02	2.631 − 03
2.0 + 05	1.374 − 02	2.972 − 03	1.332 − 02	2.994 − 03	1.322 − 02	2.856 − 03
3.0 + 05	1.192 − 02	3.209 − 03	1.141 − 02	3.095 − 03	1.147 − 02	3.088 − 03
4.0 + 05	1.067 − 02	3.298 − 03	1.018 − 02	3.151 − 03	1.027 − 02	3.174 − 03
5.0 + 05	9.740 − 03	3.318 − 03	9.274 − 03	3.159 − 03	9.376 − 03	3.194 − 03
6.0 + 05	9.008 − 03	3.304 − 03	8.570 − 03	3.140 − 03	8.672 − 03	3.181 − 03
8.0 + 05	7.912 − 03	3.226 − 03	7.520 − 03	3.061 − 03	7.617 − 03	3.106 − 03
1.0 + 06	7.112 − 03	3.121 − 03	6.758 − 03	2.959 − 03	6.847 − 03	3.005 − 03
1.5 + 06	5.787 − 03	2.850 − 03	5.501 − 03	2.700 − 03	5.571 − 03	2.744 − 03
2.0 + 06	4.963 − 03	2.619 − 03	4.732 − 03	2.487 − 03	4.778 − 03	2.522 − 03
3.0 + 06	3.972 − 03	2.282 − 03	3.826 − 03	2.191 − 03	3.822 − 03	2.196 − 03
4.0 + 06	3.390 − 03	2.055 − 03	3.307 − 03	2.002 − 03	3.261 − 03	1.977 − 03
5.0 + 06	3.005 − 03	1.894 − 03	2.970 − 03	1.874 − 03	2.889 − 03	1.820 − 03
6.0 + 06	2.732 − 03	1.775 − 03	2.738 − 03	1.784 − 03	2.626 − 03	1.706 − 03
8.0 + 06	2.371 − 03	1.613 − 03	2.440 − 03	1.667 − 03	2.227 − 03	1.548 − 03
1.0 + 07	2.147 − 03	1.508 − 03	2.263 − 03	1.598 − 03	2.060 − 03	1.446 − 03
1.5 + 07	1.840 − 03	1.361 − 03	2.040 − 03	1.508 − 03	1.763 − 03	1.304 − 03
2.0 + 07	1.693 − 03	1.290 − 03	1.948 − 03	1.474 − 03	1.620 − 03	1.234 − 03

[a]Multiply m²/kg by 10 to convert to cm²/g. The numbers following + or − refer to the power of 10; for example, 3.617 + 02 should be read as 3.617 × 10². *Source:* Hubbell 1982.[9] Reproduced with permission from Elsevier.

Table 6-2 Exposure-to-dose conversion factors.

Energy (keV)	F-Factors				
	Water	Muscle	Bone	Fat	Polystyrene
10	0.914	0.925	3.477	0.513	0.349
15	0.903	0.924	3.860	0.506	0.338
20	0.895	0.922	4.086	0.503	0.334
30	0.888	0.922	4.257	0.519	0.354
40	0.891	0.926	4.045	0.569	0.418
50	0.903	0.932	3.533	0.648	0.519
60	0.920	0.941	2.914	0.733	0.628
80	0.946	0.953	1.944	0.858	0.788
100	0.960	0.960	1.451	0.920	0.867
150	0.971	0.964	1.065	0.965	0.925
200	0.973	0.965	0.982	0.975	0.934
300	0.974	0.966	0.944	0.979	0.942
400	0.975	0.966	0.936	0.980	0.943
500	0.975	0.966	0.933	0.980	0.944
600	0.975	0.966	0.932	0.981	0.944
800	0.975	0.966	0.931	0.981	0.945
1000	0.975	0.966	0.931	0.981	0.945
1500	0.945	0.966	0.930	0.981	0.945
2000	0.974	0.965	0.931	0.980	0.944
3000	0.972	0.963	0.935	0.974	0.937

Alternatively:

$$D_{tissue} = X[R] \cdot f_{tissue} \cdot A_{eq}$$
$$D_{tissue} = 213 \cdot 0.94 \cdot 0.936 \cdot 1.00$$
$$D_{muscle} = 1.87 \, \text{cGy} = 1.87 \, \text{Gy}$$

Measurement in a phantom

Modern calibration protocols recommend that calibrations of megavoltage beams be performed in water rather than in air.[10–13] This practice reduces the risk that scatter from the collimator or devices in the beam might influence the measurement. At low photon energies (below about 400 kVp), procedures for measurement in air, similar to those described above, are generally used. At higher energies, however, the chamber is placed in the phantom at the desired depth and with its long axis oriented perpendicular to the beam (Figure 6-2). This is because water is readily available, practical, and does not vary in composition. Water-equivalent and tissue-equivalent plastics, on the other hand, are generally expensive and may vary in composition from one manufacturer or batch to another. Plastic

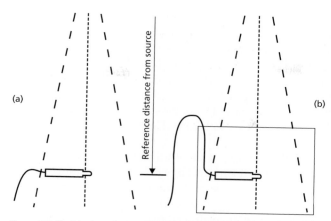

Figure 6-2 Positioning of an ionization chamber, in air (a) and in a water phantom (b), for measurements of absorbed dose.

Table 6-3 X-ray beam qualities for low energies.

Beam Code	kVp	First HVL (mm Al)	First HVL (mm Cu)	Homogeneity Coefficient (Al)
L40	40	0.50	—	0.59
L50	50	0.76	—	0.60
L80	80	1.83	—	0.57
L100	100	2.77	—	0.57
M20	20	0.15	—	0.69
M30	30	0.36	—	0.65
M40	40	0.73	—	0.69
M50	50	1.02	—	0.66
M60	60	1.68	—	0.66
M80	80	2.97	—	0.67
M100	100	5.02	—	0.73
M120	120	6.79	—	0.77
M150	150	10.2	0.67	0.87
M200	200	14.9	1.69	0.95
M250	250	18.5	3.2	0.98
M300	300	22.0	5.3	1.00

phantoms are permitted for routine beam output checks because one is only concerned with constancy in this case and plastic phantoms are convenient to use.

Most often, a depth of 2 cm to 10 cm is used. This procedure yields the dose to tissue or tissue-equivalent material that is immersed in a large volume of the same material. $f_{med} = 0.876 \frac{(\mu_{en}/\rho)\,med}{(\mu_{en}/\rho)\,air}$ for several materials expressed in [cGy/R].

Calibration of low-energy x-ray beams

Calibration procedures for low-energy x-ray beams (those from superficial and orthovoltage x-ray generators) are relatively straightforward. In part, this is because instruments used for calibration can be compared with other calibrated instruments in beams whose energies are comparable to the beam to be calibrated. A calibration procedure recommended by the AAPM states that calibrations should be performed with instruments having air-kerma calibration coefficients directly traceable to NIST.[14]

The dose to a medium is then determined by:

$$D_{med} = M N_k (\mu_{en}/\rho)_{air}^{med} \qquad (6\text{-}6)$$

where M is the instrument reading.

When the relationship between the exposure calibration coefficient and the air-kerma calibration coefficient is considered, it can be seen that Equation (6-6) is equivalent to Equation (6-4).

Beam quality

The instrument used to calibrate a low-energy x-ray beam should have a NIST-traceable calibration coefficient. It is recommended that instruments be calibrated over a range of x-ray energies spanning those of the beams to be calibrated. The HVL is generally used as a specification of beam quality.

However, HVL alone is insufficient because beams having considerably different spectra may have the same first HVL. Therefore, calibration laboratories provide exposure and air-kerma calibration coefficients as a function of HVL and kVp, to minimize this ambiguity. The *homogeneity coefficient* (HC) is the ratio of the first half-value layer to the second half-value layer and is a measure of the homogeneity of the energy spectrum of the beam. An HC with a value close to 1.00 indicates that the beam has a spectrum that is nearly monoenergetic.

A listing of x-ray beam qualities provided by NIST and the ADCLs for calibration at low-energies is shown in Table 6-3.

Ionization chamber

The instrument used for low energy x-ray calibration should be chosen carefully. In general, air-filled ionization chambers are used for reference dosimetry in such beams. Cylindrical ionization chambers are the most commonly used; however, parallel-plate chambers with thin entrance windows are recommended for x-ray beams generated at tube potentials below 70 kV. When thin-window parallel-plate chambers are employed, it may be necessary to add thin plastic foils, or plates, to the entrance window in order to remove electron contamination and provide full buildup. The total wall thickness required to provide full buildup and eliminate electron contamination when using thin-window parallel-plate chambers is shown in Table 6-4.

In addition to instrument characteristic corrections, as described earlier, ionization chambers must also be corrected for environmental conditions. The final corrected reading is the product of the individual correction factors and takes the form:

$$M = M_{raw} \cdot P_{tp} \cdot P_{ion} \cdot P_{pol} \cdot P_{elec} \qquad (6\text{-}7)$$

where M_{raw} is the ionization reading obtained with the ionization chamber. M_{raw} is determined by dividing the electrometer

Table 6-4 Total wall thickness required to provide full buildup.

Tube Potential (kV)	Total Wall Thickness (mg cm^{-2})
40	3.0
50	4.0
60	5.5
70	7.3
80	9.1
90	11.2
100	13.4

reading by the exposure time. A correction for *end effect* may be needed if the output does not reach the steady-state value simultaneously with the starting of the timer and return to zero instantaneously when the timer turns off. The end effect, δt, may be determined by plotting the electrometer reading against exposure time for several different values of exposure time and extrapolating to zero reading. The end effect may also be measured by taking electrometer readings at two exposure times, and is given by:

$$\delta t = \frac{M_2 \Delta t_1 - M_1 \Delta t_2}{M_1 - M_2}$$

where M_1 and M_2 are the electrometer readings from exposure times Δt_1 and Δt_2, respectively.[15] P_{tp} is the correction for temperature and pressure, while P_{ion} is the correction for ion recombination. Some of the ions formed by the radiation recombine with ions of the opposite sign before reaching the collecting electrode and are not measured. Several procedures have been described to estimate the actual number of ions formed by taking measurements at two voltages.[16,17] The AAPM protocol recommends that measurements be made at the normal collecting voltage and at one-half that voltage. The measured values are then compared using an expression that, for continuous beams, such as those from an orthovoltage machine or a ^{60}Co unit, assumes a nonlinear relationship between P_{ion} and voltage. P_{ion} is thus:

$$P_{ion} = \frac{1 - (V_H/V_L)^2}{(M_{raw}^H/M_{raw}^L) - (V_H/V_L)^2}$$

where M_{raw}^H and M_{raw}^L are ionization readings taken with bias voltages V_H and V_L, respectively, and $V_L \leq 0.5\, V_H$. When measuring P_{ion}, care should be taken to allow sufficient time for the instrument to stabilize at each bias voltage. It is not generally necessary to measure P_{ion} each time a beam is calibrated; it is better to measure it very carefully at the time of annual calibration.

For pulsed beams, such as those from a linear accelerator, and for values of $P_{ion} < 1.05$, P_{ion} varies linearly with voltage ratio. The appropriate expression is:

$$P_{ion} = \frac{1 - (V_H/V_L)}{\left(M\frac{H}{raw}/M\frac{L}{raw}\right) - V_H/V_L}$$

P_{ion} has also been fitted to a polynomial expression for several ratios of V_H/V_L.[18] It should be noted that P_{ion} and A_{ion} (recombination measured by an ADCL) are determined under different conditions and will not have the same value. In addition, P_{ion} is a *correction* for collection efficiency and is therefore always greater than 1. If an ion chamber exhibits P_{ion} greater than 1.05, the uncertainty of the measurement becomes unacceptably large, and another ion chamber, with P_{ion} closer to 1.0, should be used.

P_{pol} is to be used if the instrument was calibrated by the ADCL using a different polarity of bias from that used to calibrate the user's x-ray beam. This is usually not the case with low-energy x rays, and P_{pol} is generally equal to 1.0. P_{elec} is the electrometer calibration coefficient, as determined by the calibration laboratory.

Example 6-5

Ionization measurements are made in an orthovoltage beam. With a bias voltage of 300 V the reading is 1.875×10^{-8} C/min, but when the bias is reduced to 150 V the reading decreases to 1.865×10^{-8} C/min. What is the ionization recombination correction factor?

For a continuous beam, the nonlinear form of the expression must be used:

$$P_{ion} = \frac{1 - (V_H/V_L)^2}{\left(M\frac{H}{raw}/M\frac{L}{raw}\right) - (V_H/V_L)^2}$$

$$P_{ion} = \frac{1 - (2)^2}{(1.875/1.865) - (2)^2}$$

$$P_{ion} = 1.002$$

In-air calibrations

The AAPM recommends that low-energy x-ray beams be calibrated in air (see Figure 6-2). This recommendation is consistent with historical practice and represents a practical and straightforward approach to calibration. Equation (6-6) can then be used to determine the dose to an infinitesimal volume of medium suspended in air. Equation (6-6) must be modified slightly to permit determination of the dose at the surface of a phantom or patient. Regardless of whether a cylindrical or parallel plate ionization chamber is used, the AAPM protocol stipulates that the effective point of measurement is the center of the air cavity of the ionization chamber. Therefore, when calibrating a low-energy x-ray beam, the center of the ionization chamber air volume must be placed at the point of interest. This is normally the nominal treatment distance, which may also be at the end of a treatment cone. If it is not possible to position the ionization chamber at the intended reference point, an inverse-square correction may be made from the point of measurement to the reference point. When this is done, it is necessary to recognize that the inverse-square variation in beam intensity may be influenced by scattering from the cone and may not correspond to the actual distance from the x-ray target to the point of measurement.

The dose determined from a measurement of ionization in air is:

$$D_{w,0} = MN_k\,\text{BSF}\,P_{\text{stem}}(\mu_{en}/\rho)_{\text{air}}^{W} \qquad (6\text{-}8)$$

where $D_{w,0}$ is the dose to water at the surface of a phantom. M is determined according to Equation (6-7). BSF is the *backscatter factor* for the beam quality being calibrated and relates the dose at the surface of a medium to the dose to a small mass of medium suspended in air (see Chapter 7). The parameter, P_{stem}, is applied if the field size being calibrated is different from the field size in which the instrument itself was calibrated. The change in field size results in a different length of chamber stem or cable being irradiated, which may change the response of the instrument. The determination of stem correction factors is discussed in Chapter 5. The ratio of energy absorption coefficients is used to relate the dose in water to the dose determined in air at the location of the instrument. This ratio must be chosen from Table 6-1 for the energy spectrum of the beam being calibrated at the position of the ionization chamber in air. Note that Equation (6-8), in accordance with the AAPM protocol, determines the dose to water at the surface of a water phantom. The dose to tissue may be determined by substituting the energy absorption coefficient ratios for tissue and air in Equation (6-8).

In-phantom calibrations

The AAPM protocol recommends that, as an alternative, calibrations may be performed in a water phantom for beam energies > 100 kV. The recommended calibration depth is 2 cm. As indicated in Figure 6-2, the center of the ionization chamber collecting volume should be placed at 2 cm depth in the water phantom.

It is recommended that a 10 × 10 cm field be used for calibrations in a water phantom.

Under these conditions, the dose to water at 2 cm depth is:

$$D_{w,2} = MN_k P_{chbrl}^{Q} P_{\text{sheath}}(\mu_{en}/\rho)_{\text{air}}^{W} \qquad (6\text{-}9)$$

where $D_{w,2}$ is the dose at 2 cm depth in the water phantom. P_{chbrl}^{Q} is a chamber correction factor that accounts for displacement of water by the ionization chamber and the chamber stem, as well as the effects of changes in energy spectrum and angular distribution of the photon beam in the phantom compared to calibration of the chamber in air.[19] Values of P_{chbrl}^{Q} are given in Table 6-5. P_{sheath} is a correction for photon absorption and scattering in a waterproof sleeve, if used. The ratio of mass energy absorption coefficients must be chosen for the energy spectrum of the beam at the position of the ionization chamber in the water phantom. This may be different from the value that will be used for an in-air calibration of the same beam.

Calibration of megavoltage beams: The AAPM protocol

The clinical implementation of any protocol, including TG51, is a complicated procedure and deviations in beam calibrations can exist. Confusion can arise when determining appropriate calibration factors and correction factors (e.g., P_{ion}, P_{pol}) with various ion chambers.[20] Extreme care needs to be taken when calibrating the output of a linear accelerator, and this type of work should not be done at off-clinical hours such as late in the evening.

Calibration of megavoltage radiation beams involves the application of a ^{60}Co calibration coefficient to measurements in photon or electron beams of higher energies. In materials from which ionization chambers are constructed, high-energy radiations interact differently from ^{60}Co γ rays and corrections are

Table 6-5 Correction factor, P_{chbrl}^{Q} for several common chamber models and beam qualities.[19]

HVL (mm Cu)	NE2571	Capintec PR06C	PTW N30001	Exradin A12	NE2611	NE2581 or NE2561
0.10	1.008	0.992	1.004	1.002	0.991	0.995
0.15	1.015	1.000	1.013	1.009	1.007	1.007
0.20	1.019	1.004	1.017	1.013	1.017	1.012
0.30	1.023	1.008	1.021	1.016	1.028	1.017
0.40	1.025	1.009	1.023	1.017	1.033	1.019
0.50	1.025	1.010	1.023	1.017	1.036	1.019
0.60	1.025	1.010	1.023	1.017	1.037	1.019
0.80	1.024	1.010	1.022	1.017	1.037	1.018
1.0	1.023	1.010	1.021	1.016	1.035	1.017
1.5	1.019	1.008	1.018	1.013	1.028	1.014
2.0	1.016	1.007	1.015	1.011	1.022	1.011
2.5	1.012	1.006	1.012	1.010	1.017	1.009
3.0	1.009	1.005	1.010	1.008	1.012	1.006
4.0	1.004	1.003	1.006	1.005	1.004	1.003

required to determine the dose accurately. In 1971, the AAPM Subcommittee on Radiation Dosimetry (SCRAD) published a protocol describing procedures for calibrating photon and electron beams.[21] The protocol recommended the use of factors called C_λ (for photons) and C_E (for electrons) in place of the *f-factor* and A_{eq} used in Equation (6-4). The SCRAD protocol has since been superseded and is no longer in widespread use. In 1983, AAPM Task Group 21 published a protocol that enjoyed widespread use within the United States.[11] However, in 1999, it was replaced by a protocol written by AAPM Task Group 51.[10] This is the current AAPM recommendation for calibration and the TG51 protocol is described below.

Calibration of photon beams versus electron beams

Previous texts have addressed the calibration of high-energy photon beams separately from the calibration of electron beams. This was because the procedures for calibration were different. However, recent protocols for megavoltage calibrations address both photons and electrons, and the procedures are essentially identical. Therefore, this text addresses both together.

Calibration with an ionization chamber in a medium

When high-energy photons interact in a medium, they set in motion high-speed *primary* electrons (Figure 6-3). These electrons ionize the surrounding medium and generate *secondary* electrons. On the other hand, when a phantom is irradiated with an electron beam, the incident electrons may be considered the primary electrons. The electrons ionize the medium at a much higher rate than do the photons. In fact, the contribution of photons to the ion pairs produced in the air inside an ion chamber may be neglected. It is customary to think of the photons as interacting only outside the chamber, in the medium surrounding the chamber, or in the wall of the chamber itself. The electrons set in motion by these interactions penetrate the ion chamber's air volume and produce the ionization that is measured (Figure 6-4).

Dose to water from a measurement of ionization

For calibrating megavoltage beams of radiation, the point of interest is generally located within a water phantom. The measurement is made with an ion chamber immersed in the phantom. A first step in the use of the Bragg–Gray relationship is to determine the dose to the air inside the chamber. As discussed in Chapter 5, the Bragg–Gray relationship requires that several assumptions be satisfied. First, the cavity (the ionization chamber) must be sufficiently small to have a negligible influence on the electron energy spectrum and fluence at the point of

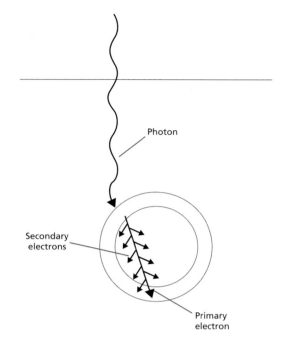

Figure 6-3 The interactions of photons and electrons in the materials surrounding the air cavity of an ionization chamber.

measurement. Second, the wall of the chamber must be constructed of material effectively identical to the medium (i.e., having the same effective atomic number), or it must be sufficiently thin that an insignificant number of photon interactions take

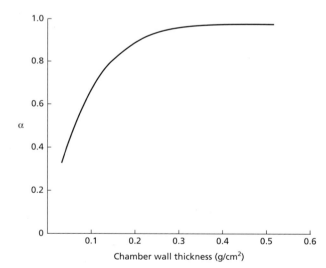

Figure 6-4 When determining the characteristics of specific ionization chambers, the spectrum of electrons passing through the air volume is important. This figure shows the fraction of electrons depositing energy in the sensitive volume of the chamber that arise in the chamber wall, during irradiation with ^{60}Co γ rays. The remaining electrons originate in the phantom material outside the chamber.
Source: Schulz et al. 1983.[11] Reproduced with permission from American Association of Physicists in Medicine.

place in the wall. A third important assumption is that the energy of a secondary electron must be deposited at the site of origin.

Few ionization chambers in use fulfill these criteria exactly (Table 6-6). To enable the collection of enough ion pairs to create a measurable signal, the chamber's collecting volume must be of at least modest size. Volumes of 0.1 to 1.0 cm³ are most common. However, the diameter of a cylindrical chamber should not exceed 1 cm. The wall thickness must be sufficiently robust for mechanical rigidity and to withstand handling. The wall material is often graphite, nylon, or a plastic, such as A-150 (a tissue-equivalent plastic) or C-552 (an air-equivalent plastic). The phantoms used by most physicists are composed either of water, polystyrene, or a water-equivalent plastic, and therefore the chamber wall is unlikely to be identical to the phantom material. Consequently, the fluence of electrons passing through the chamber is not identical to the fluence that occurs in the absence of the chamber and corrections must be applied. Finally, secondary electrons generated inside the air cavity may have sufficient energy to escape the cavity and deposit some of their energy in the medium. This has the effect of reducing the energy absorbed by the air in the chamber.

These failures of the chamber to meet the Bragg–Gray criteria mean that the Bragg–Gray relationship, $D_{medium} = D_{gas} \cdot (\bar{s}/\rho)_{gas}^{medium}$, cannot be used without modification. The AAPM protocol relies on the Spencer–Attix cavity theory,[22] which can be expressed:

$$D_{medium} = D_{gas} \cdot (\bar{L}/\rho)_{gas}^{medium} \qquad (6\text{-}10)$$

where $(\bar{L}/\rho)_{gas}^{medium}$ represents the restricted mean mass collisional stopping power averaged over the electron slowing-down spectrum in the wall material. Values of $\bar{L}/\rho$ are provided in Table 6-7. The electron slowing-down spectrum includes primary and secondary electrons with a spectrum of energies and the restricted stopping powers include only energy losses less than Δ. The formulation includes track-end corrections that account for secondary electrons that undergo inelastic collisions in which both ejected electrons have less than energy Δ. The cutoff energy is chosen to take account of the size of practical ionization chambers. Although the restricted stopping power is dependent on the choice of Δ, the Spencer–Attix cavity theory uses the ratio of restricted stopping powers, which is relatively insensitive to the choice of Δ.

The concept of restricted stopping powers is rather complicated. Consider a photon that interacts with an atom in a chamber wall, releasing an electron with several hundred keV of energy. This "primary" electron crosses the chamber air cavity and interacts multiple times with air atoms. If collisions with electrons result in the transfer of more than about 10 keV, the probability is high that the electron receiving the energy will also cross the cavity and deposit its energy in the chamber wall.

Because the energy lost in the interaction is carried out of the collecting volume, it is not measured. The probability of the interaction is not relevant when comparing the rate of local energy deposition in air to that in tissue. Therefore, only the stopping powers for interactions in which less than 10 keV (or another appropriate value, designated Δ) is transferred are considered when calculating mean restricted stopping powers.

Example 6-6

The dose to air in an ionization chamber irradiated by a 6 MV photon beam is determined to be 1 Gy. Calculate the dose to water replacing the air.

Using Equation (6-10), the dose to water is determined by multiplying the dose to air by the ratio of restricted mean mass collisional stopping powers (see Table 6-7):

$$D_{medium} = D_{gas} \cdot (\bar{L}\rho)_{gas}^{medium}$$
$$D_{medium} = 1\,\text{Gy} \cdot 1.127 = 1.127\,\text{Gy}$$

The AAPM protocol provides further corrections and procedures to account for other perturbations of the photon and electron fluence.

Dose to water calibration coefficient ($N_{D,w}$)

The AAPM calibration protocol is based upon the relationship between the dose to water at the location of the ionization chamber and the chamber's signal:

$$D_w^Q = M \cdot N_{D,w}^Q \qquad (6\text{-}11)$$

where D_w^Q is the dose to water at the point of measurement in a beam whose quality is Q. The dose to water calibration coefficient, $N_{D,w}^Q$ is determined by the calibration laboratory and is directly traceable to NIST. The corrected instrument signal M is determined as:

$$M = M_{raw} \cdot P_{tp} \cdot P_{ion} \cdot P_{pol} \cdot P_{elec} \qquad (6\text{-}7)$$

The parameters in Equation (6-7) have been described earlier. P_{ion} must be calculated using an appropriate expression for a continuous or pulsed beam (see Example 6-7). P_{pol} takes on greater significance for megavoltage calibrations as the chamber sensitivity may change with bias polarity. In this case, P_{pol} is calculated as:

$$P_{pol} = \left| \frac{M_{raw}^+ - M_{raw}^-}{2M_{raw}} \right|$$

where the superscript indicates the polarity of the charge being collected. The denominator includes either or M_{raw}^+ or M_{raw}^-, whichever polarity signal was be used for calibration. M_{raw}^+ and M_{raw}^- generally have opposite signs; these signs must be used when calculating P_{pol}. Measurement of P_{pol} is not necessary each time a beam is calibrated, but when measured, it must be done carefully with sufficient time allowed after changing the bias polarity for the instrument to stabilize. P_{pol} should be 1.0 ± 0.02 and values significantly different from unity most likely indicate an error in calculation.

Table 6-6 Physical characteristics of thimble ionization chambers commonly used for radiation therapy calibrations.

Chamber Manufacturer Description (Wall Material/Cap Material)	Thimble Wall Dimensions (cm)	Thimble Wall Dimensions (g/cm²)	Inner Axial[b] Length (cm)	Inner Diameter (cm)	Buildup Cap Thickness (cm)	Buildup Cap Thickness (g/cm²)	A_{wall}	α	$(L/\rho)_{air}^{wall} \cdot (\mu_{en}/\rho)_{wall}^{cap}$	$(L/\rho)_{air}^{wall} \cdot (\mu_{en}/\rho)_{wall}^{air}$	$N_{gas}/N_X A_{ion}$ (Gy/R)
Capintec PR-06C, PR-06G: 0.6 cm³ Farmer-type, with BC-06F cap (AE plastic/Polystyrene)	0.028	0.050	2.30	0.64	0.516	0.539	0.991	0.46	1.000	1.032	8.51×10^{-3}
Exradin Al Spokas: 0.5 cm³, tissue-equivalent, with 4 mm cap (TE plastic/TE plastic)	0.102	0.182	0.97	0.94	0.40	0.712	0.976	0.86	1.000	100	8.53×10^{-3}
Exradin T2 Spokas: 0.5 cm³, tissue-equivalent, with 4 mm cap (TE plastic/TE plastic)	0.102	0.115	0.97	0.94	0.40	0.450	0.985	0.73	1.037	1.037	8.30×10^{-3}
NEL 2505/3, 3B: 0.6 cm³ Farmer (since 1974), with 2507/3, 3A cap (Nylon 66/acrylic)	0.036	0.041	2.25	0.63	0.465	0.551	0.990	0.40	1.038	1.020	8.42×10^{-3}
NEL 2571 guarded: 0.6 cm³ Farmer (since 1979), with 2571 cap (graphite/Delrin)	0.036	0.065	2.25	0.63	0.387	0.551	0.990	0.54	1.009	1.019	8.54×10^{-3}
Nel 2581 robust: 0.6 cm³ Farmer (since 1980), with 2581 cap (TE plastic/Lucentine)	0.036	0.040	2.25	0.63	0.551	0.584	0.990	0.39	1.037	1.032	8.37×10^{-3}
PTW N23333: 0.6 cm³ Farmer-type, with NA30-387 cap (acrylic/acrylic)	0.045	0.053	2.19	0.61	0.465	0.551	0.990	0.48	1.020	1.020	8.48×10^{-3}

Table 6-7 Ratio of average, restricted collisional mass stopping powers for photon spectra, Δ = 10 keV.

Nominal Accelerating Potential (MV)	$(\bar{L}\rho)_{gas}^{medium}$							
	Water	Polystyrene	Acrylic	Graphite	A-150	C-552	Bakelite	Nylon
2	1.135	1.114	1.104	1.015	1.154	1.003	1.084	1.146
^{60}Co	1.134	1.113	1.103	1.012	1.151	1.000	1.081	1.142
4	1.131	1.108	1.099	1.007	1.146	0.996	1.075	1.136
6	1.127	1.103	1.093	1.002	1.141	0.992	1.070	1.129
8	1.121	1.097	1.088	0.995	1.135	0.987	1.063	1.120
10	1.117	1.094	1.085	0.992	1.130	0.983	1.060	1.114
15	1.106	1.083	1.074	0.982	1.119	0.972	1.051	1.097
20	1.096	1.074	1.065	0.977	1.109	0.963	1.042	1.087
25	1.093	1.071	1.062	0.968	1.106	0.960	1.038	1.084
35	1.084	1.062	1.053	0.958	1.098	0.952	1.027	1.074
45	1.071	1.048	1.041	0.939	1.087	0.942	1.006	1.061

Source: Cunningham and Schulz, 1984.[23] Reproduced with permission from American Association of Physicists in Medicine.

Example 6-7

The ionization recombination correction is determined in an accelerator beam in the manner described in Example 6-5. At 300 V, the reading is 1.624×10^{-8} C for an exposure of 100 MU, and at 150 V the reading is 1.615×10^{-8} C. What is P_{ion}?

For pulsed beams, the linear form of the equation is used:

$$P_{ion} = \frac{1 - (V_H/V_L)}{(M_{raw}^H/M_{raw}^L) - (V_H/V_L)}$$

$$P_{ion} = \frac{-1}{(1.624/1.615) - (2)}$$

$$P_{ion} = 1.002$$

Compare the ratio of ionization measurements with those given in Example 6-5.

The dose to water calibration coefficient, $N_{D,w}^Q$, must be appropriate for the beam energy, Q, being calibrated. However, it is rarely practical for calibration laboratories to attempt to provide calibrations over a range of megavoltage beam energies. Instead, NIST and the ADCLs provide dose to water calibration coefficients determined in a ^{60}Co beam. The ^{60}Co calibration coefficient is then related to the calibration coefficient at beam quality, Q, by a quality conversion factor, k_Q:

$$N_{D,w}^Q = N_{D,w}^{60Co} \cdot k_Q \qquad (6\text{-}12)$$

For x-ray beams, the quality conversion factor is a function of beam quality and varies smoothly over a small range for a wide variety of ionization chambers. The quality conversion factor may be calculated as the ratio of energy-dependent chamber characteristics for the user's beam energy and for ^{60}Co. Specifically:

$$k_Q = [(\bar{L}/\rho)_{air}^{water} \cdot P_{repl} \cdot P_{wall} \cdot P_{cel}]\frac{Q}{^{60}Co}$$

where P_{repl}, P_{wall}, and P_{cel} are the chamber's replacement correction, wall correction, and central electrode correction,

respectively. These parameters are defined in the AAPM TG21 calibration protocol.[11] Values of k_Q are provided in Table 6-8. It is possible to estimate a value for k_Q for a chamber that is not listed by selecting a listed chamber that has (1) the same wall material, (2) the same central electrode material, and (3) approximately the same wall thickness. In addition, the listed chamber should have a collecting volume with similar length and diameter as the user's instrument, although the dependence of k_Q on these parameters is weak.

Effective point of measurement

As discussed at the beginning of this chapter, the effective point of measurement of an ionization chamber used in air is considered to be its axis (see Figure 6-2). When used in a phantom, however, the effective point of measurement may move upstream from the axis of the chamber. As shown in Figure 6-5, a beam of electrons traveling along parallel paths strikes the wall of a cylindrical ion chamber at different distances upstream from the chamber center. Through an averaging procedure, the effective point of interaction can be found. In a phantom, scattering of electrons modifies the calculations. As a result, the AAPM[10,17] has recommended that the effective point of measurement be located 0.6 of the inner radius, r_{cav}, upstream from the chamber axis when measuring in megavoltage photon beams, and 0.5 r_{cav} for electron beams. Note that the correction for the location of the effective point of measurement is to be used only when determining relative depth doses. The correction is not to be applied during calibration measurements in either photon beams or electron beams.

The depth dose in low-energy ($\leq$ 6 MeV) electron beams changes rapidly. The use of a cylindrical ionization chamber for electron-beam measurements is not recommended by the AAPM because the size of the cavity of many chambers is large relative to the dose gradient.[10] Instead, the AAPM recommends the use of a parallel-plate chamber.

Table 6-8 Values of $k'_{R_{50}}$ R_{50} for selected values of R_{50} and a few commonly used ionization chambers.

R_{50} (cm)	Exradin A1, Capintec PR-05, Capintec PR-05P	NE 2505-3, -3A, 2571, 2577, 2581 Capintec PR-06C, -0G, PTW N30001	PTW N31003	Exradin A12, PTW N30002, N30004 Wellhofer IC 10/5	Exradin P11, Holt MPPK, PTB Roos, NACP	Markus PTW N23343	Capintec PS O33
2.0	1.039	1.033	1.035	1.032	1.055	1.041	1.016
2.5	1.032	1.027	1.030	1.026	1.047	1.036	1.014
3.0	1.027	1.022	1.025	1.021	1.040	1.032	1.012
3.5	1.022	1.018	1.020	1.017	1.034	1.028	1.011
4.0	1.018	1.015	1.017	1.013	1.028	1.024	1.010
4.5	1.015	1.012	1.014	1.011	1.023	1.020	1.009
5.0	1.012	1.010	1.011	1.009	1.019	1.016	1.008
5.5	1.009	1.007	1.008	1.006	1.012	1.013	1.006
6.0	1.007	1.005	1.006	1.005	1.011	1.010	1.005
6.5	1.004	1.003	1.003	1.003	1.007	1.006	1.004
7.0	1.002	1.001	1.001	1.002	1.003	1.003	1.001
7.5	1.000	1.000	1.000	1.000	1.000	1.000	1.000
8.0	0.998	0.999	0.999	0.999	0.997	0.997	0.998
8.5	0.996	0.997	0.997	0.998	0.994	0.994	0.996
9.0	0.994	0.996	0.995	0.996	0.991	0.992	0.994
9.5	0.992	0.994	0.993	0.994	0.988	0.990	0.992
10.0	0.990	0.993	0.992	0.993	0.986	0.988	0.990

As shown in Figure 6-5, the effective point of measurement of a parallel-plate chamber is at the inside surface of the entrance window when the chamber is used in a phantom. Therefore, no adjustment of depth and no calculation of P_{gr}^Q is required for parallel-plate chambers. An exposure or dose-to-water calibration coefficient assigned to a parallel-plate chamber by an ADCL is valuable for verifying the constancy of chamber response, and for satisfying state and federal regulations, but should not be used for calibration.

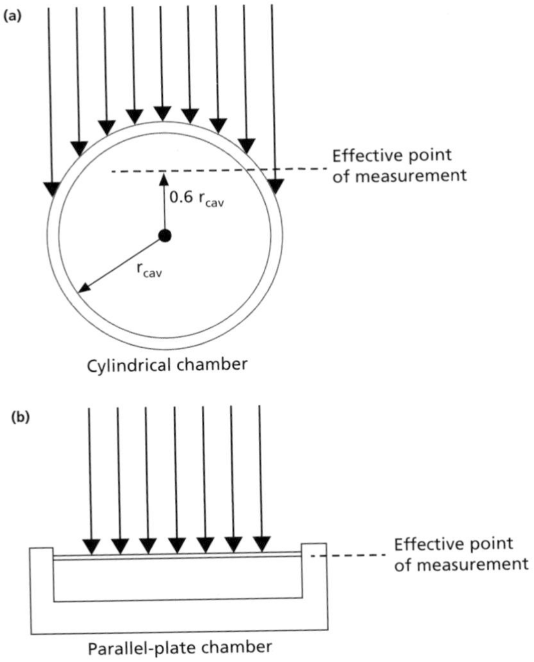

Figure 6-5 Location of the effective point for (a) a cylindrical ionization chamber and (b) a parallel-plate ionization chamber. Measurements were made with a cylindrical chamber.[10] Data were shifted upstream by 0.6 r_{cav} for photon beams (Figure 6-5a) and 0.5 r_{cav} for electron beams (Figure 6-5b). In both figures, curve I (dashed) indicates raw data while curve II (solid) indicates shifted data. The short-dashed line in the lower figure indicates percentage depth dose.
Source: Almond et al. 1999, by permission.[10]

Beam quality specification

For photon beams, the quality, Q, of the beam is determined from the percent depth dose (%D_n) at 10 cm depth in a 10 cm × 10 cm field. This is a departure from the earlier AAPM calibration protocol, and also from several international protocols, in which the beam quality is related to a ratio of percent depth dose values or tissue maximum ratios. The AAPM protocol recognizes that measurement of percent depth dose is complicated by the possibility that electron contamination will influence the measurements at the depth of maximum dose, d_{max}. Therefore, the AAPM protocol specifies that, at energies of 10 MV or above, the percent depth dose must be measured using a technique that removes contaminant electrons originating in the accelerator head and that introduces a known quantity of contaminant electrons for which mathematical corrections may be made. The procedure involves inserting a lead foil 1 mm in thickness into the beam and making measurements of percent depth dose at 100 cm SSD. Through a mathematical manipulation described below, the percent depth dose due to x rays alone, %$D(10)_X$, is determined. For x-ray energies below 10 MV, %$D(10)_X$ is simply the %D_n at 10 cm depth in a 10 cm × 10 cm field at 100 cm SSD. The values of k_Q that are reproduced in Table 6-6 are related to %$D(10)_X$.[24]

At x-ray energies above 10 MV, %$D(10)_x$ is determined from a measurement in water of %$D(10)_{Pb}$, made with a 1 mm thick lead foil in the beam. The field size must be 10 cm × 10 cm, the

SSD must be 100 cm, and the depth (corrected by 0.6 r_{cav}) must be 10 cm. The conversion from $\%D(10)_{Pb}$ to $\%D(10)_x$ depends on the location of the lead foil. If the lead foil is 50 cm $\pm$ 5 cm from the water phantom surface, then the conversion is:

$$\%D(10)_X = [0.8905 + 0.00150\%D(10)_{Pb}] \times \%D(10)_{Pb}$$

If the lead foil is at 30 cm $\pm$ 1 cm from the water phantom surface, then the conversion is:

$$\%D(10)_X = [0.8116 + 0.00264\%D(10)_{Pb}] \times \%D(10)_{Pb}$$

If the lead foil is not available, then $\%D(10)$ is measured and $\%D(10)_x$ is:

$$\%D(10)_X = [1.267\%D(10)] - 20.0.$$

When calculating $\%D(10)_x$ from $\%D(10)_{Pb}$, it is essential to use values of *percent* depth dose. The use of *fractional* depth dose will lead to large errors. $\%D(10)_x$ should be between 0 and 2.5% larger than $\%D(10)_{Pb}$.[25]

Example 6-8

Determine the beam quality, Q, for an x-ray beam of nominal energy 18 MV. A lead foil 1 mm thick is placed at 50 cm from the water surface, and ionization measurements are made at 100 cm SSD in a 10 cm $\times$ 10 cm field.

At the depth of maximum ionization, an exposure of 100 MU yields an electrometer reading of 1.901. At 10 cm depth (with the axis of the chamber positioned at 10 cm + 0.6 r_{cav}) the reading is 1.498.

Under these circumstances:

$$\%D(10)_X = [0.8905 + 0.00150\%D(10)_{Pb}]\,\%D(10)_{Pb}$$

where:

$$\%D(10)_{Pb} = 1.498/1.901 \times 100$$
$$= 78.8\%$$

Then:

$$\%D(10)_x = 79.5\%$$

For electron beams, k_Q is likewise related to the beam quality. Electron beam quality is characterized by a parameter, R_{50}, the depth at which the dose falls to 50% of the maximum dose. R_{50} is measured in a field large enough to provide full sidescatter. For $R_{50} \leq 8.5$ cm, a 10 cm $\times$ 10 cm field is used; for $R_{50} > 8.5$ cm, a 20 cm $\times$ 20 cm field is used. R_{50} is actually determined from a measurement of I_{50}, the depth at which the measured ionization falls to 50% of the maximum ionization value. If the ioniza-

tion is measured with a cylindrical chamber, the depth must be adjusted by 0.5 r_{cav}. For electron beams in which I_{50} is ≤ 10 cm, R_{50} is calculated as:

$$R_{50} = 1.029 \cdot I_{50} - 0.06$$

where R_{50} and I_{50} are expressed in cm.

The determination of k_Q for electron beams is addressed later in this chapter.

Calibration of photon beams

The dose to water in a photon beam is determined through a measurement of ionization under reference conditions. Reference conditions recommended by the AAPM protocol are at 10 cm depth in a 10 cm $\times$ 10 cm field. Calibration may be performed for either an SSD setup (nominally 100 cm to the surface of the water phantom) or a source–axis distance (SAD) set up (normally 90 cm from the source to the surface of the water phantom, so that the ionization chamber at 10 cm depth is positioned at the accelerator axis of rotation.) Under these circumstances, the dose to water D_W^Q at the position of measurement is determined by combining Equations (6-11) and (6-12):

$$D_W^Q = M \cdot N_{D,w}^{60Co} \cdot k_Q \qquad (6\text{-}13)$$

The parameters in Equation (6-12) have been defined earlier. Equation (6-13) yields the dose to water at the location of measurement. The AAPM protocol recommends that the measurement be transferred to d_{max} by dividing by the $\%D_n$ (or the tissue-maximum ratio (TMR) if calibration is performed at the isocenter). In this manner, the accelerator output is described in terms of cGy at d_{max} per MU. The $\%D_n$ used in this step must be the *clinical* $\%D(10)$, taken from data tables used for treatment planning. It should not be the $\%D(10)$ measured at the time of calibration and *must not* be $\%D(10)_x$ or $\%D(10)_{Pb}$. When calibrating a linear accelerator, it is customary to adjust the sensitivity of the monitor chamber to yield the desired dose rate. In most clinics, the output is adjusted to 1.000 cGy/MU at d_{max} in a 10 cm $\times$ 10 cm field at a distance from the source that is either at the isocenter or at a distance to the isocenter plus d_{max}. In some clinics, the calibrated dose rate determined in water is corrected to yield the dose rate in muscle. In an x-ray beam, this correction is $(\mu_{en}/\rho)_{water}^{muscle}$. Table 6-1 indicates that over the range of photon energies used in radiation therapy the correction is approximately 0.99.

Example 6-9

Determine k_Q for an Exradin model A-12 ionization chamber used in the x-ray beam described by Example 6-8.

In Example 6-8, $\%D(10)_x$ was determined to be 79.5%. Linear interpolation in Table 6-8 yields $k_Q = 0.975$.

Calibration of electron beams

The AAPM recommends that electron beams be calibrated at an energy-dependent reference depth. The choice of an energy-dependent reference depth for calibrating electron beams simplifies the protocol by permitting the use of stopping-power ratios computed as a function of R_{50}.[26] The reference depth, d_{ref}, may not be precisely at d_{max}, and a $\%D_n$ correction is made to relate the calibrated dose rate to d_{max}. d_{ref} is calculated from the electron beam quality as:

$$d_{ref} = 0.6\,R_{50} - 0.1\ cm$$

where R_{50} was described earlier. d_{ref} should be close to d_{max} for beam energies below 10 MeV, but will be deeper for higher energies.

As was the case with photon beams, the effective point of measurement of a cylindrical chamber is located upstream from the axis of the chamber. For electron beams, the AAPM recommends a shift of 0.5 r_{cav}. The shift in chamber depth is used only for measurements of relative ionization and not for calibrations or determination of other dosimetric parameters.

The determination of k_Q is slightly more complicated for electron beams than for x-ray beams. k_Q may be separated into a chamber-specific energy-dependent component, $k_{R_{50}}$, and for cylindrical chambers, a correction for gradient effects at the reference depth, P_{gr}^Q. Then:

$$k_Q = P_{gr}^Q . k_{R_{50}}$$

P_{gr}^Q is determined by the user at the time of calibration and is the ratio of ionization measurements made with the chamber axis at $(d_{ref} + 0.5\,r_{cav})$ and at d_{ref}. P_{gr}^Q is typically less than 1.0 for electron beams of energy greater than 10 MeV. At lower beam energies, P_{gr}^Q may equal 1.0 or even be slightly above unity. $K_{R_{50}}$ may be further separated into a chamber-specific component and an energy-dependent component:

$$k_{R_{50}} = k_{ecal} \cdot k'_{R_{50}}$$

k_{ecal} is the photon-electron conversion factor. For an electron beam energy of Q_{ecal}, k_{ecal} converts $N_{D,w}^{60Co}$ into $N_{D,w}^{Qecal}$. k_{ecal} is almost independent of chamber model. For most commonly used ionization chambers, k_{ecal} is within 1% of 0.9. The AAPM protocol defines Q_{ecal} as $R_{50} = 7.5$ cm. As will be seen later, the decision to separate k_Q in this manner facilitates the development and application of absorbed dose standards for electrons and it simplifies the determination of $N_{D,w}^{60Co}$ for parallel plate chambers. Values of k_{ecal} for commonly used cylindrical chambers are given in Table 6-9.

$K'_{R_{50}}$ is dependent on both R_{50} and chamber model. Graphs of $k'_{R_{50}}$ are provided by the AAPM protocol,[10] but selected values for a few commonly used chamber are given in Table 6-10.

Combining the equations above yields, for electron beams:

$$k_Q = N_{gr}^Q \cdot k_{ecal} \cdot k'_{R_{50}} \qquad (6\text{-}14)$$

The dose at d_{ref} is therefore:

$$D_w^Q = M \cdot P_{gr}^Q \cdot k_{ecal} \cdot k'_{R_{50}} \cdot N_{D,w}^{60\,Co}\ (Gy) \qquad (6\text{-}15)$$

The use of parallel-plate chambers is recommended by the AAPM, especially for low-energy electron beams.[10] However, experience has shown that the use of cylindrical chambers yields errors of less than 0.5% at energies as low as 6 MeV.[25] When parallel-plate chambers are used, an alternate procedure for determining calibration coefficient has been recommended.[10,11,27] The product of $k_{ecal} \cdot N_{D,w}^{60\,Co}$ is evaluated by comparison with an ADCL calibrated cylindrical ionization chamber as:

$$\left(k_{ecal} \cdot N_{D,w}^{60Co}\right)^{pp} = \left(D_w^Q\right)^{cyl} / \left(M \cdot k'_{R_{50}}\right)^{pp}$$

where the superscripts pp and cyl refer to parallel-plate and cylindrical chambers, respectively. $\left(D_w^Q\right)^{cyl}$ is obtained from Equation (6-15). The comparison should be performed in a beam with R_{50} as close to 7.5 cm possible, so that $k'_{R_{50}}$ is nearly unity.

The procedures described above for both cylindrical and parallel-plate chambers yield $\left(D_w^Q\right)$, the dose to water at the reference depth, d_{ref}. To determine the dose at d_{max}, the dose at d_{ref} must be divided by the percent depth dose at d_{ref}. The value of $\%D_n$ should be taken from the clinic's treatment-planning data, to ensure that patient dose calculations are consistent with calibration procedures. The calibrated dose rate determined in water in an electron beam can be corrected to provide the dose rate to muscle. The correction is $(S/\rho)_{water}^{muscle}$. Stopping power ratios published by the International Commission on Radiation Units and Measurements (ICRU) indicate that this ratio is approximately 0.99 over the clinically useful range of energies.[28]

Example 6-10

Determine k_Q for an Exradin model A-12 cylindrical ionization chamber when used to calibrate a 12 MeV electron beam. Measurements are as follows: $R_{50} = 4.67$ cm, $d_{ref} = 2.70$ cm, a measurement at d_{ref} yields a reading of 4.478×10^{-8} C per 200 MU, while a measurement at $(d_{ref} + 0.5\,r_{cav})$ yields 4.457×10^{-8} C.

$$P_{gr}^Q = M_{raw}(d_{ref} + 0.5r_{cav})/M_{raw}(d_{ref})$$
$$= 4.457/4.478$$
$$= 0.995$$

k_{ecal} (from Table 6-9) = 0.906
$k'_{R_{50}}$ (from Table 6-10) = 1.010

$$k_Q = P_{gr}^Q \cdot k_{ecal} \cdot k'_{R_{50}}$$
$$k_Q = 0.995 \cdot 0.906 \cdot 1.010$$
$$k_Q = 0.910$$

The IAEA calibration protocol

In 2000, the International Atomic Energy Agency (IAEA) published a calibration protocol based on dose-to-water standards.[29]

Table 6-9 Values of the photon-electron conversion factor, k_{ecal}, for commercial cylindrical chambers, based on a reference beam quality, Q_{ecal}, of $R_{50} = 7.5$ cm[10].

Chamber	k_{ecal}	Wall			
		Material	Thickness g/cm^2	Cavity Radius r_{cav} (cm)	Al Electrode Diameter (mm)
Farmer-like					
Exradin A12	0.906	C-552	0.088	0.305	
NE2505/3,3A	0.903	Graphite	0.065	0.315	
NE2561[a]	0.904	Graphite	0.090	0.370[e]	1.0
NE2571	0.903	Graphite	0.065	0.315	1.0
NE2577	0.903	Graphite	0.065	0.315	1.0
NE2581	0.885	A-150	0.041	0.315	1.0
Capintec PR-06C/G	0.900	C-552	0.050	0.320	
PTW N23331	0.896	Graphite	0.012	0.395[e]	
		PMMA	0.048		1.0
PTW N30001[b]	0.897	Graphite	0.012	0.305	
		PMMA	0.033		1.0
PTW N30002	0.900	Graphite	0.079	0.305	
PTW N30004	0.905	Graphite	0.079	0.305	
PTW N31003[c]	0.898	Graphite	0.012	0.275	1.0
		PMMA	0.066		1.0[f]
Other cylindrical					
Exradin A1[d]	0.915	C-552	0.176	0.200	
Capintec PR-05/PR-05P	0.916	C-552	0.210	0.200	
Wellhofer IC-10/IC-5	0.904	C-552	0.070	0.300	

Notes:
[a]The NE2611 has replaced the equivalent NE2561.
[b]PTW N30001 is equivalent to the PTW N23333 it replaced.
[c]PTW N31003 is equivalent to the PTW N233641 it replaced.
[d]The cavity radius of the A1 here is 2 mm although in the past Exradin has designated chambers with another radius as A1.
[e]In electron beams there are only data for cavity radii up to 0.35 cm, and so 0.35 cm is used rather than the real cavity radius shown here.
[f]Electrode diameter is actually 1.5 mm, but only data for 1.0 mm are available.

Table 6-10 Values of $k'_{R_{50}}$ for selected values of R_{50} and a few commonly used ionization chambers.

R_{50}(cm)	Exradin A1, Capintec PR-05, Capintec PR-05P	NE 2505-3, -3A, 2571, 2577, 2581 Capintec PR-06C, -0G, PTW N30001	PTW N31003	Exradin A12, PTW N30002, N30004 Wellhofer IC 10/5	Exradin P11, Holt MPPK, PTB Roos, NACP	Markus PTW N23343	Capintec PS O33
2.0	1.039	1.033	1.035	1.032	1.055	1.041	1.016
2.5	1.032	1.027	1.030	1.026	1.047	1.036	1.014
3.0	1.027	1.022	1.025	1.021	1.040	1.032	1.012
3.5	1.022	1.018	1.020	1.017	1.034	1.028	1.011
4.0	1.018	1.015	1.017	1.013	1.028	1.024	1.010
4.5	1.015	1.012	1.014	1.011	1.023	1.020	1.009
5.0	1.012	1.010	1.011	1.009	1.019	1.016	1.008
5.5	1.009	1.007	1.008	1.006	1.012	1.013	1.006
6.0	1.007	1.005	1.006	1.005	1.011	1.010	1.005
6.5	1.004	1.003	1.003	1.003	1.007	1.006	1.004
7.0	1.002	1.001	1.001	1.002	1.003	1.003	1.001
7.5	1.000	1.000	1.000	1.000	1.000	1.000	1.000
8.0	0.998	0.999	0.999	0.999	0.997	0.997	0.998
8.5	0.996	0.997	0.997	0.998	0.994	0.994	0.996
9.0	0.994	0.996	0.995	0.996	0.991	0.992	0.994
9.5	0.992	0.994	0.993	0.994	0.988	0.990	0.992
10.0	0.990	0.993	0.992	0.993	0.986	0.988	0.990

The protocol, known as *TRS-398*, is similar in many ways to the AAPM TG51 protocol. A comprehensive comparison of TRS-398 with TG51 indicates that, with few exceptions, the two protocols yield nearly identical results.[30]

The TRS-398 protocol determines dose in a beam of quality, Q, as:

$$D_{w,Q} = M_Q \cdot N_{D,w,Q_0} \cdot k_{Q}, Q_0 \qquad (6\text{-}16)$$

where Q_0 indicates a reference beam quality. When the reference beam quality is ^{60}Co, the subscript Q_0 is dropped. TRS-398, unlike TG51, permits the use of reference beam qualities other than ^{60}Co. Some PSDLs have developed dose-to-water calibration standards in accelerator beams. In rare cases, ionization chambers are calibrated in a reference beam quality Q_0 equivalent to the user's beam quality, Q. In this circumstance, $k_{Q,Q_0} = 1.0$ and Equation (6-16) is simplified. Otherwise, k_{Q,Q_0} is calculated in a similar fashion as k_Q.

$$k_{Q,Q_0} \cdot (S_{air}^{w})_{Q_0}^{Q} \cdot \frac{P_Q}{P_{Q_0}} \qquad (6\text{-}17)$$

The superscript Q and subscript Q_0 indicate that the stopping-power ratio, the work function, and a perturbation correction are to be evaluated at Q and Q_0 and the ratios of the quantities determined. W_{air} has generally been assumed to be independent of beam quality, but TRS-398 leaves open the possibility that this is not the case. TRS-398 uses the symbol S to represent the mean restricted collisional mass stopping power, a quantity for which TG51 uses the symbol L/ρ.

The perturbation correction P_Q is:

$$P_Q = \left[P_{dis} P_{wall} P_{cav} P_{cel} \right]_Q$$

where P_{wall} and P_{cel} are correction factors for the chamber wall and central electrode material, respectively, as described in the AAPM TG21 protocol.[11] P_{dis} corrects for the displacement of the effective point of measurement upstream from the axis of a cylindrical chamber. P_{cav} corrects for the perturbation of electron fluence due to differences between air and the water medium, and it is equivalent to P_{repl} used in TG51.

TRS-398 describes the quality, Q, of a photon beam in terms of the ionization ratio, or the ratio of TMR_{20}/TMR_{10}. For electron beams, TRS-398 describes Q in terms of R_{50} in exactly the same fashion as TG51. Both protocols accommodate the use of parallel plate chambers, but TRS-398 requires their use below 10 MeV.

Summary

- Instruments used to calibrate clinical x- and γ-ray beams in the United States are assigned calibration coefficients by an ADCL.
- The dose to tissue is related to the dose to air by the ratio of the mass-energy absorption coefficients.
- Measurements with an ionization chamber must be corrected for environmental conditions, electrical effects, and recombination of ions.

- The effective point of measurement of a cylindrical ionization chamber is displaced a small distance toward the source from the chamber axis.
- The effective point of measurement is considered for relative measurements of beam characteristics, such as percent depth dose.
- The chamber axis is used as the reference point for radiation beam calibrations.

Problems

6-1 An ADCL-calibrated chamber has an air-kerma calibration coefficient $N_K = 4.33 \times 10^7$ Gy/C, and it is used with an electrometer whose correction factor is 1.006. This system is used to measure the dose rate to water in a 250 kVp orthovoltage x-ray beam (HVL = 1.0 mm Cu) for which this value of N_K is appropriate. A 10 cm × 10 cm field at 50 cm SSD is used. An exposure of 1 minute yields an electrometer reading of 1.517×10^{-8} C. What is the exposure rate at the location of the chamber? What is the dose rate to water at the surface of a patient or phantom?

6-2 Compare the dose to bone with the dose to muscle for 250 kVp x rays. For 100 kVp x rays. For ^{60}Co γ rays.

6-3 The depth of 50% ionization R_{50} in an electron beam of nominal energy 9 MeV is 3.8 cm of water. How much uncertainty is there in the determination of k_Q for an Exradin P11 chamber if R_{50} is known with an uncertainty of 1 mm?

6-4 An ionization chamber was calibrated by an ADCL with negative bias, but measurements are made in the user's electron beam with both positive and negative bias settings. Positive bias yielded a reading of 4.45×10^{-8} C, while negative bias gave -4.49×10^{-8} C. Determine P_{pol}.

6-5 Determine P_{ion} for an ionization chamber that gives the following readings in a 6 MeV electron beam: At 300 V, 4.442×10^{-8} C; and at 150 V, 4.403×10^{-8} C.

6-6 Depth dose measurements are made in a 10 cm × 10 cm photon beam at 100 cm SSD with a 1 mm thick lead sheet at 30 cm above the water phantom surface. The reading at d_m is 0.953×10^{-8} C; and with the chamber at 10 cm + 0.6 r_{cav}, it is 0.754×10^{-8} C. Determine $\%D(10)_X$ and k_Q for a NE model 2571 chamber.

References

1 Criteria for accreditation of dosimetry calibration laboratories by the American Association of Physicists in Medicine, AAPM, January 2002.

2 ISO Report 31-0: Quantities and Units: Part O: General Principles. International Organization for Standardization, Geneva, 1992. Amendment 1, 1998.

3 Ibbott, G. S., Attix, F. H., Slowey, T. W., Fontenla, D. P., and Rozenfeld, M. Uncertainty of calibrations at the Accredited Dosimetry Calibration Laboratories. *Med. Phys.* 1997; **24**(8):1249–1254.

4 Blackwell, C. R., and McCullough, E. C. A chamber and electrometer calibration factor as determined by each of the five AAPM accredited dosimetry calibration laboratories. *Med. Phys.* 1993; **19**:207–208.

5 Report of the 17th Meeting of the Consultative Committee for Ionizing Radiation (CCRI). Published by the Bureau International des Poid set Mesures, available at www.bipm.org.

6 International Commission on Radiation Units and Measurements. *Average Energy Required to Produce an Ion Pair*, Report no. 31. Washington, DC, ICRU, 1979.

7 Niatel, M. T., Perroche Roux, A. M., and Boutillon, M. Two determinations of W for electrons in dry air. *Phys. Med. Biol.* 1985; **30**:67–75.

8 Johns, H., and Cunningham, J. *The Physics of Radiology*, 3rd edition. Springfield, II, Charles C. Thomas, 1969.

9 Hubbell, J. H. Photon mass attenuation and energy-absorption coefficients from l keV to 20 MeV. *Int. J. Appl. Radiat. Isot.* 1982; **33**:1269–1290.

10 Almond, P. R., Biggs, P. J., Coursey, B. M., Hanson, W. F., Huq, M. S., et al. AAPM's TG-51 protocol for clinical reference dosimetry of high-energy photon and electron beams. *Med. Phys.* 1999; **26**:1847–1870.

11 Schulz, R. J., Almond, P. R., Cunningham, J. R., Holt, J. G., Loevinger, R., et al. A protocol for the determination of absorbed dose from high-energy photons and electron beams. *Med. Phys.* 1983; **10**:741–771.

12 International Atomic Energy Agency. *Absorbed dose determination in external beam radiotherapy: An International Code of Practice for Dosimetry Based on Standards of Absorbed Dose to Water*, Technical Reports series no. 398, Vienna, IAEA, 2000.

13 Hospital Physicists Association Protocol: Code of practice for high-energy photon therapy dosimetry based on the NPL absorbed dose calibration service. *Phys. Med. Biol.* 1990; **35**:1355–1360.

14 Ma, C.-M., Coffey, C. W., DeWerd, L. A., Liu, C., Nath, R., et al. AAPM Protocol for 40–300 kV x-ray beam dosimetry in radiotherapy and radiobiology. *Med. Phys.* 2001; **28**(6).

15 Attix, F. H. *Introduction to Radiological Physics and Radiation Dosimetry*. New York, John Wiley & Sons, Ltd., 1986, pp. 358–360.

16 Boag, J. W. The recombination correction for an ionisation chamber exposed to pulsed radiation in a "swept beam" technique: I. Theory. *Phys. Med. Biol.* 1983; **27**:201–211.

17 Boag, J. W., and Curran, J. Current collection and ionic recombination in small cylindrical ionization chambers exposed to pulsed radiation. *Br. J. Radiol.* 1980; **53**:471–478.

18 Weinhous, M. S., and Meli, J. A. Determining Pion: The correction factor for recombination losses in an ionization chamber. *Med. Phys.* 1984; **11**:846–849.

19 Seuntjens, J. P., Van der Zwan, L., and Ma, C. M. Type dependent correction factors for cylindrical chambers for in-phantom dosimetry in medium-energy x-ray beams. *Proceedings Kilovoltage X-Ray Beam Dosimetry for Radiotherapy and Radiobiology*, C. M. Ma, and J. P. Seuntjens, (eds.). Madison, MPP, 1999, pp. 159–174.

20 Tailor, R. C., Hanson, W. F., and Ibbott, G. S. TG-51: Experience from 150 institutions, common errors, and helpful hints. *J. Appl. Clin. Med. Phys.* 2003; **4**(2):102–111.

21 SCRAD. Protocol for the dosimetry of x- and gamma-ray beams with maximum energies between 0.6 and 50 MeV. *Phys. Med. Biol.* 1971; **16**:379–396.

22 Burlin, T. E., *Radiation Dosimetry*, vol. 1. New York, Academic Press, 1968.

23 Cunningham, J. R., and Schulz, R. J. On the selection of stopping-power and mass energy-absorption coefficient ratios for high-energy x-ray dosimetry. *Med. Phys.* 1984; **11**:618–623.

24 Rogers, D. W. O., and Lang, C. L. Corrected relationship between $\%dd(10)x$ and stopping-power ratios. *Med. Phys.* 1999; **26**:538–540.

25 Tailor, R. C., Hanson, W. F., and Ibbott, G. S., TG-51 Experience from 150 institutions, common errors, and helpful hints. *J. Appl. Clin. Med. Phys.*, 2003; **4**:102–111.

26 Burns, D. T., Ding, G. X., and Rogers, D. W. O. R50 as a beam quality specifier for selecting stopping-power ratios and reference depths for electron dosimetry. *Med. Phys.* 1996; **23**:383–388.

27 Almond, P. R., Attix, F. H., Goetsch, S., Humphries, L. J., Kubo, H., et al. The calibration and use of plane-parallel ionization chambers for dosimetry of electron beams: An extension of the 1983 AAPM protocol: Report of AAPM Radiation Therapy Committee Task Group 39. *Med. Phys.* 1994; **21**:1251–1260.

28 International Commission on Radiation Units and Measures. *Stopping Powers for Electrons and Positrons*. ICRU Report 37. Washington, DC, ICRU, 1984.

29 International Atomic Energy Agency. *Absorbed Dose Determination in External Beam Radiotherapy*. IAEA Technical Report Series No. 398. Vienna, 2000.

30 Andreo, P., Huq, M. S., Westermark, M., Song, H., Tilikidis, A., et al. Protocols for the dosimetry of high-energy photon and electron beams: A comparison of the IAEA TRS-398 and previous International Codes of Practice. *Phys. Med. Biol.* 2002; **47**:3033–3053.

CENTRAL-AXIS POINT DOSE CALCULATIONS

Objectives

After studying this chapter, the reader should be able to:
- Calculate machine settings (monitor units) with the intent of delivering a specified dose to a small mass of tissue at a specified point within the patient given a set of physical beam parameters.
- Recognize the influence of radiation energy, depth, field size, and source–surface distance on depth dose and related parameters.

Introduction

The amount of radiation delivered to a location of interest in a patient by a radiation beam traversing the patient often is estimated from radiation doses measured with the radiation beam incident on a device filled with a homogeneous medium, such as water. The device is referred to as a *patient-simulating (tissue-equivalent) phantom*. Measurements are usually made with a small ionization chamber, although semiconductor diodes, thermoluminescent dosimeters, other small point detectors, or x-ray film can be used. Often the measurements are obtained at incremental depths along the central axis of the radiation beam and expressed as fractions of the amount of radiation measured at a reference location, also on the beam axis. Depending on the location of the reference dose, these fractions are described as fractional (or percent) depth doses, tissue-air ratios (TAR), tissue-phantom ratios (TPR), or tissue-maximum ratios (TMR). This chapter presents a methodology for the calculation of machine settings for the delivery of a prescribed dose of radiation, given an initial set of calibration measurements.

Hendee's Radiation Therapy Physics, Fourth Edition. Todd Pawlicki, Daniel J. Scanderbeg and George Starkschall.
© 2016 John Wiley & Sons, Inc. Published 2016 by John Wiley & Sons, Inc.

Dose calculation model

It is important to recognize that different institutions have different methods of specifying machine output. Rather than specifying a particular formula, or method, for calculating machine settings, this chapter will attempt to provide a consistent methodology that allows selection of a particular set of measurement conditions to ensure consistency in the machine setting calculations. This will allow the reader to perform a set of point dose calculations irrespective of the particular methods used to specify machine output in the radiation oncology clinic.

The goal of these calculations is to determine the machine setting that will deliver a specified dose to a small mass of tissue at a specified point within the patient, given a set of physical beam parameters. These machine parameters may include the type of radiation produced by the machine, the output of the machine, the field size, the depth of the calculation point, and the presence of any one of a number of beam modifiers.

In order to achieve this goal, the dose to a small mass of tissue in the patient is related to some sort of reference dose. This reference dose has been measured when the machine is calibrated (and verified on a regular basis). With this information, it is then possible to calculate the desired dose.

The machine setting, M, expressed either in monitor units (MU) or treatment time, is given by the equation:

$$M = \frac{D_{ref}}{\dot{D}_{ref}} + EEC$$

In this equation D_{ref} is the dose that, if delivered to a specified reference point by a specified reference field, would satisfy the goals of the prescription, $\dot{D}_{ref}$ is the dose rate (cGy/min or cGy/MU) at the reference point, and EEC is an end-effect correction.

Some examples of D_{ref} are as follows:

1 For an isocentric treatment, D_{ref} is typically the prescription dose, D_{prescr}, for the specific field.
2 For a treatment at fixed source–surface distance (SSD), D_{ref} is typically the given dose for the specific field. The given dose is the dose delivered to a point on the central axis of the beam and the depth of maximum dose, d_{max}. D_{ref} is obtained from D_{prescr} by the equation:

$$D_{ref} = \frac{D_{prescr}}{PDD(d, S, SSD)}$$

where $PDD(d,S,SSD)$ is the percent depth dose at the depth, d, of the dose prescription point, the field size, S, is defined at the patient surface a distance, SSD, from the radiation source. Percent depth doses will be described later in this chapter. The percent depth dose has been divided by 100% so it is expressed as a decimal.

3 For isocentric treatments in which the isocenter has been blocked, for example, by a multileaf collimator, D_{ref} might be the dose delivered to a point in the unblocked region of the field at the same depth as the isocenter.

4 If the machine setting is to be calculated from output from a treatment planning system, D_{ref} might be the dose delivered to a specified reference point by a specified reference field. For example, D_{ref} might be the dose delivered to the central-axis d_{max} by an open field with the SSD equal to the source–isocenter distance.

D_{ref} can be a wide variety of quantities, and it is important to determine what D_{ref} is in a particular planning situation.

Example 7-1

A dose of 200 cGy is to be delivered to the isocenter using three beams, weighted 2:1:1 at the isocenter. What is D_{ref} for each beam?

Weighting the beams 2:1:1 at the isocenter means that for every 2 Gy delivered to the isocenter from beam 1, beams 2 and 3 deliver 1 Gy each. Consequently, to deliver 200 cGy to the isocenter from the three beams, D_{ref} for beam 1 is required to be 100 cGy, and beams 2 and 3 are each required to be 50 cGy.

The value of EEC is the measured timer correction for cobalt units, and is usually assumed to be 0.0 for linear accelerators. A timer correction is needed for a cobalt unit because the radiation source is a finite size and takes a finite amount of time to move into place.

Finally, $\dot{D}_{ref}$ can be written in the form:

$$\dot{D}_{ref} = CDO\left(d_{cal}, CS_{cal}, SD_{cal}\right) \times FSF\left(CS_{cal}, CS_{ref}, FS_{ref}\right)$$
$$\times ISF\left(SD_{cal}, SD_{ref}\right)$$
$$\times OAF\left(FS_{ref}, r_{ref}\right)$$
$$\times BMF\left(FS_{ref}, d_{ref}\right)$$
$$\times TR\left(FS_{ref}, d_{ref}\right)$$

where the factors comprising $\dot{D}_{ref}$ are defined as follows:

$CDO(d_{cal}, CS_{cal}, SD_{cal})$ is the calibration dose output
$FSF(CS_{cal}, CS_{ref})$ is the field size factor
$ISF(SD_{cal}, SD_{ref})$ is the inverse square factor
$OAF(FS_{ref}, r_{ref}, d_{ref})$ is the off-axis factor
$BMF(FS_{ref}, d_{ref})$ is the beam modification factor
$TR(FS_{ref}, d_{ref})$ is the tissue ratio.

The discussion that follows defines each factor and shows how each factor is determined.

Machine calibration

The first factor, $CDO(d_{cal}, CS_{cal}, SD_{cal})$, is the calibration dose output. Recall that a previous chapter describes the calibration of megavoltage beams. Using an appropriate calibration protocol, such as the AAPM TG 51 protocol,[1] the calibration dose output is determined to be the output of the radiation machine at a specified point under a specified set of calibration conditions. The calibration dose output is generally expressed either in cGy/MU or in cGy/min.

The amount of radiation emitted by teleisotope machines, such as cobalt-60 units, is constant over the time required to treat a patient. Consequently, the calibrated dose output, and hence the machine setting, is expressed as the time the machine is on. For a linear accelerator, a monitor ionization chamber measures the amount of radiation emitted by the machine, so the calibration dose output and machine setting are expressed in terms of a specified number of MUs. For many linear accelerators $CDO(d_{cal}, CS_{cal}, SD_{cal})$ is set to be 1.0 cGy/MU. The calibration conditions may be different from the specific conditions under which the calibration has been determined; these conditions may be specified by the individual institution and may be different in different institutions.

The calibration dose output is typically specified in water at a depth, d_{cal}, for a calibration collimator setting, CS_{cal}, and a calibration distance from the source SD_{cal}. With this specification, the calibration depth, d_{cal}, is usually at d_{max}, although it may be at some other depth (e.g., at 10 cm depth to make the depth consistent with the TG51 calibration depth). The calibration collimator setting is usually 10 cm × 10 cm. The calibration distance from the source is typically either the source to the source–axis distance (SAD), or a distance equal to SAD + d_{cal}.

Corrections for field size

Because the calibration dose output is usually specified for a 10 cm × 10 cm radiation field, and a different field size is typically used for treatment, the output for the different field size needs to be determined. Changes in the collimator setting that determine the field size affect the dose to the calculation point in several ways. First, a change in collimator setting affects the output of the linear accelerator. As the collimators are opened up, more radiation comes out of the linear accelerator. Second, a change in collimator setting affects the radiation scattered into the monitor chamber, affecting the reading in the monitor chamber. Finally, a change in collimator setting affects the field size in the patient, thus affecting the amount of radiation scattered to the reference point.

The impact of field size on reference dose rate can be expressed in several ways. In one approach, the field size factor is explicitly decoupled as the product of a collimator scatter factor, $S_c(CS_{cal}, CS_{ref})$, and a phantom scatter factor, $S_p(FS_{cal}, FS_{ref})$. If the calibration dose output is expressed in air, then the collimator scatter factor is the ratio of doses measured at the same point as that for which the calibration dose output has been specified. The numerator is the in-air dose with a collimator setting CS_{ref}, while the denominator is the in-air dose with a collimator setting CS_{cal}. If the calibration dose output is expressed in water, then the collimator scatter factor is the ratio of doses measured at depth with the two collimator settings as specified, but the radiation fields are also blocked so that the field sizes are the same. If the calibration dose output is expressed in air, there is no phantom scatter factor. For calibration dose output expressed in water, the phantom scatter factor is determined as the ratio of

doses measured at the same point in water, with the same collimator setting, but the radiation fields are blocked to give the two different field sizes.

An alternative approach writes the field size factor as the product of an output factor, $OF(CS_{cal}, CS_{ref})$, and a peakscatter factor ratio, $PSF(CS_{ref}, FS_{ref})$. In this approach, the output factor accounts for the difference between the collimator setting for the reference field, CS_{ref}, and the calibration collimator setting, CS_{cal}. If the calibration dose output is expressed in air, then the output factor is the ratio of doses measured at the same point as that for which the calibration dose output has been specified. The numerator is the in-air dose with a collimator setting CS_{ref}, while the denominator is the in-air dose with a collimator setting CS_{cal}. If the calibration dose output is expressed in water, then the output factor is the ratio of doses measured at depth with the two collimator settings as specified above. The two depths may be different. For example, the depths may be specified to be the values of d_{max} for the two collimator settings. If the values of d_{max} are different for the two collimator settings, then the physicist has the option of selecting either the collimator-setting specific d_{max} or the d_{max} for the calibration collimator setting. It should be noted, then, that these values of d_{max} must also be the values used in the measurement of TR (the tissue ratio). If the collimator-specific d_{max} is used, then the tissue ratio becomes the TMR (the tissue-maximum ratio), while if the d_{max} for the calibration collimator setting is used, then the tissue ratio becomes the TPR (the tissue-phantom ratio). Note that the output factor combines factors due to collimator scatter as well as phantom scatter.

The peakscatter factor ratio accounts for differences between the field size determined by the collimator setting and the actual treatment field size. The differences in field size may be due either to the presence of secondary blocking or a reference dose specified at a different distance from the source than that of the calibration dose output. The peakscatter factor ratio is the ratio of either the peakscatter factors or the normalized peakscatter factors at FS_{ref}, the reference field size, and CS_{ref}, the reference collimator setting. The advantage of this second approach using a peakscatter factor ratio over the first approach is that systematic errors in measurement of the ratio of peakscatter factors may not have as deleterious effect on the machine setting calculation as if phantom scatter factors alone were used.

For high-energy (> 10 MV) photons, one can set the PSF (peakscatter factor) equal to 1.0 without significant loss of accuracy. If the conditions under which D_{ref} is specified are those that include an unblocked field, then the peakscatter factor ratio is 1.0, because the field size for the unblocked field is the same as the collimator setting.

If the output factor is defined at a depth other than at d_{max}, then the peakscatter factor ratio is replaced by a TAR.

Inverse square correction

The inverse square factor, $ISF(SD_{cal}, SD_{ref})$, corrects for the beam intensity from the dose calibration point, at a distance

SD_{cal} from the source, to the dose reference point, at a distance SD_{ref} from the source. If the dose calibration point is at the isocenter of the radiation machine, and the dose reference point is also at the isocenter, then the inverse square factor is 1.0. If the dose calibration point is at the SAD plus d_{max}, and the dose reference point is at the isocenter, then the inverse square factor is given by:

$$ISF\left(SD_{cal}, SD_{ref}\right) = \left(\frac{SAD + d_{max}}{SAD}\right)^2$$

In general, the inverse square factor is given by:

$$ISF\left(SD_{cal}, SD_{ref}\right) = \left(\frac{SD_{cal}}{SD_{ref}}\right)^2$$

Corrections for beam modifiers

The beam modification factor, $BMF(FS_{ref}, d_{ref})$, corrects for the presence of any and all beam modifiers such as trays, hard wedges, and compensating filters. It is important that the beam modifiers be the correct ones for the reference field regardless of the beam modifiers used for the actual treatment field, even if a wedge is used. For example, in some older treatment planning systems, the reference field is an unwedged field even if a wedge is used. In such a case, the beam modification factor should not include a wedge factor even if the actual treatment field has a hard wedge. In this case, the presence of the hard wedge is reflected in the reference dose, and inclusion of a wedge factor in the beam modification factor would result in the wedge being accounted for twice.

Each beam modification factor may or may not be dependent on field size and depth. Whether or not to incorporate these dependencies is a decision to be made by the individual physicist, but the dependencies of the beam modification factors on field size and depth should be determined. For example, the tray factor for 6 MV x-rays from a particular linear accelerator varies by 0.5% from a 5 cm × 5 cm field to a 40 cm × 40 cm field, and the wedge factor for a 60° hard wedge varies by 4% from a 4 cm × 4 cm field to a 25 cm × 25 cm field.

Corrections for patient attenuation

The final factor, $TR(FS_{ref}, d_{ref})$, is called the *tissue ratio*, and corrects for the presence of the patient. The specific ratio to be used depends on the calibration conditions. If the calibration dose output is specified in air, then the tissue ratio is the tissue-air ratio (TAR) evaluated at the field size and depth appropriate to the reference dose. If the calibration dose output is specified in water and the reference depth for the output factor is a field-size independent depth, then the tissue ratio is the tissue-phantom ratio (TPR) evaluated at the field size and depth appropriate to the reference dose and relating to the depth at which the output factor is specified. Finally, if the calibration dose output is specified in water and the reference depth for the output factor is

d_{max}, which may be field-size dependent, then the tissue ratio is the tissue-maximum ratio (TMR) evaluated at the field size and depth appropriate to the reference dose.

The actual influence of the patient on the radiation beam is quite complicated, because it includes both absorption and scatter. The absorption of photon radiation is somewhat straightforward, being described by exponential attenuation (see Chapter 2), but made somewhat more complex by the fact that the radiation beam is typically polyenergetic, with each energy component of the beam having a different attenuation coefficient. Moreover, multiple types of interactions may take place, including Compton interactions, photoelectric interactions, and pair production, resulting in different amounts of absorption and scatter. Add to this the effects of the interactions involving secondary electrons, and the resulting calculations can get very complicated.

Rather than attempt to calculate the effects of the patient on the radiation beam, one typically makes measurements of the dose distribution of the photon beam in a water phantom both as a function of depth and of field size and uses these tabulated values to calculate the dose to the patient.

Percent depth dose

Various corrections are used to take into account the influence of the patient on the radiation beam. The specific correction depends on the configuration of the patient setup. The first of these corrections for the influence of the patient on the radiation beam is the quantity referred to at the beginning of the chapter, the percent depth dose.

The central-axis depth dose, D_n, is the absorbed dose along the central axis of the radiation beam at a specified depth in the medium. The ratio of D_n to the maximum dose D_0 along the central axis is termed the *fractional depth dose*, or the *percent depth dose* $\%D_n$ if the ratio is multiplied by 100% (Figure 7-1):

$$\%D_n = (D_n/D_0) \times 100$$

For x rays generated at voltages below 400 kVp, the maximum dose occurs at the surface of the phantom, and the reference dose is measured on the central axis at the phantom surface. For higher-energy photons, the reference dose is determined on the central axis at the depth of maximum dose below the surface.

Example 7-2

An absorbed dose of 2 Gy is desired each day at a depth of 7 cm below the surface. An 8 cm × 8 cm 6 MV x-ray beam is used at 100 cm source–skin distance (SSD). With $\%D_n = 77.7\%$, what is

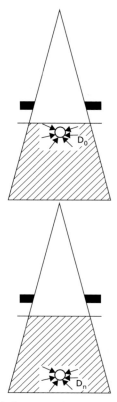

Figure 7-1 Percent depth dose. D_n is the central axis absorbed dose delivered at some depth within a patient or tissue-equivalent phantom. D_0 is the central axis absorbed dose at the depth of maximum dose. The percent depth dose is $(D_n/D_0) \times 100$.

the dose per treatment at the depth of maximum dose 1.5 cm below the surface?

$$\%D_n = (D_n/D_o) \times 100$$
$$D_o = (D_n/\%D_n) \times 100$$
$$= (2\,\text{Gy}/77.7) \times 100$$
$$= 2.57\,\text{Gy}$$

Influence of depth and radiation quality

Percent depth doses of x- and γ-ray beams of various energies are plotted in Figure 7-2 as a function of depth in millimeters below the surface of a tissue-equivalent phantom. For low-energy x-ray beams, $\%D_n$ *decreases* rapidly with depth because the low-energy x rays are rapidly attenuated in the medium. For photons of higher energy, $\%D_n$ initially increases rapidly below the surface until the depth of maximum dose is attained. Beyond this depth, the dose decreases slowly with depth. The region between the surface and the depth of maximum dose is termed the *region of dose buildup*.

For a beam of high-energy x or γ rays, the region of dose buildup provides a *skin-sparing advantage* that should be preserved in all therapeutic applications of high-energy photons except when the skin or superficial tissues are to be treated.

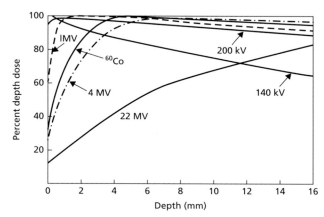

Figure 7-2 Percent depth dose for different x-ray and γ-ray beams over the first few millimeters below the surface of a tissue-equivalent phantom. All fields are 10 cm × 10 cm. For photons of higher energy, $\%D_n$ is 100 at the depth of maximum dose below the surface.
Source: Johns and Cunningham 1983[2]

To retain the skin-sparing advantage, the surface of the patient should be uncovered at the beam-entrance port (i.e., where the radiation beam enters the patient). Any material (e.g., clothing, bolus, satellite collimators, or beam-shaping blocks) on or near the beam entrance surface increases the skin dose and compromises the skin-sparing advantage. To prevent this problem, materials used to shape the radiation beam or flatten the beam-entrance port should be placed several centimeters above the skin rather than on the patient. It should be noted that there may be specific cases (e.g., post-mastectomy chest-wall irradiation) for which increased dose to the skin is desirable. In such cases, specified thicknesses of tissue-equivalent bolus are placed on the skin to raise the skin dose.

Percent depth doses for x- and γ-ray beams of different energies are shown in Figure 7-3 as a function of depth in water.

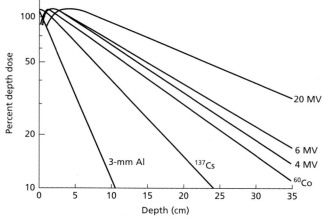

Figure 7-3 Percent depth dose for 10 cm × 10 cm area x-ray and γ-ray beams of different energies as a function of depth in water. The SSD is 100 cm for all beams except the 3.0 mm Al. (SSD = 15 cm) x-ray beam and the ^{137}Cs beam (SSD = 35 cm).
Source: Hendee 1970.[3]

Beyond the region of dose buildup, $\%D_n$ falls at a rate that varies inversely with the beam energy. Each $\%D_n$ curve reflects the contributions of (1) the inverse square decrease in dose with distance from the radiation source, (2) the attenuation of primary photons in the medium, and (3) the presence of scattered photons in the medium.

Effect of field size and shape

For an x- or γ-ray beam with small area, the central-axis depth dose is delivered almost entirely by primary photons that have traversed the overlying medium without interacting. For larger radiation fields, photons are scattered to every location on and below the surface, including those along the central axis. The relative contribution of scattered radiation to the absorbed dose increases more rapidly at depth than at locations on or near the surface because photons used in radiation therapy tend to be scattered in the forward direction. At any particular depth, the contribution of primary photons does not change with field size. Therefore, D_n increases more rapidly than D_0 as the size of the radiation field is increased, and $\%D_n$ increases with field size. This effect is demonstrated in Figure 7-4.

As the photon energy increases, the increase in $\%D_n$ with field size becomes less pronounced because higher-energy photons are scattered increasingly sharply in the forward direction, and photons scattered near the periphery of the radiation field do not reach the central axis. For example, scattered radiation contributes about 71% of the central axis dose at 10 cm depth for an x-ray beam of 2.0 mm Cu half-value layer (HVL), 10 cm × 10 cm area, and 50 cm SSD (Example 7-2). For a ^{60}Co beam of similar area and 80 cm SSD, scattered radiation contributes only about 26% to the central axis dose at 10 cm depth. At 6 MV, for a 10 cm × 10 cm field at 100 cm SSD, the contribution from

scatter at 10 cm depth is only about 22%. For fields of 10 cm × 10 cm area, scattered radiation contributes 3.6% to the dose at the depth of maximum dose for ^{60}Co γ rays and 29% to the surface dose for x rays of 2.0 mm Cu HVL. The $\%D_n$ for very high-energy photons (e.g., 18 MV x rays) is virtually unaffected by field size because the photons are scattered forward in a direction almost parallel to that of the primary photons.

For any x- or γ-ray beam of specific cross-sectional area, the $\%D_n$ decreases with increasing asymmetry of the field. Although the volume of irradiated medium may remain constant, fewer scattered photons reach the central axis of an asymmetric beam because the average distance is greater between the origin of the scattered photons and the central axis.

As an x-ray beam penetrates a medium, lower-energy photons are selectively attenuated, and the average energy of the primary beam increases (i.e., the beam is "hardened"). Except for beams of small area, however, the presence of lower-energy scattered photons more than compensates for the hardening effect, and the HVL of the beam decreases with depth. The HVL of a monoenergetic beam (e.g., ^{60}Co) also decreases with depth because the primary beam cannot be hardened, and the contribution of scattered radiation increases with depth. The reduction in HVL with depth is more pronounced for x- and γ-ray beams of large cross-sectional area because more scattered photons reach the central axis. Because of the forward direction of photons scattered from high-energy x-ray beams, the reduction in HVL with depth is less noticeable.

Example 7-3

Find the contribution of scattered radiation to the total dose at 10 cm depth for a 10 cm × 10 cm x-ray beam of 2.0 mm Cu HVL at 50 cm SSD. The $\%D_n$ at 10 cm depth is 35.5% for a 10 cm × 10 cm field and 13.4% for a field of 0 cm^2 cross-sectional area. The backscatter factors are 1.286 for the 10 cm × 10 cm field and 1.000 for the 0 cm^2 field.

The $\%D_n$ for a field of 0 cm^2 reflects the contribution of primary photons only. For a dose D_{air} of 1 Gy (100 cGy) delivered to a small mass of tissue in air at the SSD, the absorbed dose is 0.134 Gy (13.4 cGy) at a depth of 10 cm for a field of 0 cm^2 area:

$$D_n = (D_{air})(BSF)(\%D_n/100)$$
$$= (100 \text{ cGy})(1.000)(13.4/100)$$
$$= 13.4 \text{ cGy}$$

For the same absorbed dose to a small mass of tissue in air, the absorbed dose is 45.6 cGy [(100 cGy)(1.286)(35.5/100)] at a depth of 10 cm for a 10 cm × 10 cm field:

Primary radiation contributes 13.4 cGy, and scattered radiation contributes $(45.7 - 13.4) = 32.3$ cGy to the absorbed dose at 10 cm depth. The percent contributions of primary and scattered radiation to the total absorbed dose at 10 cm depth for

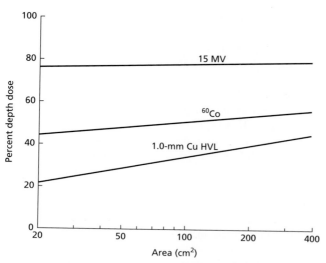

Figure 7-4 Percent depth dose at 10 cm depth as a function of field size for various x-ray and γ-ray beams with circular cross section. SSD = 100 cm for the 15 MV x-ray beam.
Source: Hendee 1970.[3]

Table 7-1 Variation in percent depth dose with field asymmetry.

Field Size (cm^2)	^{60}Co	18 MV
20 × 20	63.3	79.0
20 × 10	60.3	79.9
20 × 5	56.8	80.4

Table 7-2 HVLs of megavoltage beams have been measured in water.[4]

Energy (MV)	HVL (cm of water)
4	12.8
6	15.5
10	20.4
18	24.3

a 10 cm × 10 cm x-ray beam of 2.0 mm Cu HVL at 50 cm SSD are:

% Contribution of primary radiation = (13.4/45.7) = 29%

% Contribution of scattered radiation = (32.3/45.7) = 71%

Table 7-1 shows variation in percent depth dose, while Table 7-2 lists representative HVLs.

Example 7-4

Repeat Example 7-3 at 10 cm depth for a ^{60}Co γ-ray beam of 10 cm × 10 cm area and 80 cm SSD. The $\%D_n$ is 42.7%, and the backscatter factor is 1.000 for a field of 0 cm^2, whereas the same variables have values of 55.6% and 1.036 for a 10 cm × 10 cm field.

For a dose of 100 cGy to a small mass of tissue, the 0 cm^2 field yields:

$$D_n = (D_{air})(BSF)(\%D_n/100)$$
$$= (100\,cGy)(1.000)(42.7/100)$$
$$= 42.7\,cGy$$

and the 10 cm × 10 cm field yields:

$$D_n = (D_{air})(BSF)(\%D_n/100)$$
$$= (100\,cGy)(1.036)(55.6/100)$$
$$= 57.6\,cGy$$

The percent contributions to the total dose at 10 cm depth are:

% Contribution of primary radiation
$$= (100)(42.7\,cGy/57.6\,cGy)$$
$$= 74\%$$

% Contribution of scattered radiation
$$= (100)[(57.6 - 42.7)cGy/57.6\,cGy]$$
$$= 26\%$$

Effect of distance from source to surface

At any location in an irradiated medium, the rate of delivery of radiation is reduced by increasing the distance between the medium and the radiation source. If the radiation is emitted by a point source and attenuation of the radiation in air is ignored, the dose rate varies inversely as the distance squared. This relationship between dose rate and distance is described as an *inverse-square relationship*. It should be noted, however, that the inverse square relationship assumes a point source. For a source of finite size, the decrease in dose rate with increase in distance does not exactly obey an inverse square relationship, in particular at distances comparable to the source dimension. Except at short distances from the radiation source, however, the dose rate delivered by most photon sources used in radiation therapy may be estimated with the inverse square relationship to an accuracy of at least a few percent.

Example 7-5

Estimate the improvement in $\%D_n$ at a depth of 10 cm if the SSD is increased from 100 to 150 cm for an x-ray beam with the maximum dose at 1.5 cm below the surface:

$$(\%D_n)_{150} = (150 + 1.5\,cm)^2/[(150 + 10)\,cm]^2 e^{-\mu(10\,cm)}(100)$$
$$(\%D_n)_{100} = (100 + 1.5\,cm)^2/[(100 + 10)\,cm]^2 e^{-\mu(10\,cm)}(100)$$

The term $e^{-\mu(10\,cm)}$ describes the attenuation of the x rays in 10 cm of medium, and the squared ratio of distances represents the inverse square falloff of radiation intensity with distance. The improvement in $\%D_n$ is described by the ratio:

$$\frac{(\%D_n)_{150}}{(\%D_n)_{100}} = \left[\frac{151.5\,cm/160\,cm}{101.5\,cm/110\,cm}\right]^2$$
$$= 1.053$$

where the expressions $e^{-\mu(10\,cm)}$ and (100) cancel in the numerator and in the denominator. The $\%D_n$ at 10 cm depth is increased by the factor 1.053 (i.e., by 5.3%) in shifting the SSD from 100 to 150 cm.

As the distance increases between a radiation source and an absorbing medium, the dose rate decreases, but the $\%D_n$ increases at every location below the depth of maximum dose in the medium. The $\%D_n$ increases because the reduction in dose rate due to distance from the source is less severe for locations farther from the source. That is, the dose rate reduction at depths below the depth of maximum dose is less than the reduction in dose rate at d_{max}, and the ratio $\%D_n$ increases.

The ratio of percent depth doses at a particular depth for two SSDs is called the *F-factor* and was originally described by Mayneord.[5] The increase in $\%D_n$ with increasing SSD is accompanied by a reduction in the actual dose rate delivered to any location within the medium. In Example 7-5, for example, the dose rate at d_{max} decreases to less than half [(101.5 cm/151.5 cm)^2 = 0.45] as the SSD is increased from 100 to 150 cm. The distance from the radiation source to the patient in radiation therapy sometimes is influenced by a compromise between an increase in $\%D_n$ and a reduction in dose rate as the distance is increased.

The x-ray target of a linear accelerator behaves almost as a point source of radiation, unlike the larger source of a ^{60}Co unit. In both types of equipment, the scattering of radiation high in the collimator has the effect of broadening the source. When the divergence of the beam is measured, the radiation appears to be diverging from a *virtual source*, a point sometimes located several centimeters from the actual source. The distance from the virtual source, or *effective SSD*, should be used for inverse-square calculations. The location of the virtual source may be determined by extrapolation from a plot of $1/\sqrt{R}$ versus distance, where R is the reading from an ionization chamber with buildup in air. For x rays from most linear accelerators, the effective SSD is the same as the physical SSD, but this may not be the case with electrons.

Caution must be applied when using the inverse square relationship to determine dose rates from megavoltage photon beams at large distances. Scattered radiation from the walls, floor, or ceiling may influence the result. Extended treatment distances of 3 m or more have been used for *total body irradiation* (TBI) for ablation of bone marrow prior to transplantation. Reliance on the inverse-square law over long distances may be unwise. Instead, output measurements are generally made in a water phantom at the actual treatment distance.

Effect of depth of underlying tissue

The percent depth dose is usually measured with a thickness of underlying tissue sufficient to provide complete scatter of photons in the backward direction (backscatter). If these measurements are used to estimate the absorbed dose at locations near the beam exit surface of a patient treated with low-energy photons, the computed dose may require a correction for the absence of underlying tissue. The *exit dose* is the absorbed dose delivered to a surface where the central axis of a radiation beam emerges from the patient. The exit dose usually is estimated from central-axis depth dose data or from isodose distributions. If a scattering medium (e.g., a treatment table) is not present beyond the patient, this estimate may overestimate the actual exit dose. For high-energy radiation, corrections are rarely required, because most of the scatter occurs in the forward direction.

Tables of percent depth dose

Tables of central-axis percent depth dose are available from several sources, including Supplements 11, 17, and 25 of the *British Journal of Radiology*,[6] texts by Johns and Cunningham[2] and Khan[7], and sources cited in ICRU Report 24.[8] Published data are generally not used for patient dose calculations, because the likelihood is too great that the treatment beam characteristics are significantly different from the published data. However, published data may be valuable for comparison with measurements or to validate patient dose calculations.

Percent depth doses may not always be available for the particular radiation energy, field size, or SSD to be used. For an x-ray beam with an energy between those for which published data are available, the $\%D_n$ can be interpolated to a value intermediate between those in the published data. Usually, however, the $\%D_n$ for a particular photon beam and a particular depth is selected from data tabulated for the nearest energy, and a value is not interpolated between tables for x rays of different energies. This procedure is acceptable for validating clinical dosimetry calculations, provided that a table is available for a beam energy near that to be used clinically, because $\%D_n$ changes only gradually with photon energy.

Burns has developed a set of expressions to convert $\%D_n$ from one SSD to another.[9] These equations may be used to compute the $\%D_n$ at any SSD for which published data are not available. Burns' conversion is:

$$\%D_n(d, r, f_2) = [\%D_n(d,\ r/F, f_1)][PSF(r/F)/PSF(r)](F^2)$$

where r is the field size at the surface, f_1 is the SSD at which $\%D_n$ is known, f_2 is the SSD at which $\%D_n$ is desired, d is the depth, the PSF is the peakscatter factor (see next section) for the selected area and beam energy, and F is the Mayneord F-factor defined as (with d_m = depth of maximum dose):

$$F = [(f_1 + d)/(f_2 + d)] \times [(f_2 + d_m)/(f_1 + d_m)]$$

For high-energy x rays, the variation in $\%D_n$ with field size is small and the PSF is essentially unity. In this case, the Burns' conversion of $\%D_n$ from one SSD to another simplifies to the square of the Mayneord F-factor.

Percent depth doses usually are compiled for square fields. However, most radiation fields employed clinically are rectangular or irregularly shaped, and a method is needed to convert $\%D_n$ for square fields into values for fields of other shapes. Clarkson's method for irregular fields is discussed in the next chapter. To find the equivalent square of a rectangular field, the data developed originally by Day may be employed.[10] In this table, a rectangular field of 15 cm × 8 cm is shown to be equivalent to a square field 10.3 cm on a side.

Another approach to determining the equivalent square of a rectangular field is the use of Sterling's rule.[11] This rule states that a rectangular field is equivalent to a square field if both have the same ratio of area/perimeter (A/P). For example, a 15 cm × 8 cm field has an A/P of 2.61. A square field 10.3 cm on a side has an A/P of 2.59, a value close to 2.61. The A/P of a rectangular field is $(a \times b)/2(a + b)$, and the A/P of a square field is $a/4$, where a and b are the sides of the rectangular field, and $a = b$ for the square field. Because Sterling's rule equates the A/P ratios, $a = 4A/P$. For a 15 cm × 8 cm field, the equivalent square is $4 \times 2.61 = 10.4$ cm on a side, a value close to the 10.3 cm computed previously.

Example 7-6

An orthovoltage x-ray beam with an HVL of 2.0 mm Cu is calibrated in units of exposure rate (R/min) in air. Determine the treatment time to deliver a dose of 200 cGy to a tumor at 8 cm depth for the following data: exposure rate 80 R/min at 50 cm SSD, field size = 6 cm × 6 cm, $\%D_n = 37.8$ at 8 cm, BSF = 1.201, and f-factor (cGy/R conversion) = 0.957:

$$\text{Dose rate at tumor} = (\text{R/min})(\text{BSF})(\%D_n/100)(f\text{-factor})$$
$$= (80\,\text{R/min})(1.201)(37.8/100)(0.957)$$
$$= 34.8\,\text{cGy/min}$$

$$\text{Treatment time} = \frac{\text{Dose desired to tumor}}{\text{Dose rate at tumor}}$$
$$= \frac{200\,\text{cGy}}{34.8\,\text{cGy/min}} = 5.75\,\text{min}$$

Sterling's rule is widely used in radiation therapy to find the equivalent square of a rectangular field. It is an empirical rule, however, and does not apply to irregular (nonrectangular) or circular fields. To find the radius, r, of a circular field equivalent to a rectangular field, the following expression may be used:

$$r = (4/\sqrt{\pi})(A/P)$$

Example 7-7

The tumor described in Example 7-6 is to be treated with 18 MV x rays. The dose rate to a small mass of tissue is 1 cGy/MU at a distance of 100 cm SSD + 3.0 cm d_m. The $\%D_n$ for a 6 cm × 6 cm field is 86.1%. How many MUs are required to deliver 200 cGy to the tumor?

$$\text{Dose rate at tumor} = 1.0\,\text{cGy/MU} \times \%D_n/100$$
$$= 0.861\,\text{cGy/MU}$$

$$\text{Treatment time} = 200\,\text{cGy}/0.861\,\text{cGy/MU}$$
$$= 232\,\text{MU}$$

MUs are generally rounded to the nearest whole MU.

Tissue-air ratio

A somewhat simpler quantity than $\%D_n$ is the TAR, defined as:

$$\text{TAR} = D_d/D_{\text{air}}$$

where D_d is the absorbed dose at some location in a medium and D_{air} is the absorbed dose to a small mass of tissue suspended in air at the same location. D_{air} is sometimes described as the dose in free space, D_{fs}. The TAR is usually determined at the depth along the central axis where the rotational axis of the treatment unit is centered (i.e., the *isocenter*). D_{air} is sometimes described as the *dose to air*. This description is incorrect; D_{air} is properly

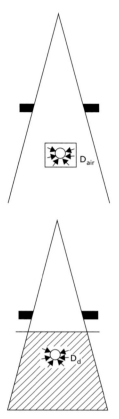

Figure 7-5 The tissue-air ratio. Both D_d and D_{air} are measured at the same distance from the source. However, the conditions for absorption and scattering differ.

defined as the absorbed dose to a small ("equilibrium") mass of tissue suspended in air.

The relationship between D_d and D_{air} is illustrated in Figure 7-5. Because the doses are measured at the same distance from the radiation source, the TAR is independent of SSD, and corrections are not required for varying SSD during therapy with multiple fields, provided that the point of calculation remains positioned at the axis of rotation of the therapy unit. The definition of TAR is essential to treatment planning in *isocentric radiation therapy*, in which the doses are measured and the target volume is positioned at the axis of rotation. Isocentric radiation therapy is preferred to fixed-SSD treatments for treatment with multiple fields because only a single setup is required.

Computing tissue-air ratio from percent depth dose

The TAR is similar to the fractional depth dose except that the reference absorbed dose is determined in air at the location of interest instead of at the depth of maximum dose in the medium. The location of interest usually is the axis of rotation (the isocenter) of the treatment unit, and it is at this location that the region to be treated is centered. The procedure for computing TARs from fractional depth doses is described below.

The cross-sectional area, A, of a beam of radiation impinging on the surface of a medium is:

$$A = A_I(\text{SSD}/\text{SAD})^2$$

where A_I is the cross-sectional area of the beam at the axis of rotation (the isocenter), SAD is the constant SAD, and SSD is the variable distance from the source to the surface. The absorbed dose, D_0, at the depth of maximum dose is:

$$D_0 = D_{\text{air}}[\text{SAD}/(\text{SSD} + d_m)]^2 \, \text{BSF}$$

where BSF is the backscatter factor for the size and shape of the radiation field at the surface, and the term $[SAD/(SSD + d_m)]^2$ corrects for the inverse square decrease in dose rate with increasing distance from a point source of radiation. The absorbed dose, D_d, in a medium at the axis of rotation (where d = depth of the isocenter) is:

$$D_d = D_{\text{air}}[\text{SAD}/(\text{SSD} + d_m)]^2 \, \text{BSF}(\%D_n/100)$$

The ratio D_d/D_{air} is the TAR. Hence:

$$\text{TAR} = [\text{SAD}/(\text{SSD} + d_m)]^2 \text{BSF}(\%D_n/100)$$

Tables of TARs are available in the literature.[2,6,7,12]

Example 7-8

Determine the TAR for a 10 cm × 10 cm beam of 6 MV x rays at 100 cm SAD, with 15 cm of tissue between the axis of rotation and the surface, and a d_m of 1.5 cm.

Notice that while the length of the field edge varies linearly with distance, the field area varies with the square of the distance. The field area, A, at the surface is:

$$A = A_I \left(\frac{\text{SSD}}{\text{SAD}} \right)^2$$

$$= (10 \text{ cm})^2 \left[\frac{100 \text{ cm} - 15 \text{ cm}}{100 \text{ cm}} \right]^2$$

$$= 72.3 \text{ cm}^2 \text{ or } 8.5 \text{ cm} \times 8.5 \text{ cm}$$

From the literature, the $\%D_n$ at 15 cm depth is 48.3% for an 8.5 cm × 8.5 cm field of 6 MV x rays at 80 cm SSD and 48.9% when corrected to an SSD of 85 cm by the procedure illustrated earlier. The backscatter factor is 1.01. The TAR is:

$$\text{TAR} = \left(\frac{\text{SAD}}{\text{SSD} + d_m} \right)^2 (\text{BSF})(\%D_n/100)$$

$$= \left(\frac{100 \text{ cm}}{(15 + 1.5) \text{ cm}} \right)^2 (1.01)(48.9/100)$$

$$= 0.660$$

Influence of field size and source–axis distance on tissue-air ratio

The absorbed dose measured in air, D_{air}, increases slowly with the size of the radiation field at the axis of rotation. The dose measured in a medium, D_d, increases more rapidly because more radiation is scattered in the medium than in air. Consequently, the ratio D_d/D_{air} (the TAR) increases with field size. The absorbed doses D_d and D_{air} are measured at the same distance from the radiation source, and the TAR is independent of SAD for all practical purposes.

Influence of radiation energy and depth

Beams of x and γ rays are attenuated by tissue between the surface of the patient and the axis of rotation. Hence the dose rate D_d at the axis decreases with increasing thickness of overlying tissue. Because D_{air} is constant, TAR also decreases with increasing thickness of overlying tissue (Figure 7-6).

Example 7-9

Determine the treatment time to deliver 200 cGy to a tumor placed at the isocenter (100 cm SAD) of an isocentric ^{60}Co unit. The field size is 6 cm × 6 cm at the isocenter, the thickness of overlying tissue is 8 cm, and the corresponding TAR is 0.736.

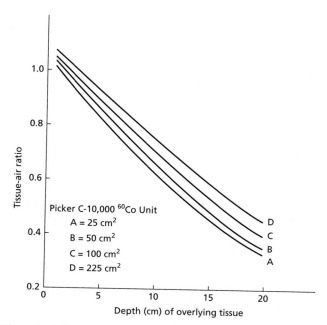

Figure 7-6 Influence of the depth of overlying tissue on the tissue-air ratio for ^{60}Co γ-ray beams of various sizes at the isocenter. *Source:* Hendee 1970.[3]

The dose rate is 80 cGy/min to a small mass of tissue at the isocenter:

$$\text{TAR} = D_d/D_{\text{air}}$$

$$D_d = (D_{\text{air}})(\text{TAR})$$

$$= (80 \text{ cGy/min})(0.736)$$

$$= 58.9 \text{ cGy/min}$$

$$\text{Treatment time} = \frac{\text{Dose desired to tumor}}{\text{Dose rate at tumor}}$$

$$= \frac{200 \text{ cGy}}{58.9 \text{ cGy/min}}$$

$$= 3.40 \text{ min}$$

Because it is essentially independent of distance, TAR (or a similar parameter) is often used for calculations of dose at extended distances.

Backscatter

When the isocenter is positioned at the depth of maximum dose, $D_d = D_0$ and the TAR are defined as the backscatter factor (BSF):

$$\text{BSF} = D_0/D_{\text{air}}$$

The percent backscatter, %BSF, is:

$$\%\text{BSF} = 100(D_0 - D_{\text{air}})/D_{\text{air}}$$

$$= 100(\text{BSF} - 1)$$

The number of photons scattered at the depth of maximum dose, d_m, in a medium depends on the amount of underlying medium and the size, shape, and quality of the x- or γ-ray beam. Because D_0 and D_{air} are measured at the same location when the isocenter is placed at the depth of maximum dose, the BSF is essentially independent of the distance from the radiation source to the surface (SSD). As the depth of underlying tissue increases, the BSF also increases until a depth is attained from which a negligible number of scattered photons reaches d_m. Photons are scattered with increased energy as the quality of the incident radiation increases, and greater depths are required to provide an infinite thickness. The thickness of most patients is adequate to provide an infinite thickness and maximum backscatter. In certain treatment situations, however (e.g., treatment of head and neck tumors), an infinite thickness may not be present, and the dose computed for the tumor may be lower than that estimated with the assumption of infinite thickness.

For high-energy photons that yield a maximum dose below rather than on or near the surface, the increase in dose as the field size expands is due to forward scatter and sidescatter as well as backscatter. In this case, the term *backscatter factor* is inappropriate and is replaced by the expression *peak scatter factor* (PSF). Note that the PSF, like the BSF, has a value of unity at a field size of 0 cm × 0 cm. The PSF is most often normalized to its value at a 10 cm × 10 cm field size and referred to as the *normalized peak scatter factor* (NPSF). The NPSF is also known

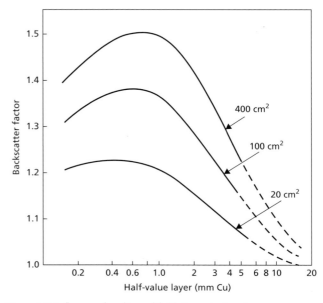

Figure 7-7 Influence of quality and field size on backscatter. *Source:* Hendee 1970.[3]

as the *phantom scatter factor* (S_p) and is useful when separating the influence of collimation and field blocking on the depth dose and dose rate. The dependence of the BSF (or the PSF) on the quality of incident radiation is illustrated in Figure 7-7. Initially, the BSF increases with increasing beam energy because more scattered photons are produced and the scattered photons are more energetic. Hence, more photons are scattered to d_m from greater depths. As the energy of incident photons continues to increase, however, photons are scattered increasingly in the forward direction, and the BSF decreases, as shown in the illustration. Maximum backscatter is achieved at HVL between 0.4 and 0.8 mm Cu, depending on the area of the radiation field. For photons of very high energy (e.g., 18 MV x rays), almost the entire scatter is in the forward direction, and the value of the BSF is close to unity.

The BSF increases with the area of the radiation field because photons are scattered toward the surface from larger volumes of tissue (Figure 7-7). For a given area, the BSF decreases with increasing asymmetry of the field because scattered photons must travel, on average, greater distances to reach d_m on the central axis. Backscatter factors for x-ray and γ-ray beams of different quality and field size are available in the literature.[2,6,7] Values of the BSF may be interpolated for photon beams with dimensions and HVLs between those listed in the literature. Backscatter factors for locations away from the central axis may be computed by a method described by Johns and Cunningham.[2]

Scatter-air ratio

For a beam of zero field size, no scattered radiation is produced in a medium, and the value of the TAR at any depth is solely a measure of the primary radiation reaching the depth. At any depth, the difference between the TAR for a field of finite size compared with that for zero field size reflects the contribution of scattered radiation at the depth. This difference is called the *scatter-air ratio* (SAR):

$$SAR = TAR(\text{finite field size}) - TAR(\text{zero field size})$$

At any location in a medium, the SAR is the dose contribution by the scattered radiation at the location expressed as a fraction of the dose delivered to a small mass of tissue in air at the same location. The value of SAR varies with the depth of overlying tissue, beam energy, and field size and shape in the same manner as the TAR.

SARs are used to calculate the dose caused by scattered radiation in a medium. They are especially useful in dose computations for irregularly shaped fields. SARs are derived from TARs and compiled as a function of depth and radius of circular fields. Compilations are available in the literature.[2,6]

Tissue-phantom ratio

In megavoltage radiation therapy, measurements are rarely made in air. Consequently, a quantity such as the TAR, which relates a dose to an in-air measurement, may not be useful. Instead a quantity such as the TPR may be used. The TPR is the ratio of the dose at a given depth in a phantom to the dose at a reference point depth, with both points equidistant from the radiation source and exposed to the same area field (Figure 7-8). The *scatter-phantom ratio* (SPR) is the ratio of the dose contribution solely by scattered radiation at a given point divided by the reference dose at a selected depth in the phantom. Although no universal agreement has been reached about the desired depth for the reference dose, a depth of 10 cm is often used in the determination of TPR and SPR.

If the reference dose is measured at the depth of maximum dose, d_m, rather than at another depth, the quantity TPR is called the *tissue-maximum ratio* (TMR). That is, the TMR is a special case of the TPR equal to the ratio of the dose at depth in a phantom divided by the maximum dose D_0. The *scatter-maximum ratio* (SMR) is defined similarly as the ratio of the dose caused solely by scattered radiation at a given point divided by the maximum dose measured at the same distance from the radiation source. Because the doses are measured at identical distances from the radiation source, they are essentially independent of distance from the source and vary only with beam energy, field size and shape, and depth of overlying tissue.

The TMR differs from the TAR because the reference dose in the TMR is measured in an extended tissue-equivalent medium, whereas the reference dose in TAR is measured to a small mass of tissue in air. Hence, the two reference doses differ by the BSF. The TMR is related to the TAR by:

$$TMR(d, r) = TAR(d, r)/BSF(r)$$

where the field size, r, is determined at depth d.

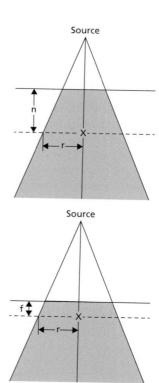

Figure 7-8 The tissue-phantom ratio is the ratio of the central axis dose, D_n, at given depth n in a tissue-equivalent phantom to the dose delivered to the same location with the same area beam but with a reference thickness, t, of overlying tissue (reference depth). If the thickness of overlying tissue equals the buildup thickness required to deliver the maximum dose, the tissue-phantom ratio is termed the *tissue-maximum ratio*.

Calculation of MUs for isocentric treatment with megavoltage beams is most easily done using TMRs.

Example 7-10

Repeat Example 7-9 for 6 MV x rays with SAD = 100 cm: the dose rate at the isocenter in a 6 cm × 6 cm field under d_{max} thickness of tissue is 0.961 cGy/MU. The TMR at 8 cm depth is 0.805.

$$TMR = D_d/D_0$$
$$D_d = D_0\, TMR$$
$$= (0.961)(0.805)$$
$$= 0.774 \text{ cGy/MU}$$

$$\text{Treatment time} = \frac{\text{Dose desired to tumor}}{\text{Dose rate to tumor}}$$
$$= \frac{200 \text{ cGy}}{0.774 \text{ cGy/MU}}$$
$$= 258 \text{ MU}$$

Monitor unit calculations for electrons

MU calculations for electrons can be performed in accordance with the report of AAPM Therapy Physics Committee Task

Group 71.[13] At standard (typically 100 cm) SSDs, the monitor unit setting (*MU*) for an electron beam is given by:

$$MU = \frac{D}{D'_0 \cdot \left(PDD\left(d, r_a, SSD_0\right) /100\% \right) \cdot S_e\left(r_a, SSD_0\right)}$$

In this expression, *D* is the absorbed dose at the point of interest from the individual field under calculation, D'_0 is the dose per MU under calibration conditions, *PDD* is the percent depth dose, evaluated at depth *d*, with applicator size r_a, and the standard SSD_0, and S_e is the output factor for the electron beam for the given applicator size and the standard SSD. The PDD is dependent on the insert size,[14] but if skin collimation is used, the PDD field size should be the skin collimation field size rather than the applicator size.

For calculating MUs for treatments at nonstandard SSDs, two approaches can be used. The effective SSD technique uses an inverse square correction based on an effective SSD in the following manner:

$$MU = \frac{D}{\begin{array}{c}D'_0 \cdot \left(PDD\left(d, r_a, SSD\right) /100\% \right) \cdot S_e\left(r_a, SSD_0\right) \\ \times \left[\left(SSD_{eff}\left(r\right) + d_0\right) / \left(SSD_{eff}\left(r\right) + d_0 + g\right) \right]^2 \end{array}}$$

whereas the air-gap technique uses an inverse square correction based on the true standard SSD with the addition of an air-gap factor in the following manner:

$$MU = \frac{D}{\begin{array}{c}D'_0 \cdot \left(PDD\left(d, r_a, SSD\right) /100\% \right) \cdot S_e\left(r_a, SSD_0\right) \\ \times \left[\left(SSD_0\left(r\right) + d_0\right) / \left(SSD_0\left(r\right) + d_0 + g\right) \right]^2 \\ \cdot f_{air}(r_a, SSD) \end{array}}$$

To determine the field size for a rectangular field, the TG71 report recommends that the square root method be used.[15] That is:

$$S_e\left(r_a, L \times W\right) = \left[\left(S_e\left(r_a, L \times L\right)\right) \cdot \left(S_e\left(r_a, W \times W\right)\right)\right]^{1/2}$$

The report also recommends that the same approach be used to determine the PDD for rectangular fields. For an irregular field, the report recommends either measuring the output factor, determining it from an analytic algorithm, or approximating the irregular field by a rectangle and using the square root method to determine the output factor.

Summary

- Percent depth dose ($\%D_n$) is the ratio of dose at depth to dose at the surface, expressed as a percentage for a constant SSD.
- $\%D_n$ is frequently used for calculating patient treatment times for treatments at fixed SSD.
- $\%D_n$ varies with beam energy, depth, field size, and SSD.
- Tissue-air ratio (TAR) is the ratio of dose at depth in tissue to the dose to an equilibrium mass of tissue suspended in air.
- TAR can be computed from $\%D_n$.

- The backscatter factor (BSF) is equivalent to the TAR at d_{max}.
- The scatter-air ratio (SAR) is determined by subtracting the zero field size TAR from the TAR for finite field size.
- The tissue-phantom ratio (TPR) is the ratio of dose at depth to dose at a reference depth.
- The tissue-maximum ratio (TMR) is a special case of the TPR where the reference depth is set equal to the depth of d_{max}.
- Treatment time calculations for isocentric treatments are most easily performed using TAR, TPR, and TMR.

Problems

7-1   The backscatter factor is 1.282 for a 7 cm × 7 cm x-ray beam with HVL of 1.0 mm Cu. What is the percent backscatter? What is the absorbed dose at the surface of a patient for an exposure to 105 R (*f*-factor = 0.957)?

7-2   The backscatter factor is 1.256 for a 7 cm × 7 cm x-ray beam with HVL of 1.5 mm Cu. Estimate the backscatter factor for a 7 cm × 7 cm x-ray beam with an HVL of 1.2 mm Cu.

7-3   The $\%D_n$ is 70.7 at 9 cm depth for a particular 6 MV x-ray beam. What dose is required at the 1.5 cm d_m to deliver 250 cGy to a tumor at 9 cm depth?

7-4   Determine the treatment time (MU setting) to deliver 200 cGy to a tumor 8 cm below the surface of a patient exposed to a 10 cm × 10 cm 6 MV field at 100 cm SSD. The accelerator is calibrated to deliver 1 cGy/MU at d_m, 10 cm × 10 cm, 100 cm SSD. What is the dose per treatment at d_m? Determine the exit dose for a patient thickness of 20 cm.

7-5   Determine the contributions of primary and scattered radiation at 16 cm depth for a 10 cm × 10 cm field of 10 MV x rays (SSD = 100 cm).

7-6   Determine the equivalent square of an 8 cm × 14 cm 10 MV x-ray beam. Estimate the absorbed dose delivered by this field at the depth of maximum dose and at the beam exit surface of a patient receiving 200 cGy to a tumor at 10 cm depth. The patient is 26 cm thick and the SSD is 100 cm.

7-7   At a depth of 10 cm and an SSD of 100 cm, the $\%D_n$ is 67.0% for a 10 cm × 10 cm beam of 6 MV x rays. The $\%D_n$ for the field increases to 70.6% if the SSD is increased to 150 cm. What change in MU setting is required to deliver the same dose at 10 cm depth with the increased SSD?

7-8   The TMR is 0.756 for an 8 cm × 8 cm beam of 6 MV x rays with 10 cm of overlying tissue. If the dose rate at d_{max} is 1.009 cGy/MU at the axis of rotation, what is the dose rate at the isocenter of an 8 cm × 8 cm beam with 10 cm of overlying tissue? Determine the monitor setting to deliver 200 cGy at the isocenter.

7-9   Determine the time required to deliver 200 cGy with a ^{60}Co γ-ray beam 6 cm × 6 cm in area at the isocenter positioned at the center of a water-filled cylinder with a radius of 11 cm. The dose rate is 61.3 cGy/min at the isocenter in air.

7-10 Determine the TAR for a 7.5 cm × 7.5 cm beam of 4 MV x rays at 100 cm SAD, with 16 cm of tissue between the isocenter and the surface. The $\%D_n$ at 16 cm depth is 37.8% for a 6 cm × 6 cm field at 80 cm SSD, and the backscatter factor is 1.01.

7-11 At 10 cm depth, $\%D_n = 58.5$ for a 10 cm × 10 cm ^{60}Co beam at 80 cm SSD. Estimate $\%D_n$ at 10 cm depth for a 10 cm × 10 cm ^{60}Co beam at 100 cm SSD.

References

1 Almond, P. R., Biggs, P. J., Coursey, B. M., Hanson, W. F., Huq, M. S., et al. AAPM's TG-51 protocol for clinical reference dosimetry of high-energy photon and electron beams. *Med. Phys.* 1999; **26**:1847–1870.

2 Johns, H. E., and Cunningham, J. R. *The Physics of Radiology*, 4th edition. Springfield IL., Charles C. Thomas, 1983.

3 Hendee, W. R. *Medical Radiation Physics*, 1st edition. Chicago, Mosby–Year Book, 1970.

4 Tailor, R. C., Tello, V. M., Schroy, C. B., Vossler, M., and Hanson, W. A generic off-axis energy correction for linac photon beam dosimetry. *Med. Phys.* 1998; **25**(5):662–667.

5 Mayneord, W., and Lamerton, L. A survey of depth dose data. *Br. J. Radiol.* 1941; **14**:255–264.

6 Central axis depth dose data for use in radiotherapy. *Br. J. Radiol.* 1961; **34**(suppl 11):1–114. 1972; **45**(suppl 17):1–147. 1983; **56**(suppl 25):1–148.

7 Khan, F. M. *The Physics of Radiation Therapy*. Baltimore, Williams & Wilkins, 4th edition, 2010.

8 International Commission of Radiation Units and Measurements. *Determination of Absorbed Dose in a Patient Irradiated by Beams of x- or γ rays in Radiotherapy Procedures*. Recommendations of ICRU, Report 24, Washington, DC, 1976.

9 Burns, J. Conversion of percentage depth doses from one FSD to another, and calculation of tissue/air ratios. *Br. J. Radiol.* 1961; **34**(suppl 10):83–85.

10 Day, M. The equivalent field method for axial dose determinations in rectangular fields, *Br. J. Radiol.* 1961; **34**(suppl 10):95–100.

11 Sterling, T., Perry, H., and Katz, L. Automation of radiation treatment planning: IV: Derivation of a mathematical expression for the percent depth dose surface of cobalt 60 beams and visualization of multiple field dose distributions. *Br. J. Radiol.* 1964; **37**:544–550.

12 Jani, S. K. *Handbook of Dosimetry Data for Radiotherapy*. Boca Raton, FL, CRC Press, 1993.

13 Gibbons, J. P., Antolak, J. A., Followill, D. S., Huq, M. S., Klein, E. E. et al. Monitor unit calculations for external photon and electron beams: Report of the AAPM Therapy Physics Committee Task Group No. 71, *Med. Phys.* 2014; **41**(3).

14 Shiu, A. S., Tung, S. S., Nyerick, C. E., Ochran, T. G., Otte, V. A., et al. Comprehensive analysis of electron beam central axis dose for a radiotherapy linear accelerator. *Med. Phys.* 1994; **21**:556–566.

15 Mills, M. D., Hogstrom, K. R., and Almond, P. R. Prediction of electron beam output factors. *Med. Phys.* 1982; **9**:60–68.

8

EXTERNAL BEAM DOSE CALCULATIONS

Objectives

By studying this chapter, the reader should be able to:
- Describe the complexities related to patient-specific dose calculations.
- Describe various photon beam dose calculation algorithms and recognize their approximations and sources of uncertainty.
- Understand methods of heterogeneity corrections.
- Describe methods of calculating electron beam dose distributions.

Introduction

Broadly speaking, the term *treatment planning* refers to all processes and decisions that lead to a plan of action for treating a patient with radiation. Central to the process of treatment planning is the calculation of the radiation dose and the implementation of the algorithms upon which the dose calculation is based. Early treatment-planning computers simply reproduced manual methods of calculation. As more powerful computers became available, increasingly complex techniques were implemented, leading to greater accuracy and reliability of the calculated dose in most clinical situations. With this increased accuracy has come increased confidence in the ability to deliver high radiation doses to target organs while sparing sensitive normal structures.

Algorithms for dose calculation have evolved over the years, from the very simple to the very complex.[1] The choice of algorithm can be of critical importance. A reduction in tumor control has been observed if an inappropriate (or incorrectly commissioned) algorithm was used.[2] Since all dose calculation algorithms contain approximations, it is necessary to understand the systematic and random errors and uncertainties in the calculated dose distributions. This applies both to the dose distribution seen on the computer monitor and to the beam-on time calculated for each treatment field. Catastrophic errors,

Hendee's Radiation Therapy Physics, Fourth Edition. Todd Pawlicki, Daniel J. Scanderbeg and George Starkschall.
© 2016 John Wiley & Sons, Inc. Published 2016 by John Wiley & Sons, Inc.

affecting many patients, have resulted from not understanding these details.[3]

In this chapter, external beam photon calculations are covered in some detail while electron beam calculations are briefly addressed.

Dose calculation challenges

The development of modern algorithms for calculating dose distributions has faced several challenges due to the complexity of contemporary radiation treatment. Several of these challenges include the need to model sophisticated methods of beam delivery, the need to consider cases in which lateral disequilibrium occurs for high-energy photon fields, as well as the need to account for interface effects (two related dose calculation issues).

Treatment fields

Modern radiotherapy equipment is equipped with capabilities far more sophisticated than the equipment commonly used for radiation therapy in the 1960s and 1970s. As an example, the use of asymmetric collimators requires computational techniques to consider the variation of dose with off-axis distance.[4–6] Incorporation of multileaf collimators (MLCs) has created an additional demand for the development of more sophisticated calculation methods, particularly for static and dynamic intensity-modulated radiation therapy (IMRT), to fully account for the dosimetric influence of the MLC.[7] The use of very small radiation fields as seen in stereotactic radiosurgery also requires special considerations.[8] In particular, dose calculations for radiosurgery must be carried out at high resolution in order to accurately account for the steep dose gradients. Radiosurgery beam data for algorithm development and treatment planning system validation is similarly demanding to acquire, as measurements of very high precision are needed.[9]

Lateral disequilibrium in high-energy beams

A phenomenon described as *lateral electronic disequilibrium*[10,11] occurs as high-energy photons interact with tissue to yield high-energy Compton electrons that may travel several centimeters through tissue. Some of these electrons deposit dose outside of the open photon beam (see Figure 8-1). As a result, the dose within the field is reduced and the dose deposition outside the field edges is increased, resulting in a broadening of the penumbra. This effect is more pronounced in low-density tissue such as lung, where the Compton electrons can travel correspondingly larger distances than in high-density tissue.[12] Only some of the most advanced computational techniques, such as the convolution/superposition algorithms and Monte Carlo methods, can model the behavior of electrons under these conditions. Lateral disequilibrium also exists in very small fields

(e.g., for stereotactic radiosurgery) due to the out-scatter of electrons.

Interface effects

The deposition of dose in the region of tissue interfaces is also complex. The sudden change in the probability of interaction of photons with the medium, combined with the transport of high-energy Compton electrons across the boundary, yields complex changes in the dose distribution. This effect may present a significant problem for accurate dose calculation in the vicinity of air cavities such as the nasal sinuses. Dose calculation algorithms older than those developed in the 1980s cannot address the transport of electrons. Modern three-dimensional techniques are able to address this problem with some accuracy.[13–15] Monte Carlo methods are also able to effectively compute the dose across an interface.[16,17]

Aspects of clinical photon beams

Manual calculations of dose to selected points in a patient are sometimes performed to determine the treatment time or monitor unit (MU) setting. *Monitor unit* refers to a number that is set on the treatment machine console to deliver the intended treatment for a given beam. It is typically related through machine calibration to the radiation dose administered to a simulated patient. For example, 1 MU for a 6 MV x-ray beam may be set to equal 1 cGy for a 10 cm × 10 cm field at the point of maximum dose along the central beam axis in a water phantom set up at either 98.5 cm source–distance (SAD calibration) or 100 cm source–surface distance (SSD calibration). The MU came into use with modern linear accelerators in the 1960s to replace timer settings used with cesium and cobalt teletherapy machines.

True three-dimensional calculation of the absorbed radiation dose is accomplished by considering radiation interactions and the scattering of radiation throughout the patient volume, including the effects of heterogeneities on both primary and scattered radiation. Although considerably more complex and demanding of computer resources, three-dimensional treatment planning is both cost-effective and practical in modern radiation oncology departments.[18] The ability to use sophisticated, computationally intensive dose calculation algorithms in routine clinical use has also been facilitated by improved computer hardware (as described in Chapter 13).

The components of a clinical photon beam that must be modeled for accurate dose calculation are shown in Figure 8-1. In a modern linear accelerator, the photon beam is created when high-energy electrons are directed toward a high-Z target (usually tungsten). The resulting interactions of the electrons with the target produce photons that are primarily forward-directed and resemble the shape of a teardrop. The clinical photon beam is created in one of two ways: (1) the photons interact with a flattening filter that flattens the peak of the teardrop lobe of photons

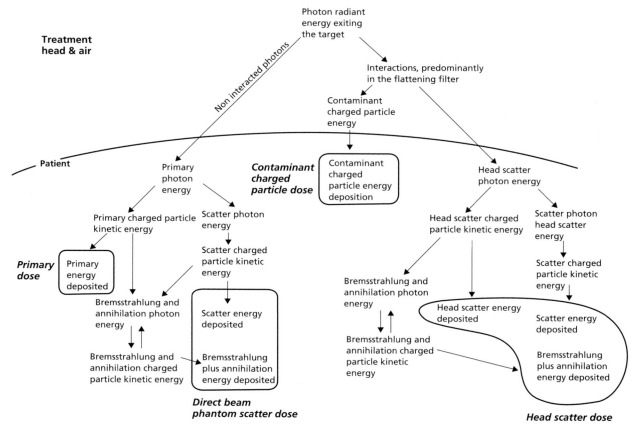

Figure 8-1 Interaction components of a clinical photon beam with the patient.
Source: Ahnesjö and Aspradakis 1999.[1] Reproduced by permission of IOP Publishing.

coming from the target, or (2) the photons coming from the target do not interact with a flattening filter (i.e., flattening-filter-free beam) and the peaked teardrop lobe is used for treatment.

The majority of photons coming from the target interacts directly with the patient and appears to originate from a point source of radiation. About 10% of the photons reaching the patient appear to originate from other locations in the linac head.[19] These photons are primarily created in the flattening filter and are called *head scatter* or *extra-focal photons*. For flattening-filter-free beams, these photons (and the subsequent particles) are largely nonexistent and do not need to be modeled for accurate dose calculation. Another component that needs to be modeled in dose calculation algorithms is the electron contamination. Electron contamination consists of electrons that are generated in the linac head from photons interacting with the high-Z components of the linac head (e.g., ion chamber, jaws, MLCs, etc.). These are mostly low-energy electrons that deposit their energy near the surface in the buildup region of the photon beam depth dose curve and are particularly difficult to model accurately. Electron contamination can also deposit appreciable dose in some clinical situations such as into the contralateral breast when a physical wedge is used on the medial tangent beam.[20,21]

Photons are known as *indirectly ionizing radiation* in part because they do not deposit significant amounts of energy by themselves. Rather, when the photons do interact with a medium, they set high-energy electrons into motion that deposit the majority of energy to the patient from a clinical photon beam. The electrons depositing dose can also create new photons (called *secondary photons*) that travel far distances from the primary interaction site before interacting with the patient and generating electrons, which then deposit dose. Each subsequent interaction generates photons and electrons of lower energy, thus depositing dose closer to the interaction site.

Head scatter also needs to be modeled. The sequence of events for head-scattered photons is the same as that for primary photons. The difficulty in modeling head scatter is that these photons do not simply appear to originate from a point source. Flattening-filter-free beams generate fewer head-scattered photons compared to flattened beams. As a result, flattening-filter-free beams are easier to model than flattened beams.

Electron transport is more difficult to model than photon transport because electrons in motion are continuously interacting in the material, changing direction, and losing energy. In contrast, a photon travels in a straight line with constant energy until it interacts with an orbital electron or nucleus of an atom in the material. To further complicate the situation, high-energy photons set high-energy electrons into motion, which can travel some distance from the primary interaction site. Electrons and photons interact differently with a material depending on its density. Therefore, heterogeneous material of the human body (e.g., bone, muscle, lung, etc.) adds another layer of complexity to achieve accurate dose calculation results.

Beam data

Most treatment planning systems require the entry of data that describe the radiation beam. The amount of data required depends on the computational algorithm, varying from almost none to thousands of measurements that completely map the radiation beam for a variety of field sizes. Systems that require the entry of a reduced amount of measured beam data rely upon a detailed description of the design of the accelerator head, collimator, and accessories. The accuracy of any treatment planning system is ultimately determined by comparison with measured data. Complete validation of a treatment planning system requires comparison between calculations and measurements over a wide variety of treatment conditions, necessitating a large volume of measured data.[22] Hence, it is unrealistic to expect that the choice of algorithm or commercial treatment planning computer can completely eliminate the need for measured data.

In situations where small amounts of measured data are required, it may be practical to enter measured values through a keyboard. The most common method of data transfer used currently, however, is to transfer the measured data electronically from a beam scanning system directly into the treatment planning computer. This capability is available from many manufacturers of treatment planning and beam scanning systems. An example of measured beam profiles of the type entered into many treatment planning systems is shown in Figure 8-2. The acquisition of beam data and treatment planning system commissioning are safety-critical activities. Incorrectly measuring these data can lead to errors in dose calculation and/or beam-on time calculations that harm many patients. An incorrectly commissioned system may go unnoticed for many months or until patients start appearing with unexpected outcomes.[3]

Patient data

Corrections for inhomogeneous tissues cannot be made unless the location and composition of such tissues are known. Various systems for obtaining patient anatomical information have been investigated. Primary among these systems is the use of CT images.[23] CT images are attractive for treatment planning for two primary reasons: (1) CT produces high-resolution images with minimal distortions, and (2) there is a near one-to-one correspondence of gray scale and tissue density (i.e., bone is white and air is black).

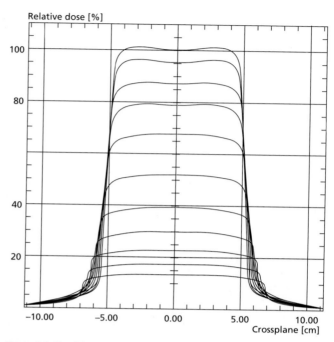

Figure 8-2 Graphic representation of several measured beam profiles of the type entered into a treatment planning computer. The illustration shows a number of profiles made along lines perpendicular to the central axis at several depths in a phantom.

The use of CT images for radiation therapy treatment planning has become widely accepted, and for many types of treatment it is considered the standard of care. Several important issues must be considered when using CT images for treatment planning. For diagnostic imaging, patients are generally positioned on a curved table top, quite unlike the flat treatment couches used in radiation therapy. The choice of couch shape can significantly alter not only the quality of the image but also the relationship of external landmarks to internal anatomy.[24] A flat table top helps in reproducing the patient position for treatment compared to the patient's position from CT simulation. Patient motion during imaging should be minimized because it can cause artifacts and reduce image quality.

Homogeneous dose calculations assume that all tissues within patients have a uniform density equal to that of water. Heterogeneous dose calculations utilize tissue densities determined by a CT scan. While it may be argued that including heterogeneities yields more accurate dose distributions, much of the historical data for determining effectiveness in radiation oncology have been based on homogeneous dose calculations. This is becoming less of an issue as calculation algorithms that accurately account for patient heterogeneities are now readily available and routinely used in the clinic.

Computed tomography also provides information about the physical density of anatomical tissues. CT images are composed of varying shades of gray, where the brightness of each pixel is related to the physical density of the tissue and to the linear attenuation coefficient of the x rays used for imaging. However,

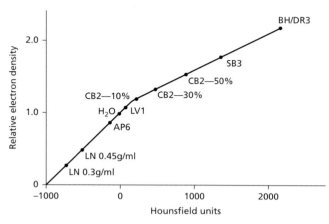

Figure 8-3 Relationship between CT number and electron density. The relationship is not necessarily a smooth function, and it may be different from one CT scanner to another.
Source: Constantinou et al. 1992.[25] Reproduced with permission from American Association of Physicists in Medicine.

the interaction of photons in a radiation therapy beam is not governed by the attenuation coefficients obtained at diagnostic x-ray energies. Instead, because the most common interaction in a therapy photon beam is Compton scattering, the frequency of photon interaction is dependent on the electron density (electrons per cubic centimeter) of the medium. Therefore, the relationship between CT number and relative electron density must be determined for each CT scanner (Figure 8-3). This relationship must be used to convert CT images into images of relative electron density.[25] All treatment planning systems include software to perform this translation. Once images of relative electron density are prepared, the computer can perform a *heterogeneity correction* with one of the methods outlined later in this chapter.

The use of attenuation coefficients determined at diagnostic energies can lead to inaccurate corrections for heterogeneities. Most treatment planning systems are capable of using patient density information in a pixel-by-pixel format. However, it is also possible to outline individual organs and assign an average (or "bulk") relative electron density to the entire organ. This can be useful when accounting for contrast agents in the treatment planning CT scan, for example. When contrast agents are used, the CT numbers will be artificially elevated. This will create unrealistic dose calculations and should be avoided. To mitigate this situation, it may be necessary to outline the region of contrast agent and manually adjust the CT numbers within the region using the functionality of the treatment planning system.

Photon beam computational algorithms

The ICRU has divided photon beam calculation methods into four classifications.[26] Listed in approximate chronological order of their development, they are *analytical* methods, *matrix*

methods, *semi-empirical* methods, and *three-dimensional integration* methods.

The analytical and matrix methods were developed when computers in radiation therapy were not very powerful. These methods permitted computation of the dose distribution in a single plane in a reasonable amount of time, making possible the development of multiple alternative plans. As more complex and accurate computational algorithms became available, they were implemented on available computer hardware. The calculation times increased, and it was common for computers to be provided with both a rapid, but less accurate, algorithm and a slow, but more accurate, algorithm. The slower algorithm could be reserved for the generation of a final treatment plan only after an acceptable beam arrangement had been determined using the faster technique. As computer speeds have increased and advances have been made in treatment planning programs, this limitation has been largely eliminated, allowing both fast and accurate dose calculation.

Analytical methods

One of the earliest analytical techniques for radiation therapy treatment planning was developed in the 1960s by Sterling et al.[27] The method is based on two equations. One equation models the central axis percent depth dose and the other models the beam profile as a function of depth and off-axis distance. The dose at any point in the irradiated volume is the product of the result of these two calculations. The analytical method was improved over time to include the effects of field blocking and wedge attenuation but is no longer used clinically.[28]

Matrix techniques

In the early 1970s, several treatment planning computer systems were developed to perform calculations based on measurements of large amounts of beam data. These measurements were stored in matrix form and aligned with rays diverging from the radiation source. A diverging matrix is illustrated in Figure 8-4. The matrix itself is formed by first drawing diverging *fan lines* that radiate from the source. In a water phantom, these fan lines intersect *depth lines* located at selected depths below the surface and drawn perpendicular to the central axis. Measurements are made along the central axis and at intersections between the depth lines and fan lines. The data are stored in two tables: a table of percent depth dose values and a table of off-axis ratios. The off-axis ratios are normalized to the central-axis value along each depth line. Both tables are compiled for representative field sizes spanning the clinical range of interest.

A treatment plan is generated by retrieving, for each beam in the treatment plan, the appropriate central axis depth dose table and appropriate set of beam profiles. The beam profiles are taken from the table that corresponds to the width of the beam

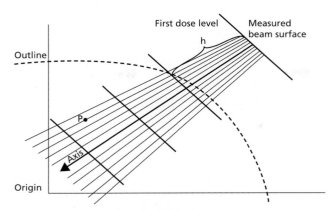

Figure 8-4 A fan-line/depth-line diverging array for representing measurements of beam characteristics. The beam array is shown superimposed upon a patient contour.
Source: Milan and Bentley. 1974.[29] Reproduced with permission from The British Institute of Radiology.

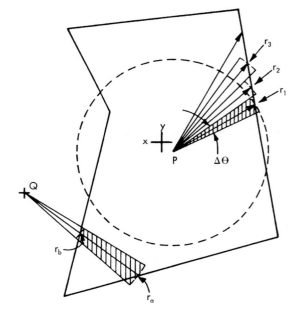

Figure 8-5 The Clarkson method. When implemented by computer, the field is generally divided into sectors that span no more than 10°.
Source: Cunningham 1989.[33] Reproduced with permission from Elsevier.

being planned (the dimension of the field shown on the plane of the treatment plan; see Figure 8-4). The central axis depth dose table is taken from the field size corresponding to the equivalent square of the treatment field. In both cases, interpolation may be used when the field dimensions fall between dimensions for which data have been compiled.

This computational technique has the advantage of speed, because data can be retrieved quickly from a mass storage device (hard drive) for each beam in the treatment plan. The method has the perceived disadvantage that a large amount of measured data must be stored before treatment planning can be performed. As mentioned earlier, however, the data required for treatment planning are generally no more than those required for the normal commissioning of a treatment unit. Another disadvantage is the relative inflexibility of calculation in handling beam configurations that are not similar to the measurement configuration, such as irregularly shaped beams, as well as heterogeneity calculations. Matrix techniques are no longer used clinically.

Semi-empirical methods

Clarkson method

It has long been recognized that the dose at a point in a patient is the sum of the dose from two contributions: primary radiation and scattered radiation. In the mid-1970s, efforts were directed to modeling the primary and scattered radiation independently to provide more accurate estimates of the dose at a point resulting from changes in field characteristics at a distance from the point. Probably the most well-known of these methods is the *Clarkson scatter integration technique*[30,31] A computer implementation of the Clarkson method incorporates several improvements over the manual calculation method.

Shown in Equation (8-1) is a general expression for calculating the dose to a point, Q, in an irregularly shaped field using the Clarkson method.

$$D_Q = D_{Primary} + D_{Scatter}$$
$$= D_C \left[f(x, y) \cdot TAR(d, 0) + \frac{\Delta\theta}{2\pi} \sum SAR\left(d, r_i\right) \right] \quad (8\text{-}1)$$

where dose due to primary radiation is given by the beam profile factor $f(x, y)$ and the zero-area tissue-air ratio (TAR) at depth d. The dose due to scatter radiation is given by the scatter-air ratio (SAR) at depth d for radius r of the sector (Figure 8-5 and Chapter 7). The component D_C is the open-field calibration factor. The scatter integration is performed by the computer in exactly the same fashion as if it were performed manually, although the field may be divided into more sectors than might be used for manual calculations.

The primary off-axis factor can be calculated with a model that considers the primary radiation to be affected by three components: penumbra, block, or collimator transmission, and flattening filter effects. The penumbra correction models the variation in primary dose rate in the penumbra region created by the shadow of the collimator jaws and by field blocking. In some implementations of the algorithm, the penumbra correction is based on the *Wilkinson extended source model*, shown in Figure 8-6.[32] This model originally described a ^{60}Co source as a broadened distribution of activity. The source activity was depicted as being greatest on the axis of the source, and decreased at distances away from the axis. As previously discussed, the presence of scattered radiation high in the collimator caused the effective source to appear wider ("extended")

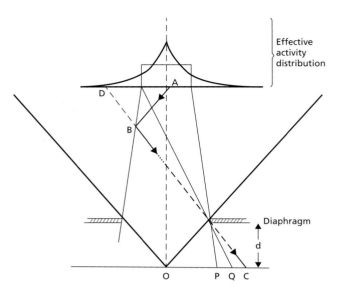

Figure 8-6 The geometry for the Wilkinson extended source model. Radiation reaching points at locations represented by P, Q, and C may appear to come from different parts of an "extended" source.
Source: Wilkinson 1970.[32]

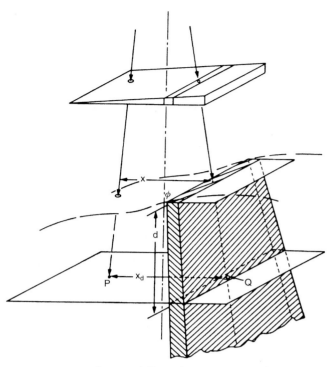

Figure 8-7 Diagram depicting differential scatter-air ratios. The crosshatched region represents a volume element of an irradiated phantom. Radiation is scattered from it to points such as P, which is at a distance x from the volume element.
Source: Cunningham 1989.[33] Reproduced with permission from Elsevier.

than the actual source (i.e., extra-focal source). The model has been applied to accelerators to describe the apparent source of radiation.

This model incorporates correction factors for the source diameter, the depth below the surface at the point of calculation, the SSD distance, and the source-to-diaphragm distance, or the distance from the source to the final field-defining aperture. A penumbra correction is calculated by integrating over the area of the extended source as observed from the calculation point. In practice, the integration is performed analytically, in a manner similar to the summation of the scatter component in Equation (8-1). The presence of blocking is taken into account by including a block or collimator transmission factor for the primary off-axis factor to yield a more accurate estimate of the dose under the blocks or collimator. The transmission term is simply equal to the block transmission factor at calculation points that fall under a block.

The original implementation of the Clarkson method was developed for cobalt units, for which the primary dose rate was quite constant from the central axis to a point near the edge of the field, where it began to decrease. In an accelerator x-ray beam, the primary dose rate may actually increase at distances away from the central axis, an effect manifested as "horns" in the isodose distributions from many linear accelerators (see the profiles in Figure 8-2). A flattening filter correction is required to model this increase in dose rate away from the central axis for linear accelerators.

For semi-empirical methods, the primary radiation is considered to be affected by three components: penumbra, block or collimator transmission, and flattening filter effects. These are combined into the primary off-axis factor used in a Clarkson

method to compute dose. The Clarkson method is largely no longer used but some systems using this method may still exist.

Differential scatter-air ratio calculation

A significant shortcoming of the Clarkson method is its assumption that scattered radiation is generated with uniform intensity throughout the field, with the exception of regions shielded by the collimator or blocks. Factors that alter the primary photon fluence at depth, such as the presence of partially transmitting filters (wedges) or non-uniform surface contours, are ignored. As shown in Figure 8-7, the *differential scatter-air ratio* (dSAR) method allows variations in the amount of scattered radiation to be considered, based on the distance from a reference point and the presence of beam modifiers, such as wedges.[33]

The dSAR method can be combined with the conventional Clarkson method, so that the scattered radiation reaching a point of interest from each of the numerous field sectors drawn around the point is integrated along each sector. The resulting dSAR is similar to a point-spread function that defines the scattered radiation from a pencil beam of photons.

The three calculation methods described above rely on data measured in homogeneous water phantoms, with the assumption that the patient also is homogeneous. Several techniques have been described for correcting for the presence of heterogeneities. These methods include the *ratio of tissue-air ratios* method, the *power law tissue-air ratio* method[34,35] and the *equivalent tissue-air ratio* method.[36] The computerized implementation of each of these methods of heterogeneity correction is essentially identical to the manual technique. Once the dose at a point has been calculated using an analytical, matrix, or semi-empirical method, a heterogeneity correction is applied to compensate for the presence of inhomogeneous tissue within the field. Both the ratio of TARs method and the power law TAR method are "one-dimensional" techniques, in that they consider only the effect of heterogeneities that fall on a line from the source to the point of calculation. Heterogeneities that lie away from this line are not considered, nor are the lateral extent of heterogeneities. The equivalent TAR technique does consider the effect of heterogeneities that fall away from the line connecting the source and the point of interest. Although this technique does not explicitly account for the dose attributed to secondary electrons, it is inherently three-dimensional. However, most of the planning systems that have implemented this algorithm collapse the three-dimensional patient volume into a two-dimensional slice through the isocenter, in order to reduce calculation time but sacrificing some accuracy. This approach makes the technique essentially a "2.5–dimensional" calculation.

Three-dimensional integration methods

Several investigators have developed proposals for full three-dimensional calculation of dose distributions.[37] The technique can be used to calculate the distribution of dose following a limited number of photon interactions within a patient. *Convolution algorithms* are based on the principle that the deposition of dose from a single photon interaction is independent of the location of the interaction.[14,38] This three-dimensional dose distribution represents the transport of photons and electrons away from the primary interaction site. It is commonly referred to as a *dose-spread array, point-spread function,* or simply a *kernel.* The dose in a treatment volume then is computed by superimposing the dose kernel throughout the three-dimensional irradiated volume, weighted by the total energy released per unit mass (*terma*) at each point. The total energy released per unit mass at any point in the patient can be simply modeled by exponential attenuation.

Monte Carlo methods (see description below) have been used to generate dose-spread arrays for monoenergetic pencil beams of photons that interact at the center of a large volume of water.[13,39] The change in dose distribution near the field boundaries is considered by modeling the change in primary photon fluence at these boundaries. The effects of heterogeneities are included by (a) determining the change in primary photon fluence as a result of passage through the heterogeneity and (b) scaling the dimensions of the dose kernel according to the density of the patient.

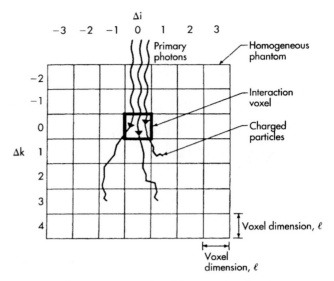

Figure 8-8 Schematic representation of the generation of a primary dose-spread array.
Source: Mackie et al. 1985.[15] Reproduced with permission from American Association of Physicists in Medicine.

Investigators have used different Monte Carlo codes to compute dose kernels.[14,15,39,40] One method by which a primary dose-spread array is computed using the EGS3 Monte Carlo code is shown in Figure 8-8. The resulting dose-spread array is depicted in an isodose format in Figure 8-9. In this illustration, only the dose distribution resulting from *first-scattered* radiation from the site of the primary interaction is shown. Because radiation is frequently scattered multiple times, the dose at any point in a patient results not only from primary interactions and from radiation that has been scattered once but also from radiation that has been scattered two or more times. The dose-spread array, point-spread function, or kernel refers to a method of characterizing dose deposition in tissue for a particular energy spectrum in the beam.

The availability of advanced computer technologies has prompted the development of treatment planning software that uses convolution techniques.[13–15,37,38,40,41] In the implementation of a pure convolution algorithm, a separate calculation is performed for each energy component of the incident photon spectrum, then summed over the photon spectrum. Several methods have been proposed to speed up the calculation. In one method, the convolution is reduced to a product by use of *Fourier transforms.*[41] In another approach, both the dose-spread array and the terma are separately averaged over the photon energy spectrum, then integrated together.[42] In a pure convolution calculation, the dose-spread array is independent of location, and Fourier transforms can speed up the calculation. However, once the dose-spread array has been averaged over the photon energy spectrum, it is no longer location-independent, and the calculation becomes more time-consuming. This technique is called the *convolution-superposition method.* The

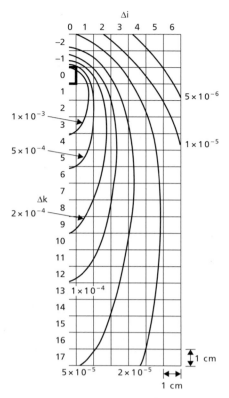

Figure 8-9 Truncated first scatter (TFS) dose-spread array in isodose format.
Source: Mackie et al. 1985.[15] Reproduced with permission from American Association of Physicists in Medicine.

calculations were time consuming when these algorithms were developed. As computing speed has increased, the algorithms have become practicable for routine clinical treatment planning. This type of calculation is the primary method used clinically today.

Monte Carlo methods

The Monte Carlo method of dose calculation is a multidimensional integration technique that randomly samples from probability distributions that govern the transport of radiation (e.g., photons and electrons) through matter. It was developed during research on neutron diffusion for the development of the atomic bomb during World War II. This calculation technique was given the code name *Monte Carlo* for the city in Monaco famous for gambling, which is also based on random events.

Dose calculation using Monte Carlo techniques involves modeling (or simulating) each individual particle from its creation until it loses all of its energy. The terminology of Monte Carlo dose calculations is shown in Figure 8-10.

Each particle simulated creates a history, or *shower*. This refers to the transport of a single primary particle and all subsequent particles that are created. The track of a particle is the

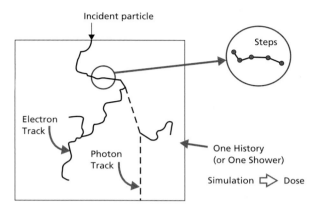

Figure 8-10 Description of the nomenclature used for Monte Carlo dose calculation.
Source: Pawlicki and Ma 2001.[43] Reproduced with permission of Elsevier.

path it takes until it loses all of its energy. A collection of all the tracks of primary and subsequent particles constitutes one history. To lend itself to computer calculation, each particle track must be divided into many individual steps. A Monte Carlo simulation is a complete set of several millions of histories in a given geometrical situation (e.g., linear accelerator and patient) for the purpose of dose calculation. Every time a particle takes a step and loses energy, its energy loss is recorded. Summing the dose contribution (energy/mass/voxel) from the millions of individual histories results in a dose distribution.

Implementation of the Monte Carlo method includes four major aspects: generation of random numbers and random variables, development of the physical interaction model, depiction of the patient geometry, and summation of data to generate dose statistics. *Random numbers* are unitless numbers from zero to one that are generated from a computer algorithm and used to determine the particular nature of the radiation interaction. Since a computer is completely deterministic, any computer algorithm that produces a random sequence of numbers cannot, by definition, be truly random. Therefore, the term *pseudo-random numbers* is sometimes used. Random numbers are converted to random variables by transforming the random numbers to a value from a *probability density function* (PDF). The PDFs contain the physical description of radiation transport in matter (e.g., interaction type, energy losses, distance traveled between interactions) and are part of the physical interaction model of the Monte Carlo algorithm. The physical interaction model also contains the mathematical/computer method (algorithm) to describe the radiation interactions with matter. The geometry refers to the mathematical description of separate surfaces or bodies through which particles are transported.

For patient-specific Monte Carlo dose calculation, the CT scan is used to create volume elements (*voxels*). As radiation is transported through the three-dimensional CT scan, data such as energy deposition in a voxel are recorded and summed (sometimes called *scoring*). A dose distribution is built from the summation of energy deposition for all histories in the simulation. The energy deposition is converted to dose by dividing the total energy deposited in a voxel by the mass of that voxel (dose = energy/mass in units of Joule/kilogram = Gray). The dose reported by Monte Carlo calculations is the dose to the material in each voxel, which is different from other dose calculation algorithms, such as the convolution and superposition algorithms that calculate the dose to water. The reason is that the energy deposited is proportional to the stopping power of the material in the voxel. The convolution and convolution-superposition algorithms use kernels that are pre-calculated in water and simply scale the kernels based on the local density of the material in each voxel. The differences between dose to water and dose to tissue can range from 1% in soft tissue to 10% for bone. To compare Monte Carlo dose to convolution and convolution-superposition dose, one must scale the Monte Carlo dose by the stopping power ratio.[44]

Results from the Monte Carlo calculations are derived from random events. The dose deposited in a single interaction is a stochastic variable with an associated uncertainty. By collecting many histories, it is possible to minimize the uncertainty in dose and thereby improve the precision in the final result. Techniques can be applied to further reduce the uncertainty after a simulation is completed. These are generally referred to as *de-noising techniques*.[45] In Monte Carlo, it is essential to report the statistical uncertainty in the dose results; therefore, one knows how much confidence one should have that the dose from the Monte Carlo simulation is the true dose. The entire Monte Carlo simulation process is shown in Figure 8-11.

The Monte Carlo method is very accurate, but computationally intensive. Although computer hardware has improved significantly over the years, the Monte Carlo method is still not used for routine *photon* beam treatment planning. However, newer deterministic algorithms called *grid-based Boltzmann equation solvers* are being developed. Grid-based methods calculate the dose by directly solving the governing transport equations without the use of pre-calculated kernels as used in the convolution and convolution-superposition algorithms. Therefore, grid-based calculations are deterministic and are not subject to statistical uncertainty, as seen in Monte Carlo algorithms, but are just as accurate. The grid-based algorithms are still able to account for all relevant neutral and charged particle interactions. The benefit of these algorithms is shorter calculation times while retaining the accuracy of the Monte Carlo method.[46]

Electron-beam computational algorithms

A number of computational algorithms similar to those used for photon beams have been applied to electron beams, including the Monte Carlo method. The Monte Carlo method is a general-purpose algorithm. Monte Carlo electron-beam calculations are a subset of Monte Carlo high-energy photon-beam calculations. The only difference is the geometry through which the particles are transported (e.g., scattering foil and electron applicator)

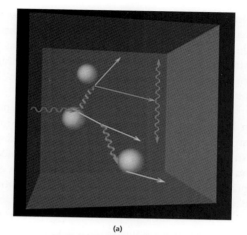

(a)

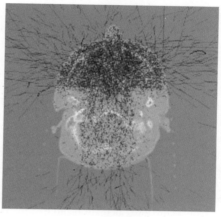

(b)

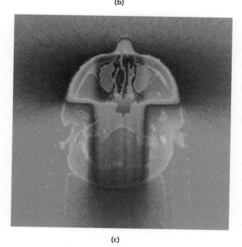

(c)

Figure 8-11 Monte Carlo example. (a) Single photon interaction. (b) 1.7×10^5 particles. (c) 6.8×10^7 particles.
Source: Nomos, Peregrine treatment planning system.

on the way to the patient. The matrix methods are also directly applicable to electron beams, provided that the location of fan lines and depth lines are adjusted to be consistent with the shape of the dose distribution for each electron beam energy. However, matrix techniques do not exactly model the unique ways in which electron beams interact with inhomogeneous tissues. For more accurate modeling, several analytical techniques have been pursued, including the use of the age-diffusion equation.[47,48] The central axis depth dose distribution for electron beams has also been modeled using an equation in the form of the Fermi-Dirac distribution function.[49]

Prior to the general use of the Monte Carlo method for electron beam dose calculations, the *pencil-beam method* demonstrated the greatest potential for accurate electron-beam dose distribution calculations.[50–53] The pencil-beam equation is based on the spread of electron dose from a narrow electron beam (pencil beam) defined at the plane of final collimation. In a high-energy electron beam, the spatial distribution of absorbed energy is dictated by the multiple scattering of electrons. The dose spread array covers a smaller area than that of a photon beam, because of the decreased range of electrons. The dose distribution in a broad beam can be generated by superposition of many electron pencil-beam distributions. An extension of the pencil-beam algorithm in which the pencil beams are redefined as they penetrate the patient (*redefinition pencil-beam equation*) has been accomplished.[53]

Electron-beam dose distributions calculated via the Monte Carlo method are the most accurate, and routinely used for electron-beam treatment planning. The calculation speed is not a significant issue as for photon-beam calculations because electrons deposit dose directly and fewer histories are needed to achieve a statistically significant result. Electron beam Monte Carlo algorithms are commercially available[54,55] and should be used for electron beam dose calculation and treatment planning.

Summary

- Challenges to accurate dose calculation include:
  - Complex field shapes and beam-defining devices
  - Lateral electronic disequilibrium
  - Interface effects
  - Patient heterogeneities.
- Some of the components of a photon beam that need to be modeled are:
  - Primary photon energy
    - Primary charged particle kinetic energy (primary dose)
    - Scatter photon energy (direct beam phantom scatter dose)
  - Head scatter photon energy (head scatter dose)
    - Head scatter charged particle kinetic energy
    - Scatter photon head scatter energy
  - Contaminant charged particle energy (contaminant charged particle dose).
- Computed tomography is used for patient-specific dose calculation because (1) CT produces high-resolution images with minimal distortions and (2) there is a one-to-one correspondence of gray scale and tissue density (i.e., bone is white and air is black).

- The ICRU has divided photon beam calculation methods into four classifications:
  - Analytical
  - Matrix
  - Semi-empirical
  - Three-dimensional integration.
- Dose computation algorithms for treatment planning systems utilize a balance between speed and accuracy. More accurate algorithms, such as convolution/superposition and Monte Carlo, are becoming commonplace with modern computing systems.
- Heterogeneity corrections have utilized corrections based on the effective depth, dose deposition kernel "stretching" (convolution/superposition), and large samples of simulated interactions (Monte Carlo).
- Monte Carlo dose calculation simulates particles and directly calculates dose to medium. It is very accurate but computationally intensive.

Problems

8-1   A three-dimensional treatment planning system utilizes a 20 cm × 20 cm × 15 cm dose calculation matrix. The dose grid resolution is 4 mm. If the matrix size is changed to 10 cm × 10 cm × 15 cm, and the resolution is changed to 5 mm, how many times faster will the calculation be?

8-2   List the components of a photon beam that must be modelled accurately in a dose calculation algorithm. In what clinical situations might dose calculation uncertainty play a role?

8-3   a) Write a simple equation for dose to a point in an open field.
b) Calculate the dose to a point in the patient if it is known that the primary component of dose is 70 cGy and the scatter component of dose to the point is 30 cGy.

8-4   For 200 cGy given to point P, estimate the dose to point Q under the block as shown in the picture. Modify your equation from Problem 8-3a to do this calculation. Explain your result.

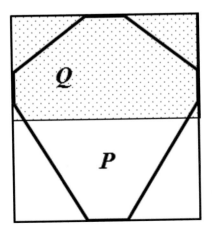

8-5 What is one aspect of a Monte Carlo calculated dose distribution that is different from any other method of calculated dose distribution?

8-6 Why might electron beam Monte Carlo dose calculations be used routinely in the clinic but photon beam Monte Carlo dose calculations might not?

References

1 Ahnesjö, A. and Aspradakis, M. M. Dose calculations for external photon beams in radiotherapy, *Phys. Med. Biol.* 1999; **44**: R99–R155.

2 Latifi, K., Oliver, J., Baker, R., Dilling, T. J., Stevens, C. W., et al. Study of 201 non-small cell lung cancer patients given stereotactic ablative radiation therapy shows local control dependence on dose calculation algorithm. *Int. J. Radiat. Oncol. Biol. Phys.* 2014;**88**(5):1108–1113.

3 Bogdanich, W. and Ruiz, R. R. Radiation Errors Reported in Missouri, *NY Times*; February 10, 2010, http://www.nytimes.com/2010/02/25/us/25radiation.html?r=0, accessed September 15, 2015.

4 Khan, F. M., Gerbi, B. J., and Deibel, F. C. Dosimetry of asymmetric x-ray collimators. *Med. Phys.* 1986; **13**:936–941.

5 Kwa, W, Kornelsen, R. O., Harrison, R. W., el-Khatib, E. Dosimetry for asymmetric x-ray fields. *Med. Phys.* 1994; **21**:1599–1604.

6 Thomas, S. J., and Thomas, R. L. A beam generation algorithm for linear accelerators with independent collimators. *Phys. Med. Biol.* 1990; **35**:325–332.

7 Chui, C.-S., LoSasso, T, and Spirou, S. Dose calculation for photon beams with intensity modulation generated by dynamic jaw or multileaf collimations. *Med. Phys.* 1994; **21**:1237–1244.

8 Peters, T. M., Clark, J. A., Pike, G. B., Henri, C., Collins, L., et al. Stereotactic neurosurgery planning on a personal-computer-based workstation. *J. Diagn. Imag.* 1989; **2**:75–81.

9 Bjarngard, B. E., Tsai, J.-S., and Rice, R. K. Doses on the central axes of narrow 6-MV x-ray beams. *Med. Phys.* 1990; **17**:794–799.

10 Haider, T K., and el-Khatib, E. E. Differential scatter integration in regions of electronic non-equilibrium. *Phys. Med. Biol.* 1995; **40**(1):31–43.

11 Woo, M., Cunningham, J. R., and Jezioranski, J. J. Extending the concept of primary and scatter separation to the condition of electronic disequilibrium. *Med. Phys.* 1990; **17**:588–595.

12 Young, M. E., and Kornelsen, R. O. Dose corrections for low-density tissue inhomogeneities and air channels for 10-MVx rays. *Med. Phys.* 1983; **10**(4):450–455.

13 Mohan, R., Chui, C., and Lidofsky L. Differential pencil beam dose computation model for photons. *Med. Phys.* 1986; **13**:64–73.

14 Ahnesjo, A. Collapsed cone convolution of radiant energy for photon dose calculation in heterogeneous media. *Med. Phys.* 1989; **16**:577–592.

15 Mackie, T. R., Scrimger, J. W., and Battista, J. J. A convolution method of calculating dose for 15-MVx rays. *Med. Phys.* 1985; **12**:188–196.

16 Ma, C. M., Li, J. S., Pawlicki, T., Jiang S. B., Deng, J., et al. A Monte Carlo dose calculation tool for radiotherapy treatment planning. *Phys. Med. Biol.* 2002; **47**(10):1671–1689.

17 DeMarco, J. J., Solberg, T. D., and Chetty, I. Monte Carlo methods for dose calculation and treatment planning: A revolution for radiotherapy. *Adm. Radiol. J.* 1999; **18**(8):24–27.

18 Perez, C. A., Purdy, J. A., Harms, W. B., et al. Three-dimensional treatment planning and conformal radiation therapy: Preliminary evaluation. *Radiother. Oncol.* 1995; **36**:32–43.

19 Ahnesjö, A. Analytical modeling of photon scatter from flattening filters in photon therapy beam. *Phys. Med. Biol.* 1994; **21**:1227–1235.

20 Weides, C. D., Mok, E. C., Chang, W. C., Findley, D. O., and Shostak, C. A. Evaluating the dose to the contralateral breast when using a dynamic wedge versus a regular wedge. *Med. Dosim.* 1995; **20**(4):287–293.

21 Warlick, W. B. Dose to the contralateral breast: A comparison of two techniques using the enhanced dynamic wedge versus a standard wedge. *Med Dosim.* 1997; **22**(3):185–191.

22 Kutcher, G. J., et al. Comprehensive QA for radiation oncology: Report of AAPM Radiation Therapy Committee Task Group 40. *Med. Phys.* 1994; **21**(4):581–618.

23 Stewart, J. R., et al. Computed tomography in radiation therapy, *Int. J. Radiat. Oncol. Biol. Phys.* 1978; **4**:313–324.

24 Hobday, P., et al. Computed tomography applied to radiotherapy treatment planning: Techniques and results. *Radiology* 1979; **133**:477–482.

25 Constantinou, C., Harrington, J. C., and DeWerd, L. A. An electron density calibration phantom for CT-based treatment planning computers. *Med. Phys.* 1992; **19**:325–327.

26 International Commission on Radiation Units and Measurements, Report No. 42: *Use of Computers in External Beam Radiotherapy Procedures with High-Energy Photons and Electrons.* Washington, DC, ICRU, 1987.

27 Sterling, T. D., Perry, H., and Katz, L. Automation of radiation treatment planning, *Br. J. Radiol.* 1964; **37**:544–550.

28 Van de Geijn J, et al. *A unified 3-D model for external beam dose distributions.* Computers in Radiation Therapy. Proceedings of the 7th International Conference on the Use of Computers in Radiotherapy, Tokyo, 1980.

29 Milan, J., and Bentley, R. E. The storage and manipulation of radiation dose data in a small digital computer. *Br. J. Radiol.* 1974; **47**:115–121.

30 Clarkson, J. A note on depth doses in fields of irregular shape. *Br. J. Radiol.* 1941; **14**:265.

31 Cundiff, J. H., et al. A method for the calculation of dose in the radiation treatment of Hodgkin's disease. *Am. J. Roentgenol. Radium Ther. Nucl. Med.* 1973; **117**(l):30–44.

32 Wilkinson, J. M., Rawlinson, J. A., and Cunningham, J. R. *An extended source model for the calculation of the primary component of a cobalt-60 radiation beam in penumbral regions.* Presented at American Association of Physicists in Medicine Workshop, Chicago, September 17, 1970.

33 Cunningham, J. R. Keynote Address: Development of computer algorithms for radiation treatment planning, *Int. J. Radiat. Oncol. Biol. Phys.* 1989; **16**:1367–1376.

34 Cassell, K. J., Hobday, P. A., and Parker, R. P. The implementation of a generalized Batho inhomogeneity correction for radiotherapy planning with direct use of CT numbers. *Phys. Med. Biol.* 1981; **26**(5):825–833.

35 Wong, J. W, and Henkelman, R. M. Reconsideration of the power-law (Batho) equation for inhomogeneity corrections. *Med. Phys.* 1992; **9**:521–530.

36 Sontag, M. R., and Cunningham, J. R. The equivalent tissue–air ratio method for making absorbed dose calculations in a heterogeneous medium. *Radiology* 1978; **129**:791–794.

37 Webb, S. *The Physics of Three-Dimensional Radiation Therapy: Conformal radiotherapy, radiosurgery and treatment planning.* Bristol, Institute of Physics Publishing, Ltd., 1993.

38 Boyer, A. L., and Mok, E. C. A photon dose distribution model employing convolution calculations. *Med. Phys.* 1985; **12**: 169–177.

39 Pijpelink, J., Van den Temple, Y., and Hamers, R. *A pencil beam algorithm for photon beam calculations.* Nucletron-Oldelft Activity Report No. 6, 21–32, 1995.

40 Mackie. T. R., et al. Generation of photon energy deposition kernels using EGS Monte Carlo code, *Phys. Med. Biol.* 1988; **33**: 1–20.

41 Boyer, A. L., et al. Fast Fourier transform convolution calculations of x-ray isodose distributions in homogeneous media. *Med. Phys.* 1989; **16**:248–253.

42 Papanikolaou, N., Mackie T. R., Wells, C., Gehring, M., and Reckwerdt, P. Investigation of the convolution method for polyenergetic spectra. *Med. Phys.* 1993; **20**(5), 1327–1336.

43 Pawlicki, T. and Ma, C.-M. Monte Carlo simulation for MLC-based intensity-modulated radiotherapy. *Med. Dosim.* 2001;**26**(2):157–168.

44 Siebers, J. V., et al. Converting absorbed dose to medium to absorbed dose to water for Monte Carlo based photon beam dose calculations. *Phys. Med. Biol.* 2000; **45**(4):983–995.

45 El Naqa, I., et al. A comparison of Monte Carlo dose calculation denoising techniques. *Phys. Med. Biol.* 2005; **50**(5):909–922.

46 Vassiliev, O. N., et al. Validation of a new grid-based Boltzmann equation solver for dose calculation in radiotherapy with photon beams. *Phys. Med. Biol.* 2010; **55**(3):581–598.

47 Ayyangar, K., Leonard, C., and Suntharalingam, J. Computerization of electron beams for treatment planning. *Med. Phys.* 1980; **7**:440.

48 Kawachi, K. Calculation of electron dose distribution for radiotherapy treatment planning. *Phys. Med. Biol.* 1975; **20**:571–577.

49 Shabason, L., and Hendee, W. R. An analytic expression for central axis electron depth dose distributions. *Int. J. Radiat. Oncol. Biol. Phys.* 1979; **5**:263–267.

50 Hogstrom, K. R., Mills, M. D., and Almond, P. R. Electron beam dose calculations. *Phys. Med. Biol.* 1981; **26**:445–459.

51 Lillicrap, S. C, Wilson, P., and Boag, J. W Dose distributions in high energy electron beams: Production of broad beam distributions from narrow beam data. *Phys. Med. Biol.* 1975; **20**:30–38.

52 Mah, E., et al. Experimental evaluation of a 2D and 3D electron pencil beam algorithm. *Phys. Med. Biol.* 1989; **34**:1179–1194.

53 Shiu, A. S. and Hogstrom, K. R. Pencil-beam redefinition algorithm for electron dose distributions. *Med. Phys.* 1991; **18**(1): 7–18.

54 Fragoso, M., et al. Experimental verification and clinical implementation of a commercial Monte Carlo electron beam dose calculation algorithm. *Med Phys.* 2008; **35**(3):1028–1038.

55 Hu, Y. A., et al. Evaluation of an electron Monte Carlo dose calculation algorithm for electron beam. *J. Appl. Clin. Med. Phys.* 2008; **9**(3):2720.

EXTERNAL BEAM TREATMENT PLANNING AND DELIVERY

Objectives

After studying this chapter, the reader should be able to:
- Identify the major steps in the treatment planning process.
- Describe the role of virtual simulation in radiation therapy treatment planning.
- Differentiate between immobilization and localization, and describe current techniques for both.
- Identify the various definitions of target volumes.
- Differentiate between serial and parallel organs at risk.
- Describe the process of inverse planning and identify several optimization algorithms used in inverse planning.
- Give examples of cases favorable to either forward planning or inverse planning.
- Define intensity modulated radiation therapy.
- Describe intensity modulated radiation therapy delivery methods.
- Describe serial tomotherapy and helical tomotherapy.
- Describe robotic treatment delivery.

Introduction

Treatment planning involves many processes and decisions leading to the treatment of a patient. Dose calculation is just one of the processes in this chain of events and is described in Chapter 8. However, other processes include a physician's analysis and interpretation of diagnostic procedures, consultations with other specialists, decisions supporting treatment with external radiation, and simulation of proposed treatment fields.

The treatment planning process can be described in the following manner:

1 The physician determines the *target volume* to be irradiated on the basis of physical examination, pathology results, and imaging studies. Computed tomography (CT) is one of the most commonly used imaging techniques for treatment planning, although magnetic resonance imaging (MRI),

Hendee's Radiation Therapy Physics, Fourth Edition. Todd Pawlicki, Daniel J. Scanderbeg and George Starkschall.
© 2016 John Wiley & Sons, Inc. Published 2016 by John Wiley & Sons, Inc.

radiography, angiography, radionuclide (metabolic) imaging, and other techniques can be used.

2 The physician then specifies the dose to be delivered to the target volume. This "dose prescription" is generally based on the physician's experience and on published reports and recommendations. In some cases, the dose prescription is dictated by the requirements of a clinical trial. The clarity of the prescription may be improved through use of the terminology recommended by the International Commission on Radiation Units and Measurements (ICRU).[1] The ICRU is an international group of volunteer experts that publishes reports and guidance on a wide variety of topics related to ionizing radiation.

3 The physician often will also identify sensitive normal tissues, or *organs at risk* (OAR), and specify dose-volume constraints for these OAR. These constraints may take the form of an upper limit of dose for tissues such as the spinal cord. This upper limit may be specified either as maximum dose to any point in the region or as maximum dose to a specified volume in the region. For other tissues, such as lungs or parotids, the constraints may take the form of a mean dose or a maximum dose to a specified volume in the region. These limiting doses are based on the physician's experience, as well as on the determination of *tolerance doses* for the organs, above which an unacceptable frequency of complications might be expected.

4 Through consultation with a medical physicist and/or a dosimetrist, the physician selects treatment beams and energies to be used. In some circumstances, the choice of beam modality and energy may be guided by the location of the target organ or by the maximum depth of the target tissue.[2]

In more complicated cases, the beam modality and energy are chosen by comparing alternate treatment plans generated as described in Step 5.

5 Finally a treatment plan is generated and optimized. The procedure is guided by a number of goals[3] such as:
   • The dose gradient throughout the tumor should be minimal.
   • The tumor dose should be significantly greater than the dose anywhere else in the irradiated volume.
   • The *integral dose* should be kept as low as possible.
   • The shape of the high-dose volume should conform to the *planning target volume* (PTV).
   • The dose to OAR should be kept below levels that have a significant probability of causing damage.
   • The dose distribution should consider regions of possible tumor extension or lymphatic spread (these should be included in the PTV).

Early treatment-planning computers simply reproduced manual methods already in use. As more powerful computers have become available, increasingly complex techniques have become practical, such as implementation of Monte Carlo calculations (described in Chapter 8).

During the 1980s and early 1990s, a transition occurred from two-dimensional (2D) planning to systems that began to encompass the three-dimensional (3D) nature of the patient and certain aspects of treatment planning. The term *three-dimensional treatment planning* describes current clinical treatment planning systems. All systems permit the entry of image data, such as that from a CT scanner, which is then manipulated and displayed in other orientations to demonstrate the 3D nature of the patient's anatomy. True 3D calculation of the absorbed radiation dose is performed. Three-dimensional treatment planning allows physicians to simulate the delivery of radiation directly on an image-based model of the patient. This advance has increased accuracy in treatment field design. Although considerably more complex and demanding of computer resources, 3D treatment planning is both cost-effective and practical in modern radiation oncology departments.[4]

Techniques of shaping radiation dose distributions to the target volume are referred to as *conformal therapy* (Figure 9-1).[5]

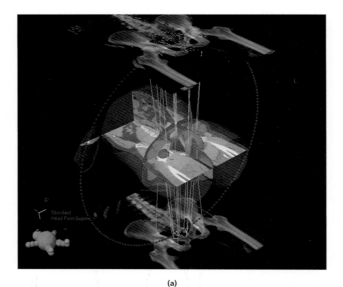

(a)

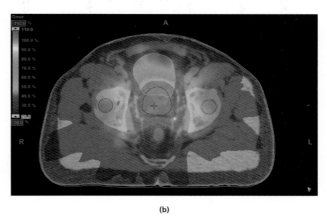

(b)

Figure 9-1 (a) CT image obtained through the pelvis of a patient undergoing radiation therapy. (b) The prostate, rectum, and bladder are outlined, and a planning target volume is drawn around the prostate to include a margin. Conformal shaped beams are placed to deliver a uniform dose to the target. For a color version of this figure, see the color plate section.

The term was coined in 1961 by Takahashi to connote techniques to match the high-dose region of treatment to the irregular 3D shape of the treatment volume. Most people refer to it as 3D conformal radiotherapy (3DCRT). The increased use of conformal therapy permits the delivery of higher doses to the target volume while maintaining acceptable doses to adjacent normal tissues. This capability improves the probability of tumor control without a corresponding increase in treatment complications.[4] As technology has continued to improve with both hardware and software advances, *intensity-modulated radiation therapy* (IMRT) has allowed for even higher conformal doses with acceptable normal tissue doses.

Virtual simulation techniques

The *simulator* is a device that mimics the geometry of the treatment unit. It is used to position the patient for treatment and to determine the location of the central beam axis (isocenter). In the past, this had been accomplished with a physical device in which the patient was positioned under fluoroscopic guidance and planar x-ray films were taken to define the treatment field. Conventional simulators have been superseded by the use of CT simulators, in which the simulation x-ray image is replaced by a *digitally reconstructed radiograph* (DRR), calculated by casting rays from a virtual source and calculating the attenuation of these rays through the 3D CT image data set. To obtain the resolution typical of a conventional simulation x-ray film, virtual simulation studies may require transverse images every few millimeters. Also, to provide sufficient patient anatomy superior and inferior to the target, the length of the patient scanned may extend well above and below the target. A 30 cm length scanned in 0.2 cm increments yields 150 CT images that must be fed into the planning computer. The images must be thin (i.e., small slice thickness) and contiguous for best results. In the computer workstation, the image information is reformatted and reconstructed to yield 3D representations of the patient. In this process of *virtual simulation*, a conventional CT scanner is used to (a) produce images comparable to those generated by a radiation therapy simulator and (b) to duplicate the patient-alignment functions of an analog simulator.[6–9]

A full set of parallel CT images contains an enormous amount of data, the presentation of which can be complicated and confusing. To address this difficulty, different methods of displaying 3D information have been developed.[10] They include the use of selective *volume rendering* techniques,[11–13] in which only tissues corresponding to a selected range of densities are displayed and the use of semitransparent structures so that other structures can be seen through them (Figure 9-2).

To enable the visualization of patient anatomy with respect to the proposed treatment beam, a technique known as *beam's eye view* (BEV) has been developed. BEV replaces the conventional simulation image. By moving the CT data set relative to the beam and updating the BEV in real time, *virtual fluoroscopy* can be

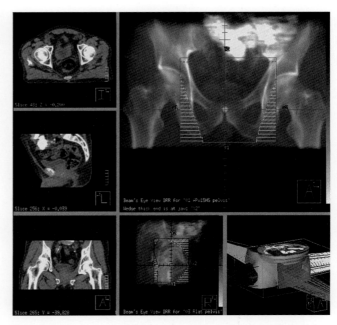

Figure 9-2 Reconstruction of CT images can present patient information in a variety of ways. **Counterclockwise from top left:** Transverse, sagittal, coronal, lateral DRR, 3D reconstruction, and anterior DRR.

performed that allows the physician to accurately position the isocenter in the virtual patient. In this approach, patient anatomy is displayed as if it were being viewed from the source of radiation. The central axis of the beam is identified, typically appearing as a dot or cross in the center of the image, and the edges of the field are shown as a rectangle at the location of the isocenter of the treatment unit. Through the use of real-time 3D display techniques, patient anatomy can be rotated and translated to simulate gantry rotation and couch motion, and the rectangle representing the radiation beam can be rotated to simulate collimator rotation. Finally, beam-shaping blocks, or the leaves of a *multileaf collimator* (MLC), are drawn to indicate the shape of the field.

As a final step in the virtual simulation procedure, a DRR is generated (Figure 9-3).[14,15] The result is an image comparable to a simulator film, and many systems include additional features to enhance the DRR image. The CT images contain soft tissue and bony information in a matrix format and the computer can reconstruct this information in ways to provide the physician with valuable information.

All systems also permit multi-modality image fusion, such as superimposing MR images on CT images. In this way the physician can use the increased tissue contrast provided by MR images to aid in the design of the treatment fields. Image registration, once tedious and time-consuming, is now an automated process utilizing techniques such as *mutual information*, which translates and rotates (and possibly distorts) one image until maximum correlation with the second image is achieved.[16,17] The physician or physicist can then fine-tune the fusion based

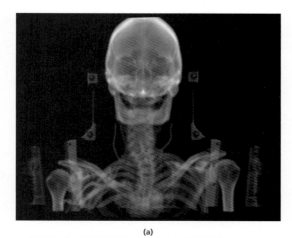

(a)

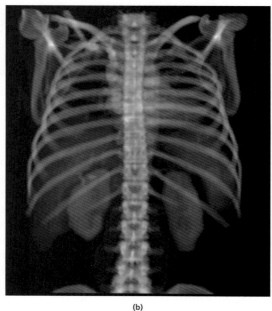

(b)

Figure 9-3 Digitally reconstructed radiographs for a head treatment (a) and gastroesophageal (GE) junction (b). Thin slices provide detail similar to that of conventional simulation films.

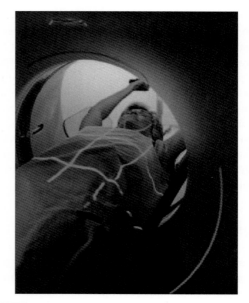

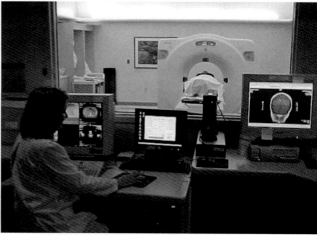

Figure 9-4 CT simulation, showing patient setup to fit easily through the bore of the scanner, and lasers used to mark setup points. The console area has the CT control console, laser positioning system, and viewing workstation.

on experience. Although CT and MR images may display pixel values using different lookup tables, the similarities in anatomy are characterized as mutual information. The process of correlating and aligning the anatomy yields an accurate image fusion.

Many centers have abandoned conventional simulators and are using the space to house a CT scanner to achieve virtual simulations (Figure 9-4). A few issues must be considered when using a CT simulator in place of a conventional simulator:

1 Differences in geometry between the virtual simulator and the treatment machine. The principal limitation here is the physical bore size of the CT scanner, typically around 70 cm, compared with the relatively unobstructed treatment setup on the linear accelerator. This is particularly a problem for breast treatments in which the arm is raised above the patient's head

and may not be very mobile after surgery. For large patients, the field of view of the scanner may not be great enough to provide the patient's external contour. Larger-bore scanners exist to solve these problems (e.g., 85 cm), but budget constraints for many departments limit their availability, particularly if the scanner is shared with the radiology department.

2 Inability of the couch to move laterally and vertical limits of couch movement. Most scanners have an internal laser system, but it often does not perform at the exacting levels required for radiation therapy, because the lasers are mounted on the moving gantry. Fixed wall lasers have to be shifted out of the isocenter of the CT scanner, since that point is within the bore of the scanner. In addition, the bore limits couch movement compared with conventional simulation, with no

lateral movement or rotation and limited vertical movement. To solve these problems, movable lasers are available which are shifted a known distance out of the bore. These lasers can be programmed directly from the virtual simulation software to indicate isocenter position.

3 Philosophy of technique. There are two schools of thought with regard to virtual simulation. The first is to use the simulator to create a 3D model of the patient, with the actual simulation performed as a post-processing procedure that does not require the patient to stay on the table. In this way, the time of the simulation (and one of the patient's first experiences in treatment) is kept to a minimum. This approach requires the patient to be marked with reference points prior to leaving, and any shift in the actual treatment isocenter must take place at a later time. The second school of thought is to follow the traditional simulation technique, which requires the patient to be present until the simulation is complete. In this case, the isocenter can be marked directly on the patient, avoiding any future shift. With the additional contouring on the CT images, however, this process can often take much longer than a traditional simulation, thereby causing discomfort to the patient. Some centers accept a compromise in which the physician sets the isocenter, but all contouring and beam placement take place after the patient has left.

Defining the target and other structures precisely on the CT images with the patient in the treatment position allows the beam portals to be precisely aligned. This provides many options, such as reduced margins and dose escalation, to increase the success of the radiation treatment.

Immobilization and localization

Consistency is critical in patient setup between virtual simulation and treatment, as well as in localization of the target. Two key concepts in creating reproducible patient setups are *immobilization* and *localization*. Immobilization devices position the patient and restrict motion and are created at the time of the simulation. Localization techniques use information obtained at the time of simulation to accurately position the isocenter and are typically applied at the time of treatment. Immobilization and localization devices to achieve this goal come in two principal varieties: (a) external fixation and localization devices and (b) internal image-based localization.

Common external fixation and localization devices include molds and masks shaped to the patient's external surface to provide a reproducible setup from treatment to treatment (Figure 9-5). Fine tolerances on couch position for these systems can be achieved by using devices that are locked to the treatment couch in positions to match the virtual simulation. Optical imaging can be used to recreate the patient's external surface for positioning the patient (Figure 9-6). In this case, two or three room cameras compare the difference between images taken at the time

of treatment to a reference image, and real-time patient monitoring can be achieved with this method. Hence, respiratory motion can be monitored in this manner and gated treatments are possible. Additionally, accuracy sufficient for cranial stereotactic radiosurgery (SRS) can be achieved with such a monitoring system.

A similar concept is to use a camera system with external fiducials to position the patient. External fiducials commonly employ markers, such as reflective balls, with a camera system used to monitor their position. This information can be used to position the patient and accurately localize the target. In addition, the fiducial locations can be used to trigger the beam on and off in response to patient motion such as breathing. If the balls are referenced to a fixed part of patient anatomy (e.g., the hard palate, by mounting the fiducials on a custom dental bite block), setup accuracy required for stereotactic radiotherapy can be achieved. The fiducials can be monitored during treatment to ensure that the patient does not move.

Internal or image-based localization is used to reduce setup error between treatments, based on image information available at the time of treatment. Internal fiducials are also commonly used, either implanted in the skull for SRS and radiotherapy or implanted in the target itself (e.g., prostate) (Figure 9-7).

Segmentation of the CT image data set

As was described previously in the treatment planning process, the CT image data set needs to be segmented and the physician needs to delineate the target volume to be treated. This is typically done via manual contouring. Two broad categories of structures need to be defined: target and OAR. The target can be further broken down into various components:[1,18]

- Gross tumor volume (GTV): The GTV is the region of demonstrable disease and is delineated by the physician based on any palpable mass or visible observation of mass on imaging, such as CT, MRI, PET, US.
- Clinical target volume (CTV): The CTV is the volume that must be irradiated to the desired prescription dose and is defined by the physician as the GTV plus a margin that includes microscopic disease not visible on imaging based on knowledge of tumor spread. For example, a margin of 6–8 mm is typically used in planning non-small-cell lung cancer. This margin is based on pathology studies.[19]

Both the GTV and CTV are oncological entities that must be defined prior to treatment planning and are independent of the specific treatment modality.

- Internal target volume (ITV): The ITV is the volume that incorporates the CTV and accounts for intrafractional tumor motion and interfractional anatomic variation. The ITV is determined by the physicist based on knowledge of intrafractional tumor motion and interfractional anatomic variation. This is an expansion for internal changes or motion.

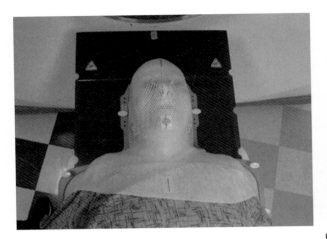
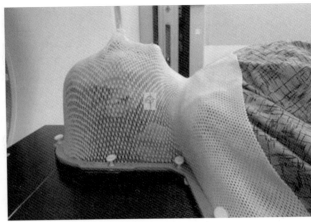

(a)

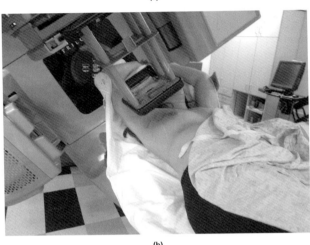

(b)

Figure 9-5 (a) Immobilization of patient for head and neck treatment. This system incorporates shoulder immobilization and extends beyond the end of the treatment couch. (b) Immobilization for breast treatment with both arms extended above the patient's head and uses a commercial breast board for repositioning. For a color version of this figure, see the color plate section.

- Planning target volume (PTV): The PTV is a geometrical concept used to add additional margin to ensure the target receives the prescribed dose, taking into consideration patient setup inaccuracies. The PTV is determined by the physicist based on the immobilization technique for the patient. It should be noted that the ITV and PTV cannot be changed after treatment planning unless there is a physical justification for their change, such as a different immobilization technique.

A variety of methods can be used to contour normal tissue anatomy, including manual delineation, threshold-based segmentation, and model-based segmentation. Manual segmentation is the most time-consuming as it requires the user to manually delineate each structure, as is done for the target volume. Threshold-based segmentation is one of the simplest types of segmentation tools and works well for lung and bony anatomy as it segments pixels depending on their intensity value. Lung and bone have sharp large intensity differences compared to surrounding tissue and steep gradients at their boundaries and are

completely surrounded by surrounding tissue. Model-based segmentation starts with a model of anatomic structures from a library of models and then deforms the organ model to fit the current CT image dataset.[20,21]

Selection of ideal treatment plan

Development of the ideal treatment plan requires a process for altering treatment planning parameters (either manually or automatically) to yield an optimal dose throughout the PTV, while keeping the dose low to OAR.[22] For conventional treatment planning, the alteration of treatment parameters is conducted by trial and error and is influenced by the combined experience of the planner and the physician. Alternative treatment plans are generated sequentially, and the improvement or deterioration of the plan is noted, until an ideal plan is reached,

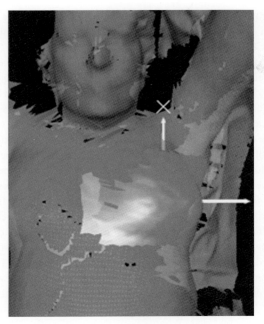

Figure 9-6 Optical surface imaging used for positioning or patient monitoring. For a color version of this figure, see the color plate section.

when the PTV is adequately covered and the OAR doses are within tolerance.

Optimization and evaluation of a treatment plan includes the review of isodose curves on images as well as analysis of statistical information about the treatment plan. An isodose curve

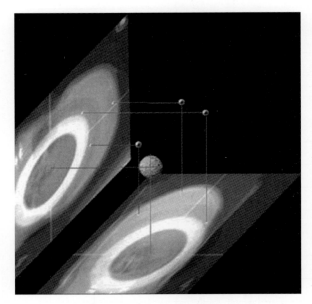

Figure 9-7 X-ray localization utilizing implanted fiducials. Two orthogonal films are taken, and the gold fiducials (three small spheres) are digitized from each image. By triangulation and with known positions of the markers relative to the target (larger sphere), the target can be accurately positioned for treatment.

is analogous to a topographic map with contour lines denoting areas with the same altitude, or elevation. Similarly, an isodose distribution displays areas receiving the same radiation dose. This can be visually displayed as isodose lines or as a dose color-wash. A visual check of the isodose distribution can quickly give information about target coverage and organ sparing.

To improve the process of optimizing a treatment plan, several computational techniques are available that yield useful statistical information about the plan. A histogram is one of these methods. A histogram is used to show the distribution of data in a graphical representation with the data first divided up into bins (x-axis) and the number of counts of a certain value, for each bin, on the y-axis. In radiation therapy, a useful histogram is the *dose–volume histogram* (DVH). A DVH is a graphic representation that relates the dose received by the patient (x-axis) to the volume of tissue receiving the dose (y-axis).[23–25]

Dose–volume histograms

Figures 9-8 through 9-12 illustrate the step-by-step procedure for developing a DVH for a simple example of a treatment of the target with an adjacent OAR, using an equally weighted *4-field box* technique. Figure 9-8 shows a rectangular PTV and OAR.

The dose received is indicated within each square and is a function of dose deposition as a function of depth. Figure 9-9 shows the photon beam percent depth dose curve that is used for calculating the dose delivered to each square in this plan.

Figure 9-10 shows the calculated dose distribution, mapped onto the square array, and binned in each box.

Figure 9-11a and b show the cumulative dose distribution and cumulative dose matrix for the equally weighted 4-field box treatment, respectively. Another way to present the data shown in Figure 9-11a is to normalize the dose matrix. This is shown

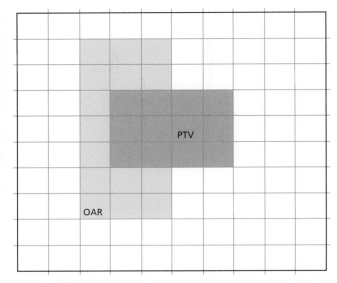

Figure 9-8 Schematic diagram showing rectangular PTV adjacent to OAR.

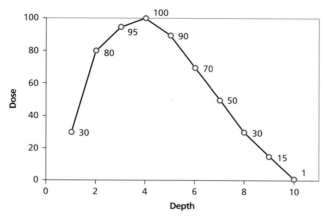

Figure 9-9 Percent depth dose curve used in this example to calculate dose to each square in the plan.

in Figure 9-11b. Here, the dose has been normalized to the maximum dose in Figure 9-11a, which is 320. This is accomplished by dividing all the values shown by 320.

There are two types of DVHs: differential and cumulative. The differential DVH is a histogram of dose bins and the frequency with which each dose occurs in each bin. The differential DVH for the dose distribution and structures shown in Figure 9-11 is illustrated in Figure 9-12.

The differential DVH is peaked for the PTV at the maximum dose of 100. The skin also shows a peak at 100 because the PTV is included in the skin, but the skin differential DVH is peaked at lower doses because most of the skin is getting a low dose. The DVH for the OAR has a peak at the lower dose of about 40 and the skin also shows a corresponding peak at that dose level.

Differential DVHs have not been routinely used in the clinic. However, calculating the differential DVHs is the first step toward calculating the cumulative DVH, and cumulative DVHs are considered more valuable for routine treatment plan evaluation. When most individuals refer to a DVH, they are referring

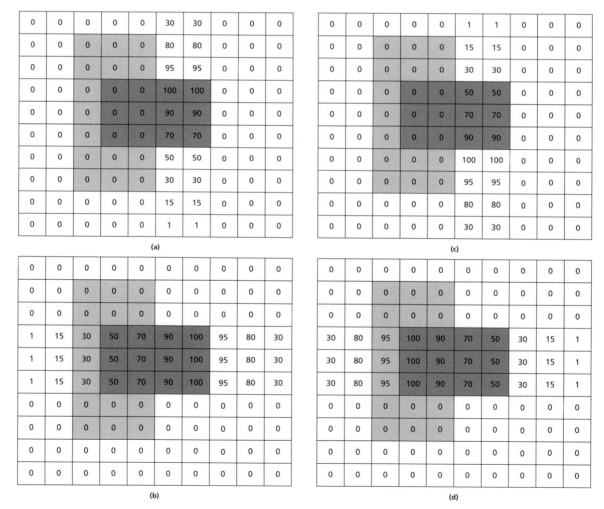

Figure 9-10 Four dose matrices corresponding to each of the fields in a 4-field box treatment. (a) Dose matrix for AP treatment field. (b) Dose matrix for PA treatment field. (c) Dose matrix for left lateral treatment field. (d) Dose matrix for right lateral treatment field.

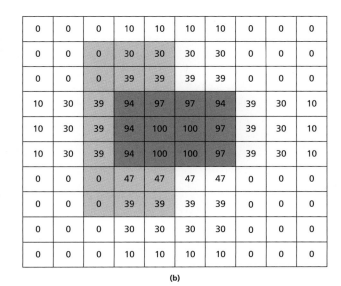

0	0	0	31	31	31	31	0	0	0
0	0	0	95	95	95	95	0	0	0
0	0	0	125	125	125	125	0	0	0
31	95	125	300	310	310	300	125	95	31
31	95	125	310	320	320	310	125	95	31
31	95	125	310	320	320	310	125	95	31
0	0	0	150	150	150	150	0	0	0
0	0	0	125	125	125	125	0	0	0
0	0	0	95	95	95	95	0	0	0
0	0	0	31	31	31	31	0	0	0

(a)

0	0	0	10	10	10	10	0	0	0
0	0	0	30	30	30	30	0	0	0
0	0	0	39	39	39	39	0	0	0
10	30	39	94	97	97	94	39	30	10
10	30	39	94	100	100	97	39	30	10
10	30	39	94	100	100	97	39	30	10
0	0	0	47	47	47	47	0	0	0
0	0	0	39	39	39	39	0	0	0
0	0	0	30	30	30	30	0	0	0
0	0	0	10	10	10	10	0	0	0

(b)

Figure 9-11 (a) Cumulative dose matrix. (b) Normalized dose matrix.

to a cumulative DVH. A cumulative DVH is determined in a similar fashion as the differential DVH. A cumulative DVH for the 4-field box treatment of the target described above is shown in Figure 9-13.

The cumulative DVH plots the volume as a function of cumulative dose received. That means it represents the volume of a structure that receives a dose equal to or greater than a particular dose. The horizontal axis (dose) is labeled in units of cumulative dose and the vertical axis (volume) of a cumulative DVH graph can be labeled as either an absolute volume or normalized volume, as shown in Figure 9-13. Cumulative DVHs are often used to compare competing treatment plans and the best plan is often selected from the DVH.

The example shown above is for a case where the main objective is to treat the PTV and obtain maximum coverage of the PTV. This can be observed in the cumulative DVH with normalized values as the PTV line is pushed out to the far right,

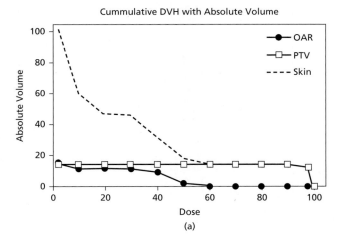

(a)

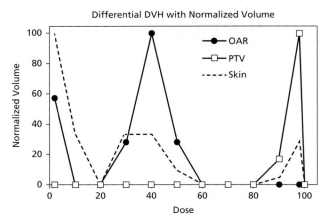

Figure 9-12 Differential dose–volume histogram of the dose distribution shown in Figure 9.11.

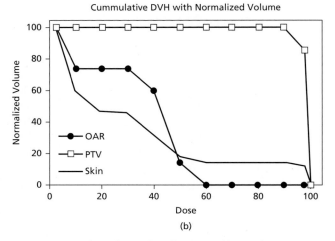

(b)

Figure 9-13 Cumulative dose–volume histogram. (a) Cumulative dose–volume histogram with absolute volumes displayed. (b) Cumulative dose–volume histogram with normalized volumes displayed.

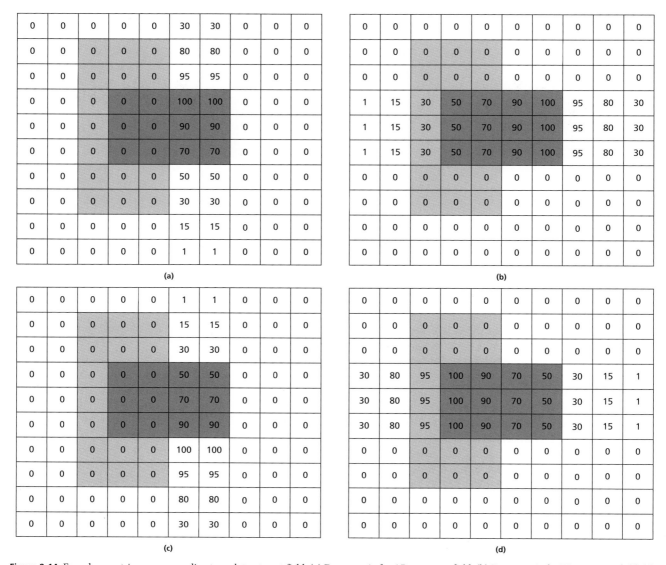

Figure 9-14 Four dose matrices corresponding to each treatment field. (a) Dose matrix for AP treatment field. (b) Dose matrix for PA treatment field. (c) Dose matrix for left lateral treatment field. (d) Dose matrix for right lateral treatment field.

indicating that 100% of the dose is covering a large percentage of the volume. In other words, a large percentage of the target volume is being covered by 100% of the prescribed dose. A perfect DVH for a target would be flat and then have a straight vertical drop at 100% of the dose. However, that is an ideal case, and there is usually a small shoulder in the upper right of the curve along with a small tail in the lower right (Figure 9-13b). These indicate a small deficiency in covering the target completely along with some volume of the target getting more than the prescribed dose (hot spots), respectively.

OAR for an ideal plan will have a small percentage of volume receiving a high dose. An ideal plan would also demonstrate a straight vertical drop along the vertical axis, toward the origin, for the OAR, in which 100% of the OAR volume receives none of the dose. Again, this would be for an ideal case

and more often we have something similar to that shown in Figure 9-13b, where the DVH curve slowly decreases to zero. Plans that are effective at sparing OARs have DVH curves that are pushed to the bottom left of the figure. Figure 9-14 illustrates the DVH curve of the same treatment where the OAR have been spared more than the previous example. The figure shows the dose distribution that is used for the AP, PA, left lateral, and right lateral beams in the same 4-field box plan. Figure 9-15a, b, and c show the cumulative dose matrix, normalized dose matrix, and normalized cumulative DVH, respectively.

As can be seen in Figure 9-15c, the DVH for the PTV has a large dip due to the sacrifice of coverage in order to spare the OAR. Care should be taken when analyzing DVHs to ensure adequate target coverage along with OAR sparing.

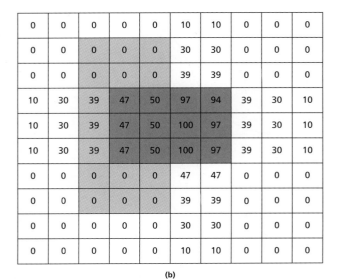

(a)

(b)

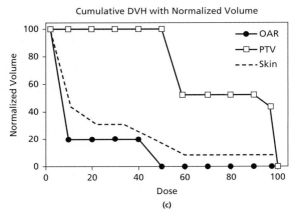

Cumulative DVH with Normalized Volume

(c)

Figure 9-15 (a) Cumulative dose matrix. (b) Normalized dose matrix. (c) Normalized cumulative dose–volume histogram.

Biological modeling

The technique of *biological modeling* in radiation therapy involves maximizing the *tumor control probability* (TCP) and minimizing the *normal tissue complication probability* (NTCP). It has long been recognized that the distribution of absorbed dose is not the only criterion that might be used to select a superior treatment plan from several alternatives. Because biological response is probably not a linear function of dose, factors such as variable sensitivities of different tissues, effects of fractionation, and the possible use of biological modifiers must be considered. Some of these factors have been addressed through the development of models for TCP and NTCP.[26–30] Both quantities are sigmoidal functions of dose. That is, for low doses, the curves of TCP and NTCP versus dose are relatively flat indicating a relative insensitivity to dose. At some value of dose, the curves rise steeply until a value of 100% is reached. At this value of dose, the probability of either tumor control or normal tissue complications is near 100%. Beyond this dose, the curve is flat. Representative graphs of TCP and NTCP are shown in Figure 9-16. The product of TCP and (1-NTCP) yields the probability of *uncomplicated tumor control*. A representative graph is shown in Figure 9-17. As of this date, however, only limited efforts have been made to correlate these biological models with clinical outcome data.

Forward planning

The concept of *forward planning* (Figure 9-18 and Figure 9-19) involves the modification of beam parameters based on observed isodose distributions or patient geometry.[32] Typically, forward planning begins by setting up a common beam arrangement for the site being treated. Then the dose is computed, and *hot spots* or *cold spots* are detected in the dose distribution. Next, a set of sub-beams (also known as segments or control points) are generated to reduce the hot spots and increase dose to the hot spots. Finally, the weighting of the beams is adjusted to provide a uniform dose across the treated region, either manually or automatically.

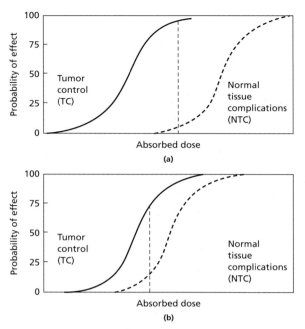

Figure 9-16 A schematic showing the tumor control probability and normal tissue complication probability as a function of dose. (a) A favorable situation in which a high tumor control probability can result with a small complication probability. (b) A less favorable situation where a high tumor control probability would result in a larger complication probability. *Source:* Wambersie et al. 1988.[31]

Forward planning techniques may be utilized to achieve a more uniform dose to the target volume. It requires an initial calculation of dose with subsequent beam modifiers to adjust various dose levels. Most treatment planning systems can accommodate some form of forward planning. Several advantages are achieved by using a forward planning technique. First, the resulting beams are rather intuitive since they are based on observed dosimetry. Second, there are relatively few control points when compared with intensity modulation techniques. Third, quality assurance can often be accommodated by using the current clinical techniques in use. This approach can often save time in treatment planning and delivery, by eliminating trial-and-error approaches such as multiple wedge angles and/or

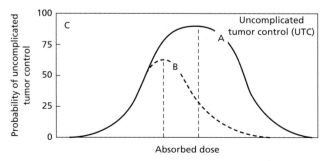

Figure 9-17 The "mantelpiece clock" overlap curve of TCP and (1-NTCP). Curves A and B correspond with use of the curves from Figure 9.10. This shows the probability of uncomplicated tumor control (P_{UTC}). *Source:* Wambersie et al. 1988.[31]

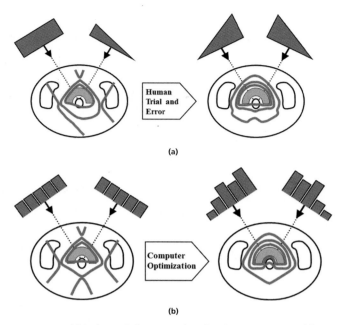

Figure 9-18 (a) In forward planning, a dose distribution is computed for external beams of specified size, direction, and weighting. (b) In inverse planning, the size, direction, intensity modulation, and weighting of external beams are computed to deliver a predetermined dose distribution.

orientations. In the case of tangential fields for treating the breast, for example, the dosimetrist may have to try a number of wedges and wedge orientations to get the best treatment plan. Beam modification can take the form of wedges, blocks, compensators, beam weighting, or fluence editing. Wedges, blocks, and compensators can alter the isodose distribution through attenuation of the radiation beam. Beam weighting also modifies the isodose distribution; however, this is done through placement of a weight factor on each beam such that more dose is delivered through one beam angle than another.

Fluence editing can also modify the isodose lines by using the MLCs to attenuate the beam. One example of the use of fluence editing would be for a breast treatment where the forward planning technique can use a standard wedge in one field and the segments on the other field effectively "clean up" the dose distribution. With this approach, the radiation therapists do not have multiple wedges and wedge orientations to contend with during treatment, thereby shortening the overall treatment time.

Inverse planning

Inverse planning is the name given to a prescribed technique of treatment optimization by automated methods.[33,34] For radiation therapy, it involves development of a treatment plan whereby the planning computer is given a set of objectives and beam parameters to adjust in an iterative fashion to arrive at a satisfactory dose distribution. For example, the treatment planning computer could iteratively adjust the weights of the beams to provide the most uniform dose to the target. In

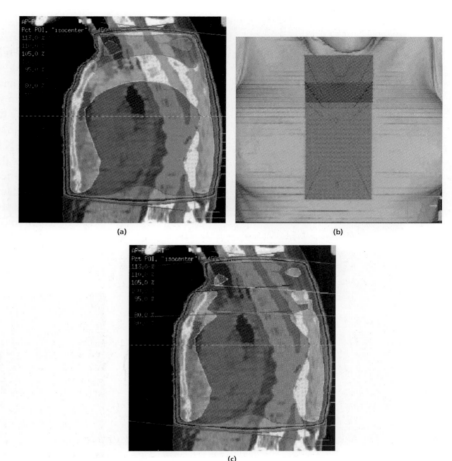

Figure 9-19 Forward planning example for AP/PA treatment of the mediastinum. (a) Sagittal view of AP/PA treatment plan with open fields and no wedges. (b) Anterior surface rendering showing the original field and two smaller fields (*subfields* or *segments*) with the superior jaw position reduced to block higher dose levels in thinner parts of the patient. (c) By adjusting the weights of the segments, a uniform dose throughout the entire region is obtained.

this case, the objective is uniform dose to the target, and the adjustable beam parameter is the weight of each beam. Iterative problem-solving techniques in inverse planning, particularly with complex objective functions, is an ideal application for fast treatment planning computers. A disadvantage of inverse planning is that there are often multiple objective functions, and the relative weighting of importance of the various objectives adds an additional level of complexity and variability to the planning process.

Individual beams can be divided into small (e.g., 5 mm × 5 mm) beamlets, and the weight of each beamlet can be adjusted to provide a uniform dose to the target, while at the same time limiting the dose to normal tissues. This technique is known as *intensity-modulated radiation therapy* (IMRT).[35–38] In the case of a seven-beam arrangement of 10 cm × 10 cm fields broken into 5 mm × 5 mm beamlets, the result is 400 beamlets for each beam, or a total of 2800 adjustable parameters!

Intensity modulated radiation therapy

The advantage of intensity modulation is that it allows the delivery of uniform dose distributions to concave target volumes, which is not possible with unmodulated beams. Beam direction can be important in the optimization process.[39,40] The beam direction may be set by the operator, positioned at predetermined angles, or in some cases there is a separate optimization process that selects optimal beam angles for treatment. The computer then adjusts the beamlet weights to find the optimum solution (Figure 9-20).[41,42]

Treatment planning techniques

IMRT requires the clinician to accurately define the treatment objectives. This task can be quite involved, because choices must be made not only about what occurs within the target but also about what happens anywhere the beams intersect. Routinely, more beams are required in IMRT than with other techniques, such as 3D conformal treatment planning, and these beams may be irradiating tissues that previously were outside the fields. For example, head and neck portals typically utilize lateral fields, but with IMRT, it is common to use seven or nine beams around the circumference of the patient, causing irradiation of tissues, such as the anterior portion of the mouth and the cerebellum that were previously blocked.[43] While it is true that the dose to these structures is significantly less than the target dose, these

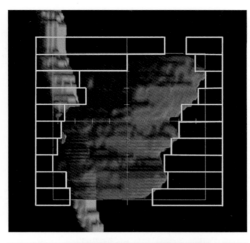

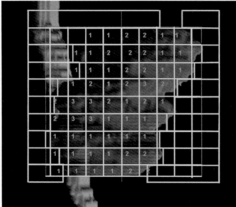

Figure 9-20 Initialization of optimization by defining field limits (top image), and creating beamlets with adjustable weights (bottom image).

structures must be identified and included in the inverse planning process and evaluated by the physician and monitored during treatment to quickly detect unanticipated side effects. Although dose can be highly conformal compared with even 3DCRT, IMRT has its advantages and disadvantages. The major advantage is the highly conformal nature of the dose delivery; however, a disadvantage is the low dose smearing around the target area. Due to the large number of treatment fields needed for IMRT, large regions that would have received little to no dose with 3DCRT receive low doses in IMRT.

There are three general classifications of anatomical structures in IMRT planning:

1 Target volumes. Target volumes in IMRT should follow ICRU 50 and 62 definitions described previously. The GTV is contoured manually by the physician to include all palpable or visible disease on imaging studies. The GTV is expanded to create the CTV based on microscopic disease that is not visible on imaging based on knowledge of disease spread. The CTV can then be expanded to create an ITV and PTV by the physicist to include intra- and interfractional motion and setup uncertainty.

2 Critical structures or OARs. With IMRT, defining critical structures becomes very important, because the beams are likely to be converging from many directions, and more OARs will be irradiated. Also, if the computer does not know that a structure is present, it will not be able to avoid it. Since it is possible to obtain steep dose gradients with IMRT, adequate margins must be defined around critical structures such as the spinal cord to account for patient setup uncertainty and motion.[44,45] The ICRU defines the *planning organ at risk volume* (PRV) to be the OAR plus this margin.[18]

3 Dose shaping structures. To obtain the desired dose distribution and beam characteristics, it may be advantageous to utilize hypothetical structures that control the geometry of the dose distribution (Figure 9-21). These structures may or may not relate to actual patient anatomy. A rather simple example is to define normal tissue as everything that is not included in the target(s) and critical structures.

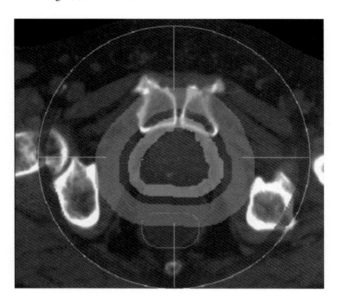

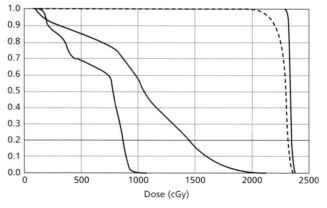

Figure 9-21 Dose-shaping structures and corresponding dose–volume histogram for a 3-D conformal treatment to be used in designing dose–volume-based objectives for IMRT. Each ring has a corresponding dose–volume histogram, with the outermost ring having the lowest dose and progressing inwards.

Setting the objective function

Objective functions used in IMRT can be determined from published clinical data, from experience from other institutions, and from current planning techniques. Objective functions can be either dose-based or dose–volume-based.[46–49] For example, "give a minimum dose of 5000 cGy to the PTV" is an example of a dose-based objective, whereas "keep the dose below 2000 cGy to 50% of the parotid volume" is an example of a dose–volume-based objective, because it includes information on how much of the volume can receive a given dose. The objectives are entered into the planning system by defining the name of the structure, dose level to achieve or avoid, fraction or percent of volume, and importance relative to other clinical objectives. The values are often displayed on a DVH to yield a graphical representation of the objectives.

In developing objectives to be used clinically, physicians can refer to previous experience by looking at DVHs from similar cases and making improvements. One of the primary goals of IMRT for prostate cancer, for example, is to lower the rectal dose. Previous DVHs for prostate patients provide a good baseline for how to set objectives to achieve that goal (Figure 9-22). Alternatively, clinicians may set objectives by utilizing published clinical data or experience from other institutions with IMRT capability (Figure 9-23). Many clinicians made use of the paper by Emami, et al.,[50] and now more recent data have come from

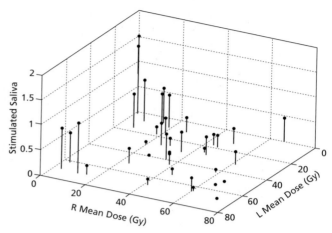

Figure 9-23 Stimulated saliva as a function of parotid dose. Either sparing one parotid or keeping the mean parotid dose less than 25 Gy should reduce the amount of xerostomia in patients.
Source: Chao, et al 2001[52] Reproduced with permission of Elsevier.

the Quantitative Analysis of Normal Tissue Effects in the Clinic (QUANTEC)[51].

In the development of dose-shaping objectives, trial and error may be used to obtain desirable dose distributions that satisfy physicians and physics staff. For example, if it is desired to keep overall beam weights similar for all fields, a ring structure at a large distance from the target can be utilized. The DVH for this structure is computed using uniform open fields of equal weight. This DVH is then used to create dose–volume objectives for that structure (see Figure 9-21).

Optimization

The objectives are combined to define an *objective function* or *cost function*, a measure of the disagreement between the desired dose distribution and the calculated distribution. A cost function is a way to mathematically describe the desired result and to assign "penalties" for not achieving the desired result. The objective function may be focused on achieving a uniformly homogeneous dose in the PTV and minimizing the integral dose to OAR. This function is iteratively optimized using one of several techniques that search for a minimum value of the objective function, depending upon the planning system in use. One of the dangers of using some optimization algorithms is the risk of being trapped in a local minimum of the objective function, not recognizing that the local minimum is some distance from the global minimum (Figure 9-24). The technique of *simulated annealing* allows one to escape a local minimum in the search for the global minimum of the cost function.[53]

The result of the optimization process is a *fluence map* for each beam. A fluence map (or intensity map) is a 2D matrix of beamlet intensity for each beam. It has been given other names, such as *intensity map*, *fluence matrix*, and *opening density matrix*. These matrices are commonly displayed as a

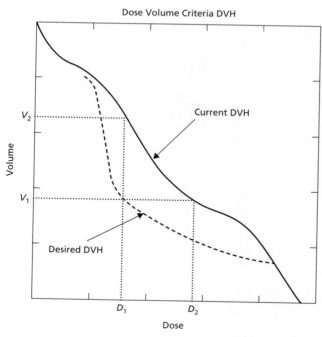

Dose Volume Criteria DVH

Figure 9-22 Dose–volume-based objective to make an improvement on the existing DVH. Generally, this technique is useful to lower the dose to a critical structure.
Source: Wu and Mohan 2000.[49] Reproduced with permission from American Association of Physicists in Medicine

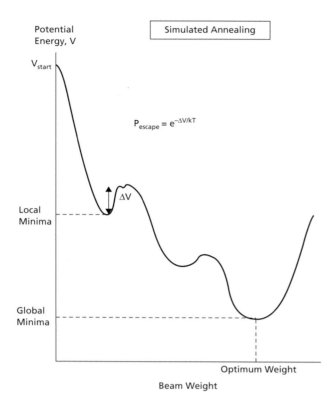

Figure 9-24 Optimization technique to prevent settling on a local minima solution. The optimizer has enough "energy" to escape small local traps to find a global solution.

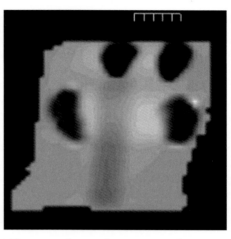

Figure 9-26 Fluence map for nasopharynx patient. The positions of the eyes and parotids are easily seen. The spinal cord is the slightly darkened region running vertically in the center of the image. Note the brighter area between the cord and parotids to make up for these areas being blocked from other beam directions.

2D gray scale image, or a 3D map, as shown in Figure 9-25 and Figure 9-26.

Conversion to deliverable treatment

The solution to the optimization of the objective function presents the ideal fluence to treat the patient. However, physical

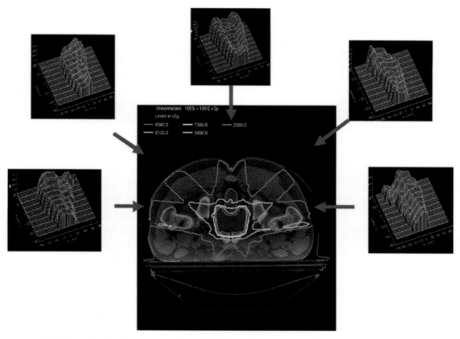

Figure 9-25 Five-field prostate IMRT showing 3D fluence maps for each field and the corresponding dose distribution in the patient. Although fluence maps appear to be complex, persons with experience can see common trends to assist in evaluating a treatment plan. These trends may include (a) a noticeable decrease in intensity in areas intersecting critical structures, (b) an increase in intensity outside a critical structure in the plane of gantry rotation to compensate for other beams with reduced intensity to avoid critical structures, and (c) an increase in intensity for projections that have the best view of the target.

restrictions of the treatment unit usually require conversion of the ideal fluence map to a fluence that can actually be delivered. The closest match to the ideal fluence map is achieved using x-ray beam compensators because they have a high resolution of the intensity map limited only by the physical properties of the machine used to mill or print the compensator. More often, MLCs are used to deliver the treatment. In this approach, the conversion process involves dividing the beam into a number of MLC patterns, or *segments*, that will deliver an approximation to the fluence map. As with the optimization process, a number of schemes have been developed for accomplishing this task and have been described in the literature.[54] The result of the optimization is a set of beam segments that approximate the fluence map according to parameters such as the minimum number of monitor units (MUs) per segment, size of segment, number of segments, and so on. When these segments are delivered by the treatment unit, a segment shape will be set, the beam will be turned on for the appropriate number of MUs, and the beam will then step to the next segment. Since the beam is off while the MLC leaves are moving, the method is commonly known as *step-and-shoot* or *static IMRT*. Once the segments have been converted, the delivered dose distribution should be evaluated, together with the final DVH, to ensure that all treatment objectives are met. In addition, the dose in areas outside the target volume should be examined closely to make sure that the dose in those areas is acceptable. It should be noted that optimization algorithms have been developed that solve directly for the MLC leaf settings. When such algorithms are used, it is not necessary to convert the fluence map to MLC leaf settings.

Dynamic delivery techniques

An alternative approach to treatment delivery involves moving the MLC leaves while the x-ray beam is on. This *sliding window* approach is more complex than step-and-shoot for the following reasons: (a) The "window" is often very narrow, resulting in narrow beam geometry and (b) the MLC quality assurance protocol for dynamic delivery is more stringent, requiring leaf speed characterization. With the sliding window method, very complex distributions can be achieved (as illustrated in Figure 9-27).

Allowing the gantry to rotate while the leaves are moving is a technique known as *volumetric modulated arc therapy* (VMAT).[55–57] This approach may require a few arc passes to completely deliver the treatment, because a given gantry angle can have only one MLC shape per arc. This method allows very complex dose distributions, but is challenging to plan and verify.

Tomotherapy

Tomotherapy is a treatment technique that combines the physical appearance and imaging capabilities similar to a CT scanner with some of the treatment capabilities of a linear accelerator.

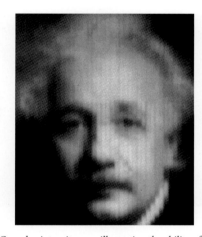

Figure 9-27 Complex intensity map illustrating the ability of IMRT to produce highly complex fields. The width of the leaves, oriented vertically, is the primary resolution limitation.
Source: Courtesy of Varian.

The treatment unit uses megavoltage x rays from a compact linear accelerator to image the patient. It then uses the same megavoltage x rays to treat the patient. The unit has a moveable couch that glides in and out of the bore of the treatment and imaging unit.

Serial tomotherapy

Serial tomotherapy (from the Greek *tomo*, meaning "slice"), has been in clinical use since 1994. The commercial system combines a narrow MLC attachment to the linac with precise couch increments to deliver a slice-by-slice treatment.[58,59] The MLC operates in binary mode, with the leaves either fully open or fully closed. Thousands of patients have been treated with this system, most of whom are patients with brain or head and neck cancers. This system has paved the way for other planning and delivery systems that are now available, because it provided much of the early clinical data demonstrating the benefits of IMRT.

Helical tomotherapy

In the same manner that CT scanners have moved from axial to helical delivery, tomotherapy has also adopted a helical delivery system.[60–63] The treatment unit looks much like a CT scanner, with a compact 6 MV linear accelerator replacing the x-ray tube. With this design, many of the components in a standard linear accelerator are not needed. For example, (a) the compact size eliminates the long cantilevered gantry and the bending magnet; (b) there are no electron energies and the target is fixed, so there is no carousel; and (c) since the beam is modulated by the MLC, there is no need for a flattening filter. The absence of a flattening filter provides a higher beam output compared with a flattened beam from a conventional linear accelerator. A binary

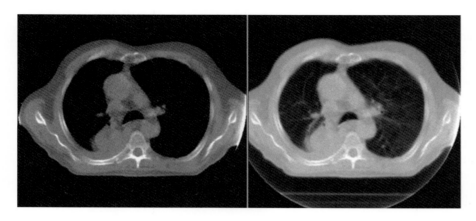

Figure 9-28 Megavoltage CT images. Both images show good contrast and resolution.

MLC is used, similar to the collimator for serial tomotherapy (mentioned above). Some additional features include:

- gantry with 360° continuous rotation and CT-like geometry
- on-board megavoltage CT imaging with a dose per scan of approximately 1.5–2.5 cGy
- maximum field size of 5 cm × 40 cm
- maximum dose rate at isocenter of 800–1100 cGy.

The clinical success of conformal (and conformal avoidance) radiotherapy relies upon the ability to accurately localize the beam on a day-to-day basis. On-board axial image information is obtained using the megavoltage beam and a bank of CT detectors. Megavoltage CT (MVCT)[64] provides good image quality and is not subject to artifact generation in high-density objects (e.g., dental fillings) that adversely affect kilovoltage CT (Figure 9-28). Also, an electron density conversion is not required, because the imaging beam and treatment beam are one and the same.

Robotic treatments

A robot-controlled linear accelerator has been developed for SRS and IMRT (Figure 9-29). Six degrees of freedom are indicated in the image. This treatment device merges state-of-the-art technology from the manufacturing industry (robotics) with advanced radiation delivery in the form of a compact linear accelerator.

At the time of this publication, the CyberKnife Robotic Radiosurgery system (Accuray Inc., Sunnyvale CA) is the only such radiosurgery system commercially available. The American Association of Physicists in Medicine published a Task Group report on the use of robotic radiosurgery systems and described the CyberKnife system in detail. The following description of the Accuray CyberKnife system is reproduced with permission from Task Group Report Number 135.[65]

The Accuray CyberKnife® Robotic Radiosurgery system is, at the time of publication, the only robotic radiosurgery device in clinical use.[66–68] It consists of a compact x-band linear accelerator mounted

on an industrial robotic manipulator arm. The manipulator arm is configured to direct the radiation beams to the region of beam intersection of two orthogonal x-ray imaging systems integrated to provide image guidance for the treatment process. The patient under

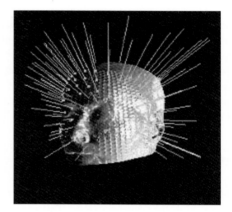

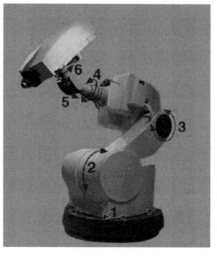

Figure 9-29 CyberKnife robotic radiotherapy machine (bottom) with a 3D head rendering displaying large number of beam angles achievable with robotic head (top).

treatment is positioned on an automated robotic couch such that the target to be treated is located within this radiation beam accessible region. The movements of the robotic manipulator arm and the robotic patient support assembly are under the direct control of a computer system that is in turn controlled by the radiation therapist (during patient treatments) or the medical physicist (for quality assurance measurement purposes).

The treatment planning system for the CyberKnife® is device-specific. It is an inverse planning system which uses linear optimization to optimize the beam angle and beam MUs. The user can select the preconfigured treatment path, collimator size, dose calculation algorithm (raytracing or Monte Carlo), and set the dose constraints.

While most CyberKnife® treatments are nonisocentric, there is a reference point in the room which serves as the origin for several coordinate systems used within the CyberKnife® application, and to which the robot and imaging calibration is defined. This point in space is defined by an "isocrystal" which is mechanically mounted on the "isopost." In this report, this point in space is defined as the "geometric isocenter." It must not be confused with the "treatment isocenter," which refers to an isocentric treatment to a target which may be located at a distance from the geometric isocenter. While a small fraction of CyberKnife® treatments are either isocentric or an overlay of isocentric shots of different collimator sizes, the majority of treatments are nonisocentric. This means that beams are pointing away from the geometric isocenter to create highly irregular target shapes that can contain surface concavities [...]

There are three targeting methods currently in use in the CyberKnife® image guidance system: bony structure tracking,[69] fiducial marker tracking,[70] and soft tissue tracking. Each of these will be discussed in the following paragraphs. Bony structure tracking includes skull tracking (6D Skull) and spine tracking (XSight® Spine).[71,72] Soft tissue tracking (XSight® Lung) uses density differences between the target and surrounding lung tissues without the need for invasive fiducial placement.

6D Skull tracking: The Skull tracking algorithm uses the entire image region to develop a targeting result. Because of the very high radiographic contrast at the boundary of the skull, steep image gradients are produced that allow the 2D/3D registration algorithm to function very reliably.[73] However, there are a few scenarios where special attention is required and the reader is referred to the AAPM task group report for further information [...]

Fiducial tracking: Tracking by locating radio-opaque markers rigidly associated with a target is one of the most accurate CyberKnife® targeting procedures. Overall accuracy is primarily dependent on the number of fiducials implanted,[74,75] their spread, and their ability to be uniquely identified on each targeting image. Among the conditions that can influence this accuracy are fiducials that move with respect to each other, fiducials that cannot be resolved on both images, fiducials that are implanted near metallic surgery clips, imagers that have severe uncorrected pixel artifacts, and CT imaging artifacts [...]

Spine tracking: Spine tracking relies on the bony structure along the spinal column. To accommodate small interfraction deformations, this algorithm performs small-image registrations at 81 points at the intersections of a rectangular tracking grid. This targeting method is influenced by initial placement of the targeting grid, inherent bony contrast (e.g., either a large patient or severe osteoporosis), x-ray technique, and initial alignment to the wrong vertebral body [...] The tracking grid size should be chosen to maximize the amount of spine within the grid. The grid should neither include too much soft tissue (in which case it should be made smaller), nor miss part of the bony spine (in which case it should be enlarged).

Additionally, it is important to verify visually that the correct level is tracked. Special attention should be paid when treating thoracic spine. Due to similarities in the bony structures at that particular region, misalignment to the incorrect vertebral body could occur. This could lead to a spatial misplacement of dose causing treatment of the wrong vertebral body. It is therefore important that after the radiation therapist has aligned the patient, the radiation oncologist and the Qualified Medical Physicist are called to verify that the correct vertebra is being treated [...]

Soft tissue (XSight® Lung) tracking: This tracking modality uses the density difference of the target to the surrounding tissue. Tumors to be treated with this algorithm must have well defined boundaries, not be obscured by radiographically dense structures (spine, heart), and be within a range of sizes that can be accommodated by the algorithm. This tracking algorithm is very susceptible to x-ray technique and targeting parameter range choices (acceptable confidence threshold, image contrast setting, search range, etc.) and is also the most difficult to verify tracking accuracy.

Summary

- Treatment planning includes two general aspects: (1) acquisition of image data that are then manipulated and displayed to demonstrate the 3D nature of the patient's anatomy and (2) performing a 3D calculation of the absorbed radiation dose.
- Conformal radiation therapy involves techniques of shaping radiation dose distributions to the target volume, usually based on axial CT images.
- With the availability of tissue density information from CT, the ability to perform heterogeneity corrections has gained increasing use in clinical treatment planning. Although many of the historical data are based on homogeneous calculations, the complexity of 3D and IMRT planning techniques often requires heterogeneity corrections, particularly when used to modify observed isodose distributions.
- Virtual simulation involves creating a 3D model of the patient, usually from a contiguous CT scan data set. Isocenter placement, beam arrangement, and dose calculation can then take place on the imaging data set.
- Immobilization involves techniques to minimize patient motion during treatment in order to ensure accurate and reproducible setup for each treatment.

- Increased attention is being directed at target localization to improve accuracy and limit uncertainty in mobile structures, such as the prostate. Techniques include real-time imaging with ultrasound and tomotherapy. Positioning may be relative to anatomical structures or fiducials, either implanted or external.
- DVHs are graphical depictions of radiation dose to various structures of interest for the treatment plan.
- The biological response of tumors and critical structures has been addressed through the development of models for TCP and NTCP.
- Intensity modulated radiation therapy involves three general steps:
  1 Setting dose or dose-volume objectives, based on accurate and detailed structure definition.
  2 Iterative optimization using any of a number of available mathematical techniques to accomplish the objectives.
  3 Conversion to a deliverable treatment, such as step-and-shoot MLC segments or dynamic sliding window.
- Serial tomotherapy involves incremental slice-by-slice treatments, and helical tomotherapy involves overlapping helical treatments on a device that looks much like a conventional CT scanner.

Problems

9-1 Identify five immobilization or localization devices used at your institution/clinic. List them and describe their clinical uses (sites treated).

9-2 Describe at least one difference and one similarity between forward planning and inverse planning.

9-3 What is a DRR and how is it created?

9-4 Describe what is meant by BEV.

9-5 Briefly describe the following acronyms: GTV, CTV, PTV, ITV, and PRV.

9-6 Given the dose matrices below, representing each of the four treatment fields, calculate the cumulative dose matrix and the normalized dose matrix. Also, use a spreadsheet program (e.g., Microsoft Excel) to create cumulative DVHs for the normalized dose matrix, including the OAR, PTV, and Skin.

0	0	0	0	0	10	10	0	0	0
0	0	0	0	0	20	20	0	0	0
0	0	0	0	0	40	40	0	0	0
0	0	0	0	0	80	80	0	0	0
0	0	0	0	0	100	100	0	0	0
0	0	0	0	0	80	80	0	0	0
0	0	0	0	0	40	40	0	0	0
0	0	0	0	0	20	20	0	0	0
0	0	0	0	0	5	5	0	0	0

0	0	0	0	0	10	10	0	0	0
0	0	0	0	0	25	25	0	0	0
0	0	0	0	0	50	50	0	0	0
0	0	0	0	0	85	85	0	0	0
0	0	0	0	0	100	100	0	0	0
0	0	0	0	0	85	85	0	0	0
0	0	0	0	0	50	50	0	0	0
0	0	0	0	0	25	25	0	0	0
0	0	0	0	0	10	10	0	0	0

0	0	0	0	0	0	0	0	0	0
0	0	0	0	0	0	0	0	0	0
0	0	0	0	0	0	0	0	0	0
5	10	40	60	80	95	100	90	70	35
5	10	40	60	80	95	100	90	70	35
5	10	40	60	80	95	100	90	70	35
0	0	0	0	0	0	0	0	0	0
0	0	0	0	0	0	0	0	0	0
0	0	0	0	0	0	0	0	0	0

0	0	0	0	0	0	0	0	0	0
0	0	0	0	0	0	0	0	0	0
0	0	0	0	0	0	0	0	0	0
30	55	80	100	95	70	50	30	15	5
30	55	80	100	95	70	50	30	15	5
30	55	80	100	95	70	50	30	15	5
0	0	0	0	0	0	0	0	0	0
0	0	0	0	0	0	0	0	0	0
0	0	0	0	0	0	0	0	0	0

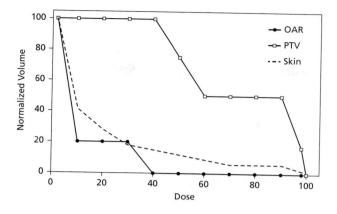

9-7 What is an objective or cost function? What are two general categories of optimization algorithms?

9-8 For a head and neck treatment plan, the field size is 15 cm × 15 cm. If there are nine fields and the pencil-beam algorithm uses 5 mm beamlets, how many adjustable intensity parameters are there?

9-9 What are the QUANTEC dose limit recommendations for the brain, spinal cord, cochlea, larynx, and parotids for a patient with conventional fractionated treatment? What are the recommendations for a single fraction SRS treatment?

References

1 International Commission on Radiation Units and Measurements. Report No. 50: *Prescribing, Recording and Reporting Photon Beam Therapy*. Washington, DC, ICRU, 1993.

2 Laughlin, J. S., Mohan, R., and Kutcher, G. J. Choice of optimum mega-voltage for accelerators for photon beam treatment. *Int. J. Radiat. Oncol. Biol. Phys.* 1986; **12**(9):1551–1557.

3 Hope, C. S., Laurie, J., Orr, J. S., and Halnan, K. E. Optimization of x-ray treatment planning by computer judgment. *Phys. Med. Biol.* 1967; **12**:531–542.

4 Perez, C. A., Purdy, J. A., Harms, W., Gerber, R., Graham, M. V., et al. Three-dimensional treatment planning and conformal radiation therapy: Preliminary evaluation. *Radiother. Oncol.* 1995; **36**: 32–43.

5 Purdy, J. A., and Starkschall, G. (eds.). *A Practical Guide to 3-D Planning and Conformal Radiation Therapy*. Madison, WI, Advanced Medical Publishing, 1999.

6 Sherouse, G. W., and Chaney, E. L. The portable virtual simulator. *Int. J. Radiat. Oncol. Biol. Phys.* 1991; **21**:475–482.

7 Sherouse, G. W., Bourland, J. D., Reynolds, K., McMurry, H. L, Mitchell, T. P., and Chaney, E. L. Virtual simulation in the clinical setting: Some practical considerations. *Int. J. Radiat. Oncol. Biol. Phys.* 1990; **19**:1059–1065.

8 Jani, S. *CT Simulation for Radiotherapy*. Madison, WI, Medical Physics Publishing, 1993.

9 Coia, L., Shultheiss, T., and Hanks, G. *A Practical Guide to CT-Simulation*. Madison, WI, Advanced Medical Publishing, 1995.

10 Rosenman, J., Sherouse, G. W., Fuchs, H., Pizer, S. M., Skinner, A. L., et al. Three-dimensional display techniques in radiation therapy treatment planning. *Int. J. Radiat. Oncol. Biol. Phys.* 1989; **16**:263–269.

11 Lee, J. S., Jani, A. B., Pelizzari, C. A., Haraf, D. J., Vokes, E. E., et al. Volumetric visualization of head and neck CT data for treatment planning. *Int. J. Radiat. Oncol. Biol. Phys.* 1999; **44**(3):693–703.

12 Gehring, M. A., Mackie, T. R., Kubsad, S. S., Paliwal, B. R., Mehta, M. P., and Kinsella, T. J. A three-dimensional volume visualization package applied to stereotactic radiosurgery treatment planning. *Int. J. Radiat. Oncol. Biol. Phys.* 1991; **21**(2):491–500.

13 Reynolds, R. A., Sontag, M. R., and Chen, L. S. An algorithm for three-dimensional visualization of radiation therapy beams. *Med. Phys.* 1988; **15**(1):24–8.

14 Sherouse, G. W., Novins, K., and Chaney. E. L. Computations of digitally reconstructed radiographs for use in radiotherapy treatment design. *Int. J. Radiat. Oncol. Biol. Phys.* 1990; **18**:651–658.

15 Webb, S. *The Physics of Three-Dimensional Radiation Therapy: Conformal Radiotherapy, Radiosurgery and Treatment Planning*. Bristol, Institute of Physics Publishing, Ltd., 1993.

16 Collignon, A., Maes, F., Delaere, D., Vandermeulen, D., Suetens, P., and Marchal, G. Automated multi-modality image registration based on information theory. In *Information Processing in Medical Imaging (Brest)*. Y. Bizais, C. Barillot, and R. Di Paola (eds.). Dordrecht, The Netherlands, Kluwer Academic, 1995.

17 Viola, P., and Wells III, W. M. Alignment by maximization of mutual information. *Proc. 5th Int. Conf. on Computer Vision (Boston)*. IEEE, 1995.

18 International Commission on Radiation Units and Measurements. *International Commission on Radiation Reports and Measurements: Prescribing, Recording and Reporting Photon Beam Therapy* (Supplement to ICRU Report 50); Report #62. Bethesda, MD, ICRU, 1999.

19 Giraud, P., Antoine, M., Larrouy, A., et al. Evaluation of microscopic tumor extension in non-small-cell lung cancer for three-dimensional conformal radiotherapy planning. *Int. J. Radiat. Oncol. Biol. Phys.* 2000; **48**(4): 1015–1024.

20 Pekar, V., McNutt, T. R., and Kaus, M. R. Automated model-based organ delineation for radiotherapy planning in prostatic region. *Int. J. Radiat. Oncol. Biol. Phys.* 2004; **60**(3): 973.

21 Kaus, M. R., Brock, K. K., Pekar, V., Dawson, L. A., Nichol, A. M., and Jaffray, D. A. Assessment of a model-based deformable image registration approach for radiation therapy planning. *Int. J. Radiat. Oncol. Biol. Phys.* 2007; **68**(2), 572–580.

22 McDonald, S. C., and Rubin, P. Optimization of external beam radiation therapy. *Int. J. Radiat. Oncol. Biol. Phys.* 1977; **2**:307–317.

23 Drzymala, R. E., Mohan, R., Brewster, L., Chu, J., Goitein, M., et al. Dose–volume histograms. *Int. J. Radiat. Oncol. Biol. Phys.* 1991; **21**(1):71–78.

24 Drzymala, R. E., Holman, M. D., Yan, D., Harms, W., Jain, N. L., et al. Integrated software tools for the evaluation of radiotherapy treatment plans. *Int. J. Radiat. Oncol. Biol. Phys.* 1994; **30**(4): 909–919.

25 Lawrence, T. S., Tesser, R. J., and Ten Haken, R. K. Application of dose volume histograms to treatment of intrahepatic malignancies with radiation therapy. *Int. J. Radiat. Oncol. Biol. Phys.* 1990; **19**:1041–1047.

26 Kutcher, G. J., and Burman, C. Calculation of complication probability factors for non-uniform normal tissue irradiation: The effective

volume method. *Int. J. Radiat. Oncol. Biol. Phys.* 1989; **16**:1623–1630.

27 Lyman, J. T. Complication probability as assessed from dose volume histograms. *Radiat. Res.* 1985; **104**:S13–S19.

28 Martel, M. K., Ten Haken, R. K., Hazuka, M. B., Kessler, M. L., and Turrisi, A. T. Analysis of tumor dose-volume histograms in relationship to local progression free survival for lung cancer patients. *Int. J. Radiat. Oncol. Biol. Phys.* 1993; **27**(suppl 1):238.

29 Niemierko, A., and Goitein, M. Implementation of a model for estimating tumor control probability for an inhomogeneously irradiated tumor. *Radiother. Oncol.* 1993; **29**:140–147.

30 Niemierko, A., and Goitein, M. Optimization of 3D radiation therapy with both physical and biological end points and constraints. *Int. J. Radiat. Oncol. Biol. Phys.* 1992; **23**:99–108.

31 Wambersie, A., Hanks, G., and Van Dam, J. Quality assurance and accuracy required in radiation therapy: Biological and medical considerations. In *Selected Topics in Physics of Radiotherapy and Imaging*, U. Madhvanath, K. S. Parthasarathy, and T. V. Venkateswaran (eds.). New Delhi, McGraw-Hill, 1988.

32 Xiao, Y., Galvin, J., Hossain, M., and Valicenti, R. An optimized forward-planning technique for intensity modulated radiation therapy. *Med. Phys.* 2000; **27**(9):2093–2099.

33 Hristov, D., Stavrev, P., Sham, E., and Fallone, B. G. On the implementation of dose-volume objectives in gradient algorithms for inverse treatment planning. *Med. Phys.* 2002; **29**(5):848–856.

34 Chui, C. S., and Spirou, S. V. Inverse planning algorithms for external beam radiation therapy. *Med. Dosim.* 2001; **26**(2):189–197.

35 IMRT Collaborative Working Group. Intensity modulated radiotherapy: Current status and issues of interest. *Int. J. Radiat. Oncol. Biol. Phys.* 2001; **51**(4):880–914.

36 Webb, S. *The Physics of Conformal Radiotherapy*. Bristol, Institute of Physics Publishing Ltd., 1997.

37 Purdy, J., Grant III, W. H., Palta, J. R., Butter, B., and Perez, C. A. *3D Conformal and Intensity Modulated Radiation Therapy: Physics and Clinical Applications*. Madison, WI, Advanced Medical Publishing, 2001.

38 Brokaw, M. *Intensity Modulated Radiation Therapy. Optimizing Clinical Quality and Financial Performance*. Oncology Roundtable, The Advisory Board Company, 2002.

39 Brahme, A. Optimization of radiation therapy. *Int. J. Radiat. Oncol. Biol. Phys.* 1994; **28**:785–787.

40 Soderstrom, S., and Brahme, A. Selection of suitable beam orientations in radiation therapy using entropy and Fourier transform measures. *Phys. Med. Biol.* 1992; **37**:911–924.

41 Oldham, M., and Webb, S. The optimization and inherent limitations of 3D conformal radiotherapy treatment plans of the prostate. *Br. J. Radiol.* 1995; **68**:882–893.

42 Starkschall, G., and Eifel, P. J. An interactive beam-weight optimization tool for three-dimensional radiotherapy treatment planning. *Med. Phys.* 1992; **19**:155–163.

43 Eisbruch, A., Ten Haken, R. K., Kim, H. M., Marsh, L., and Ship, J. A. Dose, volume and function relationships in parotid salivary glands following conformal and intensity modulated irradiation of head and neck cancer. *Int. J. Radiat. Oncol. Biol. Phys.* 1999; **45**(3):577–587.

44 McKenzie, A., van Herk, M., and Mijnheer, B. Margins for geometric uncertainty around organs at risk in radiotherapy. *Radiother. Oncol.* 2002; **62**(3):299–307.

45 Wu, Q., Manning, M., Schmidt-Ullrich, R., and Mohan, R. The potential for sparing of parotids and escalation of biologically effective dose with intensity-modulated radiation treatments of head and neck cancers: A treatment design study. *Int. J. Radiat. Oncol. Biol. Phys.* 2000; **46**(1):195–205.

46 Chao, K. S., Ozyigit, G., Low, D.A., Wippold, F. J., and Thorstad, W. L. *Intensity Modulated Radiation Therapy for Head and Neck Cancers*. Philadelphia, Lippincott, Williams and Wilkins, 2002.

47 Zelefsky, M., Fuks, Z., Happersett, L., Lee, H. J., Ling, C. C., et al. Clinical experience with intensity modulated radiation therapy (IMRT) in prostate cancer. *Radiother. Oncol.* 2000; **55**:241–249.

48 Sternick, S. (ed.). *Theory & Practice of Intensity Modulated Radiation Therapy*. Madison, WI, Advanced Medical Publishing, 1997.

49 Wu, Q., and Mohan, R. Algorithms and functionality of an intensity modulated radiotherapy optimization system. *Med. Phys.* 2000; **27**(4):701–711.

50 Emami, B., Lyman, J., Brown, A., Cola, L., Goitein, M., et al. Tolerance of normal tissue to therapeutic radiation. *Int. J. Radiat. Oncol. Biol. Phys.* 1991; **21**(1):109–122.

51 Quantitative Analysis of Normal Tissue Effects in the Clinic. *Int. J. Radiat. Oncol. Biol. Phys.* 2010; **76**(3):S1–S160.

52 Chao, K. S., Deasy J. O., Markman, J., Haynie, J., Perez, C. A, Purdy, J. A., Low, D. A. A prospective study of salivary function sparing in patients with head-and-neck cancers receiving intensity-modulated or three-dimensional radiation therapy: Initial results. *Int. J. Radiol. Oncol. Biol. Phys.* 2001; **49**(4):907–916.

53 Mageras, G. S., and Mohan, R. Application of fast simulated annealing to optimization of conformal radiation treatments. *Med. Phys.* 1992; **20**:639–647.

54 Que, W. Comparison of algorithms for multileaf collimator field segmentation. *Med. Phys.* 1999; **26**(11):2390–2396.

55 Yu, C. X., Li, X. A., Ma, L., Chen, D., Naqvi, S., et al. Clinical implementation of intensity-modulated arc therapy. *Int. J. Radiat. Oncol. Biol. Phys.* 2002; **53**(2):453–463.

56 Wong, E., Chen, J. Z., and Greenland, J. Intensity-modulated arc therapy simplified. *Int. J. Radiat. Oncol. Biol. Phys.* 2002; **53**(1):222–235.

57 Ma, L., Yu, C. X., Earl, M., Holmes, T., Sarfaraz, M., et al. Optimized intensity-modulated arc therapy for prostate cancer treatment. *Int. J. Cancer.* 2001; **96**(6):379–384.

58 Salter, B. J. NOMOS Peacock IMRT utilizing the Beak post collimation device. *Med. Dosim.* 2001; **26**(1):37–45.

59 Low, D. A., and Mutic, S. A commercial IMRT treatment-planning dose-calculation algorithm. *Int. J. Radiat. Oncol. Biol. Phys.* 1998; **41**(4):933–937.

60 Mackie, T. R., Holmes, T., Swerdloff, S., Reckwerdt, P., Deasy, J. O., et al. Tomotherapy: A new concept for the delivery of dynamic conformal radiotherapy. *Med. Phys.* 1993; **20**(6):1709–1719.

61 Olivera, G. H., et al. Tomotherapy. In *Modern Technology of Radiation Oncology*. J. Van Dyk (ed.). Madison, WI, Medical Physics Publishing, 1999.

62 Shepard, D. M., Olivera, G. H., Reckwerdt, P. J., and Mackie, T. R. Iterative approaches to dose optimization in tomotherapy. *Phys. Med. Biol.* 2000; **45**(1):69–90.

63 Kapatoes, J. M., Olivera, G. H., Ruchala, K. J., Smilowitz, J. B., Reckwerdt, P. J., and Mackie, T. R. A feasible method for clinical

delivery verification and dose reconstruction in tomotherapy. *Med. Phys.* 2001; **28**:528–542.

64 Ruchala, K. J., Olivera, G. H., Kapatoes, J. M., Schloesser, E. A., Reckwerdt, P. J., and Mackie, T. R. Megavoltage CT image reconstruction during tomotherapy treatments. *Phys. Med. Biol.* 2000; **45**(12):3545–3562.

65 Dieterich, S., Cavedon, C., Chuang, C. F., Cohen, A. B., Garrett, J. A., et al. Report of AAPM TG 135: Quality assurance for robotic radiosurgery. *Med. Phys.* 2011; **38**(6):2914–2936.

66 Adler, Jr., J. R., Chang, S. D., Murphy, M. J., Doty, J., Geis, P., and Hancock, S. L. The CyberKnifeVR: A frameless robotic system for radiosurgery. *Stereotact. Funct. Neurosurg.* 1997; **69**:124–128.

67 Kuo, J. S., Yu, C., Petrovich, Z., and Apuzzo, M. L. The CyberKnifeVR stereotactic radiosurgery system: Description, installation, and an initial evaluation of use and functionality. *Neurosurg.* 2003; **53**:1235–1239; discussion 1239.

68 Quinn, A. M. CyberKnifeVR: A robotic radiosurgery system. *Clin. J. Oncol. Nurs.* 2002; **6**:149, 156.

69 Fu, D., and Kuduvalli, G. A fast, accurate, and automatic 2D–3D image registration for image-guided cranial radiosurgery. *Med. Phys.* 2008; **35**:2180–2194.

70 Mu, Z., Fu, D., and Kuduvally, G. A probabilistic framework based on hidden Markov model for fiducial identification in image-guided radiation treatments. *IEEE Trans. Med. Imaging* 2008; **27**:288–1300.

71 Muacevic, A., Staehler, M., Drexler, C., Wowra, B., Reiser, M., and Tonn, J. C. Technical description, phantom accuracy, and clinical feasibility for fiducial-free frameless real-time image-guided spinal radiosurgery. *J. Neurosurg. Spine.* 2006; **5**:303–312.

72 Fu, D., and Kuduvalli, G. Enhancing skeletal features in digitally reconstructed radiographs. In *Medical Imaging 2006: Image Processing*, Vol. 6144, J. M. Reinhardt and J. P. Pluim (eds.). San Diego, The International Society for Optical Engineering, abstract 61442M, 2006.

73 Fu, D., and Kuduvalli, G. A fast, accurate, and automatic 2D–3D image registration for image-guided cranial radiosurgery. *Med. Phys.* 2008; **35**:2180–2194.

74 Murphy, M. J. Fiducial-based targeting accuracy for external-beam radiotherapy. *Med. Phys.* 2002; **29**:334–344.

75 West, J. B., Fitzpatrick, J. M., Toms, S. A., Maurer, Jr., C. R., and Maciunas, R. J. Fiducial point placement and the accuracy of point-based, rigid body registration. *Neurosurgery* 2001; **48**:810–816.

CHAPTER

10

THE BASICS OF MEDICAL IMAGING

Objectives

After studying this chapter, the reader should be able to:
- Identify sources of image contrast on a planar radiographic image.
- Describe the origin of the differences in image contrast between kilovoltage and megavoltage images.
- Understand how the number of bits and the binning of pixel values affect the display of a digital image.
- Understand how the pixel resolution affects the display of a digital image.
- Describe the technique of histogram equalization and how it can improve visualization.

Introduction

For several decades after the discovery of x rays, medical radiology evolved as the application of ionizing radiation to the diagnosis and treatment of human disease and injury. Over this period, radiologic specialists were trained in both diagnostic applications (diagnostic radiology) and therapeutic procedures (therapeutic radiology). In the early years, many radiologists practiced as both diagnosticians and therapists. After World War II, however, both diagnostic and therapeutic radiology grew in complexity. For example, radiation therapy became immensely

more sophisticated with the advent of ^{60}Co and its requirements for more sophisticated treatment planning and monitoring to replace visual monitoring (e.g., skin reddening and blistering) used with superficial and orthovoltage therapy. In the early 1970s, diagnostic radiology and therapeutic radiology were finally recognized as separate specialties, with separate training programs, separate accreditation committees for residencies, and separate certification procedures for specialists. Radiation therapists became known as *radiation oncologists*, and the term *radiation therapist* was transferred to the technologists who deliver treatments under the supervision of radiation oncologists. Most academic institutions established departments of radiation oncology independent of departments of (diagnostic) radiology, and physicists increasingly focused their expertise on technical challenges in a single discipline such as radiology, radiation oncology, or nuclear medicine. Residency programs in radiology included almost no training in radiation oncology, and educational programs in radiation oncology contained only a token exposure, if any, to diagnostic imaging.

Over the past several decades, treatment planning and patient position monitoring in radiation therapy have become increasingly complex. High-energy accelerators for x-ray and particle-beam treatments, computers, mathematical algorithms, software programs, the heightened presence of physicists and

---

Hendee's Radiation Therapy Physics, Fourth Edition. Todd Pawlicki, Daniel J. Scanderbeg and George Starkschall.
© 2016 John Wiley & Sons, Inc. Published 2016 by John Wiley & Sons, Inc.

computer specialists, an increased regulatory burden, and a growing demand for quality control all contribute to this complexity. Also enhancing the complexity is expanding use of imaging techniques, especially computed tomography (CT), positron emission tomography (PET), and magnetic resonance (MR) imaging for treatment simulation, treatment planning, and a three-dimensional (3D) visualization of tumors and surrounding anatomic structures. The acceptance of imaging techniques as an essential part of radiation therapy demands that radiation oncologists acquire a fundamental understanding of these techniques, their strengths and limitations, and their applications to treatment planning and monitoring in radiation therapy.

Imaging is an important component of radiation therapy for several reasons. First, imaging is used to diagnose malignant disease. Diagnosis, in fact, was the original goal of medical imaging. In contemporary medicine, and radiation therapy in particular, imaging goes much further than the diagnosis of disease. Imaging plays a major role in the design of radiation treatments. Imaging is used for the targeting of tumors. Targeting consists of localization of the tumor, of determining the extent of the tumor, and of defining the gross tumor volume (GTV). Tumor targeting in recent years has been taken to a higher level by using imaging methods for the precise setup of patients. Imaging is also used for verification of radiation treatment; that is, ascertaining that the radiation is being delivered to the precise region where it is intended, and also for monitoring of radiation treatment; that is, verifying that the treatment is having the desired effect on the patient. As imaging methods are becoming more sophisticated, imaging is likely to play an even greater role in targeting and verification.

This chapter is the first of several chapters devoted to medical imaging and its applications in radiation therapy. In this chapter, we first identify characteristics that all imaging systems have in common. We then define some features of image quality and relate these features to properties of the interaction of radiation with matter. Finally, we compare the basic concepts of analog to digital imaging and relate how these concepts affect the final images that we observe in the clinic. In Chapter 11, we describe the various types of imaging systems, and in Chapter 12 we show how image guidance can improve localization in radiation therapy.

Characteristics of imaging systems

In general, imaging systems exhibit several common characteristics. Common to all imaging systems is some sort of imaging medium. The imaging medium is that component of an imaging system that interacts with the patient. The magnitude of the interaction is a measure of what we are looking for in the patient. Examples of imaging media include x rays and ultrasound. Each imaging system has a source that produces the imaging medium. Most important are the specific interactions between the imaging medium and the patient. Sometimes we detect the result of direct interactions between the imaging medium and the patient, such as the attenuation of an x-ray beam as it passes through the patient, which we can correlate to the anatomic differences within the patient. In other techniques; for example, in nuclear medicine imaging, we determine the distribution of imaging medium within the patient and correlate this distribution with physiology inside the patient. In such cases, interactions between the imaging medium and the patient may interfere with the interpretation of the image, and have to be accounted for in some manner. Finally, we must have some sort of device that can detect the distribution of imaging medium by performing measurements external to the patient. It is the interpretation of the distribution of imaging medium that eventually is correlated to whatever we are trying to infer about the patient.

Image contrast

Image contrast is what enables us to differentiate anatomic structures on radiographic images. The discussion of image contrast begins by more precisely identifying what a radiographic image is. A radiographic image (or, more precisely, a radiographic projection image) is a map of the differential attenuation of x-ray photons as a beam of these photons passes through an absorber. Because of differences in the attenuation of the x-ray beam as it passes through an absorber, such as a patient, different numbers of x-ray photons strike a detector placed distal to the patient. These differences in the number of photons reaching the detector are displayed and correlated with differences in the anatomy inside the patient. Figure 10-1 illustrates the differential attenuation of such an x-ray beam passing through an absorber.

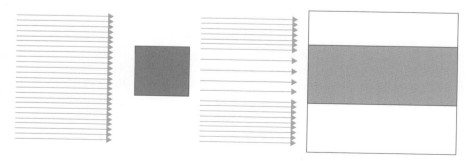

Figure 10-1 An x-ray beam, passing through an absorber, is differentially attenuated. The display of the differential attenuation on the image receptor allows us to infer the presence of an object inside the absorber that caused the differential attenuation. For a color version of this figure, see the color plate section.

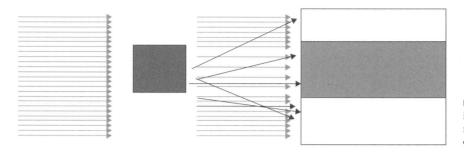

Figure 10-2 An illustration of the lack of information provided by scattered radiation reaching the image receptor. For a color version of this figure, see the color plate section.

Example 10-1

A monochromatic x-ray beam of energy 30 keV passes through 10 cm of tissue. Embedded in the tissue is 1 cm of bone. Compare the differences in attenuation of the beam passing through bone and soft tissue to attenuation of the beam passing through soft tissue alone. The linear attenuation coefficient for 30 keV x rays in soft tissue is 0.3604 cm^{-1}, whereas the linear attenuation coefficient for 30 keV x rays in cortical bone is 2.529 cm^{-1}.[1]

The relative intensity of the beam exiting the tissue is given by:

$$\frac{I}{I_0} = \exp(-\mu x)$$

For a beam passing through 10 cm of soft tissue, $\mu x = 3.604$, so $\frac{I}{I_0} = 0.02721$. For a beam passing through 9 cm of soft tissue and 1 cm of bone $\mu x = 9 \times 0.3604 + 1 \times 2.529$, or 5.773, so $\frac{I}{I_0} = 0.00311$, or almost a factor of 10 lower.

This difference in beam intensity of approximately a factor of 10 is relatively easy to detect.

Example 10-2

Repeat the previous calculation for a monochromatic x-ray beam of energy 2 MeV. The linear attenuation coefficient for 2 MeV x rays in soft tissue is 0.04893 cm^{-1}, whereas the linear attenuation coefficient for 2 MeV x rays in cortical bone is 0.08753 cm^{-1}.[1]

Repeating the calculation using the linear attenuation coefficients for 2 MV x rays, we find that for a beam passing through 10 cm of soft tissue, $\mu x = 0.4893$, so $\frac{I}{I_0} = 0.6131$. For a beam passing through 9 cm of soft tissue and 1 cm of bone, $\mu x = 9 \times 0.04893 + 1 \times 0.08753$, or 0.5279, so $\frac{I}{I_0} = 0.5898$. Here we see a difference of only about 4%.

An x-ray energy specified at 30 keV corresponds to a polyenergetic x-ray beam of approximately 100 kVp, a typical energy used in diagnostic imaging, whereas an energy of 2 MeV corresponds to a polyenergetic beam of approximately 6 MV, a typical energy used in radiation therapy. Recall that at the lower energies the photoelectric effect dominates the x-ray interactions, whereas at higher energies the Compton interaction is the dominant interaction. Attenuation due to the photoelectric effect is dependent on atomic number Z raised to the third power; attenuation due to the Compton interaction is dependent on the mass density. Bone has an effective atomic number almost twice that of soft tissue, so the probability of a photoelectric interaction in bone is almost eight times that in soft tissue; the mass density of bone is just under twice that of soft tissue, so the probability of a Compton interaction in bone is a bit under twice that of an equal thickness of soft tissue. Consequently, the contrast between bone and soft tissue displayed in a radiograph acquired at diagnostic imaging energies is significantly greater than that displayed in a radiograph acquired at therapy energies.

In addition to the differences in attenuation, an additional issue that affects the image quality when higher-energy x rays are used for imaging is the production of scattered radiation from the Compton interaction. X rays, produced via the Compton interaction and reaching the image receptor, provide little information as to their point of origin. These scattered photons add to noise on the radiographic image without providing information regarding the internal anatomy. Figure 10-2 illustrates the distribution of radiation reaching the image receptor, including the scattered radiation from the attenuator, which results in noise in the image.

As a consequence of the increased difference in differential attenuation using lower-energy x rays and the absence of scattered radiation from interactions at these energies, radiographic images acquired at diagnostic energies exhibit significantly greater image quality than those acquired at the higher energies used in radiation therapy. Figure 10-3 illustrates the differences in image quality between a digitally reconstructed radiograph, simulated using x rays of lower photon energies, compared with a portal image, acquired at megavoltage energy.

Digital imaging concepts

Dynamic range

In recent years, images have been almost exclusively acquired digitally. Consequently, it is important to introduce some of the concepts related to the quality of digital images. To begin with, a digital image is simply a display of an array of numbers, each number corresponding to a density. Arrays may be two-dimensional, in which the elements are called *pixels* (which stands for "picture elements") or they may be 3D, in which the

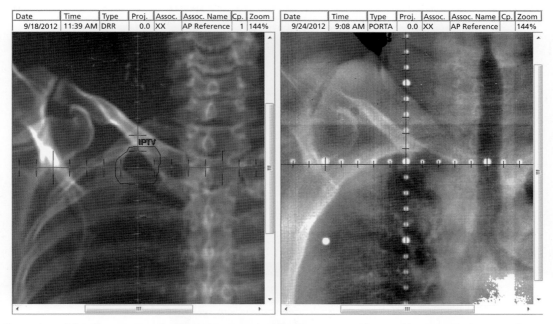

Date	Time	Type	Proj.	Assoc.	Assoc. Name	Cp.	Zoom
9/18/2012	11:39 AM	DRR	0.0	XX	AP Reference	1	144%

Date	Time	Type	Proj.	Assoc.	Assoc. Name	Cp.	Zoom
9/24/2012	9:08 AM	PORTA	0.0	XX	AP Reference		144%

Figure 10-3 Comparison of digitally reconstructed radiograph, generated at kilovoltage energy with a portal image acquired at megavoltage energy. *Source:* Courtesy of P. Balter, UT MD Anderson Cancer Center.

elements are called *voxels* (which stands for "volume elements"). In contrast to an analog image, such as a film image, in which the film density is a continuous value, in a digital image the precision of the density at a point is limited by the number of bits used to specify the value and the dynamic range of the measurement device. For example, if 8 bits are used to characterize the value of a pixel, then the value can have up to 2^8, or 256, values. The precision is then determined by dividing the dynamic range by the number of levels.

Example 10-3

Suppose we had a digital thermometer that represented temperature values by 16 bits. If the dynamic range of the thermometer is from –20° to 120°, what is the temperature resolution of the thermometer?

16 bits corresponds to 2^{16}, or 65,536 levels.

The dynamic range is 140°, so the precision is 140/65,536 = 0.002°

Clearly, increasing the number of bits used to represent a value has a significant effect on the precision.

Figure 10-4 illustrates a photograph with different numbers of bits representing the gray scale. Note how changing the bit depth has profound effects on the contrast resolution of the photograph.

Gray-scale binning

In general, images contain more bit depth than output devices are capable of representing. Historically, CT images have been

represented by 12 bit integers, thus allowing 2^{12}, or 4096, levels. However, modern devices are capable of using 16 bits or more. Most output devices display 8 bit images, consisting of 256 levels. Even so, a human observer typically is capable of discerning 6 bits, or 64 levels, of gray. Mapping the 4096 gray levels onto a 256 gray-scale display allows adjustment of the contrast and the dynamic range of an image. Figure 10-5 illustrates how a window width and window level can be determined to map an image onto a display. The original CT image contains 4000 CT values between –1000 and +3000. A window of values between P_1 and P_2 is determined so that any pixel with a CT value below that of P_1 is displayed as pure black and above P_2 is displayed as pure white. Pixel values between P_1 and P_2 are displayed as various shades of gray.

Figure 10-6 displays a set of 14 bit (16,384 levels) digital chest radiographs illustrating how varying the window level and window width changes what can be seen on the radiograph. In Figure 10-6(a) a very large window width of 11,731 pixel values is used, with the window level set at the approximate midpoint of the pixel values. Note that almost all the pixels fall at the low end of the window, which in this image displays them very close to the white end of the gray scale. Very little contrast is evident in the image, and almost the entire image appears white. In Figure 10-6(b) the window width is greatly reduced, to a value of 939 pixel values, and the window level set to a value of 802. Pixels with values less than 333 ($802 - \frac{1}{2} \times 939$) are displayed as white, and pixels with values greater than 1272 are displayed as black. In this figure, the contrast is greatly increased, but, because most of the pixels in the lung have values in excess of 1272 and are displayed as black, no detail is visible in the lung. Changing the

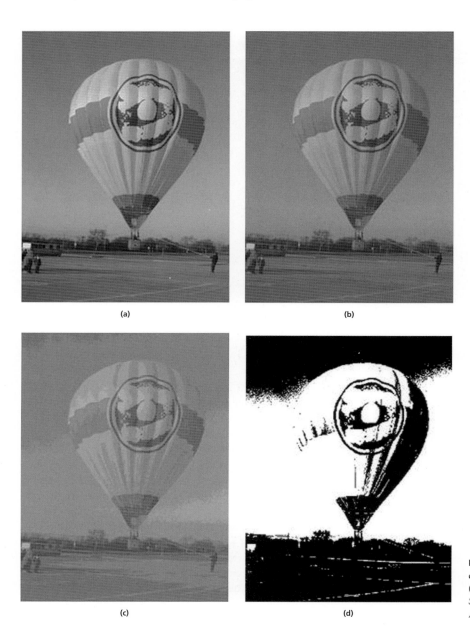

(a)

(b)

(c)

(d)

Figure 10-4 A photograph displayed with different numbers of bits: (a) 8 bits, (b) 7 bits, (c) 3 bits, (d) 1 bit.
Source: Courtesy of P. Balter, UT MD Anderson Cancer Center.

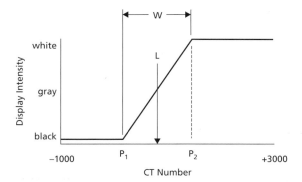

Figure 10-5 Mapping a set of CT numbers onto a display by setting a window width (W) and window level (L).

window level to 2022 and the window width to 2253, as seen in Figure 10-6(c), places most of the soft-tissue pixels below the lower window value of 895; consequently, they show up as white with very little image detail. Finally, in Figure 10-6(d), in which a window level of 1506 and a window width of 3003 are used, detail is visible in both the soft tissue and in the lung. By carefully adjusting the window level and the window width on a display of a digital image, the observer is able to select a region of interest and carefully examine detail in that region of interest.

Example 10-4

Suppose we had a 12 bit image, with pixel values ranging from 0 to 4095, which we want to map into an 8 bit display (values of

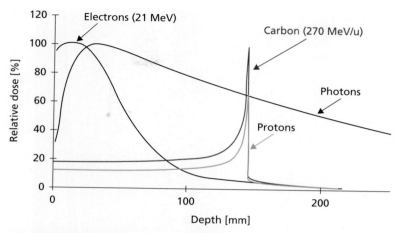

Figure 3-2 Ionization of carbon and proton beams as a function of depth in water illustrating the enhanced ionization that takes place at the end of the particle beam range.

Hendee's Radiation Therapy Physics, Fourth Edition. Todd Pawlicki, Daniel J. Scanderbeg and George Starkschall.
© 2016 John Wiley & Sons, Inc. Published 2016 by John Wiley & Sons, Inc.

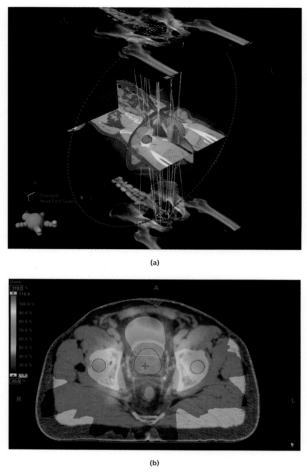

Figure 9-1 (a) CT image obtained through the pelvis of a patient undergoing radiation therapy. (b) The prostate, rectum, and bladder are outlined, and a planning target volume is drawn around the prostate to include a margin. Conformal shaped beams are placed to deliver a uniform dose to the target.

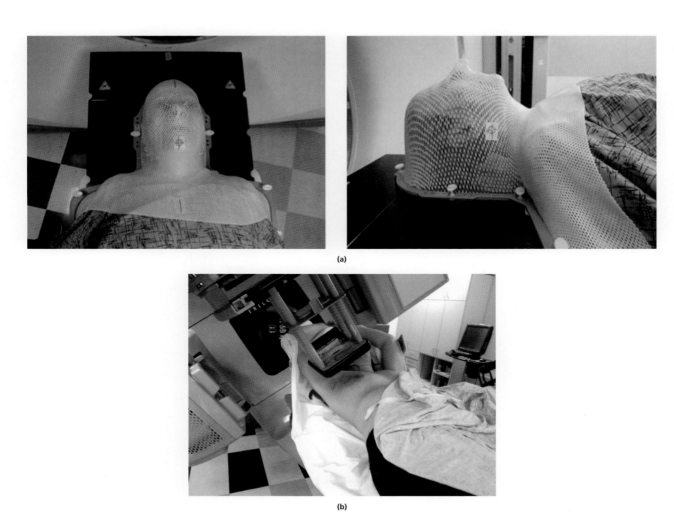

Figure 9-5 (a) Immobilization of patient for head and neck treatment. This system incorporates shoulder immobilization and extends beyond the end of the treatment couch. (b) Immobilization for breast treatment with both arms extended above the patient's head and uses a commercial breast board for repositioning.

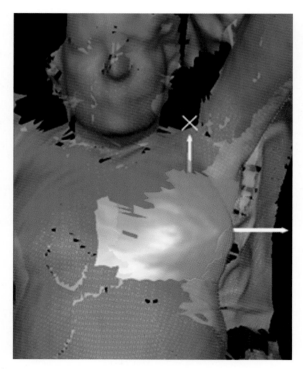

Figure 9-6 Optical surface imaging used for positioning or patient monitoring.

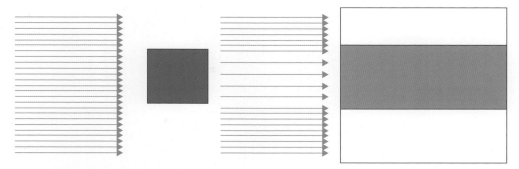

Figure 10-1 An x-ray beam, passing through an absorber, is differentially attenuated. The display of the differential attenuation on the image receptor allows us to infer the presence of an object inside the absorber that caused the differential attenuation.

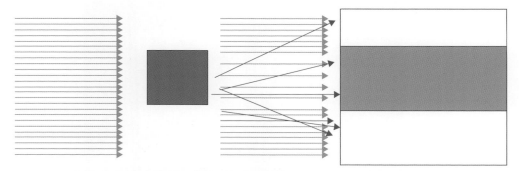

Figure 10-2 An illustration of the lack of information provided by scattered radiation reaching the image receptor.

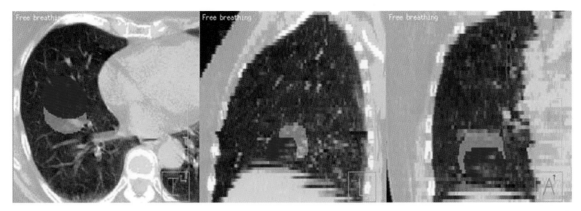

Figure 12-1 Axial, lateral, and coronal CT images of a lung illustrating tumor location at inspiration (red) and expiration (yellow). Motion of the centroid of the tumor is measured as 0.06 cm lateral, 1.37 cm anterior-posterior, 0.87 superior–inferior, and 1.62 cm total.

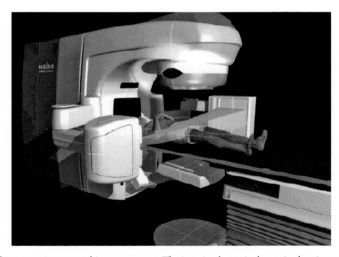

Figure 12-7 Gantry-mounted kilovoltage x-ray source and image receptor. The imaging beam is shown in the picture and the treatment beam is perpendicular to the imaging beam and straight down on the patient (not shown in the figure).
Source: Varian Medical Systems. Reproduced with permission of Varian Medical Systems.

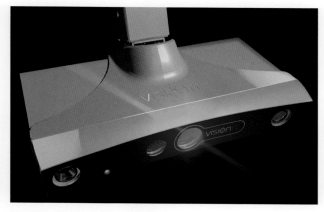

Figure 12-11 The stereoscopic camera used for surface-based patient alignment.

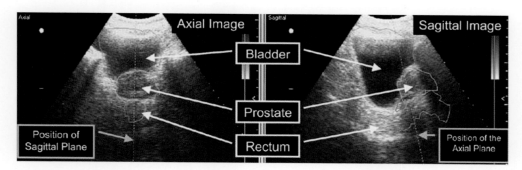

Figure 12-12 Ultrasound-guided target localization. Contours were imported from a treatment planning system and used as a reference for aligning the ultrasound images acquired in the treatment room.
Source: Kuban 2005.[31] Reproduced with permission of Elsevier.

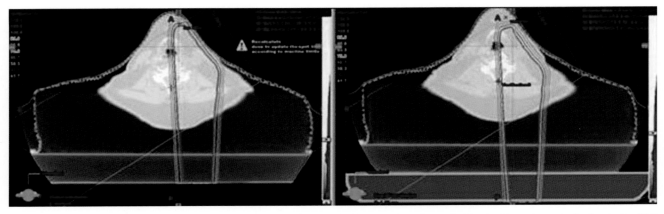

Figure 15-10 Inadvertent addition of digital couch to beam path, as shown in the figure on the right, resulted in significant change in the dose to the CTV.
Source: Richard Wu, UT MD Anderson Cancer Center. Reproduced with permission of R Wu.

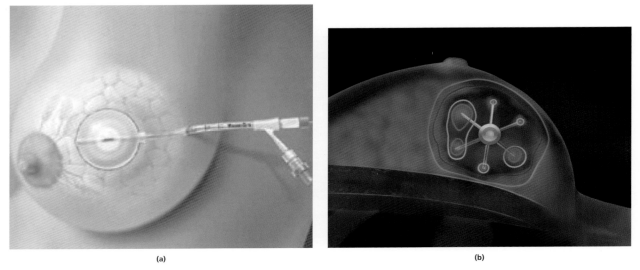

(a)   (b)

Figure 17-15 Two HDR breast applicators. (a) MammoSite single-dwell position balloon applicator. (b) SAVI (strut-adjusted volume implant) multi-dwell position cage applicator.
Source: Cianna Medical. Reproduced with permission of Cianna Medical.

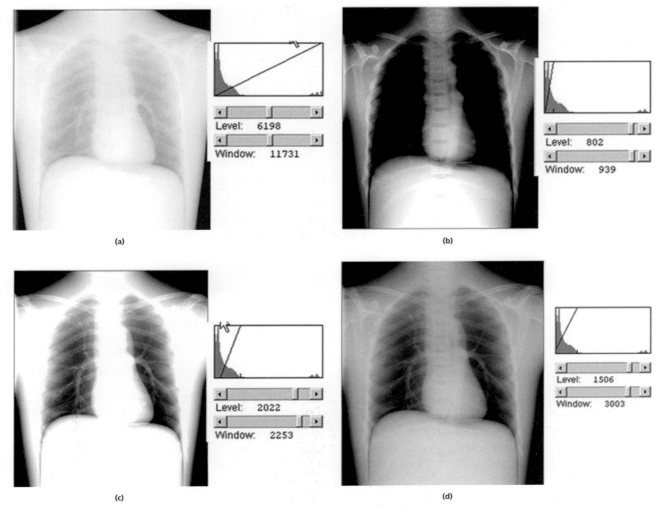

Figure 10-6 Displays of a digital chest radiograph with various window levels and window widths. (a) Level 6198, Width 11,731; (b) Level 802, Width 939; (c) Level 2022, Width 2253; (d) Level 1506, Width 3003.
Source: Courtesy of P. Balter, UT MD Anderson Cancer Center.

0 to 255). We set a window level of 1000 and a window width of 500. Pixels with values below the window are displayed as black and pixels with values above the window are displayed as white. What is the maximum pixel value displayed as black? What is the minimum pixel value displayed as white? How many pixel values are mapped into each gray-scale bin?

The maximum pixel value displayed as black is given by the window level minus half the width, or $1000 - \frac{1}{2} \times 500$, or 750.

The minimum pixel value displayed as white is given by the window level plus half the width, or $1000 + \frac{1}{2} \times 500$, or 1250.

We have 500 pixel values (the window width) that we must bin into 256 display values, so approximately 2 pixel values are placed into each gray-scale bin.

In the previous illustration and example, linear binning of pixel values into gray-scale bins has been used. That is,

approximately an equal number of pixel values were placed into each bin. Better image clarity can sometimes be obtained if the range of pixel values placed into each bin is varied. One such technique is histogram equalization, in which the bin sizes are adjusted so that an equal number of pixels is placed in each bin. Later in this chapter, we shall see how histogram equalization can improve image clarity.

Spatial resolution

Another consideration affecting the quality of digital images is the spatial resolution, which is determined by the size of the pixels. CT images, for example, are generally displayed on a 512 × 512 grid of pixels. Thus, if the field of view is 50 cm, then each pixel is approximately 1 mm × 1 mm. Figure 10-7 illustrates the effects of spatial resolution on an image. The figure of the

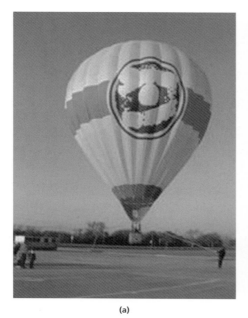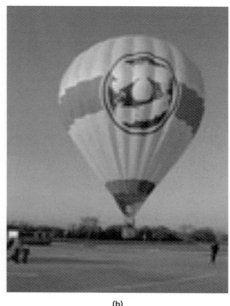

(a)   (b)

Figure 10-7 Two images displayed with different degrees of spatial resolution: (a) 600 × 800 pixels; (b) 100 × 133 pixels. *Source:* Courtesy of P. Balter, UT MD Anderson Cancer Center.

balloon on the left is obtained with a spatial resolution of 600 × 800 pixels, while the figure on the right is obtained with a spatial resolution of 100 × 133 pixels. Looking carefully at the lower-resolution image, one can actually see the pixel structure.

In generating a 3D image, it is important to note that spatial resolution in the superior/inferior direction is generally significantly lower than that in a transverse plane, being determined by the slice thickness. Digitally reconstructed radiographs (DRRs) are generated by calculating the attenuation of x rays as they travel through a 3D CT image dataset. The spatial resolution of such images is related by both the spatial resolution of the rays that are cast through the CT dataset and the spatial resolution of the CT dataset itself. Figure 10-8 illustrates the effect of changing

the CT slice thickness from 2.5 mm, which is a typical value, to 1 mm.

Image enhancement

Several techniques exist to enhance digital images used in radiation oncology. Modifying the window and level of a digital image is described earlier in this chapter. Another technique that has been used quite successfully is *histogram equalization*. To understand histogram equalization, we return to the concept of gray-scale binning. Typically, gray-scale bins are of equal width. However, if the usable range of gray-scale values falls into a rather narrow range of closely spaced pixel values,

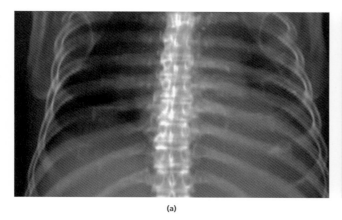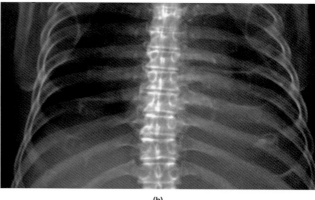

(a)   (b)

Figure 10-8 Digitally reconstructed radiographs of a thorax illustrating the effect of changing the CT slice thickness: (a) 2.5 mm slice thickness; (b) 1 mm slice thickness. *Source:* Courtesy of P. Balter, UT MD Anderson Cancer Center.

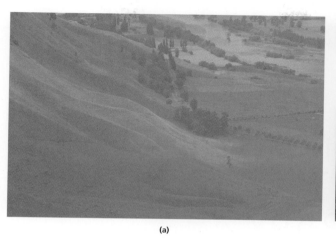
(a)

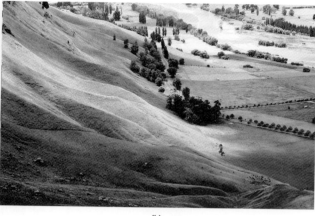
(b)

Figure 10-9 Two images of a photograph illustrating the use of histogram equalization to enhance the visualization of the image. Image (a) is the raw image, whereas image (b) has had histogram equalization applied to it.
Source: Based on photograph by Philip Capper, used in Wikipedia article http://en.wikipedia.org/wiki/Histogram˙equalization, accessed September 15, 2015.

better contrast resolution might be achieved by expanding the resolution in these regions. Rather than using gray-scale bins of equal width, histogram equalization varies the width of the gray-scale bins so that an equal number of pixels lie in each gray-scale bin. Figure 10-9 shows an example of how histogram equalization can be used to enhance an image to enable more detail to be seen.

Summary

- Medical imaging plays an ever-increasing role in radiation therapy.
- Image contrast is used to differentiate anatomic structures on radiographic images.
- The source of image contrast on radiographic images is the differential absorption of x rays resulting from differences in atomic number and mass density.
- The differences in interactions that occur between kilovoltage x rays and megavoltage x rays result in significant differences in contrast in radiographic images.
- The display of digital images is greatly affected by both the number of bits in the pixel values and the binning of the pixel values in the display device. The display is also affected by the pixel resolution.
- A more computer-oriented discussion of bits, bytes, image size, etc. is found in Chapter 13.

Problems

10-1 Consider a breast to consist of 5 cm of fatty tissue. Calculate the image contrast of a 1 mm calcification embedded in the breast using a 20 keV beam. Repeat the calculation for a 40 keV beam.

10-2 Compare the precision of digital thermometer in which temperatures are represented by 8 bits to a thermometer in which temperatures are represented by 16 bits.

10-3 Estimate the size of a typical CT image data set used in radiation treatment planning.

10-4 Compare the spatial resolution of a CT image used in treatment planning with the resolution of the matrix used to compute the dose.

Reference

1 Hubbell, J. H., and Seltzer S. M. Tables of X-Ray Mass Attenuation Coefficients and Mass Energy-Absorption Coefficients from 1 keV to 20 MeV for Elements Z = 1 to 92 and 48 Additional Substances of Dosimetric Interest, NIST Standard Reference Database #126, May 1996, http://www.nist.gov/pml/data/xraycoef/index.cfm, accessed September 15, 2015.

Objectives

After studying this chapter, the reader should be able to:

- Recognize the role of imaging in the diagnosis of malignant disease, targeting of tumors for radiation therapy, and verification of radiation treatment delivery.
- Identify the types of imaging procedures used in radiation therapy and relate the basic principles of radiation physics to these imaging procedures.
- Identify the equipment and procedures for acquiring radiographic images, as well as describe the characteristics of both analog and digital radiographs.
- Discuss the mechanism and value of x-ray and computed tomography (CT) treatment simulation in radiation therapy.
- Delineate the features of transmission CT images and the process of acquiring these images.

- Provide an in-depth explanation of the acquisition and features of ultrasound images.
- Discuss how nuclear medicine images (including single-photon emission computed tomography, or SPECT, and positron emission tomography, or PET, images) are acquired, and the attributes and limitations of these images.
- Describe magnetic resonance imaging (including fMRI) and how it contributes to treatment planning in radiation therapy.

Introduction

In the previous chapter, we identify several features common to all imaging modalities; in this chapter, we identify what

Hendee's Radiation Therapy Physics, Fourth Edition. Todd Pawlicki, Daniel J. Scanderbeg and George Starkschall.
© 2016 John Wiley & Sons, Inc. Published 2016 by John Wiley & Sons, Inc.

makes each modality different. Different modalities image different aspects of the patient. Some imaging modalities are two-dimensional (2D), imaging projections or sections of the patient, whereas others are three-dimensional (3D), imaging volumetric aspects of the patient, whereas still others are four-dimensional (4D), imaging the time evolution of 3D images. Some imaging modalities are real-time, displaying images as they are acquired, whereas others require significant amounts of time-consuming computation to present the final desired image. Some imaging modalities image anatomy, whereas others image physiology. Consequently, imaging applications are specific; we may want to identify one property or another property of the patient, and we select an imaging modality based on the property we wish to image.

The purpose of this chapter is to identify the different imaging modalities used in radiation oncology, identify features characteristic of each of these modalities, and identify the specific applications for which each modality is used.

Radiography

Radiography is the process by which information carried to an image receptor by an x-ray beam is recorded, displayed, and interpreted to yield a diagnosis or reveal the location and extent of patient disease or injury. Radiographic imaging is a form of planar 2D imaging, in which the image in a plane is a map of the transmission of x rays from a source through the patient. Regions of decreased transmission, or increased attenuation, correspond to regions of greater density or atomic number within the patient, and variations of an image, when compared with "normal," can be correlated with pathology.

In addition to identifying pathology, radiographic imaging, for many years, has been used to design radiation treatment portals. Originally, radiation therapy simulators were used to design treatment portals. A radiation therapy simulator consists of a diagnostic x-ray source mounted on an isocentric gantry that can simulate the geometries of a treatment machine. The patient was placed on a flat couch in the desired position for treatment, and the gantry, collimator, and couch were moved to the desired values for the treatment. A planar radiograph was acquired and a treatment portal was designed, often based on bony anatomy. Nowadays, computed tomography (CT) simulation is more typically used. The patient is placed on a flat couch in a CT scanner in the desired position for treatment, a CT scan is acquired, a target volume is drawn on the CT image data set, and a treatment portal is designed from a *digitally reconstructed radiograph* (DRR) based on the CT scan. The DRR can then be compared with a portal image, an image acquired using the radiation beam on the linear accelerator, and used to assess the accuracy of the treatment setup during delivery of radiation. In *image-guided radiation therapy* (IGRT), which is discussed in a later chapter, the x-ray sources are often mounted on the gantry of the linear accelerator, so images can be acquired on the treatment

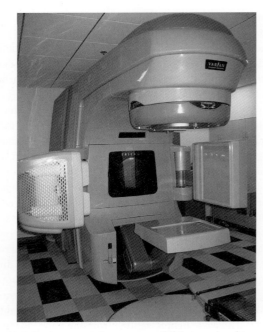

Figure 11-1 Gantry-mounted x-ray source (left in image) and image receptor (right in image) used in image-guided radiation therapy. The megavoltage image receptor is also shown in the bottom of the picture.

couch immediately prior to treatment. Figure 11-1 illustrates an onboard imager consisting of x-ray tubes and image receptors attached to the gantry of the linear accelerator.

Digital radiography

Originally, x-ray images were recorded on photographic film, with the use of intensifying screens to enhance the image. Recording x-ray images on film is considered an analog method of information acquisition because the spatial and contrast information is captured in a continuous manner. In a digital image, the spatial information is presented as a matrix of small cells (picture elements, or *pixels*), with each pixel presented as a gray level interpreted from a number for the particular pixel stored in the memory of a computer. The number is a *density value* for the tissue represented in the pixel. Several techniques are available to acquire radiographic information digitally or to convert analog images into digital format. These techniques are gradually gaining acceptance in radiology as interest grows in manipulating images by computer-based image processing programs. A second impetus for digital radiography is the desire to transmit images across *local area networks* (LANs) from their site of production to a location in the same institution where they are interpreted and used in patient care. A further incentive for digital radiology is to use *teleradiology* methods to transmit images across large distances for diagnostic interpretation and consultation. LANs are particularly useful for transmitting digital images in the hospital from the radiology department to the radiation oncology service, where they are used in treatment planning.

Such networks are often called *picture archival and communications systems* (PACS).[1].

Some digital radiography systems employ a bank of radiation detectors, such as scintillation probes, photodiodes, or semiconductor devices that scan across the patient in synchrony with a scanning fan-shaped x-ray beam. This *slit-scanning technique* yields an image with little scattered radiation.[2] The electrical signals from the detectors are converted to digital format, in which the magnitude of the signal is interpreted as a number ranging from perhaps 1 to 256 (2^0 to 2^8) and presented in the image as segmental gray levels displayed across a matrix of 512 × 512, 1024 × 1024, or 2048 × 2048 pixels. Another approach to digital radiography involves the digital conversion of the electrical signal from a television camera that views the output screen of a large image intensifier.[3]

Storage phosphor technology is one approach to digital radiography that has been deployed in many clinical settings. In this technique, the x-ray image is projected and stored on a plate containing a photostimulable phosphor, such as barium fluorobromide. When the plate is scanned some time later with an intense focused laser, visible light is emitted from the phosphor in proportion to the energy absorbed earlier from the x-ray beam. The light output from the plate is detected with a *photomultiplier tube* (PMT), or other light-sensing detector, and it is digitized to produce a signal that can be viewed as an image on a high-resolution television monitor or photographic film. Digital radiography using storage phosphor technology sometimes is referred to as *computed radiography*.

Digital x-ray detectors

In recent years, digital x-ray detectors, commonly called *electronic portal imaging devices* (EPIDs), replaced older methods of x-ray detection, such as image intensifiers and intensifying screens and film. Early forms of EPIDs used a television camera to capture the image on an image-intensifying screen and displayed this image at the viewing console. Figure 11-2 illustrates a schematic of such a device. The technology of this type of device is rather straightforward; in addition, the detector can cover a relatively large field of view. On the other hand, these devices are rather bulky, presenting an encumbrance in the vicinity of the treatment table, where therapists must physically interact with the patient. Furthermore, only a small fraction of the light generated at the image intensifier is collected in the image intensifier and reaches the viewer.

Radiographic images on film can be digitized by scanning them with a laser beam, with a light detector on the opposite side of the film used to measure the intensity of transmitted light. The signal from the detector is converted into digital form for transmission to remote locations, where it modulates the intensity of a light beam scanned across an x-ray film to reconstruct the original image. This technique can be used in teleradiology to send images to other locations in the same institution or community or across much greater distances. Once the film image is

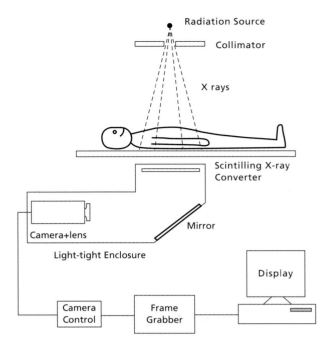

Figure 11-2 Schematic illustration of camera-based EPID. *Source:* Antonuk 2002.[4] Reproduced with permission of IOP Publishing.

digitized, it can be transmitted to remote locations over a telephone wire (twisted pair) or fiber-optic cable, or by a microwave or satellite link.

Example 11-1

What is the spatial resolution when an 8 in × 10 in radiograph is scanned into a 1024 × 1024 digital matrix?

Resolution element (pixel size) dimensions:

Horizontal (8 in)(25.4 mm/in)/1024 = 0.20 mm
Vertical (10 in)(25.4 mm/in)/1024 = 0.25 mm

Line pairs per millimeter: $1/2(1/r)$, where r = pixel dimension:

Horizontal 1/2 (1/0.20 mm) = 2.5 line pairs per mm
Vertical 1/2 (1/0.25 mm) = 2.0 line pairs per mm

The spatial resolution of the digitized image is significantly less than the 6–10 line pairs per millimeter available in the original radiograph.

Example 11-2

What is the computer storage required for the digital image in Example 11-1 if each pixel has a capacity of 256 (2^8 or 8 bits or 1 byte) of gray-scale information?

Storage = 1024 × 1024 × 8 = $8.4 × 10^6$ bits (more than one megabyte)

Computed tomography

In conventional radiography, subtle differences of a few percent in x-ray transmission through the body are not visible in the image. One reason for the failure to differentiate these subtle differences in transmission is that the projection of 3D anatomic information onto a 2D image receptor obscures the subtle differences in x-ray transmission through different structures in the body. Moreover, conventional image receptors (film, screens, image intensifiers, flat-panel imagers) are unable to resolve differences smaller than a few percent in the intensity of incident radiation. Finally, large-area x-ray beams used in conventional radiography produce significant amounts of scattered radiation that interfere with the visualization of subtle differences in x-ray transmission.

Each of these limitations in conventional radiography is significantly reduced in CT, and differences in x-ray transmission (subject contrast) of a few tenths of a percent can be revealed in the image. Although the spatial resolution of a millimeter or so provided by CT is notably poorer than that provided by conventional radiography ($\sim$0.1 mm), the superior visualization of subject contrast and the display of anatomy across planes [e.g., cross-sectional (sometimes called *transaxial*, *axial*, or *transverse*), coronal, and sagittal sections], which are not available with conventional radiography, make CT exceptionally useful for visualizing anatomy in many regions of the body.

History

The revolutionary imaging technology of CT was introduced to clinical medicine in 1972 with the announcement of the head scanner developed by Hounsfield, working at EMI, Ltd.[5] Hounsfield termed his technique *computerized transverse axial tomography*. This expression was later abbreviated to *computerized axial tomography* and was referred to as *CAT scanning*. After sufficient ridicule had been directed toward this acronym, the expression *computed tomography* (CT) was adopted by major journals in medical imaging. The technique of image reconstruction from projections employed in the EMI scanner had been used in other fields, such as radioastronomy,[6] electron microscopy[7,8] and optics[9,10] and was based on a mathematical algorithm developed by Radon in 1917.[11] The advantages of CT in clinical medicine quickly became apparent, and many companies joined the race in the mid-1970s to produce a better scanner.[12] By the end of the decade, four "generations" of CT scanners had appeared, and several of the companies had become financial casualties or had decided to redirect their attention to other ventures. Today, CT units are marketed principally by the major instrument companies servicing the medical marketplace.

CT has been a major influence on the evolution of imaging technologies in medicine over the past two decades. Some once-popular imaging techniques, such as brain scans in nuclear medicine and pneumoencephalography in radiology, have virtually disappeared, whereas others, such as cerebral angiography and myelography in radiology, have been impacted significantly. Imaging methods such as *single-photon emission computed tomography* (SPECT), *positron emission tomography* (PET), and *magnetic resonance imaging* (MRI) employ image reconstruction techniques similar to those developed for CT. Others, such as real-time and gray-scale ultrasonography, functional studies in nuclear medicine, and digital radiography, employ computer-based digital methods for data acquisition and processing that were introduced originally by CT. Treatment planning in radiation therapy has been assisted greatly by CT. Medical imaging has experienced major changes over the past four decades that were initiated with the recognition of the clinical advantages of CT in the early 1970s.

Principles of computed tomography

In early versions of the CT scanner, a narrow beam of x rays was scanned across the patient in synchrony with a radiation detector on the opposite side of the patient. The x-ray detector may be a pressurized ionization chamber, a scintillation detector, or a semiconductor diode. The transmission, I, of x rays through a patient of thickness x is given by the standard exponential attenuation equation $I = I_0 e^{-\mu x}$, with the patient assumed to have a uniform composition with linear attenuation coefficient μ. For a patient with many (n) regions, each with a different thickness and attenuation coefficient, the x-ray transmission is:

$$I = I_0 \exp(-\sum \mu_i x_i)$$

where:

$$-\sum \mu_i x_i = -(\mu_1 x_1 + \mu_2 x_2 + \cdots + \mu_n x_n)$$

and the fractional transmission is given by:

$$I/I_0 = \exp(-\sum \mu_i x_i)$$

With a single transmission measurement, the separate attenuation coefficients cannot be determined because too many unknown values of μ_i exist in the equation for fractional transmission. However, multiple measurements of x-ray transmission obtained at different orientations of the x-ray source and detector permit the computation of the separate coefficients. This computation yields a cross-sectional matrix of attenuation values corresponding to a slice of tissue through the patient. Each of the attenuation values can be expressed as a *CT number* calculated as:

$$\text{CT number} = 1000 \frac{\mu_i - \mu_w}{\mu_w}$$

where μ_i is the attenuation value of a particular volume element of tissue (voxel) and μ_w is the linear attenuation coefficient of water for the average energy of x rays in the CT beam. Each of the CT numbers can be assigned a particular shade of gray, and the matrix of CT numbers can be presented as a cross-sectional

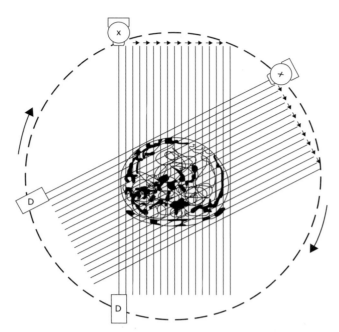

Figure 11-3 First-generation scanner using a pencil x-ray beam and a combination of translational and rotational motion.

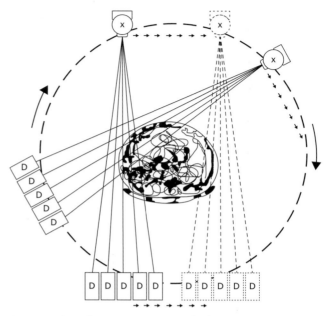

Figure 11-4 Second-generation scanner with a fan x-ray beam, multiple detectors, and a combination of translational and rotational motion.

(axial) gray-scale display. This gray-scale display constitutes the CT image. Successive CT sets of transmission measurements displaced slightly from each other through the patient yield a series of cross-sectional images representing contiguous *slices* through the body. Each slice possesses a *slice thickness* that can be varied from about 1 mm to 1 cm. Furthermore, corresponding voxels in successive slices can be combined mathematically to yield coronal and sagittal images that complement the axial images provided routinely by the CT scanner.

In first-generation CT scanners, the x-ray source provided a pencil-like x-ray beam that was scanned in translational motion across the patient at a large number (e.g., 180) of orientations that differed slightly in direction (e.g., 1°) from the preceding and succeeding scan (Figure 11-3). This translate–rotate scanning geometry required several minutes to accumulate x-ray transmission data for a single image, and patient motion interfered with image quality. The time-consuming procedure for data acquisition prevented application of the technique to areas of the body other than the head because patient motion is too severe in those areas. Succeeding generations of CT scanners have principally reflected efforts to reduce scanning times to a few seconds or less and to improve spatial resolution by introducing intrinsic methods of quality control. Second-generation scanners replaced the pencil-like x-ray beam with a fan-shaped beam that employed translate–rotate motion at angular increments of several degrees to reduce scanning times to 20 seconds or so (Figure 11-4). Third-generation scanners used a fan-shaped x-ray beam and a bank of multiple detectors that underwent purely rotational motion to reduce scan times to as short as 1 to 2 seconds (Figure 11-5). Fourth-generation scanners

use a stationary circular array of detectors and a fan-shaped x-ray beam to provide scan times comparable to those with a third-generation scanner. These scanners yield images that are restricted by image noise caused by limitations in the number of x rays used to determine the attenuation coefficients of different voxels.

Increased acquisition speed has been achieved in recent years by the introduction of *helical*, or *spiral*, *CT*, in which the gantry

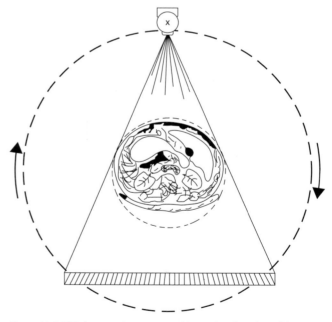

Figure 11-5 Third-generation scanner with rotational motion of the x-ray tube and detector array.

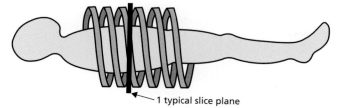

Figure 11-6 Trajectory of radiation beam in helical CT.

rotates while the patient couch translates (Figure 11-6). Even faster speeds are achieved by the use of multiple detector rings, enabling the simultaneous acquisition of several slices during each gantry rotation. Presently such systems, referred to as *multislice helical CT scanners*, with up to several hundred rows of detectors, are capable of scan times of a few seconds.

Cone-beam computed tomography (CBCT) is a technology that uses a flat-panel detector opposite the radiation source. Their major application in radiation oncology is for image guidance (see Chapter 12). In this application the kilovoltage source and flat-panel detector are both mounted on the gantry of the linear accelerator.[13] After acquisition, the CBCT image is compared with the planning CT image and adjustments are made to more accurately target the target volume.

Reconstruction algorithms

The foundation of CT is the construction of images from projections by use of a mathematical *algorithm*. Various algorithms have been used, including simple back-projection, integral equations (the *convolution method*), Fourier transformation, and series expansion.[14] Image reconstruction can be illustrated by the technique of simple backprojection applied to translate–rotate geometry.

In *simple backprojection*, each path of x-ray transmission through the body is divided into multiple, equally spaced elements, and each element is assumed to contribute equally to the total attenuation of x rays along the transmission path. In Figure 11-7, transmission path A is divided into 10 equally spaced volume elements (voxels), and each element is assumed to contribute 1% attenuation to the total 10% attenuation along the path. Path B of the x-ray transmission measured at a different orientation intersects path A at one of the voxels. The total attenuation along path B is 20%, and each of the 10 voxels along the path is assumed to contribute 2% to the attenuation. The two attenuations at the intersecting voxel are added to yield a summed attenuation of 3%. A third transmission path C also intersects the common voxel and adds an additional 3% to the summed attenuation value. For a translate–rotate geometry with 180 angular orientations, the total attenuation of the common voxel is the sum of 180 separate values, with each value measured for an x-ray path obtained at a particular angular orientation of the x-ray source and detector. Every voxel in the anatomic cross-section is intersected by 180 paths of x-ray transmission, and the

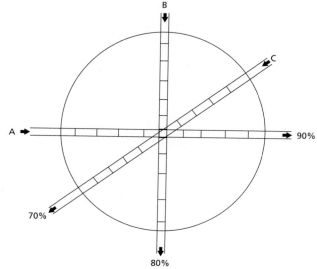

Figure 11-7 Principle of simple back construction method of image reconstruction from projections.

attenuation for each is the sum of 180 individual measurements. As a result, the cross-sectional gray-scale display of attenuation values presents picture elements (pixels) corresponding to the volume elements (voxels) of tissue in the patient, with grayness in the pixel corresponding to the attenuation in the voxel. This display constitutes the CT image compiled by the method of simple backprojection.

Simple backprojection has one major limitation: it produces images with serious blurring artifacts in regions where adjacent voxels differ significantly in their attenuation values. Suppression of these artifacts requires a modification of the simple backprojection technique in which a deblurring function is combined (convolved) with the transmission data before the transmission data are backprojected. The most common deblurring function is a *frequency ramp filter* that increases signal amplification linearly with frequency up to a cutoff frequency, where the amplification drops to zero. Because a ramp filter also amplifies the noise, an ad hoc filter such as a Hamming or Hann filter is introduced to reduce, or *roll off*, the amplification of the ramp filter at higher frequencies. Filtered backprojection removes the star-like blurring seen in simple backprojection. The technique of convolving the transmission data with a deblurring function is referred to as the *convolution method* of image reconstruction. This method is the most popular reconstruction algorithm used today in CT. One of its advantages is that the image can be compiled while x-ray transmission data are being collected.

CT is a useful imaging technique for delineating surface contours, tumor volumes, and the position of surrounding normal structures in treatment planning for radiation therapy.[15–17] It also provides attenuation values helpful in determining corrections for tissue heterogeneity during the delivery of radiation treatments.[18,19] Most commercial CT units offer software packages for extension to treatment planning applications. Many of

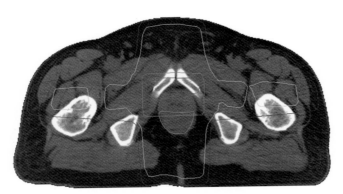

Figure 11-8 Isodose distribution superimposed on a cross-sectional CT image of the pelvis.

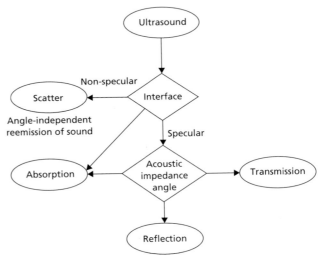

Figure 11-9 Ultrasound reflection and refraction at an interface between tissues in the body.

the packages permit direct transfer of images from the CT unit to the treatment planning computer, in which isodose distributions can be superimposed to delineate satisfactory treatment plans for the patient. An example of an isodose distribution superimposed on a cross-sectional CT image is shown in Figure 11-8.

Ultrasonography

Ultrasound imaging (*ultrasonography*) is a useful technique for delineating surface contours and internal structures important to identification of satisfactory treatment plans in radiation therapy. In this imaging method, a piezoelectric crystal at the face of an ultrasound transducer is used to generate a mechanical disturbance (pressure wave) that is propagated through tissue directly in front of the transducer. The wave is initiated by applying a momentary electrical shock to the piezoelectric crystal that sets the crystal into vibration. This vibration introduces the pressure wave into the medium. The frequency (1–10 MHz) of the pressure wave is in the ultrasound range well above the frequency range to which the human ear is responsive (20 Hz to 20 kHz).

As an ultrasound wave moves through the body, it encounters various interfaces between tissues that reflect and refract (change the direction of) the ultrasound energy (Figure 11-9). At any interface, the amount of energy reflected back toward the transducer depends on the difference in acoustic impedance across the interface. The acoustic impedance, Z, of a tissue is the product of the physical density, ρ, of the tissue and the speed, v, of ultrasound through the tissue ($Z = \rho v$).

Example 11-3

The fraction of ultrasound reflected at an interface is described by the ultrasound reflection coefficient:

$$\alpha_R = \left[\frac{Z_2 - Z_1}{Z_2 + Z_1}\right]^2$$

and Z_1 and Z_2 are the acoustic impedances of tissues on each side of the interface. What is the fraction of ultrasound energy reflected at the interface between the chest wall and lung if the ultrasound velocity is assumed to be the same in both tissues and the acoustic impedances are assumed to be approximately 1.6×10^5 g/(cm^{2}sec) in the chest wall and 0.0004×10^5 g/(cm^{2}sec) in the lung?

$$\begin{aligned} \alpha_R &= \left[\frac{Z_2 - Z_1}{Z_2 + Z_1}\right]^2 \\ &= \left[\frac{1.6 - 0.0004}{1.6 + 0.0004}\right]^2 = 0.999 \end{aligned}$$

That is, 99.9% of the ultrasound energy is reflected, and 0.001% is transmitted at the interface.

When the difference in acoustic impedance is great across an interface, most of the energy is reflected, and little is transmitted across the interface into the second medium. For this reason, ultrasonography is not useful in examining the thorax because the difference in physical density between the chest wall and the lung prevents the ultrasound from penetrating across the interface. Ultrasonography is useful for measuring the thickness of the chest wall in treatment planning because reflected ultrasound yields a clear delineation of the surface contour and the inner boundary of the chest wall. Ultrasonography also presents problems in examining structures in the shadow of bone because much of the ultrasound energy is reflected at the soft tissue–bone interface, and that which is transmitted is strongly absorbed in bone.

Ultrasonography is particularly useful for delineating tissues that differ only slightly in their acoustic impedances, provided that enough energy is reflected at the interface between the tissues to furnish a measurable signal as reflected ultrasound returning to the transducer. For example, ultrasonography is used to distinguish cysts from solid lesions in the breast following their identification as suspicious regions in mammography because enough ultrasound energy is reflected to outline the boundaries of the lesion. Furthermore a solid lesion produces additional reflections in the lesion's interior, whereas the inner region of a cyst is *anechoic* (i.e., it does not produce internal reflections, or *echoes*, of ultrasound energy). Another common application of ultrasound has been in IGRT, primarily of the prostate, in which real-time ultrasound images of the prostate, bladder, and rectum can be compared with treatment planning images of the same anatomy and adjusting the patient position based on the acquired ultrasound information.

Ultrasound energy reflected from an interface between tissues in the body returns as a pressure wave of reduced amplitude to the transducer. As it is absorbed by the piezoelectric crystal in the transducer, it generates a small electrical signal that is captured and processed. The angular orientation of the ultrasound transducer as the signal is received defines the direction of the returning pressure wave and therefore the position of the interface that produced it. The time, t, between transmission of the ultrasound energy and receipt of the returning signal defines the depth of the interface according to the expression:

$$\text{Depth} = (v \cdot t)/2$$

where v is the velocity of ultrasound. Division by 2 is required in this expression because the time, t, includes both the time to reach the interface and the time for the echo to return to the transducer. The velocity, v, of ultrasound varies slightly among different soft tissues, but a value of 1540 m/sec often is assumed in computations of the depth of reflecting interfaces.

Example 11-4

An echo is detected 130 μsec after an ultrasound pulse is transmitted into tissue. What is the depth of the interface that produced the echo?

$$
\begin{aligned}
\text{Depth} &= (v \cdot t)/2 \\
&= (154{,}000 \text{ cm/sec})(130 \times 10^{-6} \text{ sec})/2 \\
&= 10 \text{ cm}
\end{aligned}
$$

Reflected ultrasound energy is returned to the transducer most efficiently when the interface is at right angles to the ultrasound beam. However, tissue interfaces in the body can be at any angle with respect to the surface contour of the patient. To obtain images of these interfaces, the ultrasound transducer usually is rocked as it is moved across the patient's surface so that the ultrasound beam intersects interfaces at close to a right angle at least part of the time during a scan. This two-phase motion with the transducer coupled to the skin with a thin layer of gel is referred to as *compound contact scanning*.

In the early years of ultrasound imaging, a single transducer was moved manually across the body surface to obtain an ultrasound image. This process was relatively slow and required a

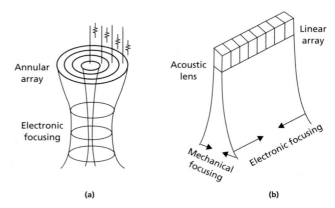

Figure 11-10 Multitransducer arrays for real-time ultrasound imaging.

highly skilled operator to acquire an acceptable image. Recent scanners provide *multitransducer arrays* that permit more rapid imaging and the acquisition of real-time images in which artifacts caused by patient motion are subdued (Figure 11-10). More complete explanations of the technology and applications of ultrasound imaging are available in standard texts on the physics of medical imaging.[20] In addition to determinations of chest wall thickness, ultrasound imaging is useful for localizing a variety of normal and abnormal structures in the head and neck, breast, upper abdomen, lower pelvis, and retroperitoneum. These applications of ultrasonography to treatment planning and delivery in radiation therapy are described in the literature.[21–23]

Nuclear medicine

Nuclear medicine is a form of functional imaging in which physiology, metabolism, and biochemistry, rather than anatomic structure, are the principal features portrayed in images. In this discipline, a radioactive nuclide (*radionuclide*) is administered to a patient, usually tagged to a specific γ-emitting radioactive pharmaceutical selected for its tendency to concentrate in a specific organ or tissue of interest in the patient. Gamma rays emitted by the nuclide escape from the body and are measured with an external detector. The measurement process yields a "map" of the accumulation, distribution, and excretion of the pharmaceutical in the organ or tissue of interest.

The use of radioactively tagged compounds as biochemical tracers has been of great importance in biology since the discovery of radioactivity. Radioactive tracers have contributed in a major way to the many advances in biology and the basic sciences underlying medicine (e.g., biochemistry, physiology, pharmacology, and cellular and molecular biology) that have occurred over this century. However, the routine use of radioactively tagged pharmaceuticals (*radiopharmaceuticals*) in clinical medicine awaited three major advances that occurred in the middle of the twentieth century. The first of these advances was the availability of nuclear reactors as sources of artificially produced radioisotopes that followed World War II and was facilitated by the Atoms for Peace program of the Atomic Energy Commission. The second advance was the development of the scintillation camera by Anger in the late 1950s,[24] while the third advance was the evolution of the radionuclide generator, specifically the ^{99}Mo-^{99m}Tc radionuclide generator, at about the same time. Today, many patients in the United States experience at least one nuclear medicine procedure, and many potential candidates for radiation therapy undergo one or more nuclear medicine procedures for purposes such as staging cancer and determining the likelihood and extent of its dissemination.

Properties of radioactive pharmaceuticals

Radionuclides are selected for diagnostic nuclear medicine based on properties that make them desirable for medical imaging. Among these desirable properties are:

- A relatively short physical half-life so that the radionuclide can be administered to the patient in sufficient activities to yield enough γ rays to produce an acceptable image, yet with little residual activity so that problems of disposing residual materials and patient wastes are reduced.
- A relatively short biological half-life so that residual activity in the patient does not produce unacceptable radiation doses.
- The emission of little particulate radiation (e.g., beta particles and conversion and Auger electrons), because these radiations do not contribute to the examination but increase the radiation dose to the patient.
- The emission of γ rays of an energy well matched to the detection efficiency of the measurement apparatus (e.g., the scintillation detector).
- The availability of a specific γ-ray energy that is well separated from γ rays of lower energy so that scattered photons can be rejected based on their lower energy.
- High specific activity so that the radionuclide can be tagged with high efficiency into the selected pharmaceutical.
- Ease of labeling of the radionuclide into the pharmaceutical.

One radionuclide that satisfies these requirements reasonably well is ^{99m}Tc, and 80% or so of all nuclear medicine procedures are performed with this material. ^{99m}Tc is produced in a radionuclide generator in which the condition of transient equilibrium (see Chapter 1) is achieved between the parent, ^{99}Mo, and the progeny, ^{99m}Tc.

Pharmaceuticals also have specific properties that make them desirable as imaging agents in nuclear medicine. Among these properties are:

- Their availability in a specific chemical form without competing chemical isomers that exhibit different physiological behaviors.
- Chemical stability *in vitro* so that the pharmaceutical can be stored before use and *in vivo* so that the radionuclide does not dissociate from the pharmaceutical once it is inside the body.
- Predictable and reproducible behavior in the body.

- A high target/non-target ratio in the body so that the radiopharmaceutical will deposit in the region of interest without delivering excessive radiation doses to other organs and tissues.
- Traceable kinetics that permit determination of quantitative parameters important to the assessment of physiological function.
- A biological half-life that is long enough to accommodate the nuclear medicine study, yet short enough to permit rapid elimination of the tagged pharmaceutical after the study has been completed.

The development of *receptor-specific radiopharmaceuticals* is one of the more promising areas of nuclear medicine today. Some of these pharmaceuticals, including radioactively tagged monoclonal antibodies, may permit identification of the presence of specific types of cancer cells at much lower concentrations than those measurable by current imaging techniques. Although much work remains to improve the sensitivity and specificity of receptor-specific radiopharmaceuticals, their appeal as a promising approach to cancer detection and staging is unmistakable.[25]

Nuclear medicine imaging

In nuclear medicine, γ rays emitted by a radionuclide tagged to a specific pharmaceutical localized in a particular organ or tissue of the patient are measured by a radiation detector positioned outside the patient. To obtain an image of the distribution of the radionuclide in the patient, the site of interaction of γ rays in the detector must be correlated with the origin of the γ rays inside the patient. To provide this correlation, a collimator is placed between the detector and the patient. Different collimators are available, including pinhole, converging, and diverging collimators. The most common collimator is the parallel multihole collimator depicted in Figure 11-11. With this collimator, the origin of a γ ray interacting in the detector is confined to a small region of the patient directly below the detector. Primary γ rays from other regions of the patient cannot reach the interaction site because they are intercepted and absorbed by the high-Z (lead or tungsten) septa in the collimator. In this manner, the collimator imposes a spatial relationship between the interaction sites in the detector and the origin of γ rays in the patient. Use of a collimator greatly restricts the efficiency of γ-ray detection in nuclear medicine because less than 1/100 of the γ rays emitted from the patient are transmitted by the collimator and reach the detector. Without a collimator, however, the sites of interaction of γ rays in the detector could not be used as a map of the distribution of radioactivity in the patient, and the acquisition of useful nuclear medicine images would be impossible.

In many applications, the radiation detector in nuclear medicine is a large (up to 50 cm diameter), relatively thin (0.6 to 1.2 cm) NaI(Tl) scintillation crystal. Mounted above the crystal are many photomultiplier tubes. When an interaction occurs in the crystal, light is released and detected by the photomultiplier

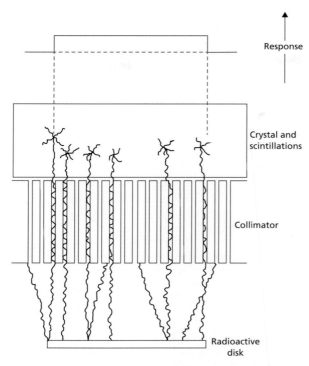

Figure 11-11 Parallel multihole collimator for nuclear medicine imaging.

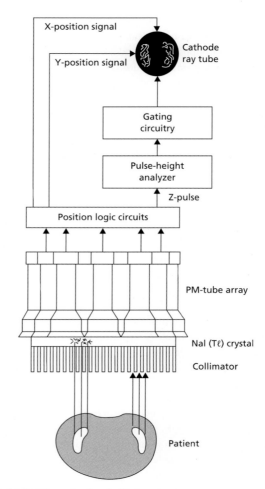

Figure 11-12 Schematic of a scintillation camera.
Source: Sorensen and Phelps 1987.[26]

tubes. The amount of light reaching each photomultiplier tube, and therefore the size of the electrical signal from it, depends on the lateral distance between the photomultiplier tube and the interaction site of the γ ray in the crystal. By electronically analyzing the relative size of the signals from the photomultiplier tubes, the location of the interaction site, and therefore the origin of the γ ray in the patient, can be identified. This analysis results in the formation of four electrical signals ($+x$, $-x$, $+y$, $-y$) that reveal the position of the interaction site in the crystal.

The γ-ray origin identified by this technique may be one of two types. It could represent the site of release of a primary γ ray from a molecule of the radiopharmaceutical deposited at the site. However, it could also represent the location where a primary photon originating elsewhere in the body is scattered toward the scintillation detector. Both the primary and scattered γ rays originating at the site could traverse the collimator and interact in the crystal. They can be distinguished, however, because a scattered photon is less energetic than a primary photon and therefore stimulates less light emission when it interacts in the crystal. To accomplish this distinction, the electrical signals from all the photomultiplier tubes are added, and the sum (the Z pulse) is compared in a *pulse height analyzer* to the size of a signal expected when a primary γ ray interacts in the crystal. If the signal is smaller than expected for a primary γ ray, interaction of a scattered photon is assumed and the pulse is rejected.

Electrical signals (Z pulses) representing interaction of primary γ rays in the NaI(Tl) crystal are transmitted to the display device in the scintillation camera. Each signal activates a short

burst of electrons from a filament. The electrons are directed toward a fluorescent screen in a *cathode-ray tube* (CRT). The four position signals ($+x$, $-x$, $+y$, $-y$) for the interaction are applied to deflection electrodes surrounding the electrons so that they strike the fluorescent screen at the location corresponding to the interaction site of the γ ray in the crystal. In this manner, an image of brief light flashes is compiled on the screen that can be photographed to reveal the distribution of sites of γ-ray interactions in the crystal and hence the distribution of radioactivity in the patient. A diagram of a scintillation camera is shown in Figure 11-12. A more complete explanation of the scintillation camera and principles of nuclear imaging in general are available in standard texts on the physics of medical imaging.[20]

Emission computed tomography

Tomography is the process of collecting data about an object from multiple views (projections) and then using these data to construct an image of a slice through the object. This approach to imaging can be applied to nuclear medicine by detecting γ rays emitted from a radiopharmaceutical distributed within the body. The term *emission computed tomography* (ECT) refers to this procedure. Tomographic images acquired by detecting annihilation photons released during positron decay are referred to as *positron emission tomography* (or *PET*). Tomographic images computed from the registration of interactions of individual γ rays are known as *single-photon emission computed tomography* (or *SPECT*).

Single-photon emission computed tomography

This nuclear imaging technique has several features in common with x-ray transmission CT. Multiple views are acquired to produce an image in one or more transverse slices through the patient. Most SPECT systems employ a rotating detector (a scintillation camera) and a stationary source of γ rays (the patient). One, two, or three scintillation cameras are mounted on a rotating gantry. Each scintillation "head" encompasses enough anatomy in the axial direction to permit acquisition of multiple image "slices" in a single scan.

One major difference between SPECT and x-ray CT is that a SPECT image represents the distribution of radioactivity across a slice through the patient, whereas an x-ray CT image reflects the attenuation of x rays across a slice of tissue. In SPECT, photon attenuation interferes with the imaging process because fewer photons are recorded from voxels at greater depths in the patient. A correction must be made for this attenuation. Methods for attenuation correction usually involve estimating the body contour, sampling the patient from both sides (i.e., 360° rather than 180° rotation), and constructing a correction matrix to adjust scan data for attenuation.

SPECT has many clinical applications, including cardiac imaging, liver/spleen studies, and chest–thorax procedures. SPECT is also important for imaging receptor-specific pharmaceuticals such as monoclonal antibodies, because it provides improved detection and localization of small sites of radioactivity along the axial dimension.

Positron emission tomography

The principle of SPECT is applicable to PET. In PET, however, the radiation detected is annihilation radiation released as positrons interact with electrons. The directionality of the annihilation photons (511 keV photons emitted in opposite directions) provides a way to localize the origin of the photons and hence the radioactive decay process that resulted in their emission. Because the directionality of annihilation photons provides information about the origin of the photons, collimators are not needed in PET imaging. This approach, referred to as *electronic collimation*, greatly increases the detection efficiency of PET imaging.

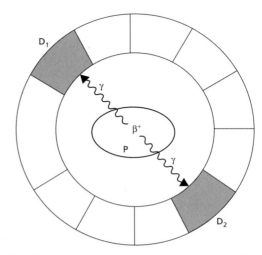

Figure 11-13 In positron emission tomography, two detectors D_1 and D_2 record the interaction of 0.511 MeV photons in coincidence, indicating that a positron decay event has taken place somewhere along a line connecting the two detectors within the patient, P.

In a typical PET system (Figure 11-13), the patient is surrounded by a ring of detectors. When detectors on opposite sides of the patient register annihilation photons simultaneously (i.e., within a nanosecond), the positron decay process that created the photons is assumed to have occurred along a line between the detectors. The PET image reveals the number of decays (counts) occurring in each of the volume elements (voxels) represented by picture elements (pixels) in the image.

Radionuclides suitable for PET imaging include ^{11}C, ^{13}N, ^{15}O, ^{18}F, ^{62}Cu, ^{68}Ga, and ^{82}Rb. Many of these nuclides have very short lives, and a cyclotron for their production must be close to the PET imager. To date, however, the most common clinical PET applications have employed ^{18}F-labeled fluorodeoxyglucose (^{18}FDG). The 1.7-hour half-life of this nuclide permits it to be obtained from a nearby supplier. PET imaging with ^{18}FDG is very useful in radiation oncology for assessing the spread of a primary cancer, detecting metastases, and monitoring the patient during and after treatment.

It is more challenging to obtain multiple image slices in PET than in SPECT. Most PET scanners use several detector rings for this purpose. Attenuation corrections are intrinsically more accurate in PET than in SPECT because the pair of annihilation photons defines a line through the patient such that the sum of the path lengths is constant irrespective of where the photons originate along the line. Originally, the attenuation correction was determined by using a γ-emitting radionuclide to obtain a transmission scan immediately after acquisition of the PET scan. In recent years, PET/CT scanners have been developed, in which a CT-scanner gantry is mounted adjacent to the PET gantry. One of the two scans is obtained, the patient table is translated, and the other scan is obtained. The information gathered from the CT scan is then used to make the attenuation correction. Figure 11-14 illustrates such a PET/CT scanner.

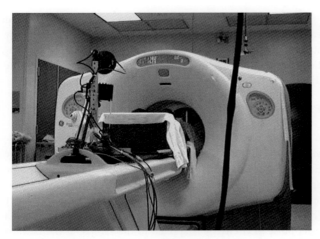

Figure 11-14 A PET/CT scanner. The gantry closer to the viewer is a CT gantry. The patient first undergoes a CT scan. The patient table is then translated a known distance, and a PET scan is acquired.

The increased efficiency in acquiring the transmission scan has enabled the PET/CT scanner to supersede the conventional PET scanner, which used the γ-emitter as the radiation source for the transmission scan. More important for radiation oncology, the PET/CT scanner enables the acquisition of a treatment planning CT scan with the physiological information from the PET scan superimposed on the CT scan. Because the radioactive fluorine isotope is bonded to a glucose molecule, it tends to collect in regions where there is increased metabolic activity, such as tumors and metastases. Figure 11-15 illustrates a PET/CT scan

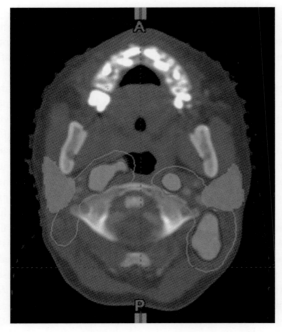

Figure 11-15 A PET scan superimposed on a CT scan used for the delineation of a target volume.

used to aid in delineating a target volume for irradiation of a head and neck tumor.

Magnetic resonance imaging

Many have viewed magnetic resonance as the most important development in medical imaging since the discovery of x rays in 1895. The technology is based on the delineation of the magnetic properties of the proton by Frisch and Stern[27] in 1933 and demonstration of the principle of magnetic resonance by Rabi[28] in 1939. The detection in 1945 by Bloch[29] and Purcell[30] of radio signals from nuclei placed in a magnetic field led to the development of the technique of nuclear magnetic resonance, which has contributed in many ways to analytical chemistry and biochemistry. In 1971, Damadian[31] employed nuclear magnetic resonance to observe differences in magnetic properties between normal and cancerous tissues in rats. Two years later, Lauterbur[32] published the first magnetic resonance image. In 2003, Lauterbur was one of the recipients of the Nobel Prize in Physiology or Medicine for his work in magnetic resonance imaging. Since that time, magnetic resonance imaging (MRI) has assumed a position of growing importance in medical imaging. Today, MRI and angiography, along with functional neuroimaging with MR techniques, hold great promise for revealing characteristics of the human body in health, disease, and injury that heretofore have been inaccessible and incompletely understood at best.

The basic requirements for MRI include nuclei with a nonzero magnetic moment, a static magnetic field, a radiofrequency field, and magnetic field gradients. Both the proton and the neutron behave like tiny magnets as a result of their spin about their own axis. Nuclei with even numbers of protons and neutrons do not exhibit magnetic properties, however, because the magnetic properties of the constituent nucleons tend to cancel out one another. In nuclei with an odd number of protons or neutrons, complete cancellation of the magnetic properties of the nucleons is not possible. Hence, these nuclei have a residual magnetic moment (i.e., they behave as a small atomic magnet). Ordinary hydrogen, ^{1}H, has the strongest magnetic moment because it contains only one nucleon, a proton, and no additional proton or neutron is available to counteract its magnetic moment. Other nuclei with an odd number of nucleons, including ^{13}C, ^{19}F, ^{23}Na, and ^{31}P, exhibit smaller magnetic moments.

Although each nucleus in a sample of hydrogen (or other material that contains nuclei with a magnetic moment) acts like a small magnet, the sample itself exhibits no net magnetism because the magnetic moments of the individual nuclei are oriented randomly and cancel each other out. If such a sample is placed in an intense magnetic field, however, the nuclei tend to align themselves either with or against the applied magnetic field. Figure 11-16 illustrates this alignment. In this orientation, the magnetic moments of the individual nuclei rotate (wobble, or *precess*) around the direction of the applied field in much the way a spinning top tends to wobble around the direction of the earth's gravitational field. This rotational frequency, ω, is known as the *Larmor frequency* and is given by:

$$\omega = \gamma B_0$$

where γ is the gyromagnetic ratio of the particular nuclei and B_0 is the strength of the magnetic field, usually described in units of Tesla. The orientation and wobbling actions produce a component vector of the magnetic moments of the nuclei in the direction of the applied field and a smaller component at right angles to the applied field. Because the magnetic moments of the sample nuclei wobble out of phase with one another, the components of the nuclear magnetic moments in a direction perpendicular to the applied field tend to cancel one another out. Hence, no net magnetic moment in a direction perpendicular to the applied magnetic field is measurable for the sample. At room temperature and with a 1.5 T magnetic field, approximately 10 per million spins will be preferentially aligned with the applied magnetic field. (See Figure 11-16.)

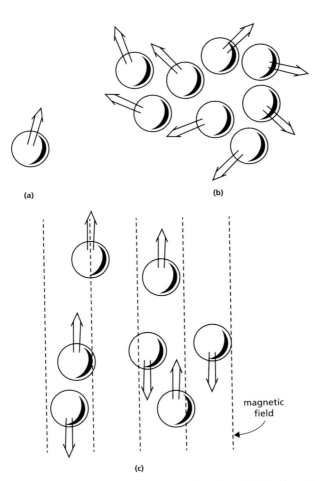

(a)

(b)

(c)

magnetic field

Figure 11-16 (a) Proton magnetic moment direction is indicated by arrow. (b) In a typical material, magnetic moments are oriented randomly. (c) If a magnetic field is applied, magnetic moments align themselves along the direction of the field. Note that some are parallel and others are antiparallel.

To generate time-dependent transverse magnetization that can be detected, transitions between the two allowed energy states must be induced. The transitions result from the application of a time-varying magnetic field with an energy equal to the difference in the energy levels, that is:

$$E = \hbar\omega = \gamma\hbar B_0$$

where $\hbar$ is Planck's constant divided by 2π. As described previously, the rotational frequency, ω, of the nuclei in a magnetic field is characteristic of the type of nuclei and the strength of the applied field. For protons in a 1.5 T field, the Larmor frequency is approximately 64 MHz. This frequency is in the radiofrequency (rf) range. This field is commonly known as the B_1 *field*. If a brief pulse of rf energy is applied to the sample at the Larmor frequency perpendicular to the static field while the nuclei are precessing, two things happen. First, the alignment of the nuclei is altered so that their magnetic component in a direction perpendicular to the applied magnetic field is changed and, second, their rotation is affected so that they precess about the applied magnetic field in phase. The result of these effects is that the sample assumes a net magnetic moment in some direction other than parallel to the applied magnetic field.

Example 11-5

Find the resonance frequency, ω, for protons ($\gamma = 42.58$ MHz/T) in a 1.5 T MRI unit.

$$\omega = \gamma B$$
$$= (42.58\,\text{MHz/T})(1.5\,\text{T})$$
$$= 63.9\,\text{MHz}$$

Immediately after application of an rf energy pulse to a sample, the nuclei begin to resume the status that they occupied before the rf was applied. In the process, the energy that was delivered to the sample by the rf pulse is released, and it can be measured with an rf antenna (a signal coil) coupled closely to the sample. The rf signal detected by the signal coil decreases (decays) over several milliseconds according to two time constants: $T1$ and $T2$. The time constant $T1$, known as the *spin-lattice* or *longitudinal relaxation time*, describes the rate of return of the magnetic moment of the sample to its original orientation before the rf pulse was applied. The time constant $T2$, known as the *spin–spin* or *transverse relaxation time*, describes the rate at which the rotating nuclei dephase to the out-of-phase condition they displayed before the rf pulse was applied. Three characteristics of the signal of radiated rf energy can be measured and used to characterize the rf signal from the sample. These characteristics are the intensity of the signal (representative of the *spin density* related to the concentration of rotating nuclei in the sample), the spin–lattice relaxation time $T1$, and the spin–spin relaxation time $T2$. These three characteristics of the sample form the basic parameters used to produce an MR image.

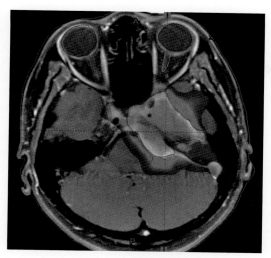

Figure 11-17 Complex isodose distribution (shown in colorwash) superimposed on a cross-sectional magnetic resonance image.

A variety of methods have been developed to apply the rf energy to a sample and to collect and measure the rf signal radiated from a sample. These methods are known as *pulse sequences* and are described in detail in texts on magnetic resonance and the physics of medical imaging.[33,34] Pulse sequences yield images with exquisite spatial and contrast information about anatomic structure and function in the patient. Included in this information are data important to delineating various

features of biologic tissue, such as the presence and extent of tumors, the shape of normal structures in the immediate vicinity of a tumor, and the distinction between recurrent tumor and radiation necrosis. An isodose distribution superimposed on an MR image is illustrated in Figure 11-17. MRI is gaining recognition as a useful adjunct to treatment planning and quality control in radiation therapy and is sure to grow in importance in the future as additional applications are identified and developed.

Functional magnetic resonance imaging

Most biological tissues exert a weak repulsive force to counteract an applied magnetic field. This effect is termed *diamagnetism*, and the tissues are said to be *diamagnetic*. Oxygenated blood (oxyhemoglobin) is diamagnetic. In tissue containing deoxygenated blood, the deoxyhemoglobin in the blood has unpaired electrons that create a highly localized region in which $T2$ is shortened. This effect is termed *paramagnetism*, and the region exhibiting the effect is typically two to three times the radius of the blood vessel nourishing the region.

Neuronal activity in a region of the brain stimulates a localized increase in blood flow, cerebral blood volume, and oxygen delivery in the region. The increased blood flow "drives out" the deoxyhemoglobin and replaces it with oxygenated blood. This process removes the $T2$-shortening effect of deoxyhemoglobin, and the change can be seen in MR images weighted to reveal $T2$

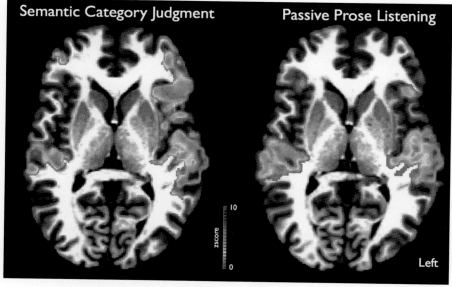

Figure 11-18 Axial images showing blood oxygenation level dependent (BOLD) activation in a single participant who took part in two standard fMRI language paradigms. The left panel shows a slice through the superior temporal gyrus and inferior frontal gyrus; the participant is using a button press to indicate whether pairs of words come from the same category (e.g., duke/king come from the same category, tree/king from a different category). The right panel shows the same participant listening to audiobook excerpts; slice plane is slightly more inferior and cuts through the body of the superior temporal gyrus. Color scale shows the z-score associated with BOLD response for task relative to resting baseline. Data were acquired on a 1.5 T Siemens Avanto with a 32-channel head coil using 4× multiband-accelerated EPI, voxel size 3 × 3 × 3 mm. Raw data were smoothed on the individual's cortical surface before analysis to increase signal-to-noise, and were analyzed in FSL. Echoplanar images and statistical maps have been resampled to 1 × 1 × 1 mm for display.
Source: Photo courtesy of Dr Frederick Dick, Birkbeck/University College London Centre for NeuroImaging.

differences. The changes in $T2$ signal can be seen within seconds after initiation of neuronal stimulation, which supports the theory that the change in MR signal is related to the movement of oxygenated blood through the capillary bed and into the venoles. That is, the oxyhemoglobin is serving as a naturally occurring contrast agent that yields MR signals corresponding to the spatial and temporal pattern of neuronal activation in the brain. Display of this pattern yields a functional map of neuronal activity in the brain. Acquisition of these maps is referred to as *functional magnetic resonance imaging* (fMRI).

Functional MRI is revolutionizing the study of brain function. Before fMRI, brain function was studied principally by analyzing neurological and behavioral abnormalities in individuals who had suffered losses in brain function through birth defects and accidents. The technique of fMRI is proving to be very useful in mapping functional areas of the brain before tumor resection, and it is helpful in the evaluation of patients following strokes and other neurovascular events. It also is adding greatly to the knowledge base of structure and function in the cognitive sciences (Figure 11-18).

Summary

- Digital x-ray detectors, including storage phosphors and charge-coupled devices, are being used with increasing frequency in radiography.
- X-ray transmission computed tomography provides planar and 3D anatomical information with exquisite contrast resolution.
- Ultrasonography reveals interfaces between tissues that differ slightly in acoustic impedance Z [Z = (velocity of ultrasound)(density of medium)].
- Nuclear medicine employs pharmaceuticals labeled with a radioactive nuclide to reveal information about the physiology metabolism, and biochemistry, as well as the anatomy of tissues.
- SPECT and PET employ single-photon and positron-emitting radioactive nuclides to produce 2- and 3D images from projections acquired with scintillation detector-based cameras.
- MRI techniques provide images with excellent contrast resolution based on subtle differences in tissue magnetization over time.
- Functional MRI reveals areas of the brain involved in sensing and responding to a variety of external and internal stimuli.

Problems

11-1 How many bytes of computer memory are used to store a 2048 × 2048 digital image that presents 256 shades of gray?

11-2 What is the spatial resolution in 1p/mm of a 4 in^2 x-ray image stored in a 512 × 512 digital matrix?

11-3 Determine the CT numbers for air ($\mu \approx 0$) and compact bone ($\mu \approx 2\,\mu_w$).

11-4 A fluid-filled cyst has an acoustic impedance of 1.50, and the liver has an acoustic impedance of 1.65. (Note the units of acoustic impedance of kg-m^2-sec$^{-1} \times 10^4$ appropriate for these values can be neglected in the computation.) Determine the percent of ultrasound reflected at the liver–cyst interface.

11-5 How much time is required for an ultrasound pulse to return to the transducer following reflection from an interface 12 cm below the surface?

11-6 What is the rotational frequency of protons in a 1.5 MRI unit?

References

1 Mun, S. K., et al. (eds.). *The First International Conference on Image Management and Communication in Patient Care: Implementation and impact*. Washington, DC, IEEE Computer Society Press, Institute of Electrical and Electronics Engineers, 1989.

2 Barnes, G., Ceare, H., and Brezovich, I. Reduction of scatter in diagnostic radiology by means of a scanning multiple slit assembly. *Radiology* 1976; **120**:691–694.

3 Smathers, R. L., and Brody, W. R. Digital radiology: Current and future trends. *Br. J. Radiol.* 1985; **58**:285–307.

4 Antonuk, L. E. Electronic portal imaging devices: A review and historical perspective of contemporary technologies and research. *Phys. Med. Biol.* 2002; **47**:R31–R65.

5 Hounsfield, G. Computerized transverse axial scanning (tomography): Part I: Description of system. *Br. J. Radiol.* 1973; **46**:1016–1022.

6 Bracewell, R. Strip integration in radio astronomy *Aust. J. Phys.* 1956; **9**:198–217.

7 DeRosier, D., and Klug, A. Reconstruction of three dimensional structures from electron micrographs. *Nature* 1968; **217**:130–134.

8 Gordon, R., Bender, R., and Herman, T. Algebraic reconstruction techniques (ART) for three-dimensional electron microscopy and x-ray photography. *J. Theor. Biol.* 1970; **29**:471–481.

9 Berry, M., and Gibbs, D. The interpretation of optical projections. *Proc. R. Soc [A]* 1970; **314**:143–152.

10 Rowley, P. Quantitative interpretation of three-dimensional weakly refractive phase objects using holographic interferometry. *J. Opt. Soc. Am.* 1969; **59**:1496–1498.

11 Radon, J. Über die Bestimmung von Funktionen durch irhe integralwerte laengs gewisser Mannigfaltigkeiten (On the determination of functions from their integrals along certain manifolds). *Ber. Saechsische Akad. Wiss. (Leipzig) Math.-Phys. Klasse* 1917; **69**:262.

12 Hendee, W. R. *Physical Principles of Computed Tomography*. Boston, Little, Brown & Co., 1983.

13 Jaffray, D. A., Siewerdsen, J. H., Wong, J. W., and Martinez, A. A. Flat-panel cone-beam computed tomography for image-guided radiation therapy. *Int. J. Radiat. Oncol. Biol. Phys.* 2002; **53**(5):1337–1349.

14 Swindell, W., and Webb, S. X-ray transmission computed tomography. In *The Physics of Medical Imaging*, S. Webb (ed.). Philadelphia: Adam Hilger, 1988.

15 Dobbs, H. J., and Parker, R. P. The respective roles of the simulator and computed tomography in radiotherapy planning: A review. *Clin. Radiol.* 1984; **35**:433–439.

16 Dobbs, J. H., and Webb, S. Clinical applications of x-ray computed tomography in radiotherapy planning. In S. Webb (ed.) *The Physics of Medical Imaging.* Philadelphia: Adam Hilger, 1988.

17 Harrison, R. M., and Farmer, F. T. The determination of anatomical cross-sections using a radiotherapy simulator. *Br. J. Radiol.* 1978; **51**:448–453.

18 Ragan, D. P., and Perez, C. A. Efficacy of CT assisted two-dimensional treatment planning in analysis of 45 patients. *AJR* 1978; **131**:75–79.

19 Silver, M. D., Nishiki, M., Tochimura, K., Arita, M., Drawert, B. M., and Judd, T. C. CT imaging with an image intensifier: Using a radiation therapy simulator as a CT scanner. In *Image Physics: Proceedings of the Society of Photo-Optical Instrumentation Engineers.* 1991; **1443**:250–260.

20 Curry, T. S., Dowdey, J. E., and Murry, R. C. *Christensen's Physics of Diagnostic Radiology,* 4th edition. Philadelphia, Lea & Febiger, 1990.

21 Carson, P. L., et al. Ultrasound imaging as an aid to cancer therapy: Part I. *Int. J. Radiat. Oncol. Biol. Phys.* 1975; **1**:119–132.

22 Carson, P. L., et al. Ultrasound imaging as an aid to cancer therapy: Part II. *Int. J. Radiat. Oncol. Biol. Phys.* 1976; **2**:335.

23 Fessenden, P., and Hand, J. W. Hyperthermia therapy physics. In *Radiation Therapy Physics,* A. R. Smith (ed.). Berlin, Springer-Verlag, 1995, pp. 315–363.

24 Anger, H. Scintillation camera. *Rev. Sci. Instrum.* 1958; **29**:27–33.

25 Srivastava, S. C., and Mausner, L. F. (ed.). Radiolabelled monoclonal antibodies: Chemical, diagnostic and therapeutic investigations. *Nucl. Med. Biol.* 1987; **13**.

26 Sorensen, J. A., and Phelps, M. E. *Physics in Nuclear Medicine.* Orlando, FL, Grune and Stratton, 1987.

27 Frisch, R., and Stern, O. Über die magnetische ablenkung von Wasserstoff-Molekulen und das magnetische moment das protons I. *Z. Physik* 1933; **85**:4–16.

28 Rabi, I. I., Millman, S., Kusch, P., and Zacharias, J. R. Molecular beam resonance method for measuring nuclear magnetic moments. *Phys. Rev.* 1939; **55**:526–535.

29 Bloch, R. The principle of nuclear induction. In *Nobel Lectures in Physics,* 1946–1962. New York, Elsevier Science Publishing, 1964.

30 Purcell, E. M. Research in nuclear magnetism. In *Nobel Lectures in Physics,* 1946–1962. New York, Elsevier Science Publishing, 1964.

31 Damadian, R. Tumor detection by nuclear magnetic resonance. *Science* 1971; **171**:1151–1153.

32 Lauterbur, P. C. Image formation by induced local interactions: Examples employing nuclear magnetic resonance. *Nature* 1973; **242**:190–191.

33 Stark, D. D., and Bradley, W. G. (eds). *Magnetic Resonance Imaging.* St. Louis, Mosby–Year Book, 1988.

34 Thomas, S. R., and Dixon, R. L. (eds.). *NMR in Medicine: Instrumentation and Clinical Applications: Medical Physics Monograph No. 14.* New York, American Institute of Physics, 1986.

12

TUMOR TARGETING: IMAGE-GUIDED AND ADAPTIVE RADIATION THERAPY

Objectives

After studying this chapter, the reader should be able to:
- Identify how intrafractional motion and interfractional variation cause uncertainty in the localization of treatment targets.
- Recognize the role of image guidance in the reduction of treatment beam portal margins.
- Identify two approaches to imaging the effects of respiratory motion.
- Identify the difference in the origin of systematic and random setup uncertainties.
- Describe the various methods of image acquisition for image-guided radiation therapy.
- Describe two-dimensional and three-dimensional methods of image alignment.
- Identify non-radiographic image alignment methods.
- Determine data requirements for image-guided radiation therapy and some of the limitations of data acquisition and transfer.

Introduction

The standard paradigm for radiation treatments is to image the patient, develop a treatment plan that irradiates a target region while sparing uninvolved tissue, transfer the plan to a treatment machine, and deliver the treatment plan. In the 20th century, patient images were acquired either using a conventional simulator or CT scanner, a few days prior to treatment. A treatment plan was developed, at first using manually obtained external contours, and later using a CT image data set. Beam parameters were transferred to the treatment machine, either manually or automatically, and the patient was treated. Images were acquired initially to verify that the treatment was delivered to the correct target volume, and then acquired on a regular (typically weekly) basis to verify the continual accurate delivery of treatment. An

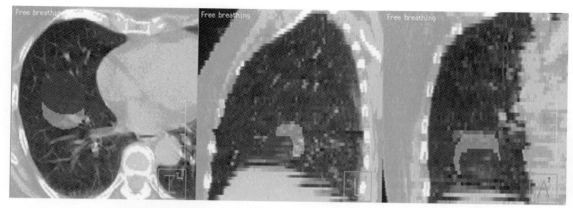

Figure 12-1 Axial, lateral, and coronal CT images of a lung illustrating tumor location at inspiration (red) and expiration (yellow). Motion of the centroid of the tumor is measured as 0.06 cm lateral, 1.37 cm anterior-posterior, 0.87 superior–inferior, and 1.62 cm total. For a color version of this figure, see the color plate section.

assumption implicit in this paradigm was that the patient information did not change during treatment, that is, there was no intrafractional motion and no interfractional variation in the patient geometry.

We now know this assumption is not true. Figure 12-1 illustrates a CT image of a lung with the tumor outline delineated on both inspiration and expiration. To account for this tumor motion, a margin of at least 1 cm was added around the *clinical target volume* (CTV) to account for respiratory motion. The magnitude of the margin was based on population studies and was isotropic, assuming that lung tumors move the same amount, irrespective of patient, location, size, etc., and that lung tumor margins expand and contract isotropically. However, neither of these assumptions is true. The extent of tumor motion has been shown to vary from zero to over 2 cm[1] and motion is more likely to be curvilinear, with the tumor trajectories most likely to be elongated ellipses[2]. By accurately assessing the extent of tumor motion, patient-specific treatment portals can be customized, reducing the amount of uninvolved tissue that needs to be irradiated.[3]

Interfractional variation is also significant. A study by de Crevoisier et al.[4] using an in-room CT scanner and acquiring scans before and after prostate treatment fractions showed statistically significant changes in bladder and rectal anatomy. A study by Barker et al.[5] using daily CT scanning of head and neck treatments with an in-room CT scanner showed median shrinkage of almost 70% of the *gross tumor volume* (GTV) as well as changes in position of the GTV with time. In both studies, modifications of treatment geometries would have been necessary to ensure optimal target coverage.

In recent years, more frequent imaging has been shown to be clinically desirable. Much of the imaging is performed immediately prior to treatment with modifications to the treatment parameters made as a result of the imaging procedure. This *image-guided radiation therapy* (IGRT) allows for more precise targeting. Moreover, as a result of this imaging, it is possible to implement *adaptive radiotherapy*, and re-plan the patient based on computation of radiation doses using the recently imaged patient anatomy.

Intrafractional motion

Intrafractional motion, motion that occurs while the radiation beam is on and the patient is being treated, or motion that occurs between beams in the same treatment session, arises primarily from respiratory motion, and is of significance in thoracic and abdominal treatments. However, intrafractional motion is also exhibited through skeletal, muscular, cardiac, and gastrointestinal motion. Most efforts to mitigate the effects of intrafractional motion, however, have addressed respiratory motion. The report of Task Group 76 of the Radiation Therapy Committee of the AAPM provides an excellent discussion of this topic.[6]

Imaging of effects of respiratory motion

During respiration, a substantial component of motion is in the superior–inferior (SI) direction, the same as the direction of motion of the CT couch. Consequently, during image acquisition different parts of the patient anatomy will move in and out of the CT slice window. This motion can give rise to artifacts in the CT image, as illustrated in Figure 12-2. These artifacts can give rise to errors in target delineation and dose calculation.

The problem with acquiring artifact-free images under respiration is that the typical respiratory period of approximately 4 to 5 seconds is approximately equal to the typical time needed to acquire a CT data set. Unless we are able to acquire a CT data set in a time period much shorter than a respiratory cycle, it is not possible to "freeze" respiratory motion in a CT scan. What makes imaging of respiratory motion possible, however, is the fact that the respiratory cycle is periodic, that is, the lungs will be in the same position repeatedly, but during different respiratory cycles. Image information over a small portion of the thorax is acquired at a specified phase of the respiratory cycle, more information

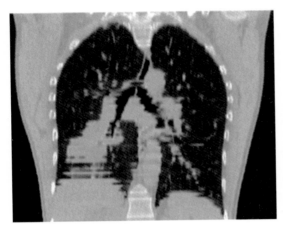

Figure 12-2 A coronal view of a free-breathing CT scan of the thorax illustrating respiration-induced artifacts, especially around the patient's diaphragm.
Source: Keall 2002.[7] Reproduced with permission of Australasian College of Physical Sciences and Engineering in Medicine.

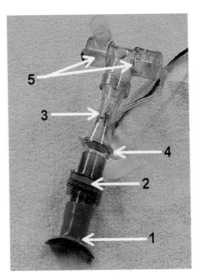

Figure 12-4 Measurement of airflow using spirometer (1) mouthpiece, (2) filter, (3) flow sensor, (4) pressure sensor, (5) occlusion valves.

is acquired at the same phase of another respiratory cycle, and so forth, until information over the desired area of the patient has been acquired of a large number of respiratory cycles. This procedure, known as *four-dimensional CT scanning* (4D-CT), replaces time as the fourth dimension with phase. A typical 4D-CT data set consists of a set of four to ten three-dimensional (3D) CT data set, each data set corresponding to a different phase of the respiratory motion.

Two technologies have made 4D-CT image acquisition possible. Multislice helical CT scanners have allowed for rapid image acquisition times, and respiratory monitors that monitor either external landmarks, airflow, or abdominal circumference are used to correlate imaging information with appropriate phases of the respiratory cycle. Figure 12-3 illustrates such a respiratory monitoring device. A reflective cube is placed on the anterior surface of the patient's abdomen, moving along with the

respiratory cycle. An infrared camera and *charged-coupled device* (CCD) detector track the motion of the cube. Figure 12-4 illustrates a spirometer, which measures airflow, while Figure 12-5 illustrates a bellows assembly, which is wrapped around the patient's abdomen and measures abdominal circumference.

Two methods have been developed for the acquisition of 4D-CT image information and are in widespread clinical use. In one method the CT scanner is operated in what is referred to as *cine mode.*[8] The CT table is kept stationary for a period of time equal to one respiratory cycle plus a gantry revolution while images are acquired. The table is then indexed a distance equal to the detector width, and image acquisition is repeated. This stationary-table image acquisition followed by table indexing is repeated until the entire data set is acquired. This technique results in the acquisition of a large number (1000–3000) of images, each

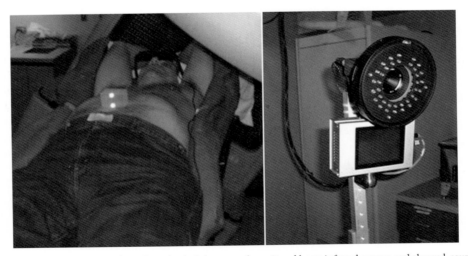

Figure 12-3 Reflectors placed on the anterior surface of a patient's abdomen and monitored by an infrared camera and charged-couple device detector.

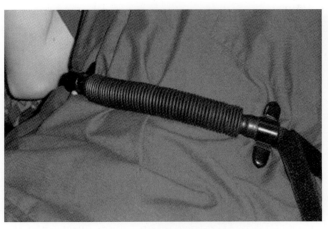

Figure 12-5 Measurement of abdominal circumference using bellows. As the patient breathes, the bellows expands and contracts.

image identified with an acquisition time obtained from the respiratory monitor. Software correlates the acquisition time of the images to the time associated with a desired phase of respiratory cycle. The projections are reconstructed and the images are then binned into the desired number of phases to obtain the 4D-CT image data set.

In an alternative method, the CT scanner is operated in helical mode with a very low pitch (typically 0.04–0.08).[9] A very large number of projection images are acquired. The software then correlates the acquisition time of the projections to the desired phase of the respiratory cycle and reconstructs the binned projections into phases. First the projections are binned and then the images are reconstructed.

The results of the two approaches to 4D-CT image acquisition are similar; one obtains several 3D CT image data sets, each data set corresponding to a different phase of the respiratory cycle.

Several other alternatives exist to image respiratory motion in CT scanning. Patients can be instructed to hold their breaths during acquisition of the CT scan. This technique is particularly useful if treatment is to be delivered during breath-hold. This technique was not possible until the multislice helical CT scanner was developed allowing for image acquisition times of a few seconds. Particularly useful in breath-hold image acquisition is providing visual feedback to patients as to the extent of their respiration. A display of respiratory tracking is often made available to the CT operators at the image acquisition console, but it is a simple matter to provide the patient with the same information, either with a monitor placed near the CT scanner or with a goggles display.

Another alternative is the use of a gated CT scan. In this technique, respiratory motion is monitored, and image data are acquired at a desired phase point in respiratory cycle.

Planning with respiratory motion

Once a 4D-CT data set is acquired, it can be used in treatment planning. Currently, most treatment planning using 4D data sets

is actually 3D planning, in which the 4D image data set is used to determine an *internal target volume* (ITV). According to the definition provided by the International Commission on Radiation Units and Measurements (ICRU), the ITV is defined to include the CTV plus an internal margin that "compensate(s) for all movements and all variations in site, size, and shape of the organs and tissues contained in or adjacent to the CTV".[10] Consequently an ITV can be extracted from a 4D-CT data set by outlining the CTV on each phase and generating an envelope of the CTV.

Because outlining the CTV on each phase of a 4D-CT data set is somewhat tedious, a good approximation to the ITV can be obtained by using a *maximum intensity projection* (MIP) to generate an envelope of motion of the GTV*. A MIP is obtained by taking the maximum value of a CT voxel over the set of phases that constitute the 4D-CT image data set. Acquisition of a MIP is possible for lung tumors because tumors typically have unit density, whereas the surrounding lung parenchyma has lower densities. The MIP is then expanded by an appropriate margin that accounts for microscopic disease to generate the ITV, which is then expanded by an appropriate margin that accounts for setup uncertainty to generate the *planning target volume* (PTV). One can then plan the treatment and calculate the dose on a CT data set obtained by taking average values of the CT voxels over the 4D-CT data set (AVG). In the case of liver tumors, which are lower in density than the surrounding parenchyma, a *minimum intensity projection* (MinIP) can be used to delineate the tumor, while performing the planning on an AVG data set.

Greater accuracy in the dose distribution can be obtained by performing a true 4D dose calculation. In a true 4D dose calculation, one delineates the GTV on each phase of the 4D-CT data set. Although this is a time-consuming procedure, software tools exist that propagate contours through each phase of a 4D-CT data set and deform them to match the images of tumors.[11] The GTV on each phase is then expanded to generate a CTV. An envelope of the CTVs produces the ITV and is expanded to obtain a PTV. So far, this procedure is just a more accurate method for generating a PTV than using a MIP image.

One phase is then selected to be a reference phase, and a beam configuration is determined to appropriately treat the PTV on the reference phase. Dose is calculated on each phase using the beam configuration thus determined. The dose matrix is then deformed from the reference phase to all other phases and the dose is accumulated over all phases of the 4D-CT data set and displayed on the reference phase.[12]

In reality, this procedure might be referred to as *3.5-D treatment planning* because the actual planning is done in three dimensions, and only the dose is calculated in four dimensions. At present, true 4D treatment planning, in which the beam configuration is determined based on the full 4D-CT data set, does

---

*This envelope of motion of the GTV has sometimes been referred to as an *internal GTV* (iGTV), but this is not standard ICRU nomenclature.

not exist for photon-beam planning, although some effort is made to use it for particle therapy.[13]

Motion mitigation

Given that respiratory motion exists, it might be desirable to mitigate the effects of such motion and reduce the size of the PTV, resulting in a reduction in dose to uninvolved tissue. Such actions may complicate the treatment delivery; consequently, if the respiratory motion is not significant, it may be better to allow for the motion to exist, and account for the motion in the treatment planning process. The AAPM Task Group 76 report recommends that mitigation be considered if the extent of respiratory-induced tumor motion exceeds 5 mm.[6] Several methods of motion mitigation include respiratory gating, breath-hold, active breathing control, abdominal compression, and tumor tracking.

Respiratory gating involves the delivery of radiation during a specified point in the patient's respiratory cycle.[14] A respiratory monitor, such as one of those described in the section on 4D imaging, is used to control the delivery of radiation. A gating window is determined, as shown in Figure 12-6. When the respiratory trace enters the window, a signal to the linear accelerator triggers the beam on, and when the trace exits the window, the signal turns the beam off. Consequently, radiation is delivered only during a specified portion of the respiratory cycle, thus "freezing" the tumor position. An important trade-off to consider in setting the window for gating is that a narrow window allows for less tumor motion, but significantly increases the time that the patient is on the treatment table, whereas a broad window allows for a greater duty cycle, but also allows for more residual motion.

An important requirement for a respiratory gating to be useful is for the patient to be able to breathe in a regular manner. Pre-treatment assessment in combination with breathing training and/or visual feedback is often very desirable.

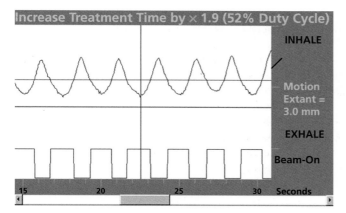

Figure 12-6 A respiratory trace from a monitor used in respiratory gating. The gating window is shown on the upper graph, and the delivery of radiation is shown in the lower graph.

Another approach to motion mitigation involves requiring the patient to undergo a breath-hold during the delivery of radiation treatment.[15] This technique, while predominantly applied to lung radiation therapy, has also been used for breast radiation therapy as a means of reducing cardiac dose. Breath-hold is most commonly implemented during deep inspiration, hence the terminology *deep inspiration breath hold* (DIBH). An advantage of DIBH is that the lungs are inflated to their greatest volume, reducing the mass of lung tissue that may be irradiated. Also, tumor motion is reduced over any sort of technique that allows free breathing. A disadvantage of DIBH is that many thoracic patients have compromised breathing abilities, and a consistent breath hold is difficult to achieve.

The difficulty of a breath hold can be ameliorated somewhat by using an occlusion spirometer to force the breath hold. This technique is known as *active breathing control* (ABC).[16] An example of a spirometer used in ABC is illustrated in Figure 12-4. After the patient has taken a breath, the occlusion valve closes the airflow for what has previously been determined to be a comfortable duration for the patient, typically 15–30 seconds, during which time radiation is delivered. Visual feedback is also desirable when using ABC.

Yet another technique for motion mitigation is *abdominal compression*.[17] Abdominal compression was first used in stereotactic irradiation. The original implementation used a stereotactic body frame with a compression plate placed against the abdomen, which reduces abdominal excursion, and hence the extent of respiratory motion.

Finally, motion mitigation can be effected by dynamically repositioning the radiation beam to track the tumor motion. This technique, known as *real-time tumor tracking*, can be achieved either by using an MLC whose motions generate a dynamic beam aperture that mimics the motion of the target volume or by using a linear accelerator attached to a robotic arm that tracks the tumor motion. The advantage of this technique is that it removes the need for a tumor motion margin in the definition of a target volume and allows for a 100% duty cycle giving rise to more efficient dose delivery. The major disadvantage of this technique is the need for real-time accurate tumor tracking. Real-time tumor tracking is a difficult problem that is currently under investigation.

Positioning uncertainties

In addition to the internal target volume, which accounts for internal motion, an additional margin must be added to the target volume to account for uncertainties inherent in the patient setup. Setup uncertainties are of two kinds: random uncertainties and systematic uncertainties.

Random uncertainties are uncertainties inherent in the patient setup; it is not possible to set the patient up in exactly the same position every time. Random uncertainties can be reduced by the use of appropriate immobilization devices including body cradles, thermoplastic masks, invasive stereotactic head frames, etc. The selection of the immobilization device is specific to the particular application and the acceptable tolerance of uncertainty.

Systematic uncertainties result from the uncertainty in the patient position during image acquisition for treatment planning. To understand the presence of a systematic uncertainty, consider a series of CT images of a patient. These images are acquired during the same session, so that the inherent patient geometry does not change measurably. Before each image acquisition, however, the patient is removed from the table and resetup. If we observe each image data set, we will find small, but observable, differences in locations of anatomic reference points or fiducial markers due to the inherent uncertainties in patient setup. The standard deviation of these locations from their mean value is a measure of the random uncertainty in the patient setup. Now, let us use one of these image data sets to plan the patient's treatment and treat the other data sets as the patient during each of the subsequent treatments. There will be a measurable deviation of the locations of reference points in the planning data set from those of the mean data set; this is a measure of the systematic uncertainty in the setup process.

Example 12-1

In a study of patient positioning, a fiducial was implanted in a patient, and the treatment isocenter was taken to be at the position of the fiducial ($x = 0$, $y = 0$, $z = 0$). Portal images were acquired of the treatment field during the first five treatments. Based on the information in the portal images, the coordinates of the fiducial were as follows:

Day	x	y	z
1	0.13 cm	−0.21 cm	−0.15 cm
2	0.05 cm	−0.13 cm	−0.21 cm
3	0.11 cm	0.05 cm	−0.25 cm
4	0.03 cm	−0.25 cm	0.11 cm
5	−0.05 cm	−0.20 cm	−0.16 cm

a. What is the systematic setup uncertainty for this patient?
We can estimate the systematic setup uncertainty for this patient by assuming that, based on the treatment plan, the isocenter was at (0, 0, 0). In that case, the systematic setup uncertainty is the distance of the mean isocenter coordinate position from (0, 0, 0).
The mean coordinate of the isocenter is (0.05, −0.15, 0.13), which gives a distance from setup of 0.21 cm.
b. What is the random setup uncertainty for this patient?
The random setup uncertainty is the standard deviation of the fiducial coordinates. This is calculated to be (0.07, 0.12, 0.14), which gives a random setup uncertainty of 0.20 cm.

Image guidance allows us to correct for the systematic uncertainty in the patient setup.

Van Herk et al. have developed a set of formulas to generate margins based on these setup uncertainties.[18] The Van Herk margin formula, which is designed to deliver at least 95% of the prescribed dose to the CTV in 90% of the population, is given as:

$$M = 2.5\Sigma + 1.64\sqrt{\sigma^2 + \sigma_p^2} - 1.64\sigma_p$$

In this equation, Σ is the standard deviation of the systematic uncertainty, σ is the standard deviation of the random uncertainties, and σ_p is the standard deviation of the dose gradient of the penumbra. Notice that the margin to account for systematic uncertainties is 50% greater than the margin that accounts for random uncertainties.

Example 12-2

In the previous example, what are the recommended margins (ignoring the penumbra)?

Using the Van Herk formula, a margin of 0.53 cm is needed to account for systematic uncertainties, and 0.33 cm is needed to account for random uncertainties, for a total margin of 0.86 cm.

The goal of *image-guided radiation therapy* (IGRT) is to remove the systematic uncertainties by imaging the patient in close temporal proximity to the actual delivery, preferably moving the patient between imaging and treatment only to correct for any deviations in measured patient position. The patient can be repositioned based on repeat imaging to remove the systematic uncertainties, but the random uncertainties cannot be removed except by modification of the immobilization methods.

Two-dimensional versus three-dimensional alignment

Image alignment in IGRT is of two types: two-dimensional (2D) alignment and three-dimensional (3D) alignment. Two-dimensional alignment is based on projection imaging, whereas 3D alignment is based on volumetric imaging, typically CT imaging.

From the very start of radiation therapy, 2D imaging was used for the verification of treatment portals. A megavoltage portal image consisting of the treatment portal and the surrounding anatomy was acquired using the treatment beam and compared to the reference image (which is usually acquired via a conventional simulator, a diagnostic radiographic x-ray machine whose geometries simulated those of the treatment machine). If it appeared that the treatment portal missed part of the tumor, adjustments were made in the patient setup to correct for the errors.

With the use of 3D conformal radiation therapy and intensity-modulated radiation therapy (IMRT), the concept of the portal image became less useful. Oblique gantry angles, oblique couch angles, and small MLC openings made it difficult to verify and correct the patient setup based solely on the treatment portal. Furthermore, beam portals were no longer based on regional bony anatomy but on the extent of observed or suspected tumor spread. Consequently, it became more convenient and reliable to acquire anterioposterior (AP) and lateral images using either the treatment beam and a megavoltage portal imager or an on-board kilovoltage portal imager, and compare these AP and lateral images to reference images acquired during simulation.

Two-dimensional alignment

2D-2D matching tools, which aid in the matching of these images, include a scale and isocenter indicator to support manual image matching, but can also include split screen and color blends allowing for combination of the reference and acquired images. Automatic alignment systems based on mutual information[19] or cross-correlations[20] can facilitate the alignment process.

In matching planar images, translations are relatively easy to interpret, but it is also possible to assess rotations, especially through the use of software tools. The major limitation is the need for radio-opaque targets for visualization. Bony landmarks are typically used, but one can also use implanted fiducials.[21]

In many IGRT systems, a kilovoltage x-ray source and image receptor are directly mounted on the gantry of the therapy unit, 90° away from the megavoltage x-ray therapy source and portal imager. Figure 12-7 illustrates such a gantry-mounted unit. The

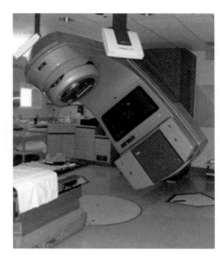

Figure 12-8 A room-mounted system with orthogonal kilovoltage imagers. Imaging sources are embedded in the floor, and image receptors are attached to the ceiling.

patient is set up on the treatment couch in the treatment position, and AP and lateral kilovoltage images are acquired. These images are compared to the simulation *digitally reconstructed radiographs* (DRRs), and adjustments are made in the patient position as needed to align the images. Because these images are AP and lateral, translational corrections can be made by lateral motions of the treatment couch. Six degree of freedom couches are available that also allow for rotational corrections.

Room-mounted orthogonal x-ray systems, as illustrated in Figure 12-8,[22] allow for real-time acquisition of images, and hence real-time adjustment of position, but because these images are not conventional AP and lateral images, software is often needed to assist in the interpretation of how adjustments need to be made. Real-time imaging of implanted fiducials using room-mounted kilovoltage imagers has also be used to assess intrafractional motion.[21]

Three-dimensional alignment

Several methods have been used for 3D alignment, including in-room CT or MR scanners, helical tomotherapy, and cone-beam CT. The CT-on-rails is a CT scanner located in the same room as the linear accelerator, using the same patient table as the linear accelerator, and is illustrated in Figure 12-9. What makes the CT-on-rails different from a conventional CT scanner is that, rather than having the patient table translate through the scanner, the CT scanner translates while the patient table remains stationary. A 3D CT data set of the patient is thus acquired and compared to the treatment planning data set. Adjustments can be made in the patient position based on alignment of the two data sets.

The helical tomotherapy system was developed by Mackie and co-workers at the University of Wisconsin in the early 1990s.[23] This device was initially designed as a means of delivering IMRT,

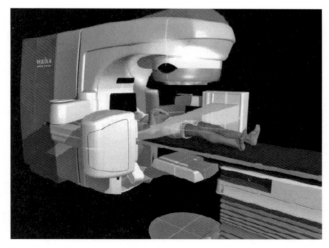

Figure 12-7 Gantry-mounted kilovoltage x-ray source and image receptor. The imaging beam is shown in the picture and the treatment beam is perpendicular to the imaging beam and straight down on the patient (not shown in the figure). For a color version of this figure, see the color plate section.
Source: Varian Medical Systems. Reproduced with permission of Varian Medical Systems.

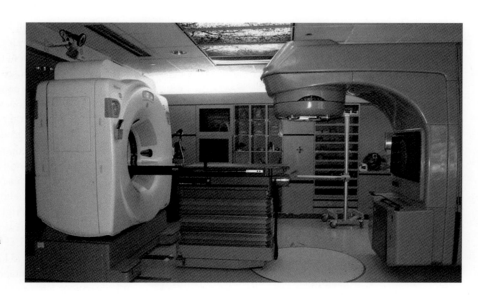

Figure 12-9 A CT scanner in the same room as the linear accelerator and using the treatment table. The CT scanner translates rather than the patient table.

and consists of a megavoltage x-ray source mounted on a ring gantry with a temporally modulated multileaf collimator. Megavoltage x-rays are delivered to treat the patient while the gantry is rotating simultaneously with table translation, much as a helical CT scanner operates. Imaging of the patient is made possible by mounting a kilovoltage x-ray source and image receptor on the gantry separated from the megavoltage source by 90°. In this manner, one has a helical CT scanner mounted on the same gantry as the megavoltage x-ray source, enabling the acquisition of CT images with the patient in the same position as for delivery of therapeutic radiation. A helical tomotherapy unit is illustrated in Figure 12-10.

Perhaps the most commonly used technology to support IGRT at present is *cone-beam computed tomography* (CBCT). In CBCT, an x-ray source, mounted on the gantry of the linear accelerator, generates a cone-shaped x-ray beam, and a 2D projection image is acquired using flat-panel detectors at a large

number of gantry angles.[24] The set of projection images are reconstructed into a 3D image data set, which is then used for patient alignment. The radiation source could be a kilovoltage x-ray tube attached to the gantry (kilovoltage CBCT) or it could be the megavoltage treatment beam (megavoltage CBCT). The 3D CT image acquired in CBCT is not necessarily of diagnostic quality, but it is adequate for localization purposes. Because rotation of the linear accelerator gantry is much slower than rotation of a conventional CT gantry (~1 minute for CBCT as compared to fractions of a second for conventional CT), motion blur can adversely affect the image quality. Moreover, because the irradiated volume is so much greater for CBCT than for conventional CT, the increase in scattered radiation leads to some image degradation. However, CBCT has several advantages over conventional CT in that the same gantry is used for image acquisition as for treatment. In addition, CBCT does not have to deal with slice thickness, so there is submillimeter spatial resolution in all three dimensions.

In a typical CBCT configuration, in which the x-ray beam and image receptor are symmetrically placed around the beam axis and a 360° gantry rotation is used, there is data redundancy, as the same projection information is acquired from gantry angles that are separated by 180°. In other words, a projection image acquired at a 0° gantry angle contains the same information as an image acquired at a 180° gantry angle. This data redundancy can be used to improve the quality of the CBCT image. Alternatively, one can displace the detector laterally to cover only half the original radiation beam, and then collimate the radiation beam by blocking half the field, thus enabling image acquisition over a much larger area of the patient while acquiring scattered radiation from a smaller volume.

CBCT is used in the manner as the CT-on-rails. Three-dimensional patient images are acquired prior to treatment and compared to the treatment planning images, and 3D-3D alignment can be used to implement changes in the patient setup if

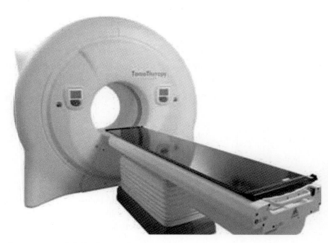

Figure 12-10 A helical tomotherapy system.

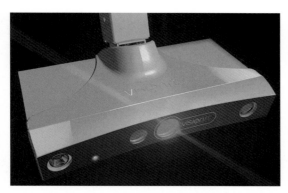

Figure 12-11 The stereoscopic camera used for surface-based patient alignment. For a color version of this figure, see the color plate section.

there is evidence of unacceptable difference in the location of the target volume.[25] 3D-3D alignment tools are similar to those used in 2D-2D alignment, but also include structure overlay. Soft-tissue targets can be visualized in 3D images, and six degrees of freedom can be determined. On the other hand, more time is required to acquire and reconstruct images, and 3D imaging results in a greater imaging dose to the patient.[26]

Non-radiographic image-guided radiation therapy

Surface-based image-guided radiation therapy

So far, we have looked at image guidance that relied on radiographic imaging to assess consistency of patient positioning. Other, less invasive, techniques have also been used. One such technique is *surface photogrammetry*, in which a stereoscopic surface view of the patient is acquired and compared to a reference surface.[27]

A reference surface is first generated, either from the planning CT scan or from the first patient treatment. The surface model consists of a set of vertices and triangular faces. After patient setup prior to treatment, a stereoscopic image of the patient surface is acquired, using a specialized camera, illustrated in Figure 12-11. The camera pod includes two *charge-coupled device* (CCD) cameras for surface image acquisition, an additional CCD camera for texture image acquisition, two flash units (one for producing a speckle pattern, the other for clear

illumination), and a slide projector for continuous speckle projection used for dynamic imaging. The cameras are calibrated to the coordinate system of the linear accelerator.

After the two stereoscopic images are acquired, the 3D locations of points on the patient surface are computed via triangulation. Skin images alone do not contain sufficient information for accurate triangulation, so a pseudorandom speckle pattern is projected during image acquisition to provide additional information to enable stereoscopic matching. Registration is then calculated using rigid-body registration, providing six degrees of freedom, three for translation and three for rotation. Because the system has been calibrated to the coordinate system of the linear accelerator, the rigid-body transformation can be applied directly to adjust the treatment couch to enable image alignment. Translational accuracy of less than 1 mm and rotational accuracy of 0.1° have been found for this type of registration.[27]

The primary advantage of surface photogrammetry for aiding in patient alignment is that it is a real-time, non-invasive method of position monitoring. However, surface photogrammetry assumes a correlation between internal anatomy and the patient surface, which may or may not be justified.[28] Therefore, early clinical use with this system has been for stereotactic radiosurgery[29] and other setups, such as breast[30].

Ultrasound systems

The use of B-mode ultrasound to support IGRT was introduced in the late 1990s, primarily as a method for image guidance in prostate radiation therapy. The system used an articulating arm and a docking tray for spatial registration. Contours of anatomic structures—including the bladder, prostate, and rectum—were imported from the treatment planning system and superimposed on axial and sagittal ultrasound images acquired in the treatment room. The contours were then used as a reference for aligning the patient. Figure 12-12 illustrates the use of B-mode ultrasound for patient alignment.

Advantages of B-mode ultrasound include the absence of ionizing radiation, the noninvasive nature of ultrasound, the ability to detect soft-tissue targets, the low cost, and the relative portability of the ultrasound unit.[31] Disadvantages include the fact that ultrasound images are often difficult to interpret and that a significant degree of operator skill is required to acquire images without tissue deformation.[32] Localization accuracy of

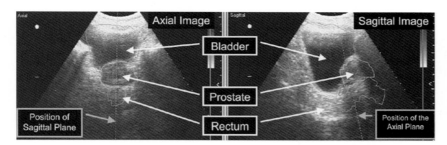

Figure 12-12 Ultrasound-guided target localization. Contours were imported from a treatment planning system and used as a reference for aligning the ultrasound images acquired in the treatment room. For a color version of this figure, see the color plate section.
Source: Kuban 2005.[31] Reproduced with permission of Elsevier.

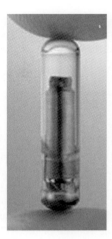

Figure 12-13 An electromagnetic transponder implanted in the region of a tumor to aid in localization.
Source: Varian Medical Systems. Reproduced with permission of Varian Medical Systems.

B-mode ultrasound was established to be within 3–5 mm compared to CT localization.[33] The accuracy of B-mode ultrasound relies on the accuracy and constancy of the speed of sound in the medium, while limitations include tissue heterogeneity, probe pressure-induced deformation, and artifacts such as reverberation and shadowing.

More recent developments include a 3D system that uses reflective markers attached to the ultrasound probe coupled with a camera-based image registration method. Image reconstruction is achieved by measuring the time-of-flight between transmitted and reflected pulses.

Electromagnetic transponder

In the early 2000s, a novel technique was developed that used radiofrequency waves for image guidance. One or more small (< 1 mm long) electromagnetic transponders (Figure 12-13) were implanted in the region of a tumor. These transponders communicated with the localization system using radiofrequency waves. This system was originally developed to improve patient positioning for prostate treatments, but was later extended to monitoring intrafractional respiratory motion.

The electromagnetic tracking system works in the following manner:[34] The wireless transponders are implanted into the patient before acquisition of the treatment planning CT data set. During treatment planning, the location of the transponders is determined relative to the isocenter on the CT data set. When the patient is positioned for treatment, magnetic source and receiver coil arrays embedded in the treatment table determine the transponder positions. The source coils generate an oscillating electromagnetic field, which induces resonance in the transponder. The source field is then switched off and the receiver coils determine the transponder position and orientation by receiving the resonance signal. This process is repeated

at a rate of 10 Hz. The coil array is tracked in real-time using infrared optical tracking. By determining the position of the coil array with respect to the room (and the linear accelerator), determining the position of the transponders with respect to the coil array, and determining the position of the isocenter with respect to the transponders, one can determine the position of the isocenter with respect to the linear accelerator. With this information, one can then make adjustments in the patient position as needed, or track the intrafractional movement of the tumor in real time.

Phantom studies have shown this technique to have submillimeter accuracy,[34] while clinical comparison of electromagnetic tracking with radiographic localization showed an average 3D difference of 1.5 mm.[35]

MR-based image-guided radiation therapy

More recently, the idea of using real-time MR to assist in image guidance has taken hold. Two potential advantages of MR image guidance include the superior soft-tissue contrast it has over CT as well as the absence of radiation dose.[36] The major obstacle that has to be overcome in incorporating real-time MR image guidance is the interference between the magnetic field in the MR scanner and the radiofrequency field of the linear accelerator.

One approach to solving this problem is the use of a low-field (0.2 T) MR scanner integrated with multiple ^{60}Co teletherapy sources.[37] However, ^{60}Co is ferromagnetic, and it was thought that the presence of ferromagnetic material could potentially affect the homogeneity of the magnetic field in the scanner. In practice, however, there does not appear to be a problem with field heterogeneity. Figure 12-14 illustrates such a device, which uses three ^{60}Co sources on a movable gantry.

A second approach uses a high-field (1.5 T) MR integrated with a 6 MV-linear accelerator.[38] The issue of magnetic interference with the linear accelerator was overcome by the use of

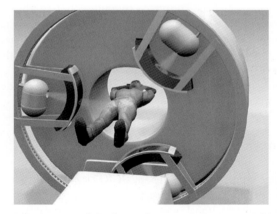

Figure 12-14 Image-guided radiation therapy system consisting of three ^{60}Co sources integrated with an MR scanner.
Source: ViewRay Incorporated. Reproduced with permission of ViewRay Incorporated.

magnetic shielding to create a zero magnetic field at the location of the accelerator gun and minimal field at the accelerator tube, whereas the issue of radiofrequency interference between the accelerator and the MR scanner was overcome by synchronizing the accelerator pulses and the MR pulses. Concern had been expressed over the possibility of dose differences due to scatter induced by beam transmission through the MR components. Furthermore, because electrons are deflected by a magnetic field, it was thought that the magnetic field from the MR scanner might affect the path of secondary electrons. Calculation-based studies have shown, however, that for clinical configurations there did not appear to be significant differences with the magnetic field.[38]

The use of MR-based image-guidance is a relatively new development in radiation oncology and it remains to have its clinical utility demonstrated.

Data requirements for image-guided radiation therapy

One of the issues that have come out of IGRT is the need to handle considerably more data than those in traditional radiation therapy. Data requirements for the traditional treatment record consisting of linear accelerator settings (i.e., MU, field sizes, couch positions, etc.) was negligible. The addition of images to the data sets increases the data load significantly. Daily orthogonal kilovoltage images add 3 MB per day; if imaging is repeated after an isocenter shift occurs, an additional 3 MB per day is required. Daily cone-beam CT imaging adds 32 MB per day. These data requirements increase if IGRT is practiced on each patient. A patient load of 40 patients per machine would result in the generation of 61 GB per year if only orthogonal images were obtained, and 325 GB per year if cone-beam CT were used for all patients.

The cost of data storage is small, and becoming less expensive all the time, but sufficient network bandwidth is required to transmit such data. The typical communication bandwidth of Ethernet inside a hospital is 100 Mbit/sec, which is likely to be adequate, but information transfer for remove viewing may be more problematic with more typical 10 Mbit/sec bandwidths or 3G bandwidth of 0.2 Mbit/sec.

The issue of data handling is covered in somewhat more depth in Chapter 14.

Summary

- Image-guided radiation therapy (IGRT) is becoming the standard of care for external beam radiation therapy.
- Both intrafractional motion and interfractional variation invalidate the traditional assumption that the images acquired of a patient prior to treatment are an accurate reflection of the patient during treatment.
- Various modalities can be used to acquire images used in IGRT, each with its own advantages and disadvantages.
- Significant bandwidth is required to handle the large numbers of images used in IGRT.

Problems

12-1 When a CT scanner is operated in helical mode for 4D image acquisition, what would happen to the images if too great a pitch were used?

12-2 Show that, by using an MIP image to delineate the ITV, one obtains an upper limit to the true ITV.

12-3 Using the data from Examples 12-1 and 12-2, estimate the reduction in the volume of the PTV if image guidance were used to remove the systematic uncertainty.

12-4 Why are limitations placed on the speed of gantry rotations in a linear accelerator, thus limiting the temporal resolution of cone-beam CT?

12-5 About how many CT scan slices are included in a typical 4D CT scan data set?

References

1 Liu, H. H., Balter, P., Tutt, T., Choi, B., Zhang, J., et al. Assessing respiration-induced tumor motion and internal target volume using four-dimensional computed tomography for radiotherapy of lung cancer. *Int. J. Radiat. Oncol. Biol. Phys.* 2007; **68**:531–540.

2 Seppenwoolde, Y., Shirato, H., Kitamura, K., Shimizu, S., Van Herk, M., et al. Precise and real-time measurement of 3D tumor motion in lung due to breathing and heartbeat, measured during radiotherapy. *Int. J. Radiat. Oncol. Biol. Phys.* 2002; **53**:822–834.

3 Butler, L. E., Forster, K. M., Stevens, C. W., Bloch, C., Liu, H. H., et al. Dosimetric benefits of respiratory gating: A preliminary study. *J. Appl. Clin. Med. Phys.* 2004; **5**:16–24.

4 de Crevoisier, R., Melancon, A. D., Kuban, D. A., Lee, A. K., Cheung, R. M., et al. Changes in the pelvic anatomy after an IMRT treatment fraction of prostate cancer. *Int. J. Radiat. Oncol. Biol. Phys.* 2007; **68**:1529–1536.

5 Barker, J. L., Garden, A. S., Ang, K. K., O'Daniel, J. C., Wang, H., et al. Quantification of volumetric changes occurring during fractionated radiotherapy for head-and-neck cancer using an integrated CT/linear accelerator system. *Int. J. Radiat. Oncol. Biol. Phys.* 2004; **59**:960–970.

6 Keall, P. J., Mageras, G. S., Balter, J. M., Emery, R. S., Forster, K. M., et al. AAPM Report 91: The Management of Respiratory Motion in Radiation Oncology. Report of AAPM Task Group 76, http://www.aapm.org/pubs/reports/RPT`91.pdf, accessed September 15, 2015. Synopsis published in *Med. Phys.* 2006; **33**:3874–3900.

7 Keall, P. J., Kini, V. R., Vedam, S. S., and Mohan, R. Potential radiotherapy improvements with respiratory gating. *Australas. Phys. Eng. Sci. Med.* 2002; **25**(1):1–6.

8 Pan, T., Lee, T.-Y., Rietzel, E., and Chen, G. T. Y. 4D-CT imaging of a volume influenced by respiratory motion on multi-slice CT. *Med. Phys.* 2004; **31**:333–340.

9 Keall, P. J., Starkschall, G., Shukla, H., Forster, K. M., Ortiz, V., et al. Acquiring 4D thoracic CT scans using a multislice helical method. *Phys. Med. Biol.* 2004; **49**:2053–2067.

10 International Commission on Radiation Units and Measurements. *ICRU Report 62. Prescribing, Recording and Reporting Photon Beam Therapy (Supplement to ICRU Report 50).* Bethesda, MD, ICRU, 1999.

11 Ezhil, M., Choi, B., Starkschall, G., Bucci, M. K., Vedam, S., and Balter, P. Comparison of rigid and adaptive methods of propagating gross tumor volume through respiratory phases of four-dimensional computed tomography image data set. *Int. J. Radiat. Oncol. Biol. Phys.* 2008; **71**:290–296.

12 Starkschall, G., Britton, K., McAleer, M. F., Jeter, M. D., Kaus, M. R., et al. Potential dosimetric benefits of four-dimensional radiation treatment planning. *Int. J. Radiat. Oncol. Biol. Phys.* 2009; **73**:1560–1565.

13 Richter, D., Schwarzkopf, A., Trautmann, J., Krämer, M., Durante, M., et al. Upgrade and benchmarking of a 4D treatment planning system for scanned ion beam therapy. *Med. Phys.* 2013; **40**:051722.

14 Ohara, K., Okumura, T., Akisada, M., Inada, T., Mori, T., et al. Irradiation synchronized with respiration gate. *Int. J. Radiat. Oncol. Biol. Phys.* 1989; **17**(4):853–857.

15 Hanley, J., Debois, M. M., Mah, D., Mageras, G. S., Raben, A., et al. Deep inspiration breath-hold technique for lung tumors: The potential value of target immobilization and reduced lung density in dose escalation. *Int. J. Radiat. Oncol. Biol. Phys.* 1999; **45**:603–611.

16 Wong, J. W., Sharpe, M. B., Jaffray, D. A., Kini, V. R., Robertson, J. M., et al. The use of active breathing control (ABC) to reduce margin for breathing motion. *Int. J. Radiat. Oncol. Biol. Phys.* 1999; **44**:911–919.

17 Lax, I., Blomgren, H., Naslund, I., and Svanstrom, R. Stereotactic radiotherapy of malignancies in the abdomen. Methodological aspects. *Acta. Oncol.* 1994; **33**:677–683.

18 Van Herk, M., Remeijer, P., Rasch, C., et al. The probability of correct target dosage: Dose-population histograms for deriving treatment margins in radiotherapy. *Int. J. Radiat. Oncol. Biol. Phys.* 2000; **47**:1121–1135.

19 Viola, P., and Wells, W. M. Alignment by maximization of mutual information. *Int. J. Comput. Vision.* 1997; **24**:137–154.

20 Murphy, M. J. An automatic six-degree-of-freedom image registration algorithm for image-guided frameless stereotaxic radiosurgery. *Med. Phys.* 1997; **24**:857–866.

21 Shimizu, S., Shirato, H., Ogura, S., Akita-Dosaka, H., Kitamura, K., et al. Detection of lung tumor movement in real-time tumor-tracking radiotherapy. *Int. J. Radiat. Oncol. Biol. Phys.* 2001; **51**:304–310.

22 Chen, G. T., Sharp, G. C., and Mori, S. A review of image-guided radiotherapy. *Radiol. Phys. Technol.* 2009; **2**:1–12.

23 Mackie, T. R., Holmes, T., Swerdloff, S., Reckwerdt, P., Deasy, J. O., et al. Tomotherapy: A new concept in the delivery of dynamic conformal radiotherapy. *Med. Phys.* 1993; **20**:1709–1719.

24 Jaffray, D. A., Drake, D. G., Martinez, A. A., and Wong, J. W. A radiographic and tomographic imaging system integrated into a medical linear accelerator for localization of bone and soft-tissue targets. *Int. J. Radiat. Oncol. Biol. Phys.* 1999; **45**:773–789.

25 Oldham, M., LeTourneau, D., Watt, L., Hugo, G., Yan, D., et al. Cone-beam-CT guided radiation therapy: A model for on-line application. *Radiother. Oncol.* **75**:271–278 (2005).

26 Murphy, M. J., Balter, J., Balter, S., BenComo, J. A., Das, I. J., et al. The management of imaging dose during image-guided radiotherapy: Report of the AAPM Task Group 75. *Med. Phys.* **34**:4041–4063 (2007).

27 Bert, C., Metheany, K. G., Doppke, K., and Chen, G. T. Y. A phantom evaluation of a stereo-vision surface imaging system for radiotherapy patient setup. *Med. Phys.* 2005; **32**:2753–2762.

28 Koch, N., Liu, H. H., Starkschall, G., Jacobson, M., Forster, K., et al. Evaluation of internal lung motion for respiratory-gated radiotherapy using MRI: Part I: Correlating internal lung motion with skin fiducial motion. *Int. J. Radiat. Oncol. Biol. Phys.* 2004; **60**:1459–1472.

29 Li, S., Liu, D., Yin, G., Zhuang, P., and Geng, J. Real-time 3D-surface-guided head refixation useful for fractionated stereotactic radiotherapy. *Med. Phys.* 2006; **33**:492–503.

30 Bert, C., Metheany, K. G., Doppke, K. P., Taghian, A. P., Powell, S. N., and Chen, G. T. Y. Clinical experience with a 3D surface patient setup system for alignment of partial-breast irradiation patients. *Int. J. Radiat. Oncol. Biol. Phys.* 2006; **64**:1265–1274.

31 Kuban, D., Dong, L., Cheung, R., Strom, E., and de Crevoisier, R. US-based localization. *Semin. Radiat. Oncol.* 2005; **15**:180–191.

32 Molloy, J. A., Chan, G., Markovic, A., McNeeley, S., Pfeiffer, D., et al. Quality assurance of US-guided external beam radiotherapy for prostate cancer: Report of AAPM Task Group 154. *Med. Phys.* 2011; **38**:857–871.

33 Lattanzi, J., McNeeley, S., Pinover, W., Horowitz, E., Das, I., et al. A comparison of daily CT localization to a daily US-based system in prostate cancer. *Int. J. Radiat. Oncol. Biol. Phys.* 1999; **43**:719–725.

34 Balter, J. M., Wright, J. N., Newell, L. J., Friemel, B., Dimmer, S., et al. Accuracy of a wireless localization system for radiotherapy. *Int. J. Radiat. Oncol. Biol. Phys.* 2005; **61**:933–937.

35 Willoughby T. R., Kupelian, P. A., Pouliot, J., Shinohara, K., Aubin, M., et al. Target localization and real-time tracking using the Calypso 4D localization system in patients with localized prostate cancer. *Int. J. Radiat. Oncol. Biol. Phys.* 2006; **65**:528–534.

36 Balter, J. M., and Cao, Y. Advanced technologies in image-guided radiation therapy. *Semin. Radiat. Oncol.* 2007; **17**:293–297.

37 Dempsey, J. F., Benoit, D., Fitzsimmons, J. R., Haghighat, A., Li, J. G., et al. A device for real time 3D image-guided IMRT. *Int. J. Radiat. Oncol. Biol. Phys.* 2005; **63**(Suppl 1): S202.

38 Lagendijk, J. J. W., Raaymakers, B. W., Raaijmakers, A. J., Overweg, J., Brown, K. J., et al. MRI/linac integration. *Radiother. Oncol.* 2008; **86**:25–29.

13

COMPUTER SYSTEMS

Objectives

After studying this chapter, the reader should be able to:
- Provide a historical perspective on the development of computers and computer networking.
- Delineate the processes and uncertainties in converting analog to digital data and vice versa.
- Demonstrate the features, advantages, and limitations of digital images.
- Discuss the characteristics and contributions of computer components, including memory, central processing unit, and input/output and mass storage devices.
- Explain the differences in various levels of software languages.
- Describe the structure and components of computer networks and their functions, including interfaces, transmission media, data compression, display stations, network standards, encryption, and security.

Introduction

The first true electronic digital computer was built in 1939 at Iowa State University by Atanasoff and Berry.[1] This device was

Hendee's Radiation Therapy Physics, Fourth Edition. Todd Pawlicki, Daniel J. Scanderbeg and George Starkschall.
© 2016 John Wiley & Sons, Inc. Published 2016 by John Wiley & Sons, Inc.

designed to help solve large arrays of linear equations in quantum mechanics. A turning point in computer technology was reached with use of the vacuum tube in computational circuits. This development allowed construction of the Electronic Numeric Integrator and Calculator (ENIAC) by Mauchly and Eckert at the University of Pennsylvania in 1945.[2] This computer was built to prepare ballistics tables for artillery in World War II. In contrast to the compact dimensions of modern computers, the ENIAC filled several large rooms.

The ENIAC was quickly found to be inadequate because it had no way of storing results or, more importantly, storing programs. A means for creating *memory* had to be developed. One early design used a delay device by which up to 500 numbers circulated through a *storage tank*. The numbers were actually represented by ultrasonic pulses traveling through a tank of mercury. A memory device of this type was built in 1947 and incorporated into the Electron Delay Storage Automatic Calculator (EDSAC), which became operational in 1949.[3]

The development of the transistor shortly after World War II brought about a revolution in the design of computers. Transistors control the flow of electricity in much the same way as vacuum tubes, but they are much smaller and use considerably less power. By the 1960s, techniques had been developed to manufacture small silicon wafers called *integrated circuits* (ICs, also known as *microchips*). These devices contained many transistors connected in complex circuits. IBM used the capability of ICs to develop a new line of computers, called the *360 series*. Other companies soon followed, including AT&T, Exxon, and Digital Equipment Corporation (DEC). Many of the early manufacturers of computers ultimately dropped out as competition became fierce and aggressive marketing strategies created giants such as IBM and DEC.

As the technology for making ICs advanced, computers could be made much more powerful. The computer industry developed large computers called *mainframes*, as well as minicomputers such as DEC's PDP-8, which was first marketed in 1965. The PDP-8 was one of the first in a long line of minicomputers marketed at a modest price. Partly inspired by a PDP-8 minicomputer handbook, Steve Wozniak created his own computer, which later evolved into the Apple Macintosh personal computer. In the late 1960s, DEC modified the PDP-8 computer to market one of the first dedicated treatment planning computers, the RAD-8.

Further reductions in the size of computer components have led to the development of tremendously powerful computers assembled into packages that fit on a desktop or even a laptop. In 1971, Intel Corporation introduced the first processor built entirely on a single silicon chip. The chip contained 2300 transistors. Because of its small size, the 4004 chip, called a *microprocessor*, could be manufactured inexpensively in bulk. Since that time, the manufacturing process has improved so much that Intel's P6 microprocessor contains 5.5 million transistors. With this smaller size has come increased speed. The P6 microprocessor can perform 133 million operations per second, and clever instruction-handling techniques increase this speed even more. Computers built around such processors are 100,000 times more powerful than the computer behemoths of the 1950s. Since the 1960s, microprocessor performance has been doubling about every two years (known as *Moore's law*).[4]

In the early 1970s, computers were introduced into radiology departments. Because of their usefulness for storing, manipulating, and displaying large amounts of data, computers were quickly incorporated into clinical nuclear medicine. They were also quickly adopted in radiation therapy, primarily for calculating and displaying isodose distributions for multifield treatments.

Terminology and data representation

Number systems

Base 10

Humans count and calculate using a base-10 number system, probably because we have 10 fingers. The term *base 10* indicates that the number system has 10 digits (0 to 9). A power of 10 is denoted by the position of a digit within a number. The base 10 number system is also referred to as the *decimal system*.

Numbers are represented by listing appropriate digits in a meaningful sequence. For example, the number 1983 actually represents $1 \times 10^3 + 9 \times 10^2 + 8 \times 10^1 + 3 \times 10^0$, where 10^0 equals 1. Multiplication or division by 10 is a simple process; it requires only that the digits in the number be shifted by one to the left of the decimal to multiply by 10, or to the right of the decimal by one digit to divide by 10. For example, $198.30 \times 10 = 1983.0$ and $198.30 \div 10 = 19.830$.

Base 2

A counting system involving only two digits (0 and 1) is used by computers because the two digits can be expressed easily by electronic means. For example, a switch in the "off" position can indicate 0, and a switch in the "on" position can indicate 1. Because this counting system has two digits, it is called *base 2* or the *binary system*. As in the decimal system, numbers in the binary system are formed by placing digits in a sequence, where the position of a digit indicates its value. The binary number 1011 actually represents $1 \times 2^3 + 0 \times 2^2 + 1 \times 2^1 + 1 \times 2^0$, where $2^3 = 8$, $2^2 = 4$, $2^1 = 2$, and $2^0 = 1$. That is, the binary number 1011 is identical in value to the decimal number 11.

Counting in the binary system is performed just as counting in the decimal system; to increment a number by 1, the digit 1 is added to the least significant (farthest to the right) digit of the number. If the least significant digit is already 1, when adding another 1, it is replaced by 0, and 1 is "carried" to the next more significant digit. The digit 0 is sometimes called the *place holder* because its function is to assist in correctly identifying the value of other digits in the number.

Table 13-1 A sequence of numbers represented in decimal and binary form.

Decimal	Binary	Decimal	Binary
1	1	11	1011
2	10	12	1100
3	11	13	1101
4	100	14	1110
5	101	15	1111
6	110	16	10000
7	111	17	10001
8	1000	18	10010
9	1001	19	10011
10	1010	20	10100

Multiplying by 2 in the binary system is analogous to multiplying by 10 in the decimal system; the digits in the number simply are shifted by one to the left to multiply by 2, and by one to the right when dividing by 2 (Example 13-1). A sequence of numbers in binary and decimal form is shown in Table 13-1.

Example 13-1

Multiply the binary number 101 by 2 twice (the equivalent of multiplying by the decimal number 4).

$101 \times 2 = 1010$ (the digits are shifted to the left one place and a zero is inserted in the least significant position)

$1010 \times 2 = 10100$ (the process is repeated)

Compare the results with the values listed in Table 13-1.

Conversion from one system to another

Conversion from the decimal system to another base requires division of the original number by powers of the new base. For example, to convert the decimal number 419 into binary form, 419 is first divided by 2^8 (or 256), then the remainder is divided by 2^7 (or 128), and so on. Conversion into decimal from any other base requires multiplication of successive powers of the base.

Example 13-2

Convert the binary number 10111 into decimal form.

Answer:

$$(1 \times 2^4) + (0 \times 2^3) + (1 \times 2^2) + (1 \times 2^1) + (1 \times 2^0)$$
$$= 16 + 0 + 4 + 2 + 1 = 23$$

Bits, bytes, and words

The fundamental unit of data in a computer is called a *bit* (for *binary* dig*it*). As a binary number, a bit can be used to represent either of two states, such as on or off. In modern computer memories, each bit is represented by a transistor, and so can indicate whether a voltage is present or absent at the transistor terminal. In magnetic storage media, such as disks and tapes, a bit represents a small area on the storage media that can be magnetized or not to indicate its state. Bits are grouped into numbers called *bytes*, each generally consisting of eight bits. Bytes, therefore, can be conveniently used to indicate numbers between 0 and $2^8 - 1$.

As will be seen later, a byte is a convenient unit of storage because it may be used to represent many types of data. Computer memory is generally described in terms of the number of available bytes. Because this number is frequently very large, the terms *kilobytes*, *megabytes*, *gigabytes*, and *terabytes* are used. The prefixes kilo-, mega-, and giga- are actually approximations, as shown below. The actual number of memory locations is only approximately a multiple of 10^3.

$$1 \text{ kilobyte (kB)} = 2^{10} \text{ bytes} = 1,024 \text{ bytes}$$
$$1 \text{ megabyte (MB)} = 2^{20} \text{ bytes} = 1,048,576 \text{ bytes}$$
$$1 \text{ gigabyte (GB)} = 2^{30} \text{ bytes} = 1,073,741,824 \text{ bytes}$$
$$1 \text{ terabyte (TB)} = 2^{40} \text{ bytes} = 1,099,511,627,776 \text{ bytes}$$

One page of a Microsoft Word document of formatted text is about 30 kB. That same page saved as an unformatted ASCII text document is about 4 kB. A single slice of a patient's CT scan is about 500 kB (or 0.5 MB) in size.

Bits are also grouped into larger units called *words*. Words are typically 16 bits (corresponding to 2 bytes), 32 bits (corresponding to 4 bytes), or 64 bits (corresponding to eight bytes). The grouping of bits into words facilitates the expression of larger integers. For example, a 32 bit word can be used to express integers between 0 and $2^{32} - 1 = 4,294,967,295$. The size of the word determines the amount of computer memory that can be accessed. A computer with 16 bit words can directly access only 65,535 memory locations ($2^{16} - 1$). Because each memory location typically stores one byte of data, this amount of memory is also known as *64 kilobytes*. Today, many computer applications require access to much larger amounts of memory, and even home computers are frequently equipped with several gigabytes of memory. Access to these large volumes of memory requires 32 bit and even 64 bit words. Large-size words permit computations with greater precision and reduced rounding errors.

Representation of data

Indication of states

Modern computers are designed to solve a variety of problems and to assist humans working in a variety of circumstances. For example, a contemporary desktop computer may be used to run a word-processing program, perform complex mathematical computations, and display images. This multitasking performance requires the computer to store and process many different types of data in digital form. The word-processing program requires the computer to present and operate on alphanumeric data (text). Programs that perform calculations require the computer to store numerical values in digital form. Earlier, it was shown how computers store integers of values ranging from 0 to a maximum dictated by the number of bits in the computer word. Computers often are required to manipulate negative numbers, fractions, and very large or very small numbers.

Numeric data

The storage of positive integers in a computer's memory has already been described. It was shown that an 8 bit binary number can easily represent numbers from 0 to 255 ($2^8 - 1$). However, it is often necessary to represent negative numbers in computer memory. To do so, the computer may reserve one bit to indicate the sign of the number, and use the remaining bits (in this case 7) to indicate the value of the number up to 127 (2^7 or $128 - 1$). Many computers today use an alternate method called *two's complement notation* to represent signed integers (i.e., 0 = positive and 1 = negative). An 8 bit binary number can therefore be used to represent numbers between –127 and +127. The binary number 0000 0001 represents the decimal number 1, whereas 0111 1111 represents positive 127. The binary number 1000 0000 represents –127, whereas 1111 1111 represents the decimal number –1. Although this notation may seem slightly awkward, it simplifies the addition of numbers in the computer's memory.

Very large and very small numbers are often required for scientific calculations. Avogadro's number (6.023×10^{23} molecules per gram-mole) and the charge on an electron (1.6×10^{-19} Coulombs) are examples. Numbers such as these may be represented in *floating point* form. Floating point is similar to exponential notation, in which a number is expressed as a decimal quantity multiplied by 10 raised to a power. Similarly, a number can be written as a binary quantity multiplied by 2 raised to a power. Typically, four 8 bit bytes are used to store floating point numbers, with one bit used to identify the sign (0 = plus, 1 = minus), 8 bits for the exponent, and 23 bits for the mantissa. While modern computer calculations are very fast, some calculations are faster than others. For example, computer instructions for floating-point computations are more time-consuming than for fixed-point (integer) computations.

Alphanumeric data

The storage of text, in the form of alphanumeric symbols, requires a conversion table between binary integers and alphanumeric symbols. The output of a computer, such as the text of a word-processor document, requires the conversion of binary integers into the shapes humans recognize as letters and symbols. The 26 letters of the alphabet, the digits 0 to 9, and a number of special symbols (such as $, !, =, etc.) are referred to collectively as the *alphanumeric character set*. With the inclusion of upper- and lowercase letters and additional symbols, the alphanumeric character set may consist of as many as 128 elements. Table 13-2 shows the American National Standard

Table 13-2 American National Standard Code for Information Interchange (ASCII).

Character	Binary Code	Character	Binary Code
A	100 0001	0	011 0000
B	100 0010	1	011 0001
C	100 0011	2	011 0010
D	100 0100	3	011 0011
E	100 0101	4	011 0100
F	100 0110	5	011 0101
G	100 0111	6	011 0110
H	100 1000	7	011 0111
I	100 1001	8	011 1000
J	100 1010	9	011 1001
K	100 1011		
L	100 1100		
M	100 1101	Blank	010 0000
N	100 1110	.	010 1110
O	100 1111	(	010 1000
P	101 0000	+	010 1011
Q	101 0001	$	010 0100
R	101 0010	*	010 1010
S	101 0011	)	010 1101
T	101 0100	-	010 1101
U	101 0101	/	010 1111
V	101 0110	,	010 1100
W	101 0111	^	011 1101
Y	101 1001		
Z	101 1010		

Code for Information Exchange (ASCII). This is one of the most widely used schemes for encoding alphanumeric information.

Analog-to-digital and digital-to-analog conversion

Measurable quantities may be displayed in one of two forms: analog and digital. The use of an analog display indicates that the quantity being measured may vary in continuous fashion. For example, a voltage may be displayed on a meter whose needle moves from zero to some maximum value. The quantity displayed may have any value within the range. Our ability to measure the quantity depends only on our ability to read the meter. A watch or clock with continuously moving hands is an example of an analog display of time. Our ability to measure time is limited only by our ability to read the position of the hands on the clock. On the other hand, a quantity may be represented digitally. Digital quantities are discrete and can assume only specific values separated by intervals. A digital voltmeter may display only integer numbers of volts (0, 1, 2, etc.), and a digital watch may display only integer numbers of minutes (e.g., 10:23).

Computers described in this chapter are digital computers. They operate only with digital quantities. However, much of the information collected in science, as well as in medicine, is presented in analog form. Therefore, conversion from analog to digital form and back again is often necessary. For example, the electrical signals from radiation detectors such as ionization chambers are in analog form. To represent the signal of an ionization

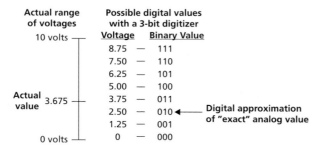

Figure 13-1 A 3 bit digitizer is used to record voltage signals over the range of 0–10 V. Because only eight digital values are possible for a 3 bit digitizer, one scheme, illustrated here, would assign all voltages between 0 and 1.25 V to the value 0 V (binary 000), all voltages between 1.25 and 2.50 V to the value 1.25 V (binary 001), and so on.

chamber in a computer requires conversion of the analog signal to digital form. Conversely, the use of a computer to control a piece of equipment (even a simple device such as a motor) may require conversion of the computer output to an analog signal. An example of an analog output from a computer is the musical sounds produced by contemporary computer systems. The representation of an analog quantity by a digital number requires that the representation be limited to a finite number of alternatives. For example, it may be desirable to represent the signal from an ionization chamber as a 3 bit binary number. This binary number can provide at most eight different values. The output of the ionization chamber may vary between 0 and 10 V. The eight available binary values can be used to display voltages between 0 and 10 V if each binary value corresponds to 1.25 V (Figure 13-1). An analog voltage between 0 and 1.25 V might be recorded as 0, whereas a value between 1.25 and 2.50 V might be recorded as 1.25 V, and so on. The error associated with this digitizing process may be as large as 1.25 V, the difference between adjacent binary values. However, the average digitization error (assuming that the analog values are uniformly distributed between 0 and 10 V) is half the digitization increment, or 0.625 V.

Such a crude digitizer may be acceptable in some circumstances, but in most scientific applications greater resolution is required. A 16 bit digitizer would be able to display voltages in the range of 0–10 V with a resolution of $10\ \text{V}/2^{16} = 0.00015$ V. The maximum error is equal to the resolution, and the average error (for analog values that are uniformly distributed between 0 and 10 V) is half of the resolution, 0.000075 V.

When digitizing an analog signal, the maximum digitization error, err_{max}, is:

$$err_{max} = R_a/N = R_a/2^n$$

and the average digitization error, err_{avg}, is:

$$err_{avg} = err_{max}/2 = R_a/2^{n+1}$$

In these expressions, R_a is the range (minimum to maximum measured analog value), and N is the number of distinct digitization increments.[3]

Example 13-3

Determine the maximum and average digitization error (in cm) of the position-sensing circuit of an isodose plotter. The detector axis is 50 cm long, and a potentiometer provides a position-dependent voltage ranging from 0 to 15 V. The voltage is monitored by a 12 bit analog-to-digital converter (ADC). The digitizer resolution is:

$$15\ \text{V}/2^{12} = 0.0037\ \text{V}$$

The maximum digitization error is therefore:

$$0.0037\ \text{V}$$

The average error is 0.00185 V, corresponding to half the digitization increment assuming that the analog values were uniformly distributed between 0 and 15 V. The problem can also be solved by noting that a 12 bit ADC is capable of 4096 values and therefore has a precision of one part in 4096.

Representation of graphic data

The set of pixels comprising an image is referred to as the *image matrix*. Matrix sizes are powers of two (e.g., 64 × 64, 512 × 512, 2048 × 2048). To store images in a computer, the image must be divided into small sections called *picture elements*, or *pixels* (Figure 13-2). Each pixel is assigned a single numeric value that denotes the color, if a color image is stored, or the shade of gray (referred to as the *gray level*), if a black and white image is stored. A digital image therefore consists of a list of binary numbers corresponding to individual pixels in the image. The number of bits used for each binary value (corresponding to each pixel) determines the number of different colors or shades of gray available. The faithfulness of the computer-rendered image to the original photograph is improved as the *bit depth* (the number of bits in the binary number used to describe the color or gray level) is increased.

Computers may generate images directly in digital form. For example, computed tomography (CT), magnetic resonance (MR), and computed radiography (CR) images are produced directly by digital computers. The number of pixels used to create an image has a profound influence on the quality of the image. The use of only a small number of pixels results in a coarse image. Likewise, a digital image produced by a computer (such as a CT image) with a large number of pixels is said to be a *high-resolution image*. The observer may not even be able to detect the individual pixels. The use of large numbers of pixels to produce images has the benefit of improved quality and

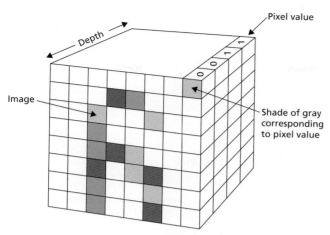

Figure 13-2 A digital image may be thought of as a three-dimensional object composed of a number of small cubes, each of which contains a binary digit (bit). The image appears on the front surface of the block. The "depth" of the block is the number of bits required to describe the color or gray level for each pixel. The total number of cubes that make up the large block is the number of bits required to store the image.

better resolution, but the disadvantage of requiring larger computer capacity to store the image. Image matrix sizes are generally powers of two, reflecting the binary nature of computer storage. For example, CT images are typically 256×256 ($2^8 \times 2^8$) pixels, or 512×512 ($2^9 \times 2^9$) pixels. If the bit depth of these images is 8 bits, the image formats would require 524,288 or 2,097,152 bits of information each, respectively. Typically, the images would be stored in bytes of 8 bits each, requiring $2^{16} = 65,536$ or $2^{18} = 262,144$ bytes, respectively.

An additional disadvantage of large image matrices is the time required to transmit an image from one computer to another. Transfer of data in serial form requires transmission of the bits of information one at a time along the connection between the two computer systems. The *transmission rate* is the number of bits of information that can be transmitted per second. Transmission rates range from a few megabits per second (Mbps) for "twisted cable" (telephone wire) to several terabits per second (Tbps) for fiber-optic cable. Clearly, larger image matrices take longer to transmit from one computer to another.

Example 13-4

The connection between two computers permits images to be transferred at a transmission rate of 9600 bits per second. Calculate the length of time required to transfer a 128×128 matrix of pixels, each consisting of 8 bit binary numbers.

The total number of bits making up such an image is $128 \times 128 \times 8 = 131,072$. At 9600 bits per second, the time required to transmit the image is 131,072/9600 = 13.65 seconds.

Computer hardware is any physical component of a computer. Computer software is any set of instructions used to

operate the computer or perform mathematical operations. A *device driver* is software that allows other higher-level software programs (e.g., word processing or spreadsheets) to use computer hardware, such as a printer or an external storage device. Some devices were standardized in the mid-1990s to use common connections and communication protocols for easy connection to any computer with additional device driver software. These devices are generally known as *USB* (Universal Serial Bus) drives.

Computer architecture

Reference has been made earlier in this chapter to computer memory. Computers actually consist of a number of components, including memory units that are linked together by pathways called *data buses* (Figure 13-3). The main memory of the computer stores the program (as a sequence of instructions) that is being executed, as well as the data being processed. A central processing unit (CPU) executes the instructions in the program to process the data. Input/output (I/O) devices are required to enable the operator to enter information into and retrieve information from the computer. Typical I/O devices include a keyboard, mouse, or other pointing device, video monitor, mass storage device, and printer or plotter. A data bus is a group of wires or fibers used to transfer data in parallel. This method is more efficient than the process of serial data transfer described earlier, in which data are transferred one bit at a time along a single connection. With parallel data transfer, bits may be transferred simultaneously along each of several connections. A data bus consisting of eight connections can transfer an 8 bit byte in the same time required for a serial interface to transfer a single bit. The speed that a user experiences when using a computer is

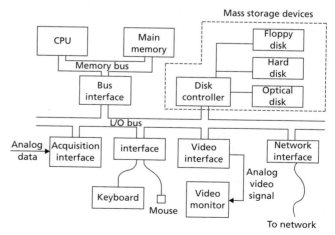

Figure 13-3 A block diagram of a modern computer. *Source:* Bushberg et al. 1994.[5]

not only dependent on the CPU but also on the bus capacity and operating system.

Memory

Computer memory provides temporary storage for the computer program (a sequence of instructions to the computer) as well as for the data currently being processed by the computer. This is not the same as where a file is stored for later use, which is a more long-term memory storage. The memory consists of a large number of data storage locations, each typically consisting of one byte. Each storage location is uniquely identified with an address. Memory addresses usually start at zero and increase sequentially. A computer having "1 megabyte" of memory actually has 1,048,576 memory locations, identified by addresses ranging from 0 to 1,048,575. Most contemporary computers have a certain amount of *random access memory* (RAM). Typical laptop computers have about 4 GB of RAM. *RAM* refers to memory into which the computer can both write and read data. A disadvantage of most modern RAM is that it is volatile, meaning that data stored in it are lost when the electrical power is switched off. To write to the memory, a computer must first send the address of the location in memory into which a datum is to be written, and then send the datum. To read from memory, the computer sends the address from which a datum is to be read and, in return, is sent the datum at that location. To be able to access a full 1 MB of memory, a computer must be able to send addresses as large a 1,048,575, or $2^{20} - 1$. This requires a word length of at least 20 bits; typically 24 or even 32 bits are used.

Another type of memory is *read-only memory* (ROM). A computer can only read data from ROM; it cannot write or alter data. The primary advantage of ROM is that data stored in it are not lost when the computer's electrical power is switched off. ROM is used to store frequently used programs provided by the manufacturer for performing important functions such as preparing the computer for operation when the power is turned on.

To provide greater flexibility and make upgrading simpler, some standardized software is provided on programmable read-only memory chips (PROMs). These chips are intended to be removed and replaced by the user as different software capabilities are required. Under some circumstances, PROMs can be reprogrammed by the manufacturer, often through a modem connection.

The amount of memory required for a computer depends on its intended applications. For example, a computer used for word processing requires sufficient memory to store the word-processing program, together with the document being written. A typical word-processing program may require megabytes of memory, while word-processing documents can be several megabytes. A computer with less available RAM may still be able to run a word-processing program, but only a portion of the program can be loaded into RAM at one time. Hence, only a subset of the available commands and functions are available at one time. Making another function available requires that another portion of the program be loaded into memory (replacing the portion previously loaded). This process delays execution of the program. Manipulation of large amounts of data, such as medical images, requires large amounts of memory to be available for the data. Modern personal computer workstations designed for handling medical images frequently have as much as 8 gigabytes of RAM.

Central processing unit

The central processing unit (CPU) is the central control mechanism of the computer. It is a collection of electronic circuits that can execute a small number of rather simple functions. For example, the CPU fetches and executes the instructions of a computer program in sequence. Typically, instructions tell the CPU to perform one of four tasks:

1 Transfer a unit of data (typically a byte or a word) from one memory location, storage register, or I/O device to another.
2 Perform a mathematical operation between two numbers.
3 Compare the value of two numbers or other pieces of data.
4 Change the address of the next instruction in the program to be executed.

For example, a program instruction may instruct the CPU to add two numbers. This operation requires the following steps.

1 Locate the first number from an I/O device or RAM.
2 Store this number in a temporary location and record the address of that location.
3 Locate the second number from an I/O device or RAM.
4 Identify the temporary storage location where the result is to be placed.
5 Perform the addition function and store the result in the identified temporary storage location.
6 Report the result of the operation back to the main program and look for the next instruction.

Most currently available computers function by using a technique called *serial processing*. This approach requires that one task is completed before another is begun. In many applications, the result of one task is the input for the next, and serial processing is necessary. In some applications, however, the completion of one task is independent of at least some other tasks. In these cases, it may be possible for one computer processor to work on one task while a separate processor works on another. This capability is known as *multitasking*. If a program is written to perform the same operation on numerous elements of data, then two processors could simultaneously operate on two pieces of data, executing the task twice as quickly. These tasks are said to be performed *in parallel*. A computer that can perform tasks in parallel is termed a *parallel processor*.

One type of parallel processor is the *array processor*. An array processor uses a single instruction to perform the same computation on all elements of a large matrix of data. Tremendous savings in computer time may be achieved by using an array processor to manipulate digital images. Such processors are routinely used in CT and MR imaging units, and they are becoming standard on all types of digital imaging systems.

Another special processor that is used routinely in radiology is the *arithmetic processor*. Many mathematical functions such as exponential quantities, square roots, and trigonometric functions can be calculated in clever but time-consuming fashion by repeated application of procedures such as addition. A faster and usually more accurate alternative involves the use of an arithmetic processor, a device that executes fewer steps in performing discrete mathematical operations. The arithmetic processor is optimized to perform mathematical functions only. It is called on by the CPU to provide these functions and return the results to memory.

The number of instructions that a computer can execute per second is a measure of the speed of the computer. The speed is usually expressed in units of *millions of instructions per second*, or MIPS.

Graphics processing unit

A graphics processing unit (GPU) is a processing unit with a highly parallel structure that makes it more effective than general-purpose CPUs for algorithms that can calculate blocks of data in parallel. A parallel calculation means that one part of the calculation does not depend on any earlier parts of the calculation. Readily parallelizable algorithms include calculation of *digitally reconstructed radiograph*s (DRRs), CT image reconstruction, and some types of dose calculation algorithms. GPUs were originally developed to support increased graphics capabilities and are found in mobile phones, personal computers, and workstations. While new to radiotherapy, GPUs are likely to play a large role in the development and clinical use of online adaptive radiotherapy techniques.

Supercomputers with parallel-processing capability can attain data-processing speeds of >300 *million floating-point operations per second* (MFLOPS). So-called massively parallel systems with several hundred microprocessors achieve giga-FLOP and tera-FLOP speeds.[6]

Input/output devices

Input/output (I/O) devices form the operator interface of a computer. Components such as a keyboard, mouse, video monitor, and printer fall into this category. These devices can send or receive data serially (using a single data line) or in parallel.

A keyboard, for example, converts each alphanumeric symbol into a digital code representing the symbol. When the letter A is struck, the keyboard transmits a sequence of voltage pulses of high (e.g., 5 V) and low (e.g., 0 V) levels. These pulses are interpreted as ones and zeroes, making up the ASCII character representation 0100 0001 (see Table 13-2).

Similarly, a printer receives a sequence of pulses, representing the ones and zeroes making up the binary code for an ASCII character. The printer interprets the code and correspondingly rotates a character wheel, squirts tiny droplets of ink, or fires a laser to deposit black powder on paper, causing the appropriate character to be printed on paper.

Mass storage devices

The programs and data used by computers are stored permanently on devices incorporating magnetic or optical encoding. The memory, or RAM, of a computer is used only to store a copy of the program being executed and the data being manipulated.

As mentioned earlier, the stored information is lost if power to the RAM is interrupted. In addition, when the memory is required to run a different program or to manipulate new data, the previous information stored in the memory may be overwritten. Before they are lost, new data created by the program should be written to a mass storage device.

Common mass storage devices include magnetic disks and optical disks. Magnetic disks and tape store data by magnetizing small regions called *domains*. When the domains are oriented together by a magnetic field, their combined magnetic fields become detectable. The local magnetic field produced by the write head of a magnetic disk drive can magnetize groups of domains in small regions of the disk. The same head, when operating in its "read" mode, can detect the pattern of magnetization. The pattern of magnetization is not lost when power is removed, so the magnetic storage devices are said to be *nonvolatile*.

Magnetic disks have been manufactured in a variety of formats. Older computer systems used flexible (or *floppy*) disks. These disks were inexpensive but held comparatively little information, typically 1.4 megabytes. The use of floppy disks has largely been superseded by CDs and, more recently, flash (USB) drives. Hard disks are available in both fixed and removable formats, with capacities from a few megabytes to a few terabytes.

Both floppy and hard disks are coated with magnetizable material. The information embedded in the disk is read with a read/write head that hovers a small distance above the disk. Data are stored along concentric *tracks*, which themselves are divided into *sectors*. The head moves radially across the disk to access different tracks. Frequently, two opposing heads are provided, and data are stored on both sides of the disk.

Data are generally written in *blocks*, and a directory stored on the disk identifies the usage of each block. A large program or data file may require a number of blocks, but, depending on the capabilities of the drive, the blocks may not have to be contiguous. Instead, the final record of each block is a *pointer* to the next block in the series used for the file. While it is potentially possible to change a single bit on a hard disk, an edited file is generally rewritten to a new location on the disk, and the previous locations are made available for new data.

The time required to move the read/write head to a desired location on the disk is called the *access time*. Typical access times range from a few milliseconds to a few hundred milliseconds. The *data transfer rate* describes the speed with which data can be written to or read from the disk. Hard disk drives can be

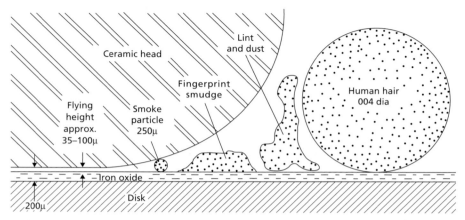

Figure 13-4 The read/write head of a hard disk drive travels only a small distance above the disk. Dirt or a hair can cause catastrophic damage. *Source:* Hendee 1985.[7]

permanently damaged if the head physically contacts the disk. Usually, before a disk drive is moved (such as the disk drive in a portable computer), a mechanism is activated to "park" the head in a secure location. Disk drives must be enclosed to protect them from dust or dirt. Because the head travels only a few micrometers above the disk, a hair or speck of dust can scratch the disk or damage the head (Figure 13-4).

Computer software

The instructions that cause computers to perform their intended functions are organized into *programs* that are collectively referred to as *software*. Software includes simple programs to add two numbers together, as well as word-processing programs, and programs to perform complex calculations with large amounts of data. Programs also exist to simplify the development of other programs.

All modern computers run a program called an *operating system*. For example, Microsoft Windows and Mac OS X are operating systems. Many computer workstations (a generation of desktop computers with fast processors and large amounts of memory) run a version of an operating system called Unix. The operating system monitors the various pieces of hardware and handles the transfer of data from one to another. It continually monitors input devices, such as a keyboard or mouse, and it interprets the instructions received from these devices. The instructions may tell the operating system to read a copy of a file into the memory, and then send the file to the printer. Initiating the operating system is termed *booting* the computer, taken from the phrase *to pull oneself up by the bootstraps*, that is, to be a self-starter.

Applications are programs developed for specific purposes such as word processing. In response to a command from the mouse or keyboard, the operating system may read an application from a disk, store it in memory, and begin executing it. Control of the computer then passes to the application.

The expression *debugging* for fixing a computer malfunction was coined in 1951 by Grace Hopper, Ph.D., a U.S. Navy admiral, after she found an actual bug (moth) in an electronic relay of a malfunctioning computer. A bug is now used to describe a problem with software when it doesn't perform as expected. In radiotherapy, most software bugs are just a nuisance but some can lead to catastrophic failures resulting in serious harm or patient death.

Programming languages

Computer languages

Instructions to a computer that enable it to perform a desired function are contained in programs. *Programs* required to make a computer function are referred to as *software* (in contrast to the *hardware*, which makes up the computer itself). A program consists of a series of instructions, arranged in a logical sequence, which when executed cause the computer to perform a set of operations. The program may be simple (e.g., instructing the computer to display a word or sentence on a monitor) or complex (e.g., word-processing and spreadsheet programs). Complicated programs often are broken up into smaller sections called *subroutines*, in which a single function or operation is handled.

The instructions that comprise a program must be written in a manner that is intelligible to the computer. Instructions that are easily interpreted by a computer are not directly translatable by humans. Consequently, several different levels of language have been developed to convert programs from the languages understood by humans to the languages understood by computers.

Low-level languages

Low-level languages are those that are understood by a computer without translation. These languages are referred to as *object code*, or *machine language*. When printed, an object code appears to be a meaningless list of numbers and letters. The

```
10 PRINT "CALCULATE POWERS of 2"
20 FOR I = 1 TO 10
    30 LET A = 2**1
    40 REM The double asterisk indicates an exponent
    50 PRINT "The" ,-I-," Exponent of 2 is ";  A
60 NEXT I
70 END
```

Figure 13-5 A simple BASIC language program.

digits and letters may be hexadecimal numbers, each representing a single instruction. For example, a particular hexadecimal code may be an instruction to the CPU to retrieve a value from memory, with the address of the value to be read given by the next instruction.

Object code is difficult for humans to interpret, even those skilled at writing programs in this language. A slightly more intelligible code is *assembly language*. This code substitutes mnemonics for each of the instructions contained in object code. These instructions, although cryptic, are at least recognizable, and they make writing programs in low-level languages a little easier. Mnemonic codes correspond one-to-one with object code instructions.

High-level languages

To facilitate the development of programs, high-level languages have been developed. These languages use commands that resemble the English language. An example of a high-level language is the BASIC program portrayed in Figure 13-5. This figure illustrates several common elements of computer programs. Instructions to the computer are listed in a logical sequence, and the sequence is defined by *line numbers*. Some instructions are intended to be repeated a selected number of times, or until some criterion is met. These instructions are placed in a *loop*. In Figure 13-5, the loop is defined by the "For" and "Next" statements (the intervening commands have been indented for clarity, a common practice by programmers). Instructions must be included to deliver the results to the person operating the program. In this example, the "PRINT" statements cause the text within quotes and the numeric values represented by the symbols "I" and "A" to be printed on an output device connected to the computer.

When a high-level programming language is used, the computer must be equipped with a program to *interpret* or *compile* programs written in the high-level language. The distinction between the two is easily made: an *interpreter* is a program that decodes the user's program (such as the BASIC program in Figure 13-5) one line at a time, acts on the instructions contained in that line, and then goes on to the next line. Each time a line is encountered, even if it falls within a loop, it must be interpreted anew. A *compiler* creates a new program in assembly language from the user's program. The assembly language program may be modified further and combined with other subroutines to finally produce a program in object code. This final version requires no interpretation and can be executed at maximum speed by the computer. However, it is almost impossible to be understood by humans, or to change. Instead, changes must be made in the original high-level program, which must then be compiled and linked once more before it is executed. The advantage is that once a program reaches its final form, the computer can execute it rapidly and as often as necessary.

An example of a section of a C program and the corresponding assembly language code generated by the compiler are shown in Figure 13-6. The program is very simple: it prompts the operator to enter two numbers, the numbers are multiplied together, and the result is displayed. The operational part of the program is contained between the brackets, and the portions offset by "/∗" are comments that are ignored by the compiler when it converts the source code to object code. The corresponding assembly code is much lengthier. Text that follows a semicolon on each line is a comment. Clearly, C code is much more compact and readable than the resulting assembly language.

A compiler is much faster than an interpreter in converting a high-level language program into object code. However, instructions in the program are almost impossible to change once the compiler has completed the translation.

In recent years, very high-level programming languages have been developed that enable the programmer to use statements that are even closer to English. Examples of such software include MATHCAD (Mathematics Computer-Aided Design) and MATLAB (Mathematics Laboratory).∗

Networking[†]

The increased use of computers in all areas of medicine, including diagnostic imaging, creates the desire to link the computers together, thereby making information present in one computer available to all computers in an institution or community This linking of computers, called *networking*, is a topic of current interest.[8–11]

In the late 1960s, the US Department of Defense wanted to develop a computer network that would survive a nuclear attack. The network would continue to deliver streams of digital data, even if a number of its components or linkages were destroyed. The solution was "packet switching," a system in which data streams are broken into smaller pieces, called *cells* or *frames*. Each cell contains not only a piece of the data, but also information such as the place of the cell in the original sequence, the priority of this stream of data compared with other data streams, and so forth. One key feature of packet switching is that

∗MATHCAD is a registered trademark of MathSoft, Inc., 201 Broadway, Cambridge, MA 02139. MATLAB is a registered trademark of The MathWorks, Inc., 24 Prime Park Way, Natick, MA 01760.
†This section on networking is taken from Hendee, W. R., and Ritenour, E. R. *Medical Imaging Physics*, 4th edition New York, John Wiley & Sons, 2001.

c program language:

```
#include <stdio.h>

main ()
    {
    float a;
    float b;
    float c;

    /*
    * Display a prompt.
    */

    printf("Enter values A, B: ");

    /*
    * Read values A and B from standard input. */

    scanf("%f,%f",&a,&b);

    /*
    * Put product of A and B in C.
    */

    c=a*b;

    /*
    * Print product on screen.
    */

    printf("The product of A and B is: %f",c);

}
```

Assembly code generated by the compiler:

```
    .SPACE     $TEXT$,SORT=8
    .SUBSPA    $CODE$,QUAD=0,ALIGN=4,ACCESS=0x2c,CODE_ONLY,SORT=24
main
    .PROC
    .CALLINFO         CALLER,FRAME=16,SAVE_RP
    .ENTRY
    STW        %r2,-20(%r30)      ;offset 0x0
    LDO        64(%r30),%r30      ;offset 0x4
    ADDIL      LR'M$2-$global$,%r27         ;offset 0x8
    LDO        RR'M$2-$global$(%r1),%r26    ;offset 0xc
    LDIL       L'printf,%r31       ;offset 0x10
    .CALL      ARGW0=GR,RTNVAL=GR              ;in=26;out=28;
    BLE        R'printf(%sr4,%r31)         ;offset 0x14
    COPY       %r31,%r2           ;offset 0x18
    ADDIL      LR'M$2-$global$+20,%r27      ;offset 0x1c
    LDO        RR'M$2-$global$+20(%r1),%r26  ;offset 0x20
    LDO        -64(%r30),%r25     ;offset 0x24
    LDO        -60(%r30),%r24     ;offset 0x28
    LDIL       L'scanf,%r31       ;offset 0x2c
    .CALL      ARGW0=GR,ARGW1=GR,ARGW2=GR,RTNVAL=GR        ;in=24,25,26;out=28;
    BLE        R'scanf(%sr4,%r31)          ;offset 0x30
    COPY       %r31,%r2           ;offset 0x34
    LDO        -48(%r30),%r1      ;offset 0x38
    FLDWS      -16(%r1),%fr4L     ;offset 0x3c
    FCNVFF,SGL,DBL             %fr4L,%fr4   ;offset 0x40
    LDO        -48(%r30),%r31     ;offset 0x44
    FLDWS      -12(%r31),%fr5L    ;offset 0x48
    FCNVFF,SGL,DBL             %fr5L,%fr5   ;offset 0x4c
    FMPY,DBL %fr4,%fr5,%fr6       ;offset 0x50
    FCNVFF,DBL,SGL             %fr6,%fr5R   ;offset 0x54
    LDO        -48(%r30),%r19     ;offset 0x58
    FSTWS      %fr5R,-8(%r19)     ;offset 0x5c
    ADDIL      LR'M$2-$global$+28,%r27      ;offset 0x60
    LDO        RR'M$2-$global$+28(%r1),%r26 ;offset 0x64
    LDO        -48(%r30),%r20     ;offset 0x68
    FLDWS      -8(%r20),%fr6L     ;offset 0x6c
```

Figure 13-6 A short section of a C language program is converted into a number of assembly language statements by the compiler.
Source: Courtesy of Yeong-Yeong Liu of Computerized Medical Systems, St. Louis, MO.

```
FCNVFF,SGL,DBL              %fr6L,%fr7    ;offset 0x70
LDIL       L'printf,%r31                  ;offset 0x74
.CALL      ARGW0=GR,ARGW2=FR,ARGW3=FU,RTNVAL=GR     ;in=26;out=28;fpin=107;
BLE        R'printf(%sr4,%r31)            ;offset 0x78
COPY       %r31,%r2          ;offset 0x7c
LDW        -84(%r30),%r2     ;offset 0x80
BV         %r0(%r2)          ;offset 0x84
.EXIT
LDO        -64(%r30),%r30    ;offset 0x88
.PROCEND  ;out=28;


       .SPACE    $TEXT$
       .SUBSPA   $CODE$
       .SPACE    $PRIVATE$,SORT=16
       .SUBSPA   $DATA$,QUAD=1,ALIGN=8,ACCESS=0x1f,SORT=16
M$2
       .ALIGN    8
       .STRINGZ  "Enter values A, B: \x00%f,%f"
       .BLOCKZ   2
       .STRINGZ  "The product of A and B is: %f"
       .IMPORT   $global$,DATA
       .SPACE    $TEXT$
       .SUBSPA   $CODE$
       .EXPORT   main,ENTRY,PRIV_LEV=3,RTNVAL=GR
       .IMPORT   printf,CODE
       .IMPORT   scanf,CODE
       .END
```

Figure 13-6 (*Continued*)

each cell also contains the address of the component to which it is being sent. Another key feature of packet switching is that the network consists of interconnected routers. Each router is a computer whose purpose is to maintain information about the addresses of surrounding routers. When a packet arrives at a router, it is automatically sent on to another router that is "closer" to its destination. Thus, if part of the network is disabled, the routers update their information and simply send cells via different routes. This earliest wide-area network was known as Arpanet, after the Department of Defense's Advanced Research Projects Administration.

The World Wide Web (WWW) was created in March 1989, at CERN, a high-energy particle physics laboratory on the Franco–Swiss border. Tim Berners-Lee, a physicist at CERN, proposed the idea of using a hypertext system that would link data from diverse information sources and different computer platforms, i.e., the WWW. In 1991, there were only 10 file servers on the WWW, at various physics laboratories. Today, the number of servers is well into the tens of millions. There is standard security when communicating between an Internet browser and a Web server. The standard security is called Secure Sockets Layer (SSL) and ensures that all data passed between a Web server and browser is secure and private.

When electronic mail (e-mail) was developed, the usefulness of Arpanet became apparent to a wider community of users in academics and in government, and the number of network users continued to grow. Arpanet was officially decommissioned in 1989. By that time, a wide community of users required that the network be continued. The administration of the network was turned over to the National Science Foundation. The network of routers, file servers, and other devices that have become the foundation of modern communications has been known as the Internet since 1989.

Network components and structure

Computer networks for medical imaging are known by many names, such as information management, archiving, and communications systems (IMACS), picture archiving and communications systems (PACS), digital imaging networks (DIN), and local area networks (LAN). These networks face some fundamental problems including (1) how to transmit images quickly, (2) how to avoid bottlenecks or "data collision" when the network is experiencing heavy use, (3) how to organize and maintain the data base or "log" that records the existence of images and their locations on the system, and (4) how to retain as many images as possible on the network for as long as necessary.

Components include image acquisition (CT, ultrasound, etc.), archiving (tape, disk, etc.), central controller, data base manager, and display station. Components that allow the network to communicate with the outside world through display and archiving techniques are referred to as *nodes*. All components are not necessarily nodes. For example, several ultrasound units might be connected to a single formatting device that translates the digital images into a standard format recognizable by the network. The formatting device communicates directly with the network and is the node for the ultrasound units.

Networks can be divided into two categories on the basis of their overall structure. Centralized networks use a single computer (a central controller) to monitor and control access to information for all parts of the network. A distributed network contains components that are connected together with no central controller. Tasks are handled as requested until a conflict arises such as more demands being placed on a component than it can handle. While it may appear chaotic, a distributed network has the advantage that other components are not affected by slowdown or stoppage of one or more components of the system. In particular, there is no central controller that would shut the whole system down if it malfunctions.

Interfaces

The interface of an imaging device such as a CT scanner with a computer network is usually a more complex matter than simply connecting a few wires. Transfer of images and other data requires that the network must be ready to receive, transmit, and store information from the device. These operations could interfere with other activities taking place on the network. Therefore, the imaging device may have to send an "interrupt" signal that indicates that a transmission is ready. The data may have to be transmitted in blocks of specified size (e.g., 256 kbyte transmission packets) that are recognizable to the network as part of a larger file of information.

The above-mentioned problems require both hardware and software solutions. Programs that control transmission of data to and from various components are called *device drivers*. The physical connectors must also be compatible with (i.e., can be attached and transmit signals to) other network components. Both hardware and software are implied in the term *interface*. Connecting a component to a computer or computer network in such a way that information may be transmitted is described as interfacing the component. There have been a number of attempts to standardize interfaces for imaging devices, including the American College of Radiology/National Electronics Manufacturers Association (ACR/NEMA) standards.[12]

Transmission media

Components of a network may be physically separated by distances varying from a few feet to several hundred miles or more. The transmission of digital information requires a transmission medium that is appropriate to the demands of the particular network. One of the most important factors to consider is the rate at which data are transmitted, measured in bits per second (bps).

Example 13-5[§]

A network is capable of transmitting data at a rate of 1 megabit per second (Mbps). If each pixel has a bit depth of 8 bits, how long will it take to transmit 50 512 × 512 images?

Since each pixel consists of 8 bits, the total number of bits is:

$$50 \left[8 \text{ bits/pixel} \times (512 \times 512 \text{ pixels}) \right] = 50 \left(2^3 \times 2^9 \times 2^9 \right) \text{ bits}$$
$$= 50 \left(2^{21} \right) \text{ bits} = 50 (2 \text{ Mbits}) = 100 \text{ Mbits}$$

The transmission time is then 100 Mbits / 1 Mbps = 100 seconds.

One of the least expensive transmission media is telephone wire (sometimes called *twisted pairs*). It is inexpensive and easy to install and maintain. However, the transmission rate does not usually exceed a few Mbps. Higher rates up to hundreds of Mbps

[§]This example is adapted from Hendee and Ritenour, 2001.

are achievable with coaxial cable. However, coaxial cable is more expensive, needs inline amplifiers, and is subject to electric interference problems in some installations. The highest transmission rates are achievable with fiber-optic cable. This transmission medium consists of glass fibers that transmit light pulses, thereby eliminating electrical interference problems. Transmission rates for fiber-optic cables are currently in the terabit per second (Tbps) range.

Data compression

Images are transmitted faster and require less storage space if they are composed of fewer bits. Decreasing the number of pixels reduces spatial resolution, however, and decreasing the bit depth decreases contrast sensitivity. It is possible, however, to "compress" image data in such a way that fewer bits of information are needed without significant loss of spatial or contrast resolution.

One way to reduce the number of bits is to encode pixel values in some sequence (e.g., row by row) to indicate the value of each pixel and the number of succeeding pixels with the same value. This decreases the total number of bits needed to describe the image, because most images have several contiguous pixels with identical values (e.g., the black border surrounding a typical CT image). Other techniques for data compression include analysis of the probability of occurrence of each pixel value, and assignment of a code to translate each pixel value to its corresponding probability. Such a "probability mapping" uses fewer bits for the more probable pixel values.[13]

In the examples above, the full information content of the image is preserved. When the image is expanded, it is exactly the same as it was before compression. These approaches to data compression are known as *lossless* (*bit-preserving*, or *nondestructive*) *techniques*. They may yield a reduction in the number of required bits by a factor of 3 or 4. When a greater reduction is needed, methods of data compression may be used that do not preserve the exact bit structure of an image, but still maintain acceptable diagnostic quality for the particular application. These techniques, known as *irreversible* (*non-bit-preserving* or *destructive*) *data compression methods*, can reduce the number of bits by an arbitrarily high factor.

An example of an irreversible data compression method involves the use of the Fourier transform to describe blocks of pixel values in the image. Some of the high- or low-frequency components of the image are then eliminated to reduce the number of bits required to store the image. When an inverse transform is used to restore the image, the loss of high or low spatial frequencies may not significantly detract from the diagnostic usefulness of the image.

Display stations and standards

The part of a computer network that is most accessible to the observer is the digital display or monitor, usually referred to as the *image workstation*. Some display stations are capable of displaying more data than are presented on the screen at one time. They may, initially, show images at reduced resolution (e.g., 1024 × 1024) while preserving the full "high-resolution" data set (e.g., 2048 × 2048) in memory. The stored data can be recalled in sections through user-selectable windows. Alternatively, only part of the image may be presented, but the part that is presented may be "panned" or moved around the full image.

Standards for digital matrix size and remote display of medical images that are acceptable for primary diagnosis from computer monitors have been established by the American College of Radiology (ACR).[12] These standards will continue to evolve as equipment performance (particularly display monitors) continues to improve. Current versions of the standards are available on the ACR web site (www.acr.org). Currently, two classes of images are recognized; small matrix systems and large matrix systems. Small matrix systems (CT, MRI, ultrasound, nuclear medicine, and digital fluoroscopy) must have a format of at least 5k × 5k × 8 bits. The display must be capable of displaying at least 5k × 0.48k × 8 bits. Large matrix systems (digitized radiographs, computed radiography) are held to a standard based upon required spatial and contrast resolution. For these imaging methods, the digital data must provide a resolution of at least 2.5 line pairs per millimeter and a 10 bit gray scale. The display must be capable of resolving 2.5 line pairs per millimeter with a minimum of 8 bit gray scale.

The industry-standard format for transferring images between components of a network is the Digital Imaging and Communications in Medicine or DICOM standard. The standard consists of specifications for various data "fields" that must occur in the image header. These fields describe attributes such as the matrix size of the image, whether it is part of a series (e.g., one slice of a multi-slice CT series), and patient demographic data. The development of the DICOM standard was initiated by the American College of Radiology (ACR) and the National Electrical Manufacturer's Association (NEMA) in 1985, and it continues to evolve as equipment capabilities change.

In 2004, the initiative known as Integrating the Healthcare Enterprise-Radiation Oncology (IHE-RO) was created to improve the functionality and data connections in radiation oncology clinics. The IHE-RO effort is collaborative between clinicians and industry representatives to develop industry standards to address issues of connectivity and other ambiguities.

Although the capabilities of "high-end" workstations are far from being standardized, some general features have been. A monitor should be able to display enough written information concerning the patient to obviate the need for transport of paper documents. The display station should be able to run image-processing software as well as provide simple display functions such as variable window level, window width, and magnification. Three dimensional reconstruction and tissue segmentation are common.

Computer requirements for treatment planning

No special or unusual requirements are imposed on computer systems for radiation therapy treatment planning. Today, treatment planning computers are assembled from components available "off the shelf" from a variety of manufacturers. Over the years, treatment planning software has been developed to run on standard high-powered desktop computers. As the capabilities of desktop computers have increased, these systems have become more powerful and suitable for treatment planning applications. Comprehensive treatment planning systems have been developed for both high-end workstations and personal desktop computers. These systems have superb graphics capabilities as well as fast processors, and they are able to handle large amounts of data. Desktop computers with GPU graphics cards can now provide equivalent or better functionality than these early workstations. For example, a number of CT or MR images can be stored. Modern 3D treatment planning computers also require large amounts of memory to store the calculated dose matrix.

Computers for treatment planning require several methods of data entry. Most systems are equipped with a *digitizer* for entering contours of anatomic structures, field shapes, and, in some cases, beam data. These systems require a mouse or some other pointing tool, as well as a keyboard. Although with the pervasive use of CT in radiation therapy, digitizers are becoming less common. To enter CT or other images, an optical disk drive or Ethernet connection will be used. A high-quality video monitor is needed, because the developing treatment plan frequently must be viewed by several people simultaneously. Finally, a laser printer is required and used for drawing the patient outline, treatment fields, and isodose curves to hardcopy. However, with electron medical records, hardcopy printouts as a method of documenting a patient's treatment plan are less and less common.

Summary

- Although computers in various forms have been available for centuries, it was the development of the transistor that ushered in the modern era of computers and information networking.
- Quantities can be expressed in many number systems; the most common systems are base 10 (decimal) and base 2 (binary).
- A single unit of information is a bit (*bi*nary digi*t*); multiples of bits make up bytes (8 bits) and words (16 or 32 bits).
- Many signal detectors and display systems are analog devices; analog-to-digital (ADCs) and digital-to-analog (DAC) converters function as interfaces between these devices and computer systems.
- Digital images are 2D matrices of pixels, with each pixel providing a bit depth for display of gray-scale information.

- Computer memory contains operational programs for the computer, and provides temporary storage for data being processed by the computer.
- The central processing unit (CPU) is the central control mechanism for the computer.
- Many input/output (I/O) devices are available, and several can serve both purposes.
- Mass data storage devices include magnetic disks and optical disks (CD-ROMS and DVDs).
- Computer languages exist at several levels, with high-level languages resembling the English language.
- Computer networks for medical imaging are frequently referred to by the acronyms IMACS, PACS, DIN, and LAN.
- Networks can be separated into two categories: centralized networks and distributed networks.
- Transmission media for information networks range from telephone lines to fiber-optic cable.
- In the transmission of digital images, data compression is usually required to reduce the data conversion and transmission time.
- Standards for transmitting images between components in a LAN are known as DICOM standards.
- Standards for image transmission from remote locations (teleradiology) have been established by the American College of Radiology.
- No special requirements are imposed on computer systems used for radiation therapy treatment planning.

Problems

13-1 Which of the following retains the information it's storing when the power to the system is turned off?
  a. ROM
  b. CPU
  c. DRAM
  d. SDRAM

13-2 What are the four essential functions of a computer?
  a. keyboard, display, memory, and disk drive
  b. word processing, spreadsheets, database, and Internet
  c. input, processing, output, and storage
  d. bits, bytes, words, and sentences

13-3 Related to protecting data sent over the Internet, what is SSL short for?
  a. Secure Socket LAN
  b. Software Security Layer
  c. Secure Software Layer
  d. Secure Socket Layer

13-4 Which storage device has the most capacity?
  a. 100 TB
  b. 100 KB
  c. 100 MB
  d. 100 GB

13-5 What does a screen resolution of 1280 × 800 measure?
  a. Pixels, height by width
  b. Pixels, width by height
  c. Millimeters, width by height
  d. Points, height by width

13-6 Convert the binary number 1110 0110 1001 1101 into decimal.

13-7 Convert the decimal number 1995 into binary.

13-8 Write 19 as a binary number. Multiply that binary number by the binary number 101. Check your answer by multiplying using the decimal system of multiplication.

13-9 You have a head and neck CT data set of 45 cm scan length and 0.5 cm slice thickness. There are 512 × 512 pixels per CT scan slide in the data set. A compression algorithm is used to reduce the "depth" of each pixel to 6 bits. How long will it take to transmit this data set from the CT scanner to the treatment planning system over a hospital network operating at 100 Mb per second (ignoring compression time and any other network delays)? How long would it take if your hospital's network was 1 Gb per second?

13-10 How many CT data sets described in Problem 13-9 (with compression) can be saved on a storage device with a capacity of 64 GB? How many for a storage device with a 1 TB capacity?

References

1 Mackintosh, A. R. The first electronic computer. *Phys. Today* 1987; **March**:25–32.

2 Mauchly, K. R. *IEEE Annals in the History of Computing*, Vol. 6. Piscataway, NJ, IEEE Computer Society, 1984, p. 116.

3 Hendee, W. R., and Ritenour, E. R. *Medical Imaging Physics*, 4th edition. New York, John Wiley & Sons, Ltd., 2001.

4 Moore, G. E. Cramming more components onto integrated circuits. *Electronics* 1965; **38**(8).

5 Bushberg, J. T., Seiberta, J. A., Leidholdt, E. M., and Boone, J. M. et al. *The Essential Physics of Medical Imaging*. Baltimore, Williams & Wilkins, 1994.

6 Glantz, J. Microprocessors deliver teraflops. *Science* 1996; **271**:598.

7 Hendee, W. R. *The Selection and Performance of Radiological Equipment*. Baltimore, Williams & Wilkins, 1985.

8 Johnson, N. D., Garofolo, G., and Geers, W. Demystifying the hospital information system/radiology information system integration process. *J. Digit. Imaging* 2000; **13**(2 Suppl. 1):175–179.

9 Langer, S. G. Architecture of an image capable, Web-based, electronic medical record. *J. Digit. Imaging* 2000; **13**(2):82–89.

10 Abbing, H. R. Medical confidentiality and electronic patient files. *Med. Law.* 2000; **19**(1):107–112.

11 Staggers, N. The vision for the Department of Defense's computer-based patient record. *Military Med.* 2000; **165**(3):180–185.

12 American College of Radiology. *Handbook of Teleradiology Applications*. Reston, VA, ACR, 1997.

13 Huang, H. K. *PACS: Basic principles and applications*. New York, John Wiley & Sons, Inc., 1999, Chapter 6.

14

RADIATION ONCOLOGY INFORMATICS

Objectives

After studying this chapter, the reader should be able to:
- Define informatics.
- Demonstrate how knowledge of informatics improves the practice of radiation oncology.
- Recognize what is an ontology and identify components of an ontology for radiation oncology.
- Identify information communication standards in radiation oncology.
- Describe the flow of information in the process of radiation therapy.

Introduction

One of the most profound, yet not widely recognized, changes in the practice of radiation oncology in the past 10–15 years has resulted from the explosion of information confronting the clinician in the management of the radiation oncology patient. The information formerly presented to the clinician was limited. Treatment plans were displayed on paper and treatment portals displayed on hardcopy radiographs. Treatment parameters were transferred manually from the hardcopy plan to the treatment machine, and radiation dose information was recorded manually on paper charts. This is no longer the case. The increased amount of information that is now acquired, transferred, and recorded far overwhelms the ability of an individual to process manually. Moreover, much of this information is now shared electronically as more institutions participate in inter-institutional protocols and clinical trials. In order to systematize the acquisition, processing, and interpretation of this information, the discipline of *informatics* has entered into the practice of radiation oncology.

Informatics, as applied to the medical domain, is the study of information in medical decision making. Such information is of various types, including textual information, such as patient demographics and physician reports; image information, such as radiographic images and histopathological images; statistical information, such as treatment records; lexicographic information, such as clinical nomenclature [Systematized Nomenclature of Medicine–Clinical Terms (SNOMED CT)][1] radiographic nomenclature (RADLEX)[2]; and other information such as genetic sequences[3].

In this chapter, the field of informatics as applied to radiation oncology will be explored. First investigated are how knowledge

---

Hendee's Radiation Therapy Physics, Fourth Edition. Todd Pawlicki, Daniel J. Scanderbeg and George Starkschall.
© 2016 John Wiley & Sons, Inc. Published 2016 by John Wiley & Sons, Inc.

in radiation oncology is represented and the way such knowledge is organized. Standards for communicating information—ensuring that information related to a patient's diagnosis, treatment, and outcome is done in a manner that is consistent and unambiguous—are explored. The next topic presented is the information flow in the course of a patient's radiation treatment, identifying what information is used and how it moves among components of the radiation treatment process. Next, the treatment planning process will be explored and the process of how information is acquired, transmitted, and applied in radiation treatment planning is explained. The chapter concludes with the identification of some potential future trends in radiation oncology informatics.

Ontologies

The first step in acquiring an understanding of how information flows through the radiation treatment process is the need for a uniform and consistent description of information flow. In order to do this an ontology is created. Ontology is defined by McShan as "a technology that is used to represent knowledge and information within a specified domain or area of interest."[4] Medical knowledge is highly structured, but representing this knowledge in natural language often hides the formalized structure.[5] An ontology provides an organized way to collect and represent medical knowledge using a database, making it easier, for example, for multiple institutions to share findings. The logic rules based on an ontology can be used to assist in clinical decision support.

In the domain of radiation oncology, one can establish an ontology for a knowledge database by the declaration of concepts, properties, relationships, and instances. Examples of *concepts* in radiation oncology include "Case," "PTV," "Treatment Beam," and "Radiation Dose."[4] These concepts have *properties* associated with them, such as "CreationDate" or "DoseUnits," and are related to other concepts via *relationships* between concepts. For example, the concept of "Treatment Plan" can be assigned a property "hasTreatmentBeam," which is a relationship to the concept "Treatment Beam." These objects can be instantiated to describe a particular *instance* of an object, that is, to provide each object with a specific value. For example, a treatment plan that consisted of parallel-opposed beams could be instantiated by creating an instance of the concept "Case" linked to an instance of the property "hasTreatmentPlan" to an instance of the concept "Treatment Plan" with the specific properties of "Name" and "Description," along with links to two instances of the object "Treatment Beam" along with the specific properties of each instance of the "Treatment Beam" object.

With the establishment of an ontology, an unambiguous understanding of concepts and their relationship can be provided, as well as enabling this knowledge to be interpreted by machine. With this information, research and clinical findings can be collected, organized, and characterized. A complete ontology for radiation oncology has not yet been developed; the magnitude of the knowledge model has so far precluded this from happening.[4]

Information standards

The communication of information among the various components of a radiation treatment system is essential for the accurate transfer of information, especially in an environment that may consist of components provided by various vendors. Although some vendors claim that a homogeneous environment with proprietary standards may result in a more accurate transfer of information, this argument is weakened when it is realized that even proprietary standards may change in time, so that an environment that is homogeneous at one time may not be so at a subsequent time. Moreover, most clinical environments are heterogeneous; users may elect to use the vendor's equipment that most closely meets their needs, and be unwilling to compromise equipment utility for ease of communication. Consequently, open information standards are necessary to ensure the accurate transfer of information among data sources and users, regardless of the environment. Recognizing this need, many vendors have adopted the Digital Imaging and Communications in Medicine (DICOM) Supplement 11, often referred to as *DICOM-RT*.

The original DICOM standard was developed to address images used in radiology; the DICOM-RT standard was developed as an extension of the DICOM Version 3.0 standard to handle the additional information in radiation oncology.[6] The RT extension defines a set of five objects associated with radiation oncology: RT Image, RT Plan, RT Dose, RT Structure Set, and RT Treatment Record. The RT Image object includes all planar images used in radiation oncology, including simulation images, portal images, and digitally reconstructed radiographs (DRRs), along with image specifications, such as pixel spacing, isocenter location, and descriptions of beam-limiting devices. The RT Plan object transfers geometric data and machine parameters from the treatment planning system to the record and verify system to the radiation delivery device and includes patient setup information, beam information, and dose prescriptions. The RT Dose object includes dose data, such as dose matrices, point doses, isodose curves, and dose-volume histograms (DVHs). The RT Structure Set object includes patient-related regions of interest and points of interest. Finally, the RT Treatment Record object includes all treatment session data, summaries of recording information, dose calculations, and dose measurements.

An important point to note is the need for consistent geometries among components in the radiation treatment process. Both the DICOM standard and the International Electrotechnical Commission (IEC) define coordinate system conventions,[7] but there is a significant difference between the two conventions for the patient coordinate system. The DICOM coordinate system is an image-based system in which the +X direction is to the right of a transverse image and the +Y direction is to the bottom

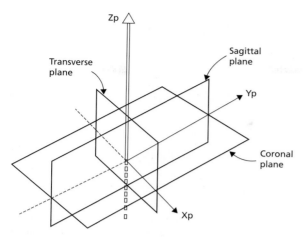

Figure 14-1 The IEC patient coordinate system.

of the image. Because it is a right-handed coordinate system, the +Z direction is toward the patient's head. In the IEC coordinate system, the +X direction is to the right of the patient, the +Y direction is toward the patient's head, and the +Z direction is toward the anterior of the patient. Figure 14-1 illustrates the IEC patient coordinate system.

Even with communication standards such as DICOM-RT, manufacturers of radiation oncology equipment still need to demonstrate that these standards allow the transfer of information among different manufacturers' platforms. To facilitate the implementation of these communication standards, a project entitled *Integrating the Healthcare Enterprise in Radiation Oncology* (IHE-RO) was developed under the sponsorship of the American Society for Radiation Oncology in collaboration with the American Association of Physicists in Medicine, the Radiological Society of North America, and the Healthcare Information and Management Systems Society. IHE-RO performs its tasks by developing and testing *IHE Integration Profiles*, which are use cases that describe solutions to specific integration problems. Participants in IHE-RO typically meet on a regular basis to test these cases in *Connectathons*, and provide regular public demonstrations of their connectivity.

Information flow in radiation oncology

Information regularly moves from one component of a radiation oncology system to another. Originally, a paper chart was used to communicate information. The paper chart will be used as a paradigm, because this model is relatively easy to understand. The paper chart has several advantages. It is fast, easy to use and modify, adaptable for the specific needs and workflow of the clinical practice, and relatively inexpensive to implement.[8] Furthermore, users have a high comfort level with this existing system. However, paper charts are not conducive to a safe communication environment, supporting real-time and team-based decision making, quality improvement, and outcome analysis.

The complexity of contemporary radiation oncology practice—combined with the aforementioned needs for supporting real-time and team-based decision making, quality improvement, and outcome analysis—have prompted the development of automated information flow systems. The simplest approach to an automated information flow system is to mimic previous processes and workflow. However, such an approach may be restrictive, lack integration, connectivity, and flexibility to modify processes. The challenge has been to establish an electronic-based information management system that meets clinical and administrative process needs, allows connectivity among multiple systems and technologies, and supports multiple workflows. Modern systems need to take into account users providing data input into the system and extract output. These users include radiation oncologists, medical physicists, dosimetrists, radiation therapists, nurses, administrative staff, and IS/IT staff. Moreover, the information management system also needs to account for interactions among users.

Information management systems need to take into account the processes that take place in a radiation oncology practice. These include the clinical and administrative activities, such as writing prescriptions, scheduling treatments, developing treatment plans, and associate these processes with the users that are involved in the processes. These processes are the fundamental elements of work in a practice. It is important to identify what information is needed for each step of a process and when this information can be captured. Consider an analogy with the paper chart: if a chart containing a treatment plan is on the physicist's desk, then the treatment plan needs to be checked. The process is the checking of a treatment plan, the user is the physicist, and the information is the treatment plan. When dealing with information transmitted electronically, it is necessary to have a well-defined workflow to ensure that each step of a process is achieved at the correct time. Figure 14-2 illustrates an example of such a workflow in radiation therapy.

The practice of radiation oncology follows a set of basic processes. In order to manage the processes effectively, it is necessary that information be available at the time of use. Nine basic processes have been defined that support clinical workflow.[8,9] These are:

- patient registration
- consultation
- departmental scheduling
- departmental charting
- set-up for treatment simulation
- treatment planning
- treatment delivery
- administrative services
- quality assurance.

The first process, patient registration, involves the acquisition of all relevant demographic information pertaining to the patient, for example, identity, insurance coverage, family members, and referring physician. In a radiation oncology information system that is integrated with the hospital information

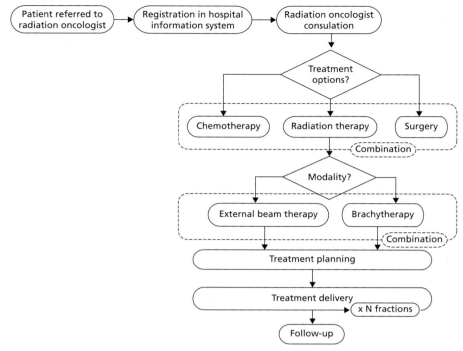

Figure 14-2 Diagram of integrated cancer treatment workflow, focusing on radiation therapy component.
Source: Courtesy of Luis Fong de los Santos, PhD, Mayo Clinic.

system such information can be readily extracted from the hospital information system. Otherwise, it needs to be entered specifically and checked against the information stored in the hospital information system.

In the consultation process, information is exchanged between the patient and the radiation oncologist, and decisions are made regarding the therapeutic plan. During the treatment, relevant information is generated and gathered to support treatment decisions, the clinical outcome is monitored and assessed, and feedback is provided to the patient. Additional information is acquired after the conclusion of treatment during follow-up examinations. Before, during, and after treatment, large amounts of information are acquired from various members of the radiation oncology team; it is highly desirable to use structured and template-based entry to assist in the analysis of these large amounts of information.

The next process, departmental scheduling, involves coordinating the time of staff members and resources. The availability of treatment machines and examination rooms must be considered, as well as that of personnel. The system needs to avoid conflicts of resources and providers. As in the case of the patient registration process, coordination with the hospital scheduling system would be an ideal, but it is rarely achievable.

The department chart is the prime location for patient treatment information. The chart records all relevant data for a single patient, for example, documentation of the patient history, results from physical examinations, pathology studies, nursing notes, records of treatment, and recording of simulation, planning, and portal images. Replacement of the traditional paper chart by an electronic chart has been a difficult transition for many radiation oncology practices. One of the primary advantages of the electronic chart is its portability. Staff does not need to search for paper charts; an electronic chart allows access for viewing and modification at multiple locations by multiple authorized users.

The process of set-up for treatment simulation involves the acquisition of two-dimensional (2D) and three-dimensional (3D) images in order to locate the target, define the isocenter, and set the patient up. Important in this process is the need to accurately transfer the coordinate system from the set-up (conventional or CT simulator) to the treatment planning computer to the treatment machine.

In the treatment planning process, simulation information is combined with information from other diagnostic imaging modalities to select the number, orientation, and characteristics of radiation beams to achieve the therapeutic goal. Once this beam information is determined, information needs to be transferred from the treatment planning to the record and verify system to the treatment delivery system. In addition, images derived from the planning system, such as DRRs, need to be transferred to the record and verify system as well.

Treatment parameters obtained by the treatment delivery system from the treatment planning system are reviewed and verified, and the treatment is delivered and recorded. With the increased use of sophisticated beam delivery systems—such as intensity-modulated radiation therapy and dynamic delivery systems—the automatic transfer of treatment parameters from the treatment planning system to the treatment delivery system is essential, as is the need for verification of the delivery.

Administrative services in a radiation oncology clinic include billing, patient education, report generation, and data collection and analysis. Linking the billing system to scheduling and code capture upon completion of tasks can improve efficiency. Automated data collection can facilitate the generation of reports that can improve the quality, safety, and efficiency of the radiation oncology practice.

The process of quality assurance was originally based on measuring and assessing the performance of radiation therapy devices and equipment in terms of predefined tolerances so as to guarantee satisfactory overall treatment delivery (e.g., within 5% of the prescribed dose)[10]. A new paradigm, however, has been developed that includes a focus on process mapping and formal risk analysis strategies.[11] Although tolerances are still a component of the new paradigm, in order to support this approach, overall information flow and workflow must now be included in the quality assurance process.

Informatics for treatment planning

The accurate flow of information is especially necessary in the process of radiation treatment planning. Mageras et al.[12] identify the following basic steps of workflow of the treatment planning process:

1 Acquisition of volumetric images.
2 Transfer of images and data to the radiation treatment planning system.
3 Definition of volumes of interest.
4 Design of treatment machine parameters.
5 Design of reference images for localization.
6 Calculation of radiation dose.
7 Review and approval of the treatment plan.
8 Transfer of the radiation treatment plan and reference images to the system that controls the localization imaging equipment and treatment machine.

Volumetric images of the patient are primarily acquired via CT scanning. In the CT image, each element of the image is represented by a pixel. The product of the pixel area and the thickness of the CT slice constitute a voxel. The digital value of the voxel is expressed as a CT number, which is related to the linear attenuation coefficient of the contents of the voxel. Although CT numbers are conventionally presented to the user in terms of Hounsfield units, ranging from −1000, representing air, through 0, which represents water, to values of 1000–2000, which represent bone, for the purposes of computation, numbers are represented as 12-bit unsigned integers, ranging from 0 to 4095.

CT images are typically acquired with a beam of energy in the range of 120–140 kVp, whereas radiation treatment is delivered with a megavoltage photon beam. The linear attenuation coefficient in the CT energy range contains a large component due to the photoelectric effect, which is highly dependent on the atomic number of the absorber, whereas the linear attenuation coefficient in the treatment energy range is almost entirely due to Compton scatter, which primarily reflects mass density; consequently, one typically incorporates a nonlinear conversion table to relate CT number to mass density.

Software systems have replaced the radiographic simulator to perform the functions of patient alignment, target and normal tissue localization, virtual fluoroscopy, definition of reference isocenter points, design of treatment portals, and generation of DRRs. One can also obtain information from MR or PET imaging; if such information is obtained, it is important to accurately register these images to the planning CT image dataset. Images acquired from CT, MR, PET, etc., are then transferred, perhaps via a picture archival and communications system (PACS), to the treatment planning system for dose calculation. In the treatment planning system, the treatment plan is generated and transferred to the treatment delivery system.

In contemporary radiation treatment planning, the required data infrastructure needs to be sufficient to handle large amounts of data. A single CT slice uses approximately 0.5 MB of space. A typical CT study with 200 slices uses 100 MB, while a 4D CT study, which typically may consist of 10 phases, uses 1 GB. Finally, a cone-beam CT image uses approximately 35 MB per scan. Moreover, the data storage needs to be redundant, which also increases storage requirements.

The treatment planning process can be viewed as a simulation of the interactions of a set of radiation beams with the patient. In addition to accurate spatial information about the patient, image information must include information about the tissue density and composition. This information must define accurate positional relationships among the images forming the 3D volume. Pixel size must be uniform, image contrast must be sufficient to discern boundaries between anatomical structures, and conversion of CT numbers to electron densities must be accurate. It is important to achieve correct spatial relationships in the display of volumetric images and the superposition of treatment planning information. Each image in the CT data set identifies an image position (the coordinates of the center of the first pixel of image) and image orientation (the orientation of first row and first column of image with patient). All images in the data set must have the same orientation. Images are ordered by the image position and CT values are mapped onto window width and window level values. All of these requirements appear to be rather straightforward, but require careful programming and quality assurance at both the manufacturer's level and the user's level to ensure that images are recorded and accurately transferred from the imaging system to the treatment planning system, and that geometric relationships are further transferred accurately to the treatment delivery device.

Image segmentation is the process of defining volumetric *regions of interest* (ROIs). This can be done either manually or automatically. Several methods are available for the representation of ROIs. One method of representing volumes is by the use of contours on axial images. A second method represents the ROIs using a polygonal mesh to define the surface of the ROI, whereas a third method encodes each voxel with a number whose nth bit is 1 if the voxel lies within the nth ROI and 0 if the voxel does not. Each representation has its own advantages. The contour representation directly acquires the ROI from segmentation on individual axial CT images and is a direct offshoot from 2D treatment planning. The mesh representation makes it easy to display the surface of ROIs. The bit coding representation makes it easier to calculate dose-volume quantities.

Image information from multiple imaging modalities can often be used to aid in the treatment planning process, often to define ROIs. In order to allow information from other imaging modalities to be incorporated into a treatment plan, image registration is required. Image registration is the determination of the geometrical transformation that maps points of an object in one image to corresponding points of that object in another image. Image registration may include translations, rotations, and scaling, as well as various forms of deformable image registration.

In order to determine treatment planning parameters, it is necessary to display the radiation beams. In a 2D display, the central axis and field edges of the beams are superimposed on axial slice. In contemporary 3D treatment planning, a *beam's-eye view* (BEV) is superimposed on a DRR. The use of the BEV display enables the treatment planning to define beam apertures to ensure that the target volume is irradiated and critical structures are shielded. The DRR is the digital equivalent of the simulation film and is used as a reference image for localization. A DRR is generated by projecting the 3D image volume onto a 2D image in which the image brightness corresponds to density-dependent attenuation. Rays are cast from the imaging source to each grid point on the DRR plane and the attenuation of the ray through the 3D CT image is calculated.

Once the treatment parameters have been determined, the radiation dose is calculated and the treatment plan is displayed. Typical display information includes dose distributions, either as 2D isodose lines or 3D dose clouds, and DVHs. The radiation oncologist reviews and approves the treatment plan. Finally, the treatment plan and reference images are archived and the information transferred to the treatment machine.

Future trends in radiation oncology informatics

Radiation oncology informatics is still a rather immature science, and there is much potential for growth in the study of information flow and its applications. Moore et al. have identified several trends in radiation oncology informatics.[13] Included among these are the use of data aggregation and cloud computing. *Data aggregation* is the ability to access and analyze data and synthesize information from many different patients over multiple institutions. Current clinical radiation therapy computation systems are being developed to take a single patient through the simulation, planning, and treatment processes with the goal of facilitating the transfer of information from one application to the next. However, such systems are not optimized for multi-patient retrospective data analyses. For example, if one needs to perform a study requiring data from treatment plans of a cohort of Stage III non-small-cell lung cancer patients, instead of retrieving a large number of treatment plans from the archives of a treatment planning system, certain to be a tedious process, a well-designed information retrieval system should be able to provide the desired information efficiently and quickly. A cloud-based system using a common server for data storage, and accessible via the Internet, can facilitate multi-institutional studies.[14] Another example in which *cloud computing* might be of use for data aggregation would be the use of accelerator log files to determine normative trends in treatment delivery. A major advantage of cloud computing is that many of the routine system maintenance tasks are shifted from the end user to the server host. Much of the software and hardware typically purchased for each user simply become a service analogous to a utility service, such as electricity or water. This results in computing models of software as a service (SaaS), platform as a service (PaaS), and infrastructure as a service (IaaS). These also include such activities as regular back up and disaster mitigation. On the other hand, the host needs to ensure that appropriate security and privacy policies are in effect.

Summary

- Informatics is the study of information in medical decision making.
- An ontology provides an organized way to collect and represent medical knowledge using a database. A complete ontology for radiation oncology does not yet exist.
- Open information standards are necessary to ensure the accurate transfer of information among data sources and users regardless of the environment. The primary standard presently used is the DICOM-RT standard.
- Information transfer using the DICOM-RT standard is frequently tested among vendors using various test cases in the IHR-RO project.
- An understanding of the information flow in the radiation oncology process is necessary to automate the information flow system.
- The application of informatics to radiation oncology is relatively immature, and many opportunities exist for its implementation in the future.

Problems

14-1 What is meant by a *database ontology*?
14-2 What is the benefit of using an ontology?
14-3 How does DICOM-RT differ from DICOM?

14-4   Radiation oncology has undergone several advancements since the DICOM-RT standard was first formulated several years ago. Can you identify quantities that are in current use in radiation oncology that are not presently included in the DICOM-RT standard?

14-5   Compare the advantages and disadvantages of presenting radiation oncology information in a structured database versus in a free-form text.

14-6   What obstacles can be anticipated in a transition from a paper chart to an electronic record-keeping system?

14-7   Related to cloud computing; what do *SaaS*, *IaaS*, and *PaaS* stand for?

References*

1 *SNOMED Clinical Terms*, https://www.nlm.nih.gov/research/umls/Snomed/snomed_main.html, accessed September 15, 2015.

2 *What is RadLex?*, http://www.rsna.org/radlex.aspx, accessed September 15, 2015.

3 Genetic Sequence Data Bank. *NCBI-GenBank Flat File Release 173.0 Distribution Release Notes: August 15 2009.* Available at ftp://ftp.ncbi.nih.gov/genbank/gbrel.txt, accessed September 15, 2015.

4 McShan D. L. Ontology for radiation oncology. In *Informatics in Radiation Oncology*, R. Alfredo C. Siochi, and G. Starkschall (eds.). Boca Raton, FL, Taylor & Francis.

5 Miller, A. A., *Developing an ontology for radiation oncology*, Master's Thesis, University of Woolongong, 2012.

6 Starkschall, G., and Balter, P., Informatics in radiation oncology. In Kagadis, G. C. and Langer, S. G. (eds.), *Informatics in Medical Imaging*, Boca Raton, FL, Taylor & Francis, 2011, pp. 325–331.

7 International Electrotechnical Commission. *IEC 61217: Radiotherapy equipment: Coordinates, movements, and scales.* Geneva: IEC, 1999.

8 Brooks, K. Radiation oncology information management system. In *The Modern Technology of Radiation Oncology*, J. Van Dyk (ed.). Madison, WI, Medical Physics Publishing, 1999, pp. 509–520.

9 Brooks, K. W., Fox, T. H., and Davis, D. L. Advanced therapy information management systems: An oncology information systems RFP toolkit. In J. D. Hazle, and A. L. Boyer (eds.). *Imaging in Radiation Therapy.* Madison, WI, Medical Physics Publishing, 1998.

10 International Commission on Radiation Units and Measurement. *Determination of absorbed dose in a patient irradiated by beams of x- or gamma-rays in radiotherapy procedures: ICRU Rep. 24.* Bethesda, MD, ICRU, 1976.

11 Huq, M. S., Fraass, B. A., Dunscombe, P. B., Gibbons, J. P., Ibbott, G. S., et al. A method for evaluating quality assurance needs in radiation therapy. *Int. J. Radiat. Oncol. Biol. Phys.* 2008; **71**(Suppl):S170–S173.

12 Mageras, G. S., Hu, Y.-C., McNamara, S., Pham, H., and Xiong, J.-P. Imaging for radiation treatment planning. In *Informatics in Radiation Oncology*, R. Alfredo C. Siochi, and G. Starkschall (eds.). Boca Raton, FL, Taylor & Francis, pp. 191–206.

13 Moore, K. L., Kagadis, G. C., McNutt, T. R., Moiseenko, V., and Mutic, S. Automation and advanced computing in clinical radiation oncology. *Med. Phys.* 2014; **41**(1).

14 Kagadis, G. C., Kloukinas, C., Moore, K., Philbin, J., Papadimitroulas, P., et al. Cloud computing in medical imaging. *Med. Phys.* 2013; **40**(7):070901.

Informatics in Radiation Oncology, edited by R. Alfredo C. Siochi, and G. Starkschall, copyright © 2013 Taylor & Francis is a good supplementary reference to this chapter.

15

PHYSICS OF PROTON RADIATION THERAPY

Objectives

After studying this chapter the reader should be able to:
- Recognize the properties of protons that make them desirable for radiation therapy.
- Identify methods for producing proton beams.
- Identify methods for generating a useful proton beam for radiation therapy.
- Differentiate between beams produced by cyclotrons versus synchrotrons.
- Differentiate between passive scattering methods and spot scanning methods for proton beam delivery and in proton treatment planning.
- Recognize the various uncertainties in proton radiation therapy and how they can be accounted for in radiation therapy.

Introduction

The idea that proton beams may have application in radiation therapy was first identified by Wilson in 1946[1] but the first clinical use of a proton beam occurred in 1954 at the Lawrence Berkeley Laboratory for irradiation of the pituitary for hormone suppression of patients with metastatic breast cancer. The first patients treated with protons at the Harvard Cyclotron laboratory were treated in 1961, also for irradiation of the pituitary gland. The first hospital-based facility was built in 1990 at the Loma Linda University Medical Center in southern California. In 2001, another hospital-based facility was established at the Massachusetts General Hospital in Boston, Massachusetts. Since that time, proton facilities have become widespread; presently about 10–15 hospital-based facilities are operational in North America with another 10–15 in the planning stage or under construction.

Several properties of protons make them desirable for radiation therapy.[1,2] As is described in Chapter 3, charged particles deposit energy approximately uniformly as they penetrate tissue, stopping abruptly after penetrating a finite range. In that way, protons are much like electrons. However, several other properties of protons make them dosimetrically more desirable than

Hendee's Radiation Therapy Physics, Fourth Edition. Todd Pawlicki, Daniel J. Scanderbeg and George Starkschall.

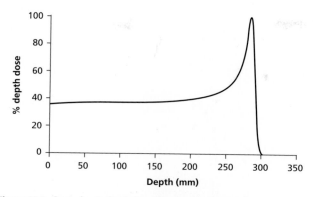

Figure 15-1 Central-axis depth dose distribution in water for a 250 MeV unmodulated proton beam.

electrons. One such property is an increase in the deposition of energy as the particle reaches the end of its range, giving rise to dose enhancement known as a *Bragg peak*. Moreover, because the proton mass is about 2000 times that of the electron, protons undergo far less scatter than do electrons. As a consequence, protons deposit very little dose beyond the range of the radiation beam. Figure 15-1 illustrates the depth dose distribution of a monoenergetic proton beam.

However, as can be seen in Figure 15-1, the *pristine Bragg peak* from a monoenergetic proton beam is too narrow to satisfactorily encompass a typical target volume. Consequently, in a typical proton treatment, monoenergetic proton beams of various energies are combined to deliver a more uniform dose to the target. This combination of energies produces a *spread-out Bragg peak* (SOBP). The addition of the lower-energy beam components increases the dose proximal to the tumor, but provides a uniform dose to the target volume. Figure 15-2 illustrates how beam components of various energies are added to the initial proton beam to generate an SOBP.

It should be noted that there is no "free lunch." Whereas a monoenergetic proton beam has a low surface dose, when the

SOBP is created to treat a clinical target volume the composite surface dose can be quite high. The significant benefit of proton beams is the dose falloff distal to the target. This, however, is also a source of uncertainty in proton therapy, as is discussed later in this chapter.

Production of proton beams

The two major types of proton accelerators in present clinical use are cyclotrons and synchrotrons. Major distinctions between the two types of accelerators are that the cyclotron has continuous output, whereas the output of the synchrotron is in packets of protons, known as *spills*. The cyclotron produces proton beams of a single, fixed-beam energy; the depth of the Bragg peak is adjusted via range modulation. Synchrotrons can vary the beam energy, allowing for *spot scanning*, a procedure in which a narrow pencil beam delivering a high dose in a Bragg peak to a single spot is moved via magnetic steering and energy variation through a target volume.

The basic principle of operation of a cyclotron is that charged particles accelerate in D-shaped electrodes (*dees*) with a high-frequency alternating voltage. Applying a static magnetic field in the direction perpendicular to the plane of the electrodes causes the charged particles to move in a spiral path until they leave the beam tube. More details of the operation of the cyclotron are given in Chapter 4.

As noted in Chapter 4, cyclotrons are not suitable for accelerating electrons, because the electrons used in therapy are relativistic; hence the synchronization between the emergence of particles from the dees and the changing polarity across the dees is lost. However, because of their greater mass, the protons used in radiation therapy are less relativistic, and can be accelerated effectively in a cyclotron. The beam extracted from the cyclotron is continuous and monoenergetic; the beam energy can be adjusted quickly using a range modulator to degrade the energy of the beam before it enters the patient. Protons are produced in a cyclotron by ionizing hydrogen gas. Features of a cyclotron include a radiofrequency (RF) system to accelerate protons, a magnetic field to keep the protons in a spiral path, and a beam extraction system.

Synchrotrons can be used to accelerate protons to energies of up to around 250 MeV, which have a maximum penetration depth of about 30 cm in tissue and are useful energies in radiation therapy. Synchrotrons use a time-dependent magnetic field, synchronized to the particle beam of increasing kinetic energy. Protons in a synchrotron are accelerated in spills until the desired energy is reached. The protons are initially accelerated in a linear accelerator to 2–7 MeV before they are injected into the synchrotron. The protons are then accelerated to the desired energy (70–250 MeV) before being extracted. Energy is then ramped down to the initial state and protons that have not been extracted into the beam line are dumped.

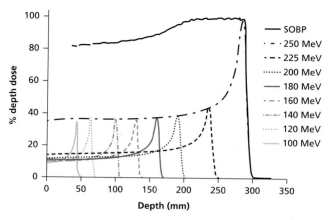

Figure 15-2 Addition of multiple beam components to initial proton beam to generate spread-out Bragg peak.

Proton Therapy

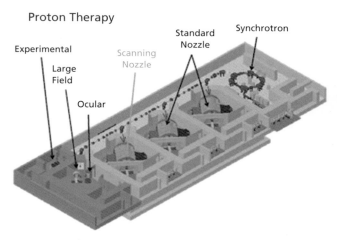

Figure 15-3 A diagram of the proton facility at The University of Texas MD Anderson Cancer Center. The synchrotron is placed at one end of the building and various beam lines are extracted, including several passively scattered beams, scanned beams, and research beams.

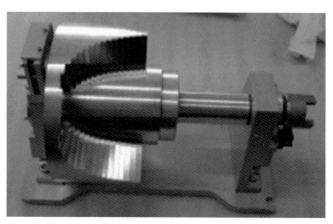

Figure 15-4 A range modulation wheel used to create an SOBP. *Source:* Courtesy of X. R. Zhu, UT MD Anderson Cancer Center.

Typical clinical accelerators have a rather small *duty cycle*. That is, the clinically useful beam is on and directed toward the patient only a small fraction of the time the patient is in the treatment room. As a consequence, proton linear accelerators do not deliver radiation beams a large percentage of the time. Because a proton beam can be magnetically steered, the accelerator can be placed in one room and the proton beam can be steered into one of several treatment rooms, allowing for multiple beam lines and a more efficient utilization of the proton accelerator. Figure 15-3 illustrates the multiple beam lines in use at a proton facility.

Machines used to generate clinical proton beams need to possess several characteristics. Generally, the proton beam exiting an accelerator is essentially monoenergetic. In order to generate an SOBP it is necessary to have some method of modulating the range of beam by varying the energy of the incident beam. Moreover, to generate a clinically useful beam, there must be a method of spreading the beam laterally. The proton beam energy can be modulated in two ways. If the beam is generated in a fixed-energy machine, for example, a cyclotron, the proton beam energy is modulated after extraction from the accelerator. This process is known as *downstream energy modulation*. A *range modulator* is used to effect downstream energy modulation. A range modulator is typically a rotating wheel of varying thickness. Passing through a specified thickness of absorber reduces the energy of the proton beam by a fixed amount. Figure 15-4 illustrates such a range modulation wheel. Alternatively, a variable energy accelerator, such as a synchrotron, can vary the proton energy prior to exiting the accelerator. This process is known as *upstream energy modulation*.

Characteristics of clinical proton beams

Several terms are used to characterize the SOBP in a clinical proton beam.[3] These include the *range*, defined as the depth of the

distal 90% dose level (d90), the *modulation width*, defined as the distance between the proximal 90 or 95% dose level (p90 or p95) and d90, and the *distal margin*, defined as the distance between d80 and d20. The distal margin is also called the *distal dose falloff* or *distal penumbra*. These terms are illustrated in Figure 15-5. Beam profile characteristics are defined based on decrements, or the percentage dose compared to the central-axis dose. The *field size* is defined to be the distance between 50% decrements, and the *lateral penumbra* is defined to be either the distance between the 20% and the 80% decrements or the distance between the 50% and the 95% decrements.

The proton beam dose monitor is typically calibrated based on the procedure outlined in IAEA Report 398[4] and is usually given in terms of the physical dose, whereas dose prescriptions are typically given in terms of cobalt gray equivalent (CGE) dose, incorporating a relative biological effectiveness (RBE) of 1.1. Because the CGE dose is different from the physical dose, it is important to clearly identify which dose is meant in a dose specification.

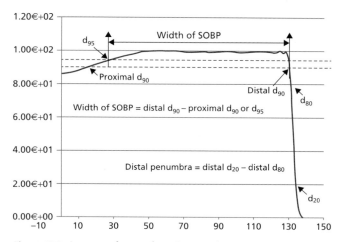

Figure 15-5 Anatomy of a spread-out Bragg peak. *Source:* Courtesy of X. R. Zhu, UT MD Anderson Cancer Center.

The beam energy is selected by determining the point of deepest penetration of the proton beam with a sufficient margin to account for both distal falloff and uncertainties in the determination of the range of the proton beam in the patient. Energies might be modified if it is necessary to prevent the overlap of matching fields, if matching fields are used. Ideally, one would use a single field, but in order to limit the dose proximal to the SOBP, it may be necessary to use multiple fields. Also due to range uncertainties, it is not always safe to point the radiation beam directly at a critical structure if insufficient margin exists between the target volume and a critical structure and target volume, that is, it is important not to place a critical structure in a region of possible distal dose falloff.

The field size of a proton beam is somewhat limited by passive scattering systems, but is typically greater for scanning systems. The lateral penumbra of a proton beam is caused both by a finite source size (geometric penumbra) and multiple Coulomb scattering. The amount of scattering increases as the protons lose energy with depth, hence the beam penumbra increases with depth. The distal penumbra is caused by range straggling, but for passively scattered beams, it is also affected by scattering in the range modulator.

Generating a clinically useful beam

Passive scattering

The beam generated from an accelerator is a monoenergetic pencil beam; both the lateral dose distribution as well as the axial dose distribution are narrow and peaked. Both dose distributions must be spread out so that the beam will be clinically useful. Earlier in the chapter, it is noted how the SOBP can be generated using range modulation; in order to spread the beam laterally, one either combines range modulation with passive scattering or uses a scanned beam. Several mechanisms are used to generate a broad, spatially uniform proton beam via passive scattering. A single scatterer of high-Z material (lead or tantalum) can spread the beam into a Gaussian-shaped peak. More efficiency can be achieved by scattering more of the central portion of beam toward the periphery; this differential scattering can be achieved by the use of a contoured scatterer that is thicker in the center than at the edges.

More commonly used is a double scattering mechanism, in which the first scatterer generates a Gaussian-shaped beam profile, spreading the beam to a second, contoured scatterer, which flattens the beam. The second scatterer includes an occluding plug to block protons in the center of the Gaussian peak. Figure 15-6 illustrates the physics of the passive scattering mode of proton beam delivery.

The region of distal falloff of the proton beam can be further modified to track the distal edge of a target volume by the use of a compensating bolus placed near the patient surface. The bolus selectively degrades the proton energy generating a beam with

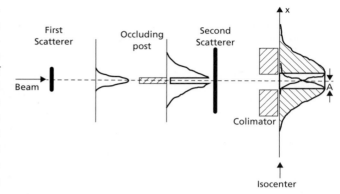

Figure 15-6 Physics of the passive scattering mode of proton beam delivery.

spatially varying range. Figure 15-7 illustrates the use of a compensating bolus to modify the region of distal falloff. Note, however, that using a compensating bolus allows sparing of distal structures but does not allow sparing of structures proximal to the target volume.

Scanning beams

The alternative to passive scattering is the use of a scanned pencil beam to generate a clinically useful dose distribution. In scanning mode, which can deliver a beam of varying energy, a pencil beam of protons is scanned across the target volume using dynamically varying scanning magnets. The energy is then changed, resulting in a change in range, and the beam is then rescanned across the target volume. Because the protons exit a synchrotron in beam spills, the combination of a pencil beam and a Bragg peak results in the dose being delivered into the target volume in the form of a small spot, hence this technique is often referred to as *spot scanning*. Table 15-1 compares passive scattering and spot scanning. Figure 15-8 illustrates the delivery of the dose into a rectangular target volume in the form of spots.

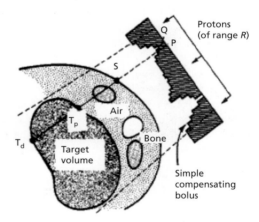

Figure 15-7 Compensating bolus used to modify the region of distal falloff. *Source:* Urie 1983.[5] Reproduced with permission from IOP Publishing.

Table 15-1 A comparison of passive scattering and spot scanning.

Passive scattering	Spot scanning
• Mature technology	• New technology
• Field-specific hardware (collimators) required	• Field-specific hardware not required
• Patient-specific aperture	• Scan defines lateral extent of beam
• Absence of proximal dose conformity	• Proximal and distal dose conformity
• Large gantry required	• Smaller gantry
• Less sensitive to organ motion	• More sensitive to organ motion
• High loss of protons	• Efficient use of protons
• Neutron produced in range modulator and scatterer	• Less neutron production
• Only supports 3D planning	• Supports intensity-modulated proton therapy (IMPT)

Table 15-2 Proton beam range as a function of field size and energy for the MD Anderson passively scattered proton beam.

Nominal energy (MeV)	Range in water (cm)		
	10 cm × 10 cm	18 cm × 18 cm	25 cm × 25 cm
100	4.9	4.3	4.3
120	6.9	6.4	6.3
140	10.2	10.0	8.4
160	13.4	13.0	11.0
180	16.9	16.1	13.7
200	21.8	19.0	16.5
225	26.9	23.6	20.6
250	32.4	28.5	25.0

Proton treatment planning

Regardless of whether passive scattering or spot scanning is used, proton-beam treatment planning is designed to take advantage of the high-dose Bragg peak and steep falloff distal to the Bragg peak. Ideally, the SOBP would cover the entire target volume; consequently, the selection of energy is based on the depth of the distal edge of the target volume.

Planning with passive scattering

In selecting an energy using a passively scattered proton beam, it is important to note that the range of the proton beam is dependent on the size of the second scatterer. For example, the passively scattered proton beam from the synchrotron at The University of Texas MD Anderson Cancer Center allows for eight nominal energies and three uncollimated field sizes, dependent on the second scatterer used for lateral spreading of the beam. These field sizes are 10 cm × 10 cm, 18 cm × 18 cm, and 25 cm × 25 cm, giving 24 possible field size and energy combinations,

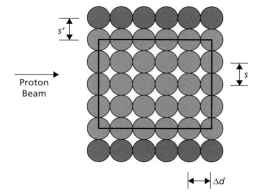

Figure 15-8 Illustrates how a target volume can be irradiated with a series of proton spots. Δd is the spot spacing in depth and is typically 0.1–0.5 cm. The spot spacings, s and s′, are typically approximately half the full width at half-maximum (FWHM) of the Gaussian pencil beam profile.
Source: Courtesy of X. R. Zhu, UT MD Anderson Cancer Center.

each with a different proton beam range. Table 15-2 illustrates the range of the proton beam as a function of size of the second scatterer and energy.

Once the energy has been selected to ensure coverage of at least the distal edge of the target volume, the beam must be shaped, both laterally and in depth. Lateral beam shaping is achieved with an aperture designed to encompass the target volume with an appropriate margin (which is discussed later in this chapter) and are fabricated out of 2 cm slabs of brass using a milling machine. Depth shaping is achieved using a compensating filter designed so that the range of the proton beam can track the distal surface of the target volume. Compensators are typically fabricated out of tissue-equivalent material such as Lucite or wax. Figure 15-9 illustrates an aperture and a compensating filter used to shape a passively scattered proton beam.

Determining appropriate margins is somewhat more complicated for a proton beam than for a photon beam. The concept of a *planning target volume* (PTV) does not apply to proton-beam treatment planning as it does for photon and electron-beam planning. The PTV, defined to be the volume that encompasses the *clinical target volume* (CTV) with margins for motion and setup uncertainty, can only be used to design the aperture margins.[6] The proximal and distal margins are beam-specific rather than setup-specific and address, in addition to uncertainties in setup, uncertainties in the conversion of CT number to stopping power leading to uncertainties in proton range. The aperture margin is designed to account for both the setup uncertainty and the penumbra. As with photon and electron beam treatments, the setup uncertainty is usually taken to be 3–5 mm depending on the treatment site and the rigidity of immobilization, whereas the penumbra is the measured distance from the 50% decrement to approximately the 95% decrement. The distal margin is determined to be equal to 0.035 times the depth of the distal edge of the CTV plus 3 mm. This margin accounts for a 3.5% uncertainty in the conversion from CT number to stopping power in addition to 3 mm to account for range uncertainty of the delivered beam and thickness of compensator.[6] A similar approach is used to determine the proximal margin.

The compensator is designed using a ray-trace algorithm to calculate the depth of the distal margin at each point across the

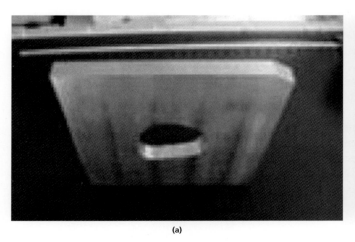
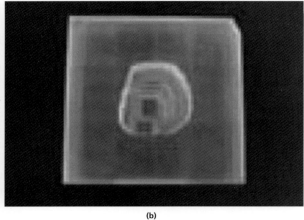

(a)

(b)

Figure 15-9 (a) Aperture and (b) compensator used for lateral and depth shaping of a proton beam.

beam grid. The appropriate amount of compensating material is then determined that will modify the range of the proton beam along each ray. In addition, the thickness of the compensating filter must be modified to account for setup uncertainties, motion, and multiple scattering of the protons by applying a *smearing radius* (SR) to the range compensator. The SR is given by the equation:

$$SR = \sqrt{(IM + SM)^2 + (0.03 \times \text{range})^2}$$

In this equation *IM* is the internal margin that accounts for internal motion, *SM* is the setup margin that accounts for setup uncertainty, and the *0.03 × range* term accounts for proton scattering. The range is calculated to be the distal CTV depth plus the thickness of any bolus. The factor of 3% times the proton range is comparable to the root-mean-square multiple scattering distance for protons.[6]

The procedure for calculating monitor units for a passively scattered proton beam is analogous to that used for calculating monitor units for a photon beam, although the factors that enter the calculation are somewhat different.[7] One first calibrates the proton beam dose monitor to deliver 1 cGy/MU at a specified set of reference conditions. For example, one set of reference conditions for calibration are a proton beam with a range of 28.5 cm [i.e., a 250 MeV beam with *range modulator wheel* (RMW) and a medium-sized second scatterer], an SOBP width of 10 cm, and an aperture that produces a 10 cm × 10 cm field at the isocenter. The point of calibration is at a depth of 23.5 cm in the center of the SOBP, and a source to calibration point distance of 270 cm. Given that set of reference conditions, one can calculate the number of monitor units (MUs) under the non-reference condition using the equation:

MU = Dose/Dose rate

where the dose rate under the non-reference condition is given by:

Dose rate = ROF × SOBPF × RSF × SOBPOCF × OCR × FSF
× ISF × CPSF

The factors that enter into the dose rate are as follows:
- ROF is the relative output factor. The ROF is the change in dose per MU for a different beam energy with a designated RMW and a second scatterer for the deepest range with no range shifter in the beam. The dose per MU changes because of the different energy distribution of the passively scattered beam.
- SOBPF is the SOBP factor, the change in dose per MU with the change in the SOBP width. The wider SOBP means the beam passes through a larger number of modulating ramp steps adding protons with shorter ranges. As the SOBP width increases, the dose per MU decreases.
- RSF is the range shifter factor. It accounts for the change in dose per MU with the thickness of the range shifter, decreasing with increasing thickness of the range shifter. The RSF also depends on the SOBP width.
- SOBPOCF is the SOBP off-center factor, accounting for the change in dose per MU with the location of the measurement point in the direction of beam away from the center of the SOBP. The SOBPOCF is given by the equation:

$$SOBPOCF = PDD \left[\frac{SSD + d_p}{SSD + d_c} \right]^2$$

where d_p is the depth of the point of interest (POI) and d_c is the depth of the center of the SOBP. For a flat SOBP, the percentage depth dose (PDD) is very close to 1.
- OCR is the off-center ratio, used when the measurement POI is located laterally from the central axis of the beam. The OCR is obtained from measured beam profiles at different depths.

- FSF is the field-size factor, which accounts for the change in the dose per MU with a change of open field size. It is significantly different from 1.0 only for small field sizes (smaller than 5 cm × 5 cm).
- ISF is the inverse square factor, a straightforward correction from reference measurement at 270 cm to actual distance of dose calculation.
- CPSF is the compensator and patient scatter factor. It accounts for the presence of the compensator as well as scatter from inhomogeneities in patient anatomy. Usually, it is calculated using the treatment planning system by taking the ratio of dose in the point of interest in the patient and dose in a homogeneous phantom for the same proton fluence and geometry without the compensator.

Planning with spot scanning

Spot scanning offers a much greater variety of beam configurations than does passive scattering. For example, a scanned proton beam at one proton facility allows for 94 energies between 72.5 and 221.8 MeV over a maximum field size of 30 cm × 30 cm. From 0.005 to 0.04 MU can be delivered per spot over a total of up to 64 layers, with a maximum number of 2,048,000 spots per field and a maximum total number of 9999.99 MU per field. Consequently, treatment planning with spot scanning is an optimization process. Spots are selected to span the target volume and the weight of each spot is optimized using an inverse planning scheme.

Optimization options include single-field optimization and multiple-field optimization. In single-field optimization each field is individually optimized to deliver the prescribed uniform dose to the target volume. Single-field optimization is generally used when critical structures are not in the beam path. Single-field optimization can be implemented to deliver either a single-field uniform dose or a single-field integrated boost. In multiple-field optimization, all spots from all fields are optimized simultaneously; another name for multiple-field optimization is intensity-modulated proton therapy (IMPT).

Single-field optimization is a simpler procedure than multiple-field optimization, with less uncertainty and less quality assurance (QA) time required than multiple-field optimization. Multiple-field optimization yields more conformal dose distributions than does single-field optimization. Using multiple-field optimization, one can avoid high doses to critical structures that may be in the beam path, and it is easier to achieve planning goals. However, multiple-field optimization yields larger uncertainties than single-field optimization, and the QA required is more time-consuming than that of single-field optimization.

Planning quality assurance

Upon completion of a proton treatment plan, review of the treatment plan is necessary. Table 15-3 identifies plan parameters that

Table 15-3 Plan parameters that need to be checked in plan review.

Parameter to check	What you're looking for
Patient photo and images	Photos in electronic medical record and CT images in treatment planning system are correct images for planning
CT scanner	Correct scanner-associated CT number to stopping power conversion table used
Immobilization and patient orientation	Correct for treatment
Body contour/Digital couch	Generously contoured
Organs with possible change (shape and density)	For example, hair of CNS and H&N patient
Patient orientation	Correctly entered in treatment planning system
Treatment site/Prescription	Site and prescription matches and prescription is normal
Critical organs	All relevant critical organs are contoured
High-Z materials and artifacts	Identified and CT numbers appropriately overwritten
Bowel gas, rectal gas	CT numbers appropriately overwritten
Target volumes	Correct volume expansions used to generate CTV and PTV
Calculation options	Correct algorithms and dose calculation grid
Beam line	Correct beam line used
Treatment table	Correct couch extension used
Uncertainty in beam path	Sharp objects, beam angle/motion/OAR on distal range
Clearances	Snout position and isocenter location
Dose distributions	Adequate individual field and combined dose coverage in 2D planes
Hot/cold spots	Unusual situations identified and physician informed
Dose-volume histograms	Consistent with plan objective and standard dose tolerance limits for OAR
Optimization options	Single-field optimization vs. multiple-field optimization
Margins	Appropriate proximal, distal, and lateral margins
Spot spacing	Appropriate spot spacing

need to be checked in a plan review. Major items to be considered in the evaluation of proton treatment plans include setup errors, effects of artifacts and implants, range uncertainty, and plan robustness. Figure 15-10 illustrates the effect of the inadvertent addition of a digital couch to the beam path. In this figure, the digital couch has been added to the imaged couch, resulting in a significant change in the range of the proton beam. Artifacts in the CT image such as those caused by dental implants can severely perturb the calculated proton beam and need to be overwritten. Uncertainties in proton planning are addressed separately in the next section.

Uncertainties in proton radiation therapy

Several points need to be made regarding uncertainties in proton radiation therapy, and one must be aware of the consequences

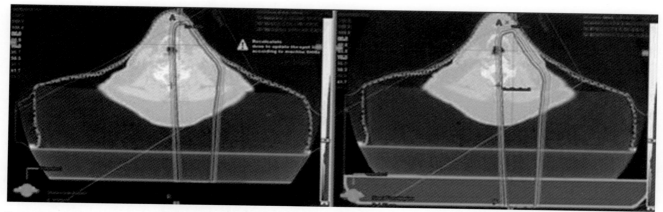

Figure 15-10 Inadvertent addition of digital couch to beam path, as shown in the figure on the right, resulted in significant change in the dose to the CTV. For a color version of this figure, see the color plate section.
Source: Richard Wu, UT MD Anderson Cancer Center. Reproduced with permission of R Wu.

of these uncertainties. Managing uncertainties is more important for proton therapy than it is for photon therapy, and it is necessary to incorporate knowledge of uncertainties in the design, optimization, and evaluation of proton treatment plans. The radiation dose distribution actually delivered may be different from the dose distribution that was planned. Consequently, treatment decisions may be suboptimal and may lead to unanticipated outcomes. Because the dose distributions upon which decisions are made may be different from the delivered dose distributions, the dose response estimates derived from treatment data may be unreliable, and future treatment decisions may be suboptimal.

It is well recognized that uncertainties exist in every step of the radiation therapy process, but uncertainties affect proton therapy quite differently from the way uncertainties affect photon therapy. For example, the sharp distal edge falloff makes proton therapy far more vulnerable to range uncertainties than photon therapy. The conversion of CT numbers to stopping powers contributes a range uncertainty of 2–3%, which needs to be accounted for in determining proximal and distal margins around the target volume (as previously discussed). For this reason, it is not advisable to aim a proton beam directly at a proximal target if a distal critical structure is directly adjacent to that target (even though the proton dose distribution is shown in the treatment planning system that it stops adequately to spare the critical structure). The presence of metal artifacts adversely affects the conversion of CT numbers and hence the range calculations. Heterogeneities in general degrade the distal falloff region, increasing the distance from the 90% to the 10% dose from 6 mm to over 32 mm.[5] Moreover intrafractional and interfractional anatomic variations can cause significant variations in the extent and location of the distal falloff region.[8]

Another serious source of uncertainties in a proton beam is uncertainty in the RBE. Normally, an RBE of 1.1 is applied to clinical proton beams, and this value appears to have some clinical justification. However, the RBE is actually a function of the energy spectra, the dose per fractions, the tissue/cell type, the alpha/beta ratio, and the end point. In particular, it should be noted that the most distal portion of the SOBP predominantly contains lower-energy, high-LET particles, whereas the most proximal portion of the SOBP contains higher-energy, lower-LET particles. Consequently, the RBE varies throughout SOBP due to the changing LET. Figure 15-11 illustrates the increase in biologically effective dose near the distal portion of the SOBP. Moreover, RBE data based on human tissue response (other than clinical data) are lacking. As a consequence of the uncertainties in RBE and range, a good mitigation strategy is to avoid allowing the proton beam to range into critical structures by choosing safe beam angles.

In addition to uncertainties in range and RBE, additional uncertainties exist in computed dose distributions. These computed dose distributions are typically based on analytic semi-empirical models, which have numerous assumptions and approximations, but this issue is not significantly different from

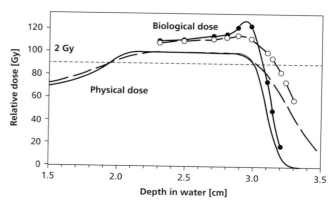

Figure 15-11 A comparison of physical dose and biologically effective dose over the SOBP of a proton beam.
Source: Paganetti and Goitein 2000.[9] Reproduced with permission of American Association of Physicists in Medicine.

uncertainties in photon dose distributions. Improved hardware and Monte Carlo dose calculations for proton beams are in development.[10]

Various approaches have been developed for proton planning to account for some of these uncertainties. For example, compensators are "smeared" to account for the effects of possible misalignment of inhomogeneity and lateral scattering.[5] Repeat imaging and adaptive replanning can mitigate the impact of interfractional variations. Appropriate optimization algorithms can generate resilient dose distributions in the face of factors that cause uncertainty. This type of optimization may not be as critical for photon planning (IMRT) as it is for proton planning (IMPT). An IMRT dose distribution remains essentially spatially unaffected by anatomic variations, so that the target is covered as long as it remains within the PTV. Such is not the case with an IMPT dose distribution, which can be greatly affected by anatomic variations, requiring anatomic variations to be incorporated into an optimization strategy. One such approach is a voxel-by-voxel worst-case approach to robust optimization.[11] In this approach multiple scenarios of maximum range and uncertainty are considered. One dose distribution is computed for each uncertainty scenario in each optimization iteration, and the worst-case dose in each voxel is selected to compute the objective function and minimize it.

Quality assurance for proton radiation therapy

Given the challenges in proton radiation therapy, it is apparent that QA plays a very important role, perhaps even more so with proton radiation therapy than with conventional (photon and electron) radiation therapy. Moreover, significant challenges exist in implementing a QA program for proton therapy.

One major issue in implementing a QA program for proton radiation therapy is that proton accelerators are far more complicated devices than linear accelerators used in conventional radiation therapy. Higher standards of practice are needed for complicated systems, such as proton accelerators, than for simpler systems, such as photon therapy machines. Moreover, the wide use of proton therapy is still relatively new; physicists have less experience with proton accelerators and are thus not as familiar with both the reliability of proton accelerators as well as the pathways of potential failure of these accelerators. Finally, because of the great expense of a proton machine, the utilization of proton accelerators may be greater than that for photon therapy machines. Whereas in many radiation oncology facilities the workload for a linear accelerator may be an 8-hour or at most a 12-hour day, allowing a significant amount of downtime for QA and maintenance activities to take place, many proton facilities are operational for longer. Typically, all QA and maintenance activities are performed after treatments are ended.

Patient QA is performed week days during a nightshift, machine QA is performed on weekends, and machine maintenance is done Saturday night and all day Sunday. Because of the very limited time available for machine QA, these activities are very carefully planned.

Patient-plan-specific quality assurance

Patient-plan-specific QA involves verifying that the plan proposed for the patient will actually deliver the desired dose distribution. It consists of generating the planned beam delivery on a phantom, and verifying that the planned beam parameters actually deliver the proposed dose distribution on the phantom. It is a very time-consuming process involving a set of measurements that must be done after treatment hours.

For a treatment plan using a passively scattered beam, the patient-specific QA procedure takes from 2.5 to 10 hours. The major contribution to the variability in the time required for patient-specific QA lies in the review of the treatment plan. Treatment plan review can take anywhere from 1 to 8 hours depending on the complexity of the treatment plan, with the longer times required for complex plans such as those for treating the craniospinal axis. The remaining QA procedures include creation of the verification plan, calculation and verification of monitor units, QA of the aperture and compensator, verification that no collisions between gantry and patient will occur during treatment, and signoff on the electronic medical record. For a treatment plan using spot scanning, patient-specific QA takes from 5 to 13 hours. QA procedures include review of the treatment plan, verifying the electronic medical record treatment delivery, creation of the verification plan, measurement of 2D dose distributions in various planes, and measurement of percent depth doses using a Markus chamber.

Machine-specific quality assurance

Machine-specific QA involves a set of procedures that are identified in ICRU Report #78.[12] Analogous to conventional QA, it consists of a set of tests that are performed daily, weekly, and annually.

Daily QA checks are performed by the radiation therapists or physicist assistants at the start of the day before any patients are treated. These checks include checks of interlocks and room lasers, if present. If an x-ray imaging system is used for patient alignment instead of room lasers, then alignment of the x-ray system is checked. For passively scattered beams, the aperture alignment is checked, while for spot scanned beams the spot position is checked, as is the dose at several spots and depth. For both types of systems the depth dose and lateral profiles are verified, as is the dose per MU under a standardized set of conditions. Finally, data flow from the electronic medical record to the delivery and imaging systems is verified.

Weekly tests are relatively straightforward. ICRU Report #78 recommends weekly tests of the patient positioning and imaging systems, but it is common practice to verify the alignment of x-ray and proton delivery systems weekly or monthly. The ICRU Report #78 recommends verifying the dose delivered to randomly selected patients, but this is not necessary if such verification is performed on every patient prior to initial beam delivery. Several checks are performed on the scanned beam. A monthly output check consisting of a single point measurement is performed for standard patterns involving all energies, calibration checks on the primary monitor are performed, and the constancy of beam flatness and symmetry is verified every month.

Annual QA is comprehensive and time-consuming; approximately 40 to 100 hours are typically required for these procedures. Annual QA tests include tests of x-ray positioning and alignment systems, calibration of CT number to stopping power conversion tables, and comprehensive tests of the therapy equipment, including monitor chambers, beam delivery termination and control interlocks, gantry isocenter, depth-dose and lateral profiles, and establishment of baseline for daily QA checks.

As physicists become more familiar with the process of proton radiation therapy and proton radiation therapy equipment, QA procedures are likely to evolve. At this stage, these procedures are extensive and time-consuming, but necessary in the interest of patient and operator safety.

Summary

- A monoenergetic beam of protons deposits approximately a uniform dose until the protons reach the end of their range, at which depth an enhanced dose is deposited (Bragg peak), beyond which very little dose is deposited.
- Clinical beam delivery of protons includes proton beams of various energies to deliver a spread-out Bragg peak (SOBP).
- Protons are typically produced either in a cyclotron, which generates a monoenergetic continuous beam, or in a synchrotron, in which the protons are delivered in beam spills, but can be delivered at varying energies.
- A clinical proton beam can be generated either by passive scattering, including the use of a range modulator and second scatterer, or by spot scanning.
- The concept of planning target volume (PTV) in proton therapy is different from that in photon therapy, because proton target volume margins also must include range uncertainties.
- In addition to range uncertainties, one must also account for relative biological effectiveness (RBE) uncertainties in proton treatment planning.
- Quality assurance (QA) for proton therapy is a much more complicated and time-consuming procedure than that for photon therapy, and adequate personnel and staff resources must be allocated for it.

Problems

15-1 Calculate the relativistic mass for a 250 MeV proton.
15-2 What energy passively scattered proton beam would be used to treat a target whose maximum depth is 8 cm with a field size of 6 cm × 8 cm?
15-3 Based on the data in Figure 15-2, estimate the relative weights of the lower-energy proton beams needed to deliver the SOBP illustrated in the figure.
15-4 a) Describe the smearing radius.
   b) Calculate the smearing radius for IM = 1.0 cm, SM = 0.5 cm, distal CTV depth of 8.0 cm.
15-5 What are the uncertainties (in %) of the CT conversion and proton scattering?
15-6 To calculate MUs for proton beams, using the MU = Dose/Dose Rate, list the factors that go into calculating the dose rate.

References

1 Wilson R. R. Radiological use of fast protons. *Radiology* 1946; **47**:487–491.
2 Allen, A. M., Pawlicki, T., Dong, L., Fourkal, E., Buyyounouski, M., Cengel, K., et al. An evidence based review of proton beam therapy: The report of ASTRO's emerging technology committee. *Radiother. Oncol.* 2012; **103**:8–11.
3 Lu, H.-M., and Flanz, J. Characteristics of clinical proton beams. In H. Paganetti (ed.), *Proton Therapy Physics*. Boca Raton, FL, CRC Press, 2012.
4 International Atomic Energy Agency. *Report 398: Absorbed dose determination in external beam radiotherapy: An international code of practice for dosimetry based on standards of absorbed dose to water.* Vienna, IAEA, 2009.
5 Urie, M., Goitein, M., and Wagner, M. Compensating for heterogeneities in proton radiation therapy. *Phys. Med. Biol.* 1983; **29**(5):553–566.
6 Moyers, M. F., Miller, D. W., Bush, D. A., and Slater, J. D. Methodologies and tools for proton beam design for lung tumors. *Int. J. Radiat. Oncol. Biol. Phys.* 2001; **49**(5):1429–1438.
7 Sahoo, N., Zhu, X. R., Arjomandy, B., Ciangaru, G., Lii, M. F., et al. A procedure for calculation of monitor units for passively scattered proton radiotherapy beams. *Med. Phys.* 2008; **35**:5088.
8 Mori, S., Dong, L., Starkschall, G., Mohan, R., and Chen, G. T. Y. A serial 4DCT study to quantify range variations in charged particle. *Radiat. Res.* 2013; **00**:1–11.
9 Paganetti, H., and Goitein, M. Radiobiological significance of beamline dependent proton energy distributions in a spread-out Bragg peak. *Med. Phys.* 2000; **27**(5):1119–1126.

10 Jia, X., Pawlicki, T., Murphy, K., and Mundt, A. J. Proton therapy dose calculations on GPU: advances and challenges. *Transl. Cancer Res.* 2012, DOI: 10.3978/j.issn/2218-676X.2012.10.03.

11 Pflugfelder, D., Wilkens, J. J., and Oelfke, U. Worst case optimization: a method to account for uncertainties in the optimization of inten-

sity modulated proton therapy. *Phys. Med. Biol.* 2008; **53**:1689–1700.

12 International Commission on Radiation Units & Measurements. *Report 78: Prescribing, Recording, and Reporting Proton-Beam Therapy.* Bethesda, MD, ICRU, 2014.

16

SOURCES FOR IMPLANT THERAPY AND DOSE CALCULATION

Objectives

After reading this chapter, the student should:
- Be able to describe the historical evolution of brachytherapy from the use of radium and radon sources to the present use of a variety of nuclides.
- Recognize the important and useful characteristics of modern nuclides used for brachytherapy.
- Be able to compute the equivalent mass of radium for a source of known activity.
- Understand the relationship between several terms for describing the strength of a brachytherapy source.
- Explain the concept of radioactive equilibrium and calculate the activities as a function of time for two sources in equilibrium.
- Compute the dose at a specified distance from a brachytherapy source.

Introduction

The implantation of sealed sources of radioactive material in, on, or around a tumor is one of the oldest methods for treating cancer with ionizing radiation, dating back to about 1900. From the inception of brachytherapy to about the 1950s, the radioactive material employed most frequently for implant therapy was radium (^{226}Ra) in secular equilibrium with its decay products. Today, radioactive sources such as cesium (^{137}Cs), iridium (^{192}Ir), iodine (^{125}I), and palladium (^{103}Pd) are being used as replacements for radium. Implant therapy is generally referred to as *brachytherapy* (from the Greek word *brachys* meaning "short"; hence, short-distance therapy) and was once called *plesiotherapy* (from the Greek word *plesios* meaning "near" or "close").

Hendee's Radiation Therapy Physics, Fourth Edition. Todd Pawlicki, Daniel J. Scanderbeg and George Starkschall.
© 2016 John Wiley & Sons, Inc. Published 2016 by John Wiley & Sons, Inc.

Techniques for implant therapy may be divided into four categories depending on placement of the source(s):

1 *Molds* or *plaques* are composed of radioactive sources that are displaced slightly above the skin in the region of a superficial lesion. The distance between the sources and the lesion is seldom greater than 1 or 2 cm. The intervening space is often filled with material such as wax or plastic and the device is placed directly on the skin surface. Radium molds were once used widely for treating superficial lesions but this technique has been superseded to a large extent by treatment with superficial x rays and electrons. Today, plaques are frequently used for the treatment of ocular tumors.

2 *Interstitial* implants are composed of radioactive needles, wires, or small encapsulated sources called *seeds* that are inserted into a lesion or into tissue in the immediate vicinity of a lesion. Interstitial implants are widely used for the treatment of intraoral and superficial lesions and for treatment of tumors in accessible areas such as the prostate, breast, cervix, and head and neck.

3 *Intracavitary* implants are composed of radioactive sources that are placed in a body cavity. Most intracavitary implants are used for the treatment of cancer of the cervix and uterus, with the sealed sources placed in the intrauterine cavity and around the cervix.

4 *Intraluminal* implants are composed of radioactive sources introduced directly into the lumen of a vessel, duct, or airway. In recent years, intravascular brachytherapy has been used for the treatment of recurrent coronary artery stenosis; however, this use has decreased dramatically with the introduction of drug alluding stents.

Techniques for implant therapy may also be divided into two categories related to duration of the implant:

1 *Temporary* implants usually require that the patient be hospitalized for the duration of treatment, which generally lasts no more than a few days. At the end of the treatment, the sources are removed. In many cases, the sources are stored for subsequent re-use.

2 *Permanent* implants are practical only for interstitial treatments and require that the sources remain in the tissue indefinitely. Sources with relatively short half-lives are used, so that the majority of the dose is delivered within a few weeks or months. Alternatively, sources that emit low-energy characteristic x rays are used for the treatment of deep-seated tumors. When such sources are used, the patient's body attenuates almost all of the radiation, and a negligible amount of radiation escapes from the patient.

Finally, techniques may also be divided by dose rate:

1 Low-dose rate (LDR): typically defined as 0.4 to 2 Gy/hr.
2 Medium-dose rate (MDR): typically defined as 2 to 12 Gy/hr.
3 High-dose rate (HDR): typically defined as > 12 Gy/hr.
4 Pulsed-dose rate (PDR): are applied at frequent intervals combining the convenience of HDR equipment with the radiobiology of LDR brachytherapy.

The choice of activity and nuclide can often yield a low dose rate at the patient's external surfaces; hence, the patient presents little or no risk of radiation exposure to others. These patients can be released from the hospital as soon as their medical condition permits. An example would be a permanent LDR prostate seed implant.

Radium sources

Radium was used in the treatment of cancer almost immediately after its discovery by Marie and Pierre Curie in 1898. Within the next two decades, the separation of radioactive radon gas from decaying radium was achieved and the radon gas, encapsulated into glass tubes, was also used for the treatment of cancer. During this time, encapsulation techniques were developed to filter beta particles from the decaying radium and radon sources, preventing tissue necrosis close to the radioactive sources.

In the decades from 1920 to 1950, much clinical experience with radium and radon was obtained. Most of the techniques used in modern brachytherapy were developed during this period. Although radium and radon are rarely used in medicine today, the techniques developed with these sources are of great importance to modern brachytherapy and are described here.

Radium sources used for implant therapy contain ^{226}Ra in secular equilibrium with its decay products. Secular equilibrium can be established for a radium source because the half-life for radioactive decay is much greater for ^{226}Ra (~1,600 years) than for any of the decay products of this nuclide. About one month is required for a new source of radium to approach secular equilibrium with its progeny. To establish secular equilibrium, the source must be sealed to prevent the escape of gaseous ^{222}Rn. The decay scheme from ^{226}Ra to stable lead (^{206}Pb) is shown in Figure 16-1. This sequence of radioactive transformations is part

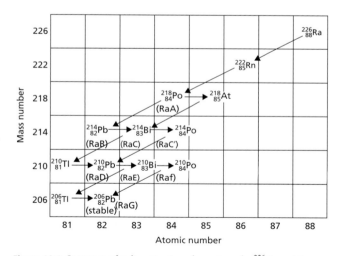

Figure 16-1 Sequence of radioactive transformations for ^{226}Ra and its decay products.
Source: Hendee 1970.[2]

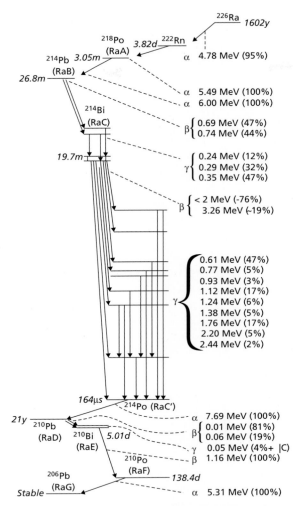

Figure 16-2 A simplified decay scheme of ^{226}Ra and its decay products showing the radiations of greatest importance in brachytherapy.
Source: Adapted from Lederer et al. 1967.[1] Reproduced with permission from John Wiley & Sons.

of the uranium decay series, of which ^{226}Ra is the sixth member. Although the γ rays used for radiation therapy are released primarily during the decay of ^{214}Pb (RaB) and ^{214}Bi (RaC) (Figure 16-2),[1] pure sources of these nuclides are not used for therapy due to their short half-lives. The γ rays of highest energy in the decay scheme are the 2.2 MeV and 2.4 MeV γ rays emitted by ^{214}Bi. The average energy is about 0.8 MeV for the γ rays emitted from a sealed source of radium (Table 16-1).[2,3] On average, 2.22 γ rays are emitted by a sealed source of radium for each decay of ^{226}Ra.

Construction of radium sources

Diagrammed in Figure 16-3 are radium needles that were historically used for interstitial implants along with radium tubes, used primarily for molds and intracavitary treatments. The radium

was supplied in the form of a salt (radium sulfate or radium chloride), which was mixed with an inert filler such as magnesium oxide or barium sulfate. The small crystals of radium salt and filler were contained within cylindrical cells about 1 cm long. The cells were made of gold foil 0.1 to 0.2 mm thick and were sealed to prevent the escape of radon gas. Each source of radium contained 1 to 3 cells surrounded by a wall of platinum, reinforced with iridium (10%). The thickness (usually 0.5 or 1 mm) of the platinum-iridium wall was sufficient to absorb alpha and beta radiation from the source. Gamma rays were attenuated only slightly by the wall.

The exposure rate from a 1 mCi point source of ^{226}Ra that is in secular equilibrium with its decay products and enclosed within a 0.5 mm Pt-Ir wall is 8.25 Röntgen per hour (R/hr) at a distance of 1 cm (or 0.825 R/hr at 1 m from a 1 Ci source).[2,4] The value of 8.25 R-cm^2/hr-mCi is referred to as the *exposure rate constant*, Γ_δ, for ^{226}Ra. The Γ_δ is related to the *specific γ-ray constant*, Γ, but includes the x rays produced following internal conversion and photoelectric absorption events in the radium salt and in the encapsulation. Until recently, it was generally assumed that 1 mCi of radium has a mass of 1 mg. It is now known that 1 mg of radium actually has an activity of approximately 0.98 mCi.

Types of radium sources

Illustrated in Figure 16-4 are three types of radium needles that were used for interstitial implants. *Uniform linear-density needles* were manufactured using full-intensity (0.66 mg/cm), half-intensity (0.33 mg/cm), or quarter-intensity (0.165 mg/cm) loadings. Needles with linear densities of 0.5 mg/cm and 0.25 mg/cm were also manufactured as they were found to be useful. *Indian club needles* had a greater activity at one end and were useful for implants with one uncrossed end. *Dumbbell needles* had a greater activity at each end and used for implants with both ends uncrossed. Tubes for intracavitary and mold therapy were typically furnished in multiples of 5 mg of radium and were usually constructed with a platinum–iridium wall 1 mm thick.

Nasopharyngeal applicators containing as much as 50–100 mg of radium in a thin capsule of 0.2–0.3 mm of metal alloy (monel metal) were also available in the past. However, these sources were found to be particularly hazardous and should be disposed of if found at an institution.

Today, radium sources are rarely found in clinical use in the United States and have been replaced with safer alternatives. However, a few sources have been retained by clinics and the accredited dosimetry calibration laboratories (ADCLs) for use as calibration standards.

Radium substitutes

The use of radium sources is associated with several hazards. Seepage of radon (^{222}Rn) from a radium source is prevented by

Table 16-1 Physical properties of radioactive nuclides used in brachytherapy.

Element	Isotope	Beta Particle Energy (MeV)[a]	Gamma-ray Energy (MeV)[b]	Exposure Rate Constant (R cm2/hr mCi)	Half-life	HVL in Water (cm)[c]	HVL in Lead (mm)[c]	Clinical Uses	Source Form
Americium	241 Am	0.0039–0.0932	0.0139–0.0595	0.1216	432.2 yr	—	1.26	Intracavitary temporary implants	Tubes
Californium	252Cf	2.13–2.15 neutrons	0.7–0.9	3.768[d]	2.645 yr	—	—	Temporary intracavitary implants	Tubes
Cesium	137Cs131Cs	0.514–1.17 None	0.662 0.029–0.034	3.28	30 yr 9.7 days	8.2	6.5	Temporary intracavitary and interstitial implants Permanent implants, many sites	Tubes, needles Seeds
Cobalt	60Co	0.313	1.17–1.33	13.07	5.26 yr	10.8	11	Temporary implants	Plaques, tubes, needles
Gold	198Au	0.96	0.412–1.088	2.327	2.7 days	7.0	3.3	Permanent implants of prostate and other sites	Seeds
Iodine	125I	None	0.0355	1.45[e]	59.6 days	2.0	0.02	Permanent interstitial implants of prostate, lung, and other sites, temporary implants of eye	Seeds
Iodine	131I	0.25–0.61	0.08–0.637	2.2	8.06 days	5.8	3.0	"Cocktail" for thyroid therapy	Liquid, capsules
Iridium	192Ir	0.24–0.67	0.136–1.062	4.62[f]	74.2 days	6.3	3.0	Temporary interstitial implants of Head, neck, breast, and other sites	Wires, seeds
Palladium	103Pd	—	0.020–0.0227	1.48	17 days	—	0.01	Permanent implants of prostate	Seeds
Phosphorus	32P	1.71	None	—	14.3 days	0.1	0.1	Sodium phosphate injection, for bone and blood diseases; chromic phosphate pleural and intraperitoneal effusions	Liquid

Source	Isotope	β energy (MeV)	γ energy (MeV)		Half-life			Clinical use	Form
Radium and decay products	226Ra	0.017–3.26	0.047–2.44	8.25[g]	1622 yr	10.6	8.0	Temporary intracavitary and interstitial implants	Tubes, needles
Radon and decay products	222Rn	0.017–3.26	0.047–2.44	8.25[g]	3.83 days	10.6	8.0	Permanent implants, many sites	Seeds
Ruthenium	106Ru	3.5 MeV max.	—	—	366 days	—	—	Temporary implants of eye	Plaques
Samarium	145Sm	—	0.0382–0.0614	—	340 days	—	—	Medical uses currently under consideration	Seeds
Strontium	89Sr	1.46	None	—	50 days	—	—	Injection for widespread bone metastases	Liquid
Strontium	90Sr	0.54–2.27	None	—	28.9 yr 64 hr	0.15	0.14	Temporary application for shallow lesions	Applicator
Tantalum	182Ta	0.18–0.514	0.043–1.453	6.71	115 days	10.0	12	Temporary interstitial implants (outpatient treatments)	Wires
Ytterbium	169Yb	—	0.060–0.100	1.58[f]	32.0 days	—	—	Temporary and permanent implants	Seeds

[a] A dash separates the minimum and maximum energies of the β-particles in the spectra. All energies listed are the maximum energy of each particle.

[b] A dash separates the minimum and maximum energies of the γ rays in the spectra.

[c] Assumes narrow beam geometry, a condition usually not found in practical brachytherapy applications.

[d] For an encapsulated source with a wall thickness equivalent to 0.5 mm Pt-Ir alloy.[5] For radium and radon, the exposure rate constant is expressed in R·cm²/hr·mg.

[e] For an unfiltered point source with δ >11.3 keV.[6,7]

[f] Neutrons/fission.

[g] This value is reduced to 1.208 by the attenuation of the filtration incorporated into commercially available seeds, together with a correction for anisotropy.[8]

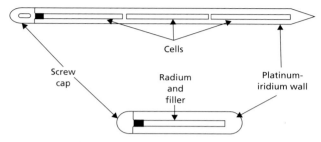

Figure 16-3 A radium needle (top) and a radium tube (bottom).
Source: Hendee 1970.[2]

enclosing the source in a doubly sealed capsule. Nevertheless, "leaky" radium sources have occurred and have caused extensive radioactive contamination. Because of the buildup of radon gas, the pressure inside a new source of radium is slightly greater than atmospheric pressure. The internal pressure continues to increase over the years because alpha particles emitted by ^{226}Ra and its decay products become gaseous atoms of helium after losing their kinetic energy, and the radiation-induced hydrolysis of water contained in the mixture of radium salt and filler produces gaseous O_2 and H_2. For this reason, care was taken to remove as much water as possible from the radium salt and filler.

Some believe that the increase in internal pressure, combined with the gradual loss of physical strength of the capsule, caused the probability of rupture of a radium source to increase with the age of the source. Users were advised not to heat radium sources above 100°C because the pressure of a gas increases with temperature (ideal gas law).[9]

Radium sources may be bent or broken by improper handling or, less frequently, by circumstances beyond the control of the user. The numerous hazards associated with the use of radium and radon prompted the development of a number of substitute sources.

Cesium-137

The most common radium substitute is ^{137}Cs. This radioisotope largely replaced radium as an implant source in the 1960s and 1970s. Cesium-137 sources were obtained as tubes or needles

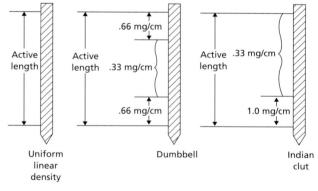

Figure 16-4 Types of radium needles.
Source: Hendee 1970.[2]

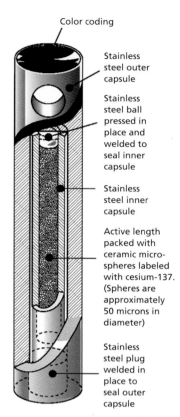

Figure 16-5 A cut-away view of a model 6D6C ^{137}Cs source.
Source: Courtesy of 3M Medical-Surgical Division, St. Paul, MN.

containing radioactive microspheres embedded in a ceramic matrix. A representative ^{137}Cs source is shown in Figure 16-5. The tubes were typically 2.65 mm in external diameter with lengths of approximately 20 mm and active lengths of 14 mm; however, larger and smaller sources were also available. Because of the experience clinicians had had with the use of radium, the activity of ^{137}Cs sources was generally described in units of mg-equivalents of radium (mg-Ra-eq). Activities ranged between 5 and 40 mg-Ra-eq. These sources were safer than radium because the radioactive material was a solid rather than a powder. Additionally, no gaseous radioactive products are produced during the decay of ^{137}Cs. The exposure rate constant for ^{137}Cs is 3.28 R-cm^2/hr·mCi. To determine the equivalent mass of radium, the activity, in mCi, is multiplied by the ratio of exposure rate constants for cesium and radium:

Equivalent mass of radium = Activity in mCi

$$\cdot \frac{3.28 \text{R} \cdot \text{cm}^2/\text{hr} \cdot \text{mCi}}{8.25 \text{R} \cdot \text{cm}^2/\text{hr} \cdot \text{mg}} \quad (16\text{-}1)$$

Example 16-1

A new ^{137}Cs source is described by its manufacturer as containing 20 mg-equivalents of radium. How many mCi of cesium are contained in the source?

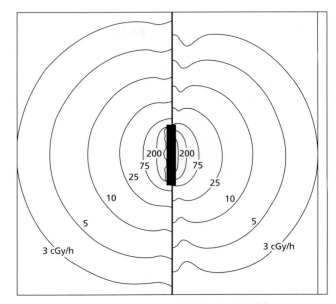

Figure 16-6 Comparison between isodose curves from a ^{226}Ra (10.7 mg) source and a ^{137}Cs source (10 mg·Ra·eq) manufactured by Oris Corporation. Both sources have an air-kerma strength of 72 μGy·m^2/hr. *Source:* Courtesy of Jeffrey F. Williamson, Ph.D., Virginia Commonwealth University, Richmond, VA.

The activity is determined from Equation (16-1) as:

$$\text{mCi of}^{137}Cs = 20 \text{ mg-Ra-eq} \cdot \frac{8.25R \cdot cm^2/hr \cdot mg}{3.28 \cdot cm^2/hr \cdot mCi}$$
$$\text{Activity} = 50.3 \text{ mCi}$$

Cesium-137 is a particularly well-suited substitute for radium, because it produces dose distributions in tissue that are virtually identical to those of radium (Figure 16-6). Furthermore, its 30-year half-life and single γ ray (0.662 MeV) help to make it a practical choice. However, cesium has widely fallen out of use, having been largely replaced by ^{192}Ir HDR remote afterloading systems.

Cobalt-60

Sources of ^{60}Co were used in the past for interstitial and intracavitary implants. Cobalt-60 emits γ rays of 1.17 and 1.33 MeV, but the short half-life of ^{60}Co (5.24 years) is an undesirable feature for a radium substitute. Sources were constructed as small wires of cobalt enclosed within a sheath of stainless steel or platinum-iridium. However, there has been a recent revival of interest in using ^{60}Co as an HDR source in remote afterloaders. Several remote afterloaders have dual sources of ^{60}Co and ^{192}Ir.

Over a distance of at least 5 cm, the variation in dose rate is about equal for sources of radium, ^{137}Cs, and ^{60}Co. This relationship is depicted in Figure 16-7.

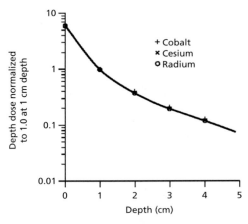

Figure 16-7 Dose falloff as a function of distance in a tissue-equivalent phantom for sources of radium (10 mg, 0.5 mm Pt (Ir)), ^{137}Cs (17.1 mg·Ra·eq, 3M model 6D6C capsule), and ^{60}Co (15.0 mg·Ra·eq, Abbott model 6796 Actacel capsule). Each source is 3.1 mm in diameter and 20 mm long, with an active length of 14 mm. Measurements are normalized to 1.00 at 1 cm depth. *Source:* Hendee 1970.[2]

Tantalum-182

Sources of ^{182}Ta were also used as brachytherapy sources in the past, but have been replaced by sources with better characteristics. Tantalum-182 sources were provided as flexible wires about 0.2 mm in diameter and encased in a platinum sheath with walls 0.1 mm thick. These sources could be inserted into locations that are not easily accessible to larger sources.[10–16] Some disadvantages included the 115-day half-life of ^{182}Ta, which is too long for this nuclide to be used as a permanent implant, and the maximum γ-ray energy of 1.45 MeV produces a less-than-desirable dose distribution. Like ^{137}Cs, ^{182}Ta has largely been replaced by ^{192}Ir.

Iridium-192

Iridium-192 has a 74-day half-life and emits γ rays with an average energy of 0.38 MeV. Iridium-192 is available either as wire or as seeds. The low energy allows for less shielding to be required, which is a nice advantage, but a key disadvantage is its short half-life, and the need for frequent exchange to keep treatment times within a reasonable range. The high specific activity of ^{192}Ir (more than 9000 Ci/g) makes it an attractive source for use when high dose rates are required. Sources with nominal activities of 10 Ci (3.7 × 10^{11} Bq or air kerma strength, S_k = 4.1 × 10^4 μGy· m^2/hr) are routinely used in HDR remote-afterloading equipment. These devices deliver dose rates as high as 700 cGy/min at 1 cm.[17–18] Consequently, HDR units must be operated in shielded rooms to avoid significant exposure to staff and other persons. A representative HDR source is shown in Figure 16-8. A representative HDR remote afterloading brachytherapy unit is shown in Figure 16-9.

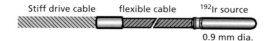

Stiff drive cable   flexible cable ^{192}Ir source

0.9 mm dia.

Figure 16-8 A representative ^{192}Ir source for HDR remote afterloading brachytherapy.
Source: Courtesy of Nucletron Corporation.

Gold-198, Iodine-125, Palladium-103, and Cesium-131

Radioactive ^{198}Au has a 2.7-day half-life and emits γ rays of 0.412 MeV. Seeds of ^{198}Au were used as a radon seed substitute for permanent implants; however, seeds of ^{125}I (half-life = 59.6 days) have essentially replaced ^{198}Au.[19]

While decaying, ^{125}I emits γ rays and x rays with energies in the range of 27–35 keV. With its low energies, ^{125}I is easily shielded with small thicknesses of lead (HVL = 0.025 mm). Numerous designs of ^{125}I seeds are available, and several are shown in Figure 16-10. Despite internal construction differences, seeds are typically 4.5 mm in length and 0.8 mm in diameter. The final panel of Figure 16-10 shows a comparison of the angular dose distribution around several iodine seeds.[20–23]

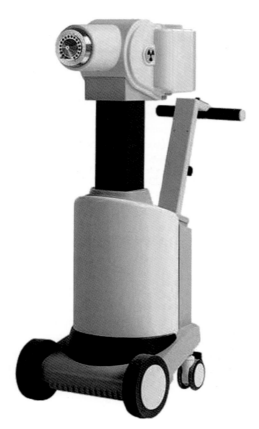

Figure 16-9 An HDR remote afterloading brachytherapy unit.
Source: Courtesy of Nucletron Corporation.

Palladium-103 is another reactor-produced nuclide with a half-life of approximately 17 days that undergoes decay by electron capture (Figure 16-11). During decay, characteristic x rays in the range of 20 to 23 keV are emitted. The low photon energy and short half-life make ^{103}Pd an attractive isotope for permanent implants in organs such as the prostate.[24] Like ^{125}I, ^{103}Pd is manufactured and sold in seed form with the same dimensions as the ^{125}I seeds (4.5 mm in length and 0.8 mm in diameter). This allows for all equipment in a permanent prostate seed implant case to be identical for either isotope.

Cesium-131 has a half-life of 9.7 days and photon energies in the range of 30 keV. It received FDA clearance for use in 2003 and has since been used to treat malignant disease of the prostate and other organs.

The difference in half-life between ^{125}I, ^{103}Pd, and ^{131}Cs leads to a difference in dose delivery in that 90% of the dose is delivered in roughly 204 days, 58 days, and 33 days, respectively.

Americium-241

Americium-241 has been considered for specific brachytherapy applications. With its long half-life (432 years) and low photon energy (60 keV), ^{241}Am shows some promise as a substitute for radium in the treatment of gynecological disease. However, the low specific activity means that sources of ^{241}Am are quite large and unsuitable for other applications. The low energy makes it plausible to construct thin foils to protect sensitive organs.

Ophthalmic irradiators

Certain ophthalmologic conditions such as pterygium, vascularization, or ulceration of the cornea, as well as certain intraorbital malignancies such as melanomas, may be treated effectively with small radioactive applicators positioned on or near the sclera for a short period of time.[25,26] Applicators for the treatment of pterygium contain ^{90}Sr in secular equilibrium with ^{90}Y. The low-energy beta particles from ^{90}Sr (0.54 MeV maximum) are absorbed by the encapsulation of the applicator, but the higher-energy betas from ^{90}Y (2.27 MeV maximum) penetrate the applicator and enter the sclera of the eye. The dose rate at the center of an applicator surface may be as high as 100 cGy/s.[27] The dose rate may vary greatly across the surface of an applicator. This dose rate may be made more uniform by constructing a compensating filter designed to fit over the end of the applicator.[28] The dose rate from a beta applicator decreases to about 5% of the surface dose rate at a depth of 4 mm, which corresponds to the depth of the lens below the cornea.[29]

Eye plaques are quite widely used to treat malignancies of the eye, such as choroidal melanoma.[30] These plaques may be loaded with γ-ray emitting sources, such as ^{125}I or ^{103}Pd, or with beta emitters, such as ^{106}Ru in equilibrium with ^{106}Rh.

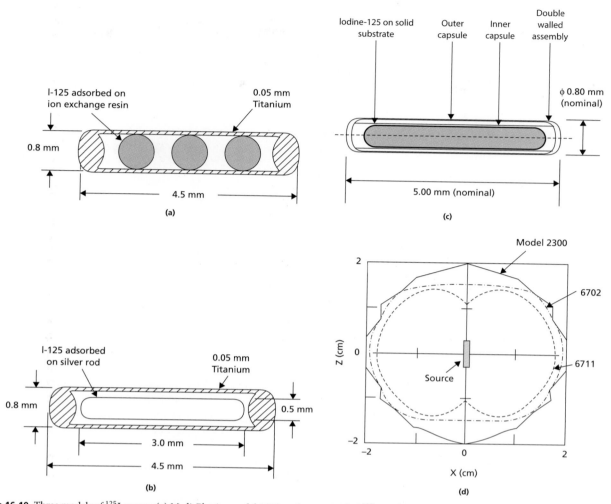

Figure 16-10 Three models of ^{125}I source. (a) Medi-Physics model 6702 seed, composed of ^{125}I adsorbed on spheres of ion exchange resin, separated by a gold sphere for radiographic localization. (b) Medi-Physics model 6711 seed containing ^{125}I adsorbed on a silver rod. (c) Best Medical International Inc. model 2300 seed containing ^{125}I adsorbed on a solid substrate. (d) Comparison of the dose distribution around these three seeds.
Source: For parts (a), (b), and (c): Weaver et al. 1990.[21] Copyright ® 1990, Elsevier. For part (d): Nath and Melillo 1993.[20] Reproduced with permission from American Association of Physicists in Medicine.

Figure 16-11 Best Industries model 200 ^{103}P seed. The ^{103}P displated on graphite pellets separated by a lead radiographic marker.
Source: Weaver et al. 1990.[21] Copyright ® 1990, Elsevier.

Implantable neutron sources

Tubes containing radioactive californium (^{252}Cf) have been investigated as a replacement for radium.[31–33] Artificially produced ^{252}Cf (half-life = 2.65 years) undergoes spontaneous fission with the release of 2.34×10^6 fast neutrons per second per microgram. Gamma rays also are emitted when ^{252}Cf undergoes spontaneous fission. The range of neutrons released during fission is short compared with the penetration of γ rays. Californium-252 sources are constructed with platinum encapsulation to attenuate and limit the γ-ray and beta-ray emissions. Consequently, sources of ^{252}Cf deliver a high tumor dose with less radiation to surrounding normal structures. Also, hypoxic tumor cells may be destroyed more efficiently with ^{252}Cf because neutrons provide an oxygen enhancement ratio near unity. The small number and high cost of ^{252}Cf sources available limit their use to experimental therapy.

Radiation safety of brachytherapy sources

Storage

Brachytherapy sources present a radiation safety hazard in radiation oncology facilities due to their small size and ease with which they may be misplaced. Consequently, secure storage facilities and meticulous inventory techniques are required. Storage in an appropriately shielded container is essential, and the shielded container itself must be stored in a locked room, with access limited to persons directly involved in brachytherapy procedures. A lead safe is required for storage of radium and cesium sources, as well as for other sources of high-activity and energetic photon emissions. Sources emitting only low-energy photons are more easily shielded, but still require secure storage.

Facilities required to handle and store brachytherapy sources in a safe manner vary with the amount of activity involved and the use of the sources. A few facilities are described in the literature.[9,34–38] Radioactive sources for implant therapy should always be handled remotely, or with forceps, and never directly with the hands. Personal dosimetry such as a ring badge should be employed while handling sources and, whenever possible, sources should be viewed indirectly with mirrors rather than by direct vision.

Test for uniform distribution of activity

An autoradiograph of a sealed radioactive source may be obtained by resting the source for a short time against an unexposed radiochromic film. Simultaneously, the film may be exposed to low-energy x rays. It is advisable to examine new brachytherapy sources radiographically before they are accepted from the manufacturer. This is particularly advisable when radium sources are used, because the distribution of activity can become nonuniform. However, nonuniform distributions of activity have been observed with ^{125}I sources, and irregular spacing of ^{192}Ir seeds within catheters has occurred. Both situations are readily detected with autoradiography (Figure 16-12).

Evaluating the safety of brachytherapy sources

Several methods have been developed for testing brachytherapy sources for leakage.[37] Two methods are described here:
- The source may be swabbed with a moistened cotton swab. Any activity present on the surface of the source will be removed by the cotton swab, which is then placed into a scintillation counter. The removed activity is determined by first calibrating the spectrometer with a known source.
- A few needles or tubes are placed in a vial containing liquid scintillation "cocktail." After 1–2 hours, the sources are

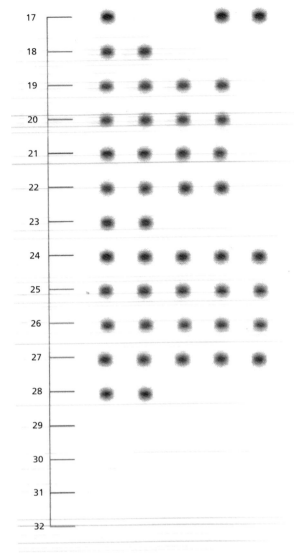

Figure 16-12 Autoradiograph of pre-loaded needles containing ^{125}I seeds for a prostate implant. Seed spacing and relative activity can be checked by analyzing the autoradiograph.

removed and residual activity is detected by analyzing the cocktail in a liquid scintillation counter. Residual activity in the vial indicates a leaking source. This method has been criticized because leaks in the source may be plugged temporarily by the liquid counting solution.

All leaking sources should be sealed in a container, removed from use, and returned to the manufacturer or disposed of properly.

Specification of brachytherapy sources

Sources used for brachytherapy may be specified in one of several ways. As indicated earlier, radium sources have been specified in terms of the mass of radium, in milligrams, incorporated into the source. To facilitate their introduction into clinical use, sources composed of nuclides intended as substitutes for radium were originally, and in some cases still are, specified in terms of milligram equivalents of radium (mg-Ra-eq). This specification is the mass of radium required to produce the same exposure rate at 1 cm from the substitute source. For radium substitutes, the relationship between mCi and mg-equivalents is determined from the ratio of the exposure rate constants for the two nuclides (Example 16-1).

Sources may also be specified in terms of their activity. The use of activity to specify a brachytherapy source is complicated by the influence of the source encapsulation on the exposure rate at some distance from the source. Sources with identical activities but with different encapsulation thicknesses may yield significantly different exposure rates at a distance. The *apparent activity*, A_{app}, of a source is determined from a measurement of the exposure rate at a distance; it describes the activity of that nuclide that would produce the same exposure rate when unencapsulated. However, the American Association of Physicists in Medicine recommends against the use of apparent activity for clinical treatment planning.[39] The National Council on Radiation Protection and Measurements Report No. 41 recommends specification of brachytherapy sources in terms of the exposure rate at 1 m from and perpendicular to the long axis of the source, at its center.[3] More recently, the American Association of Physicists in Medicine,[40] the British Commission on Radiation Units and Measurements,[41] and the Comité Francais Mesures des Rayonnements Ionisants[42] have recommended that brachytherapy sources be specified in terms of their air-kerma strength. The international community uses the term *reference air-kerma rate* (RAKR), which is defined as the air-kerma rate at 1 m from the source in μGy/hr. The air-kerma strength, S_k, is the air-kerma rate measured at a specified distance, usually 1 m. Air-kerma strength is expressed in units of μGy-m^2/hr or cGy-cm^2/hr. Air-kerma strength is related to the exposure rate, X (R/hr), at a reference point in free space by the equation:

$$S_k = X \cdot d^2 \cdot k \cdot \overline{W}/e \qquad (16-2)$$

where d is the distance along the perpendicular bisector of the source longitudinal axis to the point of measurement (usually 1 m), and the conversion from R to Gy, $k \cdot \overline{W}/e$ has the value 0.876 cGy/R for dry air. In the United States, brachytherapy sources are calibrated by the ADCLs, in terms of one or more of these units. However, manufacturers specify source calibrations in different ways and users must apply caution when converting from an unfamiliar dose rate unit to a dose prescription unit. Some treatment planning systems allow the use of multiple units; however, care must be taken when ordering sources from a manufacturer to ensure that there is no confusion among units of measurement.

Example 16-2

What is the air-kerma strength of a radium point source having an activity of 1 mg?

The exposure rate at 1 cm from a 1 mg radium point source is 8.25 R/hr. The air-kerma strength is determined from Equation (16-2) as:

$$(8.25 \text{ R/hr})(1 \text{ cm})^2(0.876 \text{ cGy/R}) = 7.23 \text{ cGy} \cdot \text{cm}^2/\text{hr}$$

Radiation dose from brachytherapy sources

Early prescriptions for brachytherapy treatments were expressed in terms of radiation exposure and they neglected the effects of photon scatter and attenuation in tissue. For many sources, the contributions of scattered radiation to a point very nearly compensate for the tissue attenuation of radiation reaching the same point. Consequently, calculations that neglect the presence of tissue can be reasonably accurate. The exposure rate (in R/hr) at some distance, r (cm), from a *point source* of radioactive material is:

$$\dot{X} = \frac{\Gamma_\delta A}{r^2} \qquad (16-3)$$

where A is the activity of the source, and Γ_δ is the exposure rate constant for the nuclide (Table 16-1). For radium filtered by 0.5 mm Pt(Ir) and in equilibrium with its decay products:

$$\Gamma_\delta = \frac{8.25 \, R \, cm^2}{mCi \times hr}$$

Example 16-3

What is the exposure rate at a distance of 100 cm from a 50 mCi point source of radium filtered by 0.5 mm of Pt(Ir)?

$$\dot{X} = (8.25 \text{ R} \cdot \text{cm}^2/\text{hr} \cdot \text{mCi})\frac{A}{r^2}$$

$$\dot{X} = (8.25 \text{ R} \cdot \text{cm}^2/\text{hr} \cdot \text{mCi})\frac{50 \text{ mCi}}{(100 \text{ cm})^2}$$

$$\dot{X} = 41.2 \frac{\text{mR}}{\text{hr}}$$

The exposure rate, $\dot{X}$, at a location, P, at a distance, r, from a radioactive source of short length, L, and linear density, ρ, is described by the equation:

$$\dot{X} = \frac{\Gamma_\delta \rho \dot{L} e^{-\mu t/\cos\theta}}{r^2} \qquad (16-4)$$

where μ is the attenuation coefficient of the wall of thickness, t, for the x and γ rays emitted by the source (Figure 16-13). The absorption of radiation from the source is greatest in directions at small angles with respect to the source axis, and least in directions perpendicular to the source axis. This *self-absorption* of radiation leads to an anisotropic dose distribution around the source. To facilitate *point-source* calculations, small sources

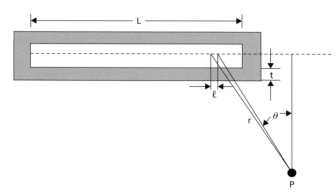

Figure 16-13 Geometry for calculating the exposure rate at location *P* near a radium source of active length *L*. *Source:* Hendee 1970.[2]

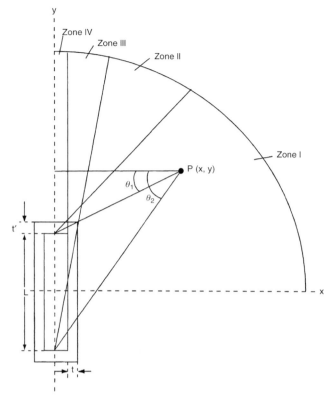

Figure 16-14 Geometry used for calculating the dose rate at a point near a line source, according to the Sievert integral.

are frequently characterized in terms of their *effective activity*, which takes into account the anisotropy.

Sievert integral

For a linear source of length *L*, the exposure rate $\dot{X}$ is computed by integrating Equation (16-4) over the length *L*. The equation cannot be integrated in closed form, but may be approximated by a technique using the Sievert integral.[43] With this approach, Meredith[44] compiled data for radium sources with different active lengths and wall thicknesses. The data describe the product of the amount of radium in milligrams and the exposure time in hours required for an exposure of 1000 R at locations along a line perpendicular to the center of a radium source. Quimby[45] expanded these data to include locations described as distances *along* (parallel with) the source axis and *away* (perpendicular to) from the source axis. The *along distance* is the distance from the center of a source to the location where a line coincident with the source axis and a line through the location of interest intersect at a right angle. The *away distance* is the distance between this intersection and the location of interest. Greenfield and associates[46] revised Quimby's tables to furnish data that describe the exposure/mg-hr at locations on a 0.5 cm grid surrounding a source of radium.

Sievert's method for calculating the dose at points around a linear source requires that the relationship between the point of interest and the source be expressed in terms of (a) the angle between a perpendicular from the point to the source longitudinal axis and (b) lines to each of the source elements. The resulting Sievert integral is shown as Equation (16-5).

$$\dot{D}\,(r, \theta) = \frac{\Gamma_\delta A f}{lr} \int_{\theta_1}^{\theta_2} e^{-\mu t / / \cos\theta} d\theta \qquad (16\text{-}5)$$

In this equation, $\dot{D}(r, \theta)$ is the dose rate at point $P\,(x, y)$, Γ_δ is the exposure rate constant, A is the activity of a source element, f is the f factor (exposure to dose conversion), l is the source element length, r is the distance from the source element to the

point $P\,(x\,y)$, a is the attenuation coefficient of the wall of thickness, t, and θ is the angle between r and a perpendicular from $P\,(x\,y)$ to the source axis.

The geometry of this integral is shown in Figure 16-14.[47] Equation (16-5) applies only in Zone I, which includes only those points that the radiation can reach without passing through an end of the source. Hence only perpendicular or oblique transmission of the radiation through the side wall of the source is considered. In Zone II transmission of radiation at an oblique angle through either the side wall or the end wall of the source is considered. At points in Zone III only the end wall is considered, while in Zone IV all of the radiation is assumed to pass perpendicularly through the end wall. In all zones an attenuation correction for the source material itself must be considered. Some contemporary calculations consider additional zones through more complex computations.

The Sievert integral, with corrections for attenuation and scatter in soft tissue around the source,[48] has been used by Shalek and Stovall[49] to compute tables of dose rates similar to those prepared by Quimby. An excerpt of these data is shown in Table 16-2 and Table 16-3. The data are corrected for oblique filtration of the γ rays in the radium salt and in the walls of the needles. Calculated dose rates around the sources can be found in the literature.[50]

Table 16-2 Dose (cGy) per mg hr in tissue delivered at various distances by linear radium sources.

Perpendicular Distance from Source (cm)	Distance Along Source Axis (cm from Center)										
	0.0	**0.5**	**1.0**	**1.5**	**2.0**	**2.5**	**3.0**	**3.5**	**4.0**	**4.5**	**5.0**
0.25	50.67	43.75	11.94	3.34	1.48	0.81	0.50	—	—	—	—
0.5	20.26	16.95	8.18	3.38	1.70	1.00	0.64	0.44	0.31	0.23	0.18
0.75	10.84	9.29	5.67	2.99	1.67	1.03	0.69	0.48	0.35	0.27	0.21
1.0	6.67	5.89	4.10	2.52	1.55	1.01	0.69	0.50	0.37	0.28	0.22
1.5	3.20	2.96	2.38	1.74	1.24	0.89	0.65	0.48	0.37	0.29	0.23
2.0	1.85	1.76	1.52	1.23	0.96	0.74	0.57	0.45	0.35	0.28	0.23
2.5	1.20	1.15	1.04	0.89	0.74	0.60	0.49	0.40	0.32	0.26	0.22
3.0	0.83	0.81	0.75	0.67	0.58	0.49	0.41	0.34	0.29	0.24	0.21
3.5	0.61	0.60	0.57	0.52	0.46	0.40	0.35	0.30	0.26	0.22	0.19
4.0	0.47	0.46	0.44	0.41	0.37	0.33	0.29	0.26	0.23	0.20	0.17
4.5	0.37	0.36	0.35	0.33	0.30	0.28	0.25	0.22	0.20	0.18	0.16
5.0	0.30	0.29	0.28	0.27	0.25	0.23	0.21	0.19	0.17	0.16	0.14

Note: Filtration = 0.5 mmPt (Ir). Active length = 1.5 cm.
Source: Shalek and Stovall 1969.[49]

Example 16-4

What is the dose rate at point *P* in Figure 16-15? The source is a 10 mg radium tube with an active length of 1.5 cm, filtered by 0.5 mm Pt(Ir). Point *P* is located at $x = 2$ cm, $y = 2$ cm (the midpoint of the source is at the origin).

The along and away distances are both 2 cm, so from Table 16-2 the dose rate = (0.96 cGy/mg hr)(10 mg) = 9.6 cGy/hr.

A Monte Carlo analysis of the Sievert integral has been performed for radium sources.[51] The analysis indicates that, while the Sievert integral overestimates dose rates in tissue per unit activity, the error is reduced if the source intensity is expressed in units of exposure rate rather than activity.

Isodose distributions from individual sealed sources

Isodose curves for a sealed source may be measured, or may be computed with data such as those in Tables 16-2 and 16-3. An isodose distribution computed for a 1 mg radium needle is shown in Figure 16-15. The dose rate is reduced near the ends of the needle because γ rays emitted at a slight angle with respect to the source axis are filtered by a greater thickness of the platinum–iridium wall. Measurement of isodose

Table 16-3 Dose (cGy) per mg hr in tissue delivered at various distances by linear radium sources.

Perpendicular Distance from Source (cm)	Distance Along Source Axis (cm from Center)										
	0.0	**0.5**	**1.0**	**1.5**	**2.0**	**2.5**	**3.0**	**3.5**	**4.0**	**4.5**	**5.0**
0.25	45.87	39.70	10.19	—	—	—	—	—	—	—	—
0.5	18.56	15.51	7.25	2.88	1.39	0.78	0.49	—	—	—	—
0.75	10.01	8.54	5.10	2.60	1.43	0.86	0.56	0.38	0.27	0.20	0.16
1.0	6.20	5.44	3.72	2.23	1.35	0.86	0.58	0.41	0.30	0.22	0.17
1.5	2.99	2.75	2.18	1.57	1.10	0.78	0.56	0.41	0.31	0.24	019
2.0	1.73	1.64	1.40	1.12	0.86	0.65	0.50	0.39	0.30	0.24	0.20
2.5	1.12	1.08	0.97	0.82	0.67	0.54	0.43	0.35	0.28	0.23	0.19
3.0	0.78	0.76	0.70	0.62	0.53	0.44	0.37	0.31	0.26	0.21	0.18
3.5	0.57	0.56	0.53	0.48	0.42	0.37	0.31	0.27	0.23	0.19	0.17
4.0	0.44	0.43	0.41	0.38	0.34	0.31	0.27	0.23	0.20	0.17	0.15
4.5	0.34	0.34	0.33	0.31	0.28	0.26	0.23	0.20	0.18	0.16	0.14
5.0	0.28	0.27	0.26	0.25	0.23	0.22	0.20	0.18	0.16	0.14	0.13

Note: Filtration = 1.0 mm Pt (Ir). Active length = 1.5 cm.
Source: Shalek and Stovall 1969.[49]

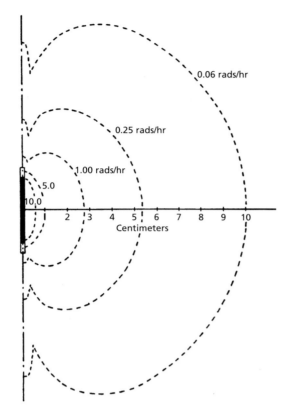

Figure 16-15 Isodose distribution for a 1 mg radium needle. *Source:* Rose et al. 1966.[47]

distributions has been accomplished using ionization chambers,[52,53] diodes,[54] thermoluminescent dosimeters,[20,55] and film dosimetry.[56] Because many brachytherapy sources emit a spectrum of x and γ rays, attention must be paid to the response of the detector to different photon energies.

Summary

- Radium and radon seeds, the original brachytherapy sources, are no longer used; they have been replaced by sources of ^{137}Cs, ^{192}Ir, ^{125}I and ^{103}Pd.
- Radioactive implants may be temporary (long-lived sources are used) or permanent (short-lived sources are used).
- Air-kerma strength (S_K with units μGy $\cdot$ m^2/hr or cGy $\cdot$ cm^2/hr) is the current preferred expression to describe brachytherapy sources.
- Early dose calculations for brachytherapy sources were based on the exposure rate at a distance from the source.
- The Sievert integral predicts the exposure at a point from a source based on source geometry, particularly oblique filtration through the jacket or wall material.

Problems

16-1 For most radioactive sources, the rate of emission of γ rays decreases continuously. However, the rate of emission of γ rays from a sealed source of radium-226 (^{226}Ra) increases to a constant value over the first 30 days or so after the ^{226}Ra is placed in the sealed container. Why?

16-2 What is the activity in mCi of ^{226}Ra, radon-222 (^{222}Rn), ^{255}Po (polonium), and ^{214}Po in a 10 mg source of radium in secular equilibrium? What is the mass in grams of ^{222}Rn in the source?

16-3 What is the volume occupied by a "carrier-free" sample of radium sulfate (RaSO$_4$) that contains 1 mg of ^{226}Ra? The density of RaSO$_4$ is 5.42 g/cm^3. Does this volume of sample fill a 1 mg needle used for interstitial implants? If not, how is a nonuniform distribution of radioactive material avoided?

16-4 What is the activity of a 1 mg-Ra-eq ^{192}Ir source? A 1 mg-Ra-eq^{60}Co source?

16-5 What is the air-kerma strength of a 1 mCi ^{125}I source?

16-6 What activity ^{125}I source will produce the same exposure rate at 10 cm distance in air as a 1 mCi ^{198}Au source?

16-7 What is the exposure rate 20 cm from a 10 mg point source of radium filtered by 1.0 mm Pt(Ir)?

16-8 For a 1 mg Ra-eq cesium source with an active length of 1.4 cm and filtered by 1 mm stainless steel, compare the dose rates at locations 2 cm and 5 cm from the source along a line perpendicular to the center of the source. Compute the dose rates

 a. using the inverse square expression and an f factor of 0.96.

 b. using the data in Table 16-2.

 Explain why the dose rates computed by the two methods do not agree.

References

1 Lederer, C. M., Hollander, J. M., and Perlman, I. *Table of Isotopes*, 6th edition. New York, John Wiley & Sons, 1967.

2 Hendee, W. R. *Medical Radiation Physics*, 1st edition. Chicago, Mosby—Year Book, 1970.

3 National Council on Radiation Protection and Measurements. *Specification of gamma ray brachytherapy sources*, Report No. 41. Washington, DC, NCRP Publications, 1974.

4 Payne, W H., and Waggener, R. G. A theoretical calculation of the exposure rate constant for radium-226, *Med. Phys.* 1974; **1**(4):210–214.

5 Pochin, E. E., and Kermode, J. C. Protection problems in radionuclide therapy: The patient as a gamma ray source. *Br. J. Radiol.* 1975; **48**:299.

6 Glasgow, G. P., and Dillman, L. T. Specific y-ray constant and exposure rate constant of ^{192}Ir. *Med. Phys.* 1979; **6**(1):49–52.

7 Glasgow, G. P. The specific y-ray constant and exposure rate constant of ^{182}Ta. *Med. Phys.* 1982; **9**(2):250–253.

8 Anderson, L. L., Kaum,H. M., and Ding, I. Y. Clinical dosimetry with I-125. In *Modern Interstitial and Intracavitary Radiation Cancer Management*, F. W. George (ed.). New York, Masson Publishing, 1981.

9 Meredith, W, and Massey, J. *Fundamental Physics of Radiology*. Baltimore, Williams & Wilkins, 1968.

10 Cohen, L. Protracted interstitial irradiation of tumors using Ta. *Br. J. Radiol.* 1955; **28**:338.

11 Haybittle, J. Dosage distributions from "hairpins" of radioactive tantalum wire. *Br. J. Radiol.* 1957; **30**:49.

12 Sakhatshiev, A., and Moushmov, M. A new type of radioactive wire source. *Radiology* 1967; **89**(5):903–905.

13 Son, Y, and Ramsby, G. Percutaneous tantalum-182 wire implantation using guiding-needle technique for head and neck tumors. *Am. J. Radiol.* 1966; **96**:37.

14 Trott, N., and Whearley, B. Tantalum-182 wire gamma ray applicators for use in ophthalmology. *Br. J. Radiol.* 1956; **29**:13.

15 VanMiert, P., and Fowler, J. The use of tantalum-182 in the treatment of early bladder carcinoma. *Br. J. Radiol.* 1956; **29**:508.

16 Wallace, D., Stapleton, J., and Turner, R. Radioactive tantalum wire implantation as a method of treatment for early carcinoma of the bladder. *Br. J. Radiol.* 1952; **25**:421.

17 Meigooni, A. S., Kleiman, M. T, Johnson, J. L., Mazloomdoost, D., and Ibbott G. S. Dosimetric characteristics of a new high-intensity Ir source for remote afterloading. *Med. Phys.* 1997; **24**(12):2008–2013.

18 Goetsch, S. J., Attix, F H., Pearson, D. W, and Thomadsen, B. R. Calibration of Ir high-dose-rate afterloading systems. *Med. Phys.* 1991; **18**(3)462–467.

19 Slanina, I., and Wannenmacher, M. Interstitial radiotherapy with Au seeds in the primary management of carcinoma of the oral tongue. *Int. J. Radiol. Biol. Phys.* 1982; **8**:1683.

20 Nath, R., and Melillo, A. Dosimetric characteristics of a double wall ^{125}I source for interstitial brachytherapy. *Med. Phys.* 1993; **20**(5):1475–1483.

21 Weaver, K. A., Anderson, L. L., and Meli, J. A. Source characteristics. In *Interstitial Brachytherapy: Physical, Biological, and Clinical Considerations*, L.L. Anderson, R. Nath, K. A. Weaver, Nori, D., Phillips, T L., Son, Y H., Chiu-Tsao, S. T, Mciqooni, A. S., Meli, J. A., and Smith, V (eds.). New York, Raven Press, 1990.

22 Gearheart, D. M., Drogin, A., Sowards, K., Meigooni, A. S., and Ibbott, G. S. Dosimetric characteristics of a new ^{125}I brachytherapy source. *Med. Phys.* 2000; **27**(10):2278–2285.

23 Hedtjarn, H., Carlsson, G. A., and Williamson, J. F. Monte Carlo-aided dosimetry of the symmetra model I25.S06 ^{125}I, interstitial brachytherapy seed. *Med. Phys.* 2000; **27**(5):1076–1085.

24 Williamson, J. F. Monte Carlo modeling of the transverse-axis dose distribution of the Model 200 ^{103}Pd interstitial brachytherapy source. *Med. Phys.* 2000; **27**(4):634–654.

25 Duggan, H. Results using strontium-90 beta-ray applicator on eye lesions. *J. Can. Assoc. Radiol.* 1966; **17**:132.

26 Friedell, H., Thomas, C, and Krohmer, J. Evaluation of clinical use of strontium-90 beta-ray applicator with review of underlying principles. *Am. J. Radiol.* 1954; **71**:25.

27 Deasy, J. O., and Soares, C. G. Extrapolation chamber measurements of ^{90}Sr^{+90}Y beta-particle ophthalmic applicator dose rates. *Med. Phys.* 1994; **21**(1):91–99.

28 Hendee, W R. Measurement and correction of nonuniform surface dose rates for beta eye applicators. *Am. J. Radiol.* 1968; **103**:734.

29 Hendee, W R. Thermoluminescent dosimetry of the beta depth dose. *Am. J. Radiol.* 1966; **97**:1045.

30 Nag, S., Quivey, J. M., Earle, J. D., Followill, D. S., Fontanesi, J., and Finger, P. The American Brachytherapy Society Recommendations for Brachytherapy of Uveal Melanomas, *Int. J. Radiat. Oncol. Biol. Phys.* 2003; **56**:544–555.

31 Oliver, G., and Wright, C. Dosimetry of an implantable ^{252}Cf source. *Radiology* 1969; **92**(1):143–147.

32 Reinig, W. Advantages and applications of ^{252}Cf as a neutron source. *Nucl. Applic.* 1968; **5**:24–25.

33 Wright, C., Boulogne, A., Reinig, W., and Evans, A. Implantable californium-252 neutron sources for radiotherapy. *Radiology* 1967; **89**(2):337.

34 Hendee, W R., and Lohlein, S. Handling radium in a hospital. *Radiol. Technol.* 1968; **39**:221.

35 Johns, H., and Cunningham, J. *The Physics of Radiology*, 3rd edition. Springfield, III, Charles C Thomas, 1969.

36 Morgan, J., and Nunnally, J. Report on a radium safe and leak testing system. *Radiology* 1969; **92**:161.

37 National Council on Radiation Protection and Measurements. *Protection against radiation from brachytherapy sources*, Report No. 40. Washington, DC, NCRP Publications, 1972.

38 Webb, H. An improved radium safe. *Br. J. Radiol.* 1960; **33**:654.

39 Williamson, J. F., Coursey, B. M., DeWerd, L. A., Hanson, W F., Nath, R., and Ibbott, G. S. On the use of apparent activity (A_{app}) for treatment planning of I and Pd interstitial brachytherapy sources: Recommendations of the American Association of Physicists in Medicine Radiation Therapy Committee Subcommittee on Low-Energy Brachytherapy Source Dosimetry. *Med. Phys.* 1999; **26**(12):2529–2530.

40 AAPM Task Group No. 32. *Specification of brachytherapy source strength*, Report No. 21, June 1987.

41 British Committee on Radiation Units and Measurements. Specification of brachytherapy sources. *Br. J. Radiol.* 1984; **57**: 941.

42 Comité Francais Mesures des Rayonnements Ionisants, *Recommendations pour La determination des doses absorbees en curietherapie*, CFMRI. Report No. 1, 1983.

43 Sievert, R. Die Gamma-strahlungsintensitatan der oberFläche and in der nachstenUmgebang von Radium-Nadeln. *Acta. Radiol.* 1930; **11**:249.

44 Meredith, W (ed.). *Radium Dosage: The Manchester System*, 2nd edition. Baltimore, Williams & Wilkins, 1967.

45 Quimby, E. Dosage table for linear radium sources. *Radiology* 1944; **43**:572.

46 Greenfield, M., Fichman, M., and Norman, A. Dosage tables for linear radium sources filtered by 0.5 and 1.0 mm of platinum. *Radiology* 1959; **73**:418.

47 Rose, J., Bloedorn, F., and Robinson, J. A computer dosimetry system for radium implants. *Am. J. Radiol.* 1966; **97**:1032.

48 Meisberger, L. L., Keller, R. J., and Shalek, R. J. The effective attenuation in water of the gamma rays of gold-198, iridium-192, cesium-137, radium-226, and cobalt-60. *Radiology* 1968; **90**:953.

49 Shalek, R. J., and Stovall, M. Dosimetry in implant therapy. In *Radiation Dosimetry*, F. H. Attixand, and E. Tochlin (eds.). New York, Academic Press, 1969.

50 Krishnaswamy, V. Dose distributions about ^{137}Cs sources in tissue. *Radiology*, 1972; **105**:181–184.

51 Williamson, J. F., Morin, R. L., and Khan, F. M. Monte Carlo evaluation of the Sievert integral for brachytherapy dosimetry. *Phys. Med. Biol.* 1983; **28**:1021–1032.

52 Baltas, D., Kramer, R., and Loffler, E. Measurements of the anisotropy of the new iridium-192 source for the microSelectron-HDR. Special Report No. 3. In *Activity selectron*, R. F. Mould (ed.). Veenendaal, Nucletron International BV, 1993.

53 Walstam, R. The dosage distribution in the pelvis in radium treatment of carcinoma of the cervix. *ActaRadiol.* 1954; **42**:237.

54 Ling, C. C, Yorke, E. D., Spiro, I. J., Kubiatowicz, D., and Bennett, D. Physical dosimetry of I seeds of a new design for interstitial implant. *Int. J. Radiat. Oncol. Biol. Phys.* 1983; **9**:1747–1752.

55 Muller-Runkel, R., and Cho, S. H. Anisotropy measurements of a high dose rate Ir-192 source in air and in polystyrene. *Med. Phys.* 1994; **21**(7):1131–1134.

56 Chiu-Tsao, S., de la Zerda, A., Lin, J., and Kim, J. H. High-sensitivity GafChromic film dosimetry for ^{125}I seeds. *Med. Phys.* 1994; **21**(5):651–657.

C H A P T E R

17

BRACHYTHERAPY TREATMENT PLANNING

Objectives

After studying this chapter, the reader should be able to:
- Describe different devices for implantation and insertion of brachytherapy sources.
- Describe different interstitial and intracavitary implant systems.
- Calculate the dose delivered for temporary and permanent implants.
- Discuss methods for localizing brachytherapy sources from planar images.
- Discuss methods of volumetric imaging techniques for high- and low-dose rate brachytherapy.

Introduction

The previous chapter describes various aspects of brachytherapy, including radioisotopes, radiation safety for brachytherapy sources, and isodose calculations and distributions around a source or sources. This chapter aims to describe the applicators and equipment used for various brachytherapy techniques as well as the historical rationale behind some of the current implant rules and reference points. Additionally, the reader will be introduced to dose calculations for permanent implants, remote afterloading systems, and localization techniques used in brachytherapy.

Design of implants

Intracavitary implant applicators

Cancer of the uterus and cervix is often treated with an applicator designed to hold sealed radioactive sources in a fixed position against the cervix and in the uterine canal. One to four

Hendee's Radiation Therapy Physics, Fourth Edition. Todd Pawlicki, Daniel J. Scanderbeg and George Starkschall.
© 2016 John Wiley & Sons, Inc. Published 2016 by John Wiley & Sons, Inc.

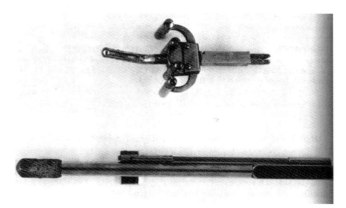

Figure 17-1 Expanding Ernst applicator for sealed source therapy of cancer of the cervix and uterus.
Source: Hendee, 1970.[2]

sealed sources are contained within a central tube (*tandem*), which is inserted into the uterine canal. Additional sources are placed in capsules, or *ovoids*, positioned against the cervix. The ovoids may be separated from each other by rubber or plastic spacers. One of the first applicators designed for treatment of the cervix is shown in Figure 17-1.[1]

Personnel involved in brachytherapy implants are potentially subject to high radiation exposures. Manual "afterloading" techniques have been developed to reduce these exposures.[3–5] Several modern afterloading applicators are shown in Figure 17-2. Sources are not introduced into the applicator until the applicator itself has been positioned inside the patient and packed into position. The sources are then installed quickly and in a manner that minimizes the radiation exposure to personnel. Additionally, remote afterloaders, which we saw in the previous chapter and are discussed again below, reduce exposure even further to effectively zero exposure for staff. Applicators are placed in the patient and connected to the remote afterloader and everyone, except the patient, leaves the room. The source(s) is then placed in position in the patient remotely, often from a shielded control room located next to the treatment room.

When cancer of the cervix or uterus is treated with sealed sources, the absorbed dose is generally calculated at points identified as A and B. The definition of points A and B is one of the most durable contributions of the Manchester system. Point A simultaneously represents two treatment-limiting conditions: (1) the lateral aspect of the target organ (the cervix) that must receive at least the minimum target dose and (2) the location of dose-sensitive normal structures, namely the ureter and the uterine artery, that limit the maximum dose tolerated. Point A is located 2 cm laterally from the uterine canal and 2 cm above the lateral fornix. Point B is located on the pelvic wall 3 cm lateral to point A (Figure 17-3). The absorbed dose to these points from each source in the applicator may be computed with data such as those in Tables 17-2, 17-3, and 17-4. The total dose to points A and B is the sum of the contributions from each source. The general location of point A often lies near a steep gradient

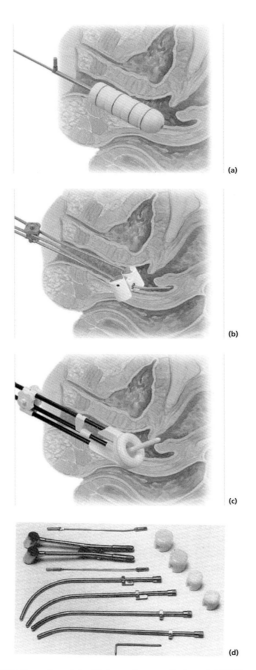

Figure 17-2 Several models of intracavitary applicators. (a) HDR segmented cylinders; (b) HDR Fletcher/Williamson tandem and ovoids; (c) HDR CT/MR compatible tandem and ring; (d) LDR Fletcher-Suit-Delclos tandem and ovoids.
Source: Parts a–c courtesy of Nucletron Corporation; Part d courtesy of Mick Radio-Nuclear Instruments Inc.

in dose rate. Hence, small changes in the definition of point A can produce large variations in the delivered dose.

The total dose also should be computed for the anterior wall of the rectum and the posterior wall of the bladder. If the computed doses are excessive, gauze inserted between the applicator and the rectum or bladder may be repacked to provide greater

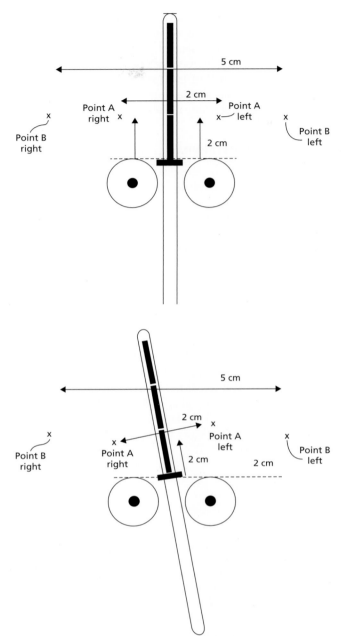

Figure 17-3 Point A is 2 cm lateral from the uterine canal and 2 cm above the lateral fornix. Point B is on the pelvic wall 3 cm lateral to point A. Note that there are two points A and two points B, with one A and one B on each side of the uterus.

separation. New high-dose rate (HDR) applicators commonly come with rectal retractors which can increase separation and decrease dose to the rectum. Dose rates along the anterior wall of the rectum and in the bladder may be measured with dosimeters such as a lithium fluoride thermoluminescent dosimeter or a cadmium sulfide probe. Some modern brachytherapy applicators incorporate lead or tungsten shielding to provide additional protection to the rectum and bladder. The influence of

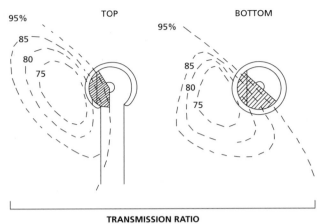

TRANSMISSION RATIO

Figure 17-4 Effect of bladder and rectal shields in the coronal plane above and below a Fletcher–Suit colpostat. The dashed curves indicate the transmission of the tungsten shielding.
Source: Haas et al. 1983.[6] Reproduced with permission of Elsevier.

the shielding material on the dose distribution has been measured (Figure 17-4), but corrections are rarely applied in clinical practice.[6,7] Recent advancements in shielded HDR applicators have provided a dynamic modulated brachytherapy (DMBT) similar to an intensity-modulated radiation therapy technique, but for brachytherapy.[8–10] Clinical techniques for low-dose rate (LDR) brachytherapy in the treatment of cervical cancer have been summarized by the American Brachytherapy Society.[11]

The procedure for identifying points A and B changed in 1953 using the external cervical os as the origin rather than the lateral vaginal fornix. On x-ray images, the ovoids often cast very little shadow, making the baseline difficult to establish. Instead of a line connecting the tops of the sources to the ovoids, the new origin became the bottom of the most inferior tandem source. Due to the construction of the spacer that separates the ovoids and holds the tandem in place, this origin usually falls near the original baseline. When afterloading tandems became prevalent, the origin frequently was defined by the position of the flange abutting the external cervical os to prevent the tandem from perforating the top of the uterus.

A recommendation for identifying reproducible calculation points is described in ICRU Report No. 38.[12] However, with the increased use of CT and MR imaging in treatment planning for brachytherapy, the Groupe Européen de Curiethérapie–European Society for Therapeutic Radiology and Oncology (GEC-ESTRO) have proposed their own definitions for target delineation and dose reporting values.[13,14] These include definitions for gross tumor volume (GTV), high-risk clinical target volume (HRCTV) and intermediate risk clinical target volume (IRCTV), as well as recommended cumulative dose-volume histogram (DVH) parameters for target volumes and organs at risk (OARs). The reader is referred to references 13 and 14 for a more thorough description and encouraged to check current literature as new recommendations have been presented in conference and publication is in progress.

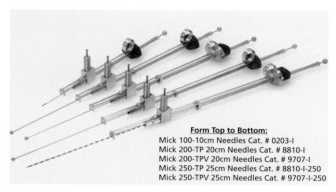

Form Top to Bottom:
Mick 100-10cm Needles Cat. # 0203-I
Mick 200-TP 20cm Needles Cat. # 8810-I
Mick 200-TPV 20cm Needles Cat. # 9707-I
Mick 250-TP 25cm Needles Cat. # 8810-I-250
Mick 250-TPV 25cm Needles Cat. # 9707-I-250

Figure 17-5 Instruments for interstitial implants.
Source: Courtesy of Mick Radio-Nuclear Instruments, Inc.

Interstitial implant applicators

Early interstitial applications were administered by inserting radium needles directly into tissue. Today, interstitial implants may be temporary (the sources are removed after a few minutes, hours, or days of treatment) or permanent (the sources remain in the patient permanently). Permanent implants are practical only when sources with either a short half-life or low energy are used. The sources are inserted directly into the tissue being treated with an applicator such as that shown in Figure 17-5. When a temporary interstitial implant is used, catheters may be introduced into the tissue and radioactive sources encased in nylon ribbons are passed through the catheters and fixed into place for the duration of treatment (LDR) or an HDR source introduced into the catheter for a few seconds or minutes for each fraction. For both permanent and temporary implants, rules are available for positioning the sources to achieve a desired dose distribution. Modern techniques include computer-aided planning, which is discussed later in the chapter.

Distribution rules for interstitial implants

Three approaches have been widely used for determining the amount and distribution of activity required for a surface mold or interstitial implant. These approaches were developed with radium sources but then continued in use for radium substitutes such as cesium and iridium. To some extent the rules were used without modification so long as the source activities were expressed in mg-Ra-eq. However, modern computer-based treatment planning techniques have permeated the field and largely eliminated their use. Hence, a brief qualitative description of the rules, their history, and significance today are described below.

The Quimby system

The Quimby system is named after Edith Quimby, who was a prominent medical physicist who worked in radiation oncology for many years at Columbia University. Using this approach, the implant was composed of one or more planes containing a uniform distribution of sealed sources. The radiation dose to tissue near the center of the plane was much greater than that delivered to tissue near the edges. With the Quimby system, a uniform distribution of sealed sources was used to produce a nonuniform distribution of radiation dose to the treated region.

The Manchester system

The Manchester system (Manchester, England) is also known as the *Paterson–Parker system* after its developers R. Paterson and H. Parker. Using the Manchester system, sealed sources were arranged in a nonuniform manner to furnish a distribution of radiation dose that varies by less than ± 10% across the implant plane(s). For a planar implant, the Manchester system always specifies the dose in a plane 0.5 cm from the plane containing the needles. British standard radium needles, those associated with the Manchester system, came in two linear radium densities: *full strength* of 0.66 mg/cm and *half strength* of 0.33 mg/cm. Rules for distributing the activity across the implant are described in Table 17-1.

More activity is required for an implant designed according to the Manchester system than for one designed by the Quimby system, provided that the doses are equal at the center of the treated area. However, the radiation dose is more uniform with the Manchester system. The Manchester system is the basis for our HDR implants today with a more uniform dose distribution across the treated area.

The Paris system

In the early 1970s, the availability of radioactive iridium wire led to the development of the Paris system for interstitial implant calculations. The system was designed originally for use with continuous wires of iridium, but was later adapted for implants constructed with iridium seeds in nylon ribbons, with the assumption that the linear activity (mCi/cm) is constant. The Paris system does not permit use of crossing sources; instead, the length of the sources is chosen to extend beyond the target volume at both ends of the implant (Table 17-1). The spacing between sources, which may vary from 5 mm to 20 mm, is kept uniform for a given implant. For volume implants, the sources are arranged in parallel planes, with the spacing between planes equal to 0.87 times the spacing between sources in a plane. The planes may be arranged so that the sources form a rectilinear pattern, or the sources in alternate planes may be offset by half the distance between sources.

Several parameters must be quantified when the Paris system is used (Figure 17-6). The *basal dose rate* is the average of the dose rates at points intermediate between the sources, in a central plane perpendicular to the sources. From this value, a *reference dose rate* is computed as 85% of the basal dose rate. If the implant is designed according to the rules of the Paris system, the

Table 17-1 Systems for interstitial brachytherapy.

	Manchester	Quimby	Paris
Representative dose and dose rate	6000–8000 R in 6–8 days 1060 R/day or 40 R/hr)	5000–6000 R in 3–4 days (60 R/hr to 70 R/hr is expected to be biologically equivalent to Manchester system)	6000–7000 cGy in 3–11 days (25–90 cGy/hr); usually in 3–6 days
Dose prescription point(s)	Effective minimum dose is 10% above the absolute minimum dose in a plane or volume	Planar implants: on the perpendicular bisector to the plane. Volume implants: to the periphery point receiving a minimum dose, the minimum in the actual implanted region	Basal dose is the average of the minimum doses in the central plane in the region defined by the source; reference dose is 85% of the basal dose and encompasses the target plane, or volume
Dose gradient	Does not vary by more than 10%, except in localized hot spots around the source	No stated goal; the intent was to determine the increased dose gradients resulting from using sources all with the same linear activity; gradient frequently approaches 100% with twice the dose in the center as at the edge of the region	15% between reference dose and basal dose (average minimum) by definition
Linear activity	Variable (0.66 mg Ra/cm, 0.50 mg Ra/cm, 0.33 mg Ra/cm)	Constant (1.0 mg Ra/cm used historically; 0.20–0.70 mg Ra eq/cm commonly used)	Constant 0.8 to 0.6 mg Ra eq/cm commonly used
Activity distribution: single plane	Areas smaller than 25 cm^2; 2/3 activity on periphery, 1/3 activity in center Areas 25–100 cm^2; 1/2 activity on periphery, 1/2 activity in center areas >100 cm^2; 1/3 activity on periphery, 2/3 activity in center	Uniform distribution over implant plane	Uniform distribution over implant plane
Activity distribution: volume	cylinder: 4/8 of the activity in the belt; 2/8 of the activity in the core; 1/8 of the activity on each end. Sphere: 6/8 of the activity in the rind; 2/8 of the activity in the core. Cube: 1/8 of the activity in each face; 2/8 of the activity in the core	Uniform distribution of activity throughout the volume	For volume, the sources are arranged in planes such that the sources in adjacent planes form either equilateral triangles or squares. Spacing between planes is about 0.87 times the spacing between sources for equivalent triangles
Source implant pattern and spacing between sources as a function of implant volume	Constant uniform spacing; 1 cm separation between sources recommended	Variable but uniform spacing with up to 2 cm separation allowed between sources; spacing between sources determined by implant target dimensions	Variable but uniform spacing. Spacing determined by implant target dimensions; larger source separation in larger volumes; 5 mm minimum to 20 mm maximum separation
Crossing needles	Perpendicular to and at the active ends of the plane of sources; if placed beyond the active ends of the needles, should be double strength. Crossing needles required; if one end uncrossed, then area of implant for calculation is decreased by 10%. Twenty percent area reduction. Correction (10% each end) for both ends uncrossed	Same as Manchester system	Not used; active sources are 20 to 30% longer than the target volume at *both* ends to compensate for uncrossed ends
Elongation factors	Area: long side/short side ratio and % correction: 2/1 (+ 5%); 3/1 (+ 9%); 4/1 (+ 12%) Volume: length/diameter ratio and % correction: 1.5/1 (+ 3%); 2/1 (+ 6%); 2.5/1 (+ 10%); 3/1 (+ 15%)	Same as Manchester system	Not used
Relation of source length to target (volume) length	Active length determines target length (or vice versa); inner needles (not periphery) determine target width	Same as Manchester system	Active source lengths 20–30% longer than the target dimensions at both ends to compensate for uncrossed ends

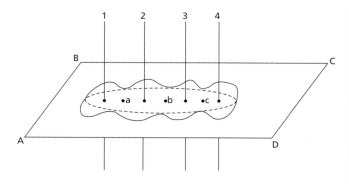

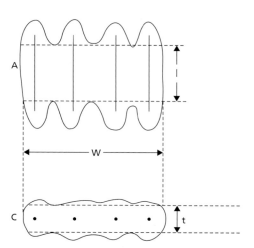

Figure 17-6 Some definitions used in the Paris system of interstitial implants. Four ribbon or wire sources (1, 2, 3, 4) transect the central plane (A, B, C, D) on which the dose calculation is carried out. The basal dose rate (BD) is the mean of the dose rates a, b, and c midway between the sources. The reference dose rate (0.85 BD) has an irregular contour (wavy line) and totally encloses the target volume. The length (l) of the treatment volume is the separation between the minimum indentations in the reference isodose curves; the width (w) is determined by the maximum extent of the reference dose rate curve. The reference dose rate and length and width are specified in the plane containing the sources.
Source: Adapted from Pierquin et al. 1978.[15]

reference dose rate corresponds to an isodose curve that encompasses the target volume. The length of the volume encompassed by the reference dose rate isodose line is shorter than the length of the sources, which should be chosen to exceed the dimensions of the target volume by 20–30%. The width and thickness of the volume encompassed by the reference dose rate isodose line are determined by the number of sources and the number of planes, respectively.[15] The Paris system has been compared with the Manchester system and offers several advantages.[16]

Remote afterloading

The benefits of brachytherapy *afterloading* are discussed earlier in this chapter. These benefits are exploited further through

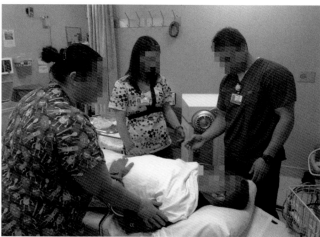

Figure 17-7 A high-dose rate remote afterloader depicting a patient setup for an endobronchial treatment.
Source: Courtesy of University of California, San Diego.

the use of *remote afterloading*. Remote afterloading devices consist of a mobile shielded safe that can be connected by a tube to an implant applicator previously placed in the patient (Figure 17-7). One or more radioactive sources can be moved by remote control from the shielded safe, through the tube, and into the implanted applicator. A programmable timer in the console of the unit causes the sources to be retracted when treatment is complete.

Remote afterloading systems may use low-activity sources that provide dose rates in the range of 0.4–2 Gy/hr. This approach is called *low-dose rate brachytherapy*. LDR systems are intended to replace conventional implants, with the added benefit that the sources can be retracted into the safe at the touch of a button, thereby permitting medical personnel to attend to the patient without risk of exposure.

High- activity sources are used in medium-dose rate (MDR) units for dose rates of 2–12 Gy/hr and in HDR units that provide dose rates greater than 12 Gy/hr, typically in the range of 150 Gy/hr. HDR units permit the delivery of brachytherapy treatments on an outpatient basis. That is, the patient is fitted with an interstitial or intracavitary applicator, and a treatment lasting only a few seconds or minutes is delivered and repeated on several occasions. The biological equivalence of HDR and LDR treatments is being evaluated.[17,18]

Pulsed dose rate (PDR) brachytherapy has been used, but is not very popular in the United States, primarily due to the regulatory requirements of the Nuclear Regulatory Commission.[19] It offers the benefits of LDR brachytherapy combined with the radiation safety advantages of a remote afterloader. Moderately high activity sources are used (typically 1 Ci of ^{192}Ir) and the dose is protracted over several days by delivering the treatment in small fractions at hourly intervals. By delivering the dose over several days, a radiobiological response similar to LDR brachytherapy is achieved, while providing almost unlimited access to the patient by healthcare staff. Monitoring of a PDR system requires the continuous availability of a knowledgeable operator to ensure safe treatment.

A remote afterloading unit offers the advantage of great flexibility in the design of the dose distribution. The unit can be programmed to position the source at a large number of locations and to pause at each location for a pre-selected time (*dwell time*). Careful selection of dwell times permits duplication of implants designed according to the Quimby system, the Manchester system, or the Paris system. Modern computer software allows for the optimization of implants using remote afterloading systems.[20]

Computer calculations

Most brachytherapy dose calculations, including those for HDR remote afterloaders and LDR permanent seed implants, are now done using computer algorithms. In 1995, the American Association of Physicists in Medicine (AAPM) published the Task Group No. 43 Report, which was a protocol (TG43) that described a dose calculation formalism for brachytherapy.[21] Since then it has been updated several times, but continues to be the recommended brachytherapy dose calculation formalism.[22,23] This formalism has been incorporated in most commercial treatment planning software that is currently available and is described more formally in the next section, on air-kerma strength calculation. One consideration to keep in mind with this dose calculation is that all material is assumed to be homogeneous. Current advances include more sophisticated dose calculation methods that are being made available in commercial modules that allow Monte Carlo-like calculations in shorter amounts of time through direct calculation of the linear Boltzmann transport equation.[24] This allows for heterogeneity

corrections to be applied; However, caution should be taken if this type of calculation is implemented into a clinic as all clinical experience is derived from doses calculated in homogenous media. AAPM Task Group 186 discusses the use and implementation of model-based algorithms.[24]

Air-kerma strength calculation

Brachytherapy sources sometimes are specified in terms of their *air-kerma strength* (S_k), expressed in units of μGy-m^2/hr or cGy-cm^2/hr. When these units are used, the dose rate, $\dot{D}(r, \theta)$, in the vicinity of the source is expressed as:[25]

$$\dot{D}(r, \theta) = S_k \cdot \Lambda \cdot \frac{G(r, \theta)}{G(r = 1\,\text{cm}, \theta = \pi/2)} \cdot g(r) \cdot F(r, \theta) \quad (17\text{-}1)$$

where Λ is the dose-rate constant for the source and surrounding medium defined at 1 cm away from the source on its perpendicular bisector.[26] The dose-rate constant is expressed in units of cGy/hr per unit air-kerma strength. In other words:

$$\Lambda = \frac{\dot{D}(1, \pi/2)}{S_k}$$

The value of the dose-rate constant Λ depends on the medium surrounding the source, because it indicates the rate at which energy is absorbed by the medium. It also depends on the design and construction of the source, because these factors influence the scattering of photons in the medium. Values of the dose-rate constant are available from the literature, source manufacturers, and calibration laboratories. Source strength conversion factors for several sources are given in Table 17-2.

$G(r, \theta)$, the *geometry function r*, with units of cm^{-2}, describes the decrease in dose as a function of distance from the source. For a point source, $G(r, \theta) = r^{-2}$. For a line source of significant length and uniform distribution of activity, $G(r, \theta) = (\theta_2 - \theta_1)/L$

Table 17-2 Source strength conversion factors for interstitial brachytherapy sources.

Sources	Source Strength Quantity	Units	Exposure Rate Constant $(\Gamma\delta)_x$ or Exposure Rate Constant for Filtration $(\Gamma\delta)_{x,t}$ R cm$^2 \cdot$ mCi$^{-1} \cdot$ hr^{-1}	Air-kerma Strength Conversion Factor (S/Quantity)[b]
All	Equivalent mass of Radium	mg $\cdot$ Ra $\cdot$ eq	8.25	7.227 U mg-Ra-eq^{-1}
All	Reference exposure rate	mR $\cdot$ m$^2 \cdot$ hr^{-1}	—	8.760 U/mR m$^2 \cdot$ hr^{-1}
		nR $\cdot$ m$^2 \cdot$ sec^{-1}	—	3.154 × 10^{-2}
		C $\cdot$ kg^{-1}	—	U/nR m^2 sec^{-1}
		m$^2 \cdot$ sec^{-1}	—	1.222 × 10^{11} U/C kg$^{-1} \cdot$ m$^2 \cdot$ sec^{-1}
^{192}Ir seed t = 0.2 mm Fe	Apparent activity	mCi	4.60	4.030 U mCi^{-1}
^{192}Ir seed t = 0.05 mm Pt-Ir	Apparent activity	mCi	4.80[a]	4.205 U mCi^{-1}
^{125}I seeds	Apparent activity	mCi	1.45	1.270 U mCi^{-1}
^{103}Pd seeds	Apparent activity	mCi	1.48	1.293 U mCi^{-1}

Notes:
[a]See the explanation for using 4.80 versus 4.60 in reference 27. Briefly, the manufacturer uses 4.80 in calibrating the sources; therefore the user must also use the same number.
[b]1 U = 1 unit of air-kerma strength = 1 μGy $\cdot$ m^2, h^{-1} = 1 cGy $\cdot$ cm$^2 \cdot$ h^{-1}.
Source: Data from Williamson and Nath 1991.[27]

Table 17-3 The geometry function, G(r, θ), for a 3.0 mm line source (^{125}I, model 6711).

θ (degrees)	r = 0.5 cm	r = 1.0 cm
0	4.396	1.023
10	4.377	1.022
20	4.23	1.019
30	4.246	1.015
90	3.885	0.993

Source: Meli et al. 1990.[25] Copyright ® 1990, Elsevier.

Table 17-4 The anisotropy factor, F(r, θ), for ^{125}I model 6711 calculated from Equation 17-5 using ling's matrix fit dose anisotropy polynomial up to a distance of 5 cm from the source.

r(cm)	0°	10°	20°	30°	90°
0.5	0.376	0.448	0.627	0.783	1.00
1.0	0.369	0.464	0.658	0.799	1.00
2.0	0.419	0.503	0.683	0.791	1.00
3.0	0.474	0.551	0.715	0.800	1.00
4.0	0.493	0.579	0.736	0.813	1.00
5.0	0.478	0.583	0.743	0.823	1.00

Source: Ling et al. 1983.[28] Reproduced with permission of Elsevier.

(see Figure 17-16). By dividing by the value of G at 1 cm and 90°, the units cancel. Representative values of G(r, θ) are shown in Table 17-3.

The *radial dose function*, g(r), accounts for absorption and scatter along the transverse axis of the source, normalized to the value at 1 cm from the source. The function g(r) is determined from depth dose measurements along the transverse axis of the source. Representative measurements are shown in Figure 17-8 for a model 6711 ^{125}I seed.

F (r, θ) is an *anisotropy factor* that accounts for absorption and scatter in the medium and in the source encapsulation. This function is obtained from relative dose measurements, and it is normalized to the measurement at θ = 90° for each value of r. Representative values of F (r, θ) are given in Table 17-4 for a model 6711 ^{125}I seed.

Example 17-1

What is the dose rate at a point near a model 6711 ^{125}I seed, if the point is located as shown in the diagram below?

$L = 0.3\,\text{cm}, \theta = 30°, y = 0.5\,\text{cm}, r = 1.0\,\text{cm}$

The air-kerma strength, S_k, of the source is 1.0 cGy-cm^2/hr. From Equation (17-1), we obtain:

$$\dot{D}(r, \theta) = S_k \cdot \Lambda \cdot \frac{G(r, \theta)}{G(1, = \pi/2)} \cdot F(r, \theta) \cdot g(r)$$

where:

$$S_k = 1.0\,\text{cGy cm}^2/\text{hr}$$
$$\Lambda = 0.847\,\text{cGy/hr per unit air-kerma strength}$$
$$G(1\,\text{cm}, 30°) = 1.015$$
$$G(1\,\text{cm}, \Pi/2) = 0.993$$
$$F(1\,\text{cm}, 30°) = 0.799$$
$$g(1\,\text{cm}) = 1.0$$

Therefore:

D(1 cm, 30°) = 0.69 cGy/hr

Dose over treatment duration

The total dose delivered over a treatment time, *t*, is determined by integrating the instantaneous dose rates over *t*, where the dose rate at a given time is simply the initial dose rate corrected for radioactive decay:

$$D = \int_0^t \dot{D}(t)dt = \int_0^t (\dot{D}_0 \cdot e^{-\lambda t})dt$$

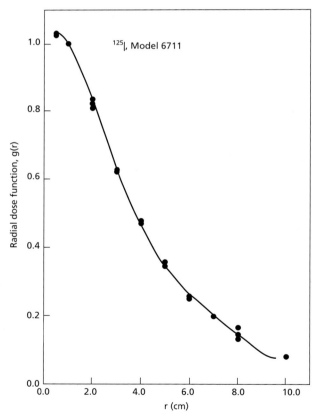

Figure 17-8 The radial dose function, g(r), for model 6711 ^{125}I seed. The solid curve is the polynomial fit to the data.
Source: Meli et al. 1990.[25] Copyright ® 1990, Elsevier.

Since the decay constant is equal to $0.693/T_{1/2}$, solving the integral gives:

$$D = 1.44 \cdot T_{1/2} \cdot \dot{D}_0(1 - e^{-0.693t/T_{1/2}})$$

In clinical practice for temporary treatments, one is often interested in finding the treatment duration. Solving for t gives:

$$t = -1.44 \cdot T_{1/2} \cdot \ln\left(1 - \frac{D}{1.44 \cdot T_{1/2} \cdot \dot{D}_0}\right) \qquad (17\text{-}2)$$

For permanent implants, the duration continues through total decay of the implanted radioactive material. Thus, $t \gg T_{1/2}$ and the equation for total dose reduces to:

$$D = 1.44 \cdot T_{1/2} \cdot \dot{D}_0$$

This equation can be solved for the initial dose rate to determine the required activity of the seeds to deliver a specified dose.

Also, for temporary applications where $t \gg T_{1/2}$, such as applications with cesium or iridium, the dose equation reduces to:

$$D = \dot{D}_0 \cdot t$$

In general practice, if the treatment duration is less than about 8% of the half-life (e.g., 5 days for ^{192}Ir), the change in dose rate due to decay is ignored, and this simpler equation is used.

Plaques

Tumors of the eye are notoriously difficult to treat effectively without injuring normal structures such as the lens, macula, and optic nerve. One approach for treating ocular tumors is use of an ophthalmic irradiator, as discussed in Chapter 16. Ophthalmologic conditions such as pterygium and vascularization or ulceration of the cornea may be treated effectively with a small radioactive applicator positioned on or near the cornea for a short period of time.[29,30] Although early applicators used sources of radium or ^{210}Pb–^{210}Bi, most applicators now contain ^{90}Y ($T_{1/2} = 64$ hr) in secular equilibrium with its parent ^{90}Sr ($T_{1/2} = 28$ yr). The front surface of the applicator absorbs most of the low-energy beta particles from ^{90}Sr (0.54 MeV $E_{\max}$), but permits the high-energy beta particles from ^{90}Y (2.27 MeV $E_{\max}$) to enter the eye. The dose rate at the center of the applicator surface may be as high as 100 cGy/s, and it may vary greatly across the surface of the applicator. The dose rate may be made more uniform by constructing a compensating filter designed to fit over the end of the applicator.[31] The dose rate from a beta applicator decreases to about 5% of the surface dose rate at a depth of 4 mm, the depth of the lens below the cornea.[32,33]

Radioactive sources contained in plaques have been used for many decades to treat superficial disease. Since the 1940s, ophthalmic plaques have been used as an attractive alternative to implantation of radioactive sources directly into the eye,[34] as

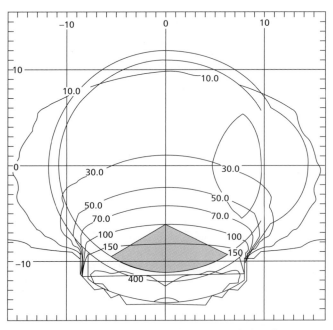

Figure 17-9 Treatment of an eye lesion about 5.5 mm thick with an eye plaque.
Source: Diagram produced using BEBIG plaque simulators V2.15, distributed by BEBIG Trade GmbH.

well as for external beam therapy with heavy charged particles.[35] A study of the effectiveness of plaque therapy compared with enucleation was conducted by the Collaborative Ocular Melanoma Study.[36] For medium-sized choroidal melanomas, it was found that there is no survival difference between brachytherapy and enucleation.[37] The plaque consists of a bowl-shaped outer shell made of an attenuating material such as a gold alloy, along with a means for attaching radioactive seeds (typically ^{125}I) inside the plaque. The gold shell is constructed to match the curvature of the orbit, and it includes eyelets to permit the plaque to be sutured to the orbit. By providing some limited collimation (Figure 17-9), the gold shell limits the dose to uninvolved structures of the eye. The plaque also protects other organs, as well as persons in the vicinity of the patient. The plaque is usually left in place for up to a week while the treatment is delivered. Often the treatment is planned with software developed for ophthalmic plaque radiotherapy.[38]

Calibration of the dose rate at the surface of beta-emitting eye applicators presents a challenge to calibration laboratories. Parallel plate ionization chambers with variable plate spacing have been used for this purpose. By decreasing the plate separation, and thus the volume, a plot of charge collected per unit chamber volume versus volume can be generated. By extrapolating to zero plate separation, the surface dose rate can be determined. Calibrated film, such as radiochromic film, can be used to calibrate the source and provide a 2D map of dose uniformity. This film is minimally sensitive to ambient light and turns blue upon exposure to radiation.

Radiographic localization of implants

In the planning of interstitial and intracavitary implants, rules and conventions are followed for placing the sources in the tissue to be treated. When the sources are inserted into tissue, however, their placement often is different from that planned. Hence, the area or volume of the actual implant may be significantly more or less than that used to compute the activity and treatment time required for the implant. After the sources have been inserted, the treatment time should be altered to correct for this difference in area or volume. Several methods have been devised for determining the actual area or volume of an implant.[39-49] One common approach to this problem is described here.

The actual area or volume of an implant may be determined from radiographs exposed at right angles to each other (*orthogonal films*). Usually, anteroposterior (AP) and lateral radiographs are used. The lengths of the borders of the implant are found by the Pythagorean Theorem. Consider a line of length L and its projections L_A and L_L on AP and lateral radiographs, respectively (Figure 17-10). L is:

$$L = \sqrt{L_A^2 + a^2}$$

or:

$$L = \sqrt{L_L^2 + b^2}$$

where a and b equal the sides of a right triangle with L_L as the hypotenuse. In Figure 17-10, a is parallel to the AP direction in the lateral radiograph and b is parallel to the lateral direction in the AP radiograph.

Projections L_A and L_L for each border of the implant are determined with the AP and lateral radiographs. The true length of each border is found by one of the expressions above. The projections of the borders must be corrected for magnification of the

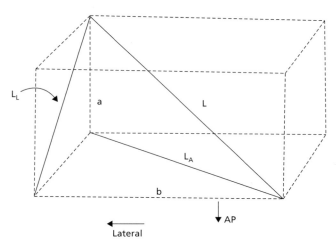

Figure 17-10 Geometry for calculating the actual borders of an interstitial implant.
Source: Hendee 1970.[2]

radiographic image. The magnification correction may be determined by placing a metal ring at the same level as the implant before each radiograph is exposed. The ratio of the largest diameter of the ring image to the actual diameter of the ring furnishes a magnification correction by which each projection of an implant border is divided before the actual border of the implant is computed.

In addition, the use of CT images to determine the locations of brachytherapy sources has been introduced, as discussed in the next section.[50]

Three-dimensional image-based implants

Prostate seed implants

Imaging methods used in external-beam treatment planning are employed in brachytherapy to aid in structure definition and catheter/source reconstruction.[51-54] One of the more commonly used methods is axial ultrasound images for planning permanent prostate seed implants. The patient is positioned in the lithotomy position and a rectal ultrasound probe is used to visualize the prostate. Axial images are obtained at fixed increments (e.g., 0.5 cm) by use of an indexed positioning system called a *stepper*. With these images, a 3D volume of the prostate is reconstructed for treatment planning. A template is used to identify needle locations in a grid pattern. The template is superimposed on the ultrasound images and the displayed positions aligned with the positions of the physical template used for the actual implant. The planning system uses the template to define allowable needle locations. Most dedicated prostate seed programs have commercially available sources characterized in terms of physical properties such as source strength, geometry, and attenuation properties. Often, they allow seeds to be automatically placed in prostate locations according to certain *rules*. Two common rules are *peripheral loading* and *modified peripheral loading* (Figure 17-11).[55] In peripheral loading, seeds are placed only on the periphery of the prostate with needles 1 cm apart. In modified peripheral loading, seeds are alternately placed on the periphery and interior of the prostate with needles often shifted by 0.5 cm in alternate slices. Compared with the peripheral loading technique, more needles are used for a modified peripheral loading implant. Clinicians can adopt either of these techniques for their patients, and they may include their own source-loading rules, such as excluding sources within 1 cm of the urethra.

Pre-loaded needles can be ordered based on the pre-plan or separate seeds and needles can be ordered and constructed in real time in the operating room. Additionally, seeds can be ordered for use with a Mick applicator for seed placement in the prostate.

At the time of implant, the physician must position the patient to match the images obtained during the volume study and also must accurately identify the base of the prostate. This is

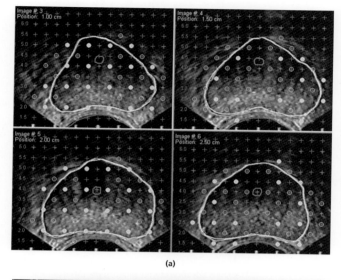

(a)

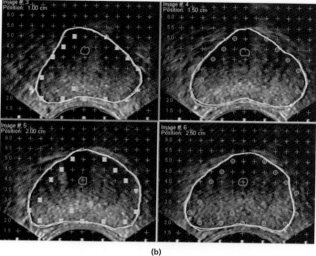

(b)

Figure 17-11 (a) Modified peripheral loading example. Planes are 5 mm apart and sources are 1 cm apart on a given plane, with an alternating pattern of needles used between planes. Loading is interior on one plane, peripheral on the next, and so on. (b) Peripheral loading example. Seeds are loaded only on the periphery of alternating planes.

especially important when a pre-plan and pre-loaded needles are used. Once the patient is prepared, special needles are inserted to anchor the prostate. To deposit the sources, the ultrasound transducer is positioned at a *retraction plane* that corresponds to the plane of the first seed in the needle. The needle is inserted until it appears on the ultrasound image and it may be further advanced slightly to account for material in the end of the needle holding the source in place (using bone wax). The needle is then retracted while holding the stylet (or plunger) in place to deposit the seeds (Figure 17-12 and Table 17-5). Cystoscopy can be used at the end of a procedure to ensure no seeds were placed into the urethra or bladder.

Example 17-2

A prostate implant patient has a transurethral resection of the prostate (TURP) procedure 6 months after a prostate seed implant. If the specimen contains 10 seeds that had an activity of 0.3 mCi each at the time of implant, what is the exposure rate to the pathologist at a distance of 50 cm from the specimen?

The specimen is taken approximately 3 half-lives after the implant, so the activity in the specimen is:

$$\text{Activity} = (10 \text{ seeds}) \times (0.3 \text{ mCi})/2^3 = 0.375 \text{ mCi}$$

For ^{125}I seeds, the exposure rate constant is 1.45 R·cm²/(mCi·hr). The exposure rate is then:

$$\dot{X} = (0.375 \text{ mCi}) \left(1.45 \frac{\text{R} \cdot \text{cm}^2}{\text{mCi} \cdot \text{hr}} \right) \left(\frac{1}{50 \text{ cm}} \right)^2$$
$$= 2.18 \times 10^{-4} \text{ R/hr} = 0.2 \text{ mR/hr}$$

Post-implant brachytherapy dosimetry often uses CT images to identify the location of the sources.[57] The sources can be clearly seen in the axial images, although there may be some uncertainty about exact location and orientation because of the finite thickness of the CT slice. Using a table increment that approximates the seed length limits duplication of sources but gives poor resolution in the axial direction. Comparison of planar film images with 3D source positions reconstructed from CT images can be helpful in evaluating the accuracy of seed location. Once structures of interest are outlined on the CT images (prostate, urethra, bladder, and rectum), then post-implant dosimetry parameters can be computed to evaluate the efficacy of the implant.

Example 17-3

A prostate gland measures 5 cm superior to inferior, 4.5 cm left to right, and 3.5 cm anterior to posterior. The treatment plan calls for 92 ^{125}I seeds, with an activity of 0.35 mCi/seed, to deliver 139 Gy to the target. How does this plan compare with the Memorial system source strength recommendations for volume implants described in Table 17-5?

The average diameter for this implant is (5.0 + 4.5 + 3.5)/3 = 4.3 cm. The total activity used is:

$$(92 \text{ seeds}) \times (0.35 \text{ mCi/seed}) = 32.2 \text{ mCi}$$

From Table 17-5 the recommended strength is:

$$A_{\text{app}} = 1.33 \, d_a^{2.2} = 1.33(4.3)^{2.2} = 33.5 \text{ mCi}$$

Thus, the treatment plan calls for about 4% less activity.

Prostate HDR

Treatment of prostate cancer with HDR remote afterloading techniques has increased dramatically, in part because of the supposition that the alpha/beta ratio for prostate tumors is lower than previously thought, particularly for high-grade tumors.

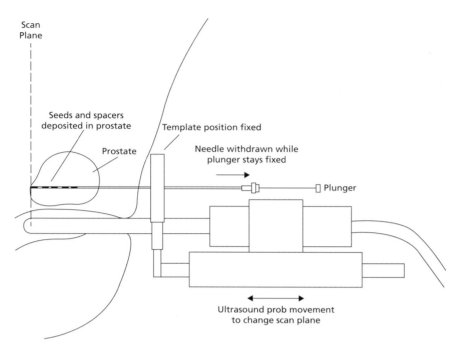

Figure 17-12 Prostate seed implant. The needle is advanced to the plane of the ultrasound image as determined from the treatment plan. The needle is retracted while the plunger stays fixed, depositing seeds and spacers in the prostate gland.

This finding means that patients with high-grade disease could potentially benefit from shorter overall treatment times. Also, use of HDR to boost the prostate dose can shorten the overall course of treatment by a few weeks. Prostate HDR involves placement of several needles in the prostate gland under ultrasound guidance, much like a permanent seed implant.[58] One technique for needle placement calls for initial needle placement halfway into the gland, which is then advanced using a flexible cystoscope that is retroflexed back to look at the wall of the bladder (Figure 17-13). When the catheters *tent* the bladder wall (the needle tips exert force on the bladder wall and deform it), the physician stops the advancement. Care has to be taken for posterior catheters because they can end up posterior to the bladder and tenting will not occur.

Modern techniques allow for ultrasound-based planning after needle insertion. This allows for a much faster patient visit.

However, if ultrasound-based planning is not available, patients are imaged with a CT scanner. A few axial cuts may help determine whether further advancement of any of the needles is desired. A complete series of axial images is then obtained and the images are transferred to the HDR treatment planning system. A CT scan that includes the template is helpful in providing information to track the catheters into the patient for proper numbering when connecting to the afterloader. With the CT images, a treatment plan is generated to produce dwell times for active dwell positions of the sources. Several methods, including inverse planning techniques based on dose objectives, are available to identify ideal dwell positions (e.g., activate all dwells within the target, but stay at least 1 cm from the urethra) and to optimize dwell times.

Example 17-4

A treatment plan using ^{192}Ir produces an isodose surface that adequately covers a target volume with 0.55 Gy/hr. Calculate the duration to deliver a 25 Gy dose.

From Equation (17-2), the time to deliver the treatment is:

$$t = -1.44 \cdot 73.8 \, \text{day} \cdot 24 \, \text{hr/day}$$
$$\cdot \ln\left(1 - \frac{25 \, Gy}{1.44 \cdot 73.8 \, \text{day} \cdot 24 \, \text{hr/day} \cdot 0.55 \, \text{Gy/hr}}\right)$$
$$= 45.9 \, \text{hr} = 1 \, \text{day} \, 21 \, \text{hr} \, 54 \, \text{min}$$

Using the simpler equation, we obtain:

$$t = \frac{D}{\dot{D}_0} = \frac{25 \, \text{Gy}}{0.55 \, \text{Gy/hr}} = 45.45 \, \text{hr} = 1 \, \text{day} \, 21 \, \text{hr} \, 27 \, \text{min}$$

Table 17-5 Memorial system source strength recommendations for a prostate seed implant.

Radionuclide	Dose (TG43) [Gy]	Range of d_a [cm]	Strength [mCi$_{apparent}$]	[U]
^{125}I	139	<3 cm	$5d_a$	$6.35(d_a)$
		>3 cm	$1.33(d_a)^{2.2}$	$1.69(d_a)^{2.2}$
^{103}Pd	120	<3 cm	$17.78(d_a)$	$23(d_a)$
		>3 cm	$3.2(d_a)^{2.56}$	$4.14(d_a)^{2.56}$
^{198}Au	$D = \dfrac{1.344}{\sqrt{V}}$	All	$50.4(d_a)$	$1.344(d_a)$

Source: Hendee 1999.[56] The recommended activity is based on the average prostate gland diameter obtained from the volume study.

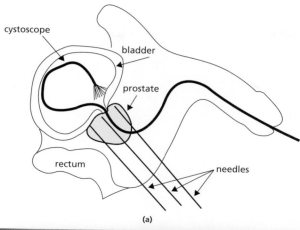

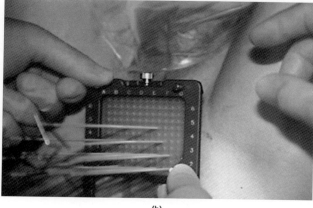

Figure 17-13 High-dose-rate prostate implant. The flexible cystoscope is inserted through the urethra and into the bladder. It is then retroflexed to observe the bladder wall as the needles are advanced to avoid puncturing the bladder.

Note that, because of the short implant duration compared with the half-life of ^{192}Ir, there is only a 1% difference between these two methods.

LDR/HDR gynecologic interstitial implant

Template-based interstitial implants for gynecologic tumors may be used when intracavitary techniques are unable to treat the full extent of the disease.[59] Image-based virtual simulation is a useful aid in determining the number, source strength, and position of needles to implant within a template. For a gynecologic implant (e.g., using a Syed implant based on a particular concentric needle geometry named for Dr. Nisar Syed), the patient is simulated with the template in position and with the vaginal obturator used to provide a reproducible position. The physician contours the tumor and other structures of interest, possibly with the aid of MR image-fusion techniques. The dosimetrist or physicist then places *virtual needles* to determine the best locations on the template to implant. Various source

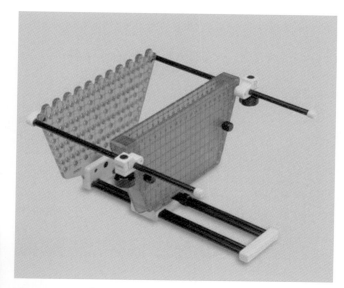

Figure 17-14 Applicator for a multiplane interstitial implant for breast cancer.

loadings can be attempted, with the resulting dose distribution presented to the physician for approval. For an LDR implant, sources are then ordered for the surgical implant. With the treatment plan as a guide, including how far to insert the needles, the physician is able to perform the implant. The patient can be imaged after surgery to verify needle placement. The planning system may allow these images to be fused into the original planning CT image for comparison. After making necessary adjustments, the clinical team can load the sources into the needles for the LDR treatment. For an HDR treatment, the patient is imaged after needle placement and planned similarly to the prostate HDR treatment described above.

Breast brachytherapy

Templates may also be used for interstitial volume implants of the breast. The treatment may be either LDR or HDR.[60–63] In some cases, a multiplane implant is used with an applicator, as shown in Figure 17-14. Cosmesis is an important consideration for these patients and dose homogeneity is a treatment planning objective. In other cases where a tumor is well localized and the margins are negative, a small single-entry device may be inserted into the tumor site for treatment with the HDR afterloader. There are a few balloon devices that can be used in these cases (one of which is shown in Figure 17-15a) as well as a cage like device (shown in Figure 17-15b).

Therapy with radiopharmaceuticals

Unsealed radioactive materials have been used in radiation therapy for many decades. Iodine-131 has long been used to treat diseases of the thyroid (hyperthyroidism and thyroid carcinoma),

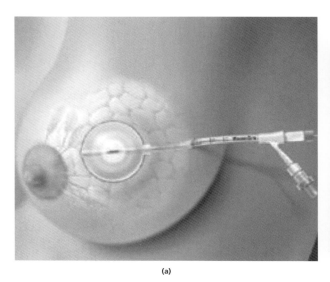
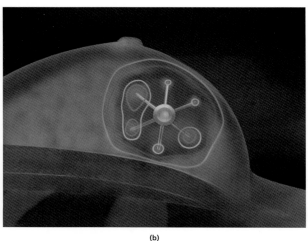

(a)   (b)

Figure 17-15 Two HDR breast applicators. (a) MammoSite single-dwell position balloon applicator. (b) SAVI (strut-adjusted volume implant) multi-dwell position cage applicator. For a color version of image (b), see the color plate section.
Source: Cianna Medical. Reproduced with permission of Cianna Medical.

and ^{32}P has been used for treatment of hematologic malignancies (polycythemia vera and leukemia) as well as malignant bone lesions. Radioactive phosphorus-32 in colloidal form has been used to treat malignancies in serosal cavities (particularly ovarian carcinoma).[64] Very little has been published regarding the dosimetry of ^{32}P used for intraperitoneal radiotherapy. Prescriptions are generally based on historical evidence showing, for example, that an activity of 15 mCi of ^{32}P sulfur colloid injected into the peritoneal cavity is effective and causes minimal complications.

Other isotopes that have been developed more recently and used for therapeutic purposes include Samarium-153 (lexidronam),[65] which is a beta emitter with a half-life of a little over 46 hours, and Radium-223 (trade name Xofigo), which is an alpha emitter with a half-life of a little over 11 days. Both isotopes are injected into the patient to treat bone metastases. Samarium-153 is a target delivery system that delivers high local doses to the bony metastasis. Likewise, Radium-223 is also a targeted drug delivery system that delivers a high localized dose to bony metastasis from prostate cancer.

Intravascular brachytherapy

Coronary artery disease is the leading cause of death in the United States and is responsible for nearly 1 million interventional procedures each year. These procedures include bypass surgery and percutaneous transluminal coronary angioplasty (PTCA). Angioplasty may include deployment of a mesh wire stent to aid in keeping the vessel open. During angioplasty, balloon inflation can cause cracks in the atherosclerotic plaque that extend into the vessel, thus damaging the vessel wall. The body's natural response is to promote smooth muscle cell growth to

repair the damage. However, the new growth (neointimal hyperplasia) can eventually result in vessel obstruction, or *restenosis*. Nearly half of the patients who receive PTCA will return within 6 months with a re-narrowing of the vessel caused by the body's response to the strain done to the vessel during angioplasty.

Ionizing radiation, on the order of 12–20 Gy, given to the vessel wall and delivered at the time of angioplasty, was an effective approach to preventing restenosis.[66-68] Several devices were used to deliver the radiation, including hand-held and remote afterloaders. Radioisotopes included both gamma and beta emitters. However, investigators looked at other methods to combat the problem of restenosis, including drug-coated stents and ultrasonic treatments. In recent times, intravascular brachytherapy procedures are not common, owing to the introduction of effective drug-eluting stents (since the early 2000s).

Summary

- Interstitial implants use needles for source placement, while intracavitary implants utilize applicators within an existing body cavity or opening.
- Implant rules or systems were developed by several institutions to aid in needle/applicator placement, source loading, and dose prescription.
- The dose for temporary implants must account for the duration of the implant and possibly source decay (unless the half-life is long compared to the implant duration).
- The dose from permanent implants is determined from the initial dose rate and the half-life of the isotope.
- Remote afterloading brachytherapy reduces the radiation exposure to staff.

- The availability of three-dimensional image-based treatment planning allows customized implants and dose distributions.
- Low-dose rate brachytherapy is characterized by dose rates on the order of Gy/hr, whereas high-dose rate brachytherapy dose rates are expressed in units of Gy/min.
- Intravascular brachytherapy is used to reduce the chance of restenosis by lowering the proliferation rate of vascular endothelial cells in response to damage during angioplasty.

Problems

17-1 The projection of a radium needle is 2.2 cm in an AP radiograph. In a lateral radiograph, the projection of the needle is 0.8 cm in the AP direction. Magnifications are 1.1 in the AP direction and 1.2 in the lateral direction. What is the true length of the needle?

17-2 A lesion is treated with 15 1 mCi ^{125}I seeds distributed uniformly over the surface of a sphere 2 cm in diameter. What is the absorbed dose at the center of the sphere during complete decay of the sources?

17-3 What is the treatment time necessary for the loaded Fletcher–Suit applicator diagrammed in Figure 17-3 to deliver 2000 cGy to point A? What is the dose at point B, 3 cm lateral to point A? All sources are cesium and are 1.4 cm in active length filtered by 0.5 mm stainless steel.

Source	Activity
1	20 mg-Ra-eq
2	15 mg-Ra-eq
3	10 mg-Ra-eq
4	15 mg-Ra-eq
5	15 mg-Ra-eq

17-4 A prostate ^{125}I implant patient has 90 seeds at 0.35 mCi/seed. Assuming that the patient's body effectively acts like two half-value layers of attenuator, determine the expected exposure rate at 1 m.

17-5 A prostate boost implant using ^{125}I is to deliver a total dose of 108 Gy. What is the initial dose rate in cGy/hr? How long does it take to deliver 90% of the dose?

References

1 Ernst, E. Probable trends in irradiation of carcinoma of cervix uteri with improved expanding type of radium applicator. *Radiology* 1949; **52**:46.
2 Hendee, W. R. *Medical Radiation Physics*, 1st edition. St. Louis, Mosby–Year Book, 1970.
3 Fishman, R., and Citrin, L. New radium implant technique to reduce operating room exposure and increase accuracy of placement. *Am. J. Radiol.* 1956; **75**:495.
4 Henschke, U., Hilaris, B., and Mahan, G. Afterloading in interstitial and intracavitary radiation therapy. *Am. J. Radiol.* 1963; **90**:386.
5 Simon, N. (ed.). Afterloading in radiotherapy. Proceedings of a conference held in New York City, May 6—8, 1971. Department of HEW Publication No. (FDA)72-8024 (BRH/DMRE 72-4).
6 Haas, J. S., Dean, R. D., and Mansfield, C. M. Fletcher—Suit—Delclos gynecologic applicator: Evaluation of a new instrument. *Int. J. Radiat. Oncol. Biol. Phys.* 1983; **9**:763–768.
7 Ling, C. C., Spiro, I. J., Kubiatowicz, D. O., Gergen, J., Peksens, R. K., et al. Measurement of dose distribution around Fletcher-Suit—Delclos colpostats using a Therados radiation field analyzer (RFA-3). *Med. Phys.* 1984; **11**(3):326–330.
8 Webster, M., Han, D., Park, J. C., Watkins, W. T., Scanderbeg, D., et al. Dynamic modulated brachytherapy (DMBT). *Med. Phys.* 2013; **40**:011718.
9 Webster, M., Devic, S., Vuong, T., Han, D., Scanderbeg, D., et al. HDR brachytherapy of rectal cancer using a novel grooved-shielding applicator design. *Med. Phys.* 2013; **40**:091704.
10 Han, D. Y., Webster, M. J., Scanderbeg, D. J., Yashar, C., Choi, D., et al. Direction Modulated Brachytherapy (DMBT) for HDR Treatment of Cervical Cancer (I): Theoretical Design. *Int. J. Radiat. Oncol, Biol. Phys.* 2014; **89**: 666–673.
11 Nag, S., Chao, C., Erickson, B., Fowler, J., Gupta, N., et al. The American Brachytherapy Society recommendations for low-dose-rate brachytherapy for carcinoma of the cervix. *Int. J. Radiat. Oncol. Biol. Phys.* 2002; **52**(1):33–48.
12 International Commission of Radiation Units and Measurements (ICRU). *Dose and Volume Specifications for Reporting Intracavitary Therapy in Gynecology: Report No. 38*. Bethesda, MD: ICRU, 1985.
13 Haie-Meder, C., Pötter, R., Van Limbergen, E., Briot, E., De Brabandere, M., et al. Recommendations from Gynaecological (GYN) GEC-ESTRO Working Group (I): concepts and terms in 3D image based 3D treatment planning in cervix cancer brachytherapy with emphasis on MRI assessment of GTV and CTV. *Radiother. Oncol.* 2005; **74**: 235–245.
14 Pötter, R., Haie-Meder, C., Van Limbergen, E., Barillot, I., De Brabandere, M., et al. Recommendations from gynaecological (GYN) GEC ESTRO working group (II): Concepts and terms in 3D image-based treatment planning in cervix cancer brachytherapy – 3D dose volume parameters and aspects of 3D image-based anatomy, radiation physics, radiobiology. *Radiother. Oncol.* 2006; **78**: 67–77.
15 Pierquin, B., Dutreix, A., Paine, C. H., et al. The Paris system in interstitial radiation therapy. *Acta. Radiol. Oncol.* 1978; **17**:33.
16 Gillin, M. T., Kline, R. W., Wilson, J. F., and Cox, J. D. Single and double plane implants: A comparison of the Manchester system with the Paris system. *Int. J. Radiat. Oncol. Biol. Phys.* 1984; **10**:921.
17 Brenner, D. J., and Hall, E. J. Fractionated high dose rate versus low dose rate regimes for intracavitary brachytherapy of the cervix. 1. General considerations based on radiobiology. *Br. J. Radiol.* 1991; **64**:133–144.
18 Orton, C. G., Seyedsadr, M., and Somnay, A. Comparison of high and low dose rate remote afterloading for cervix cancer and the importance of fractionation. *Int. J. Radiat. Oncol. Biol. Phys.* 1991; **21**:1425–1434.
19 Fowler, J. F., and Mount, M. Pulsed brachytherapy: The conditions for no significant loss of therapeutic ratio compared with traditional low dose rate brachytherapy. *Int. J. Radiat. Oncol. Biol. Phys.* 1992; **23**:661–669.

20 Edmundson, G. K. Volume optimization: An American viewpoint. In *Brachy-therapy from Radium to Optimization*, R. F. Mould et al. (eds.). Veenendaal, Nucletron International BV, 1994.

21 Nath, R., Anderson, L. L., Luxton, G., Weaver, K. A., Williamson, J. F., and Meigooni, A. S. Dosimetry of interstitial brachytherapy sources: Recommendations of the AAPM Radiation Therapy Committee Task Group No. 43. *Med. Phys.* 1995; **22**:209.

22 Rivard, M. J., Coursey, B. M., DeWerd, L. A., Hanson, W. F., Huq, M. S., et al. Update of AAPM Task Group No. 43 Report: A revised AAPM protocol for brachytherapy dose calculations. *Med. Phys.* 2004; **31**:633.

23 Rivard, M. J., Butler, W. M., DeWerd, L. A., Huq, M. S., Ibbott, G. S., et al. Supplement to AAPM TG-43 update. *Med. Phys.* 2007; **34**:2187.

24 Beaulieu, L., Tedgren, A. C., Carrier, J., Davis, S. D., Mourtada, F., et al. Report of the Task Group 186 on model-based dose calculation methods in brachytherapy beyond the TG-43 formalism: Current status and recommendations for clinical implementation. *Med. Phys.* 2012; **39**:6208.

25 Meli, J. A., Anderson, L. L., and Weaver, K. A. Dose distribution. In *Interstitial Brachytherapy*, Interstitial Collaborative Working Group (eds.). New York, Raven Press, 1990.

26 Nath, R., Anderson, L. L., Luxton, G., Weaver, K. A., Williamson, J. F., and Meigooni, A. S. Dosimetry of interstitial brachytherapy sources: Recommendations of the AAPM Radiation Therapy Committee Task Group No. 43. American Association of Physicists in Medicine. *Med. Phys.* 1995; **22**(2):209–234.

27 Williamson, J. F., and Nath, R. Clinical implementation of AAPM Task Group 32 recommendations on brachytherapy source strength specification. *Med. Phys.* 1991; **18**:439–448.

28 Ling, C. C., Yorke, E. D., Spiro I. J., Kubiatowicz, D., and Bennett S. Physical dosimetry of ^{125}I seeds of a new design for interstitial implant. *Int. J. Radiat. Oncol. Biol. Phys.* 1983; **9**:1747–1752.

29 Duggan, H. Results using strontium-90 beta-ray applicator on eye lesions. *J. Can. Assoc. Radiol.* 1966; **17**:132.

30 Friedell, H., Thomas, C., and Krohmer, J. Evaluation of clinical use of strontium-90 beta-ray applicator with review of underlying principles. *Am. J. Radiol.* 1954; **71**:25.

31 Hendee, W. R. Measurement and correction of nonuniform surface dose rates for beta eye applicators. *Am. J. Radiol.* 1968; **103**:734.

32 Coffey, C., Sayeg, J., Beach, J. L., Song, S., Landis, C., and Connor, A. Calibration of surface dose rate for a Sr-90 beta applicator: Comparison of experimental, theoretical, and biological methods. *Med. Phys.* 1981; **8**:558.

33 Hendee, W. R. Thermoluminescent dosimetry of beta depth dose. *Am. J. Radiol.* 1966; **97**:1045.

34 Stallard, H. B. Malignant melanoma of the coroid treated with radioactive applicators. *Ann. R. Coll. Surg. Engl.* 1961; **29**:170.

35 Gragoudas, E. S., Goitein, M., Verhey, L., Munzenreider, J., Urie, M., Suit, H., and Koehler, A. Proton beam irradiation of uveal melanomas: Results of a 5 1/2 year study. *Arch. Ophthalmol.* 1982; **100**:928–934.

36 Collaborative Ocular Melanoma Study, COMS Coordinating Center, The Wilmer Ophthalmological Institute, The Johns Hopkins School of Medicine, Baltimore, MD, 1989.

37 Diener-West, M., Earle, J.D., Fine, S.L., et al. The COMS randomized trial of iodine 125 brachytherapy for choroidal melanoma, III: Initial mortality findings. COMS report No. 18. *Arch. Ophthalmol.* 2001; **119**:969–982.

38 Astrahan, M. A., Luxton, G., Jozsef, G., Kampp, T. D., Liggett, P. E., Sapozink, M. D., and Petrovich, Z. An interactive treatment planning system for ophthalmic plaque radiotherapy. *Int. J. Radiat. Oncol. Biol. Phys.* 1990; **18**:679–687.

39 Egan, R., and Johnson, G. Multisection transverse tomography in radium implant calculations. *Radiology* 1956; **74**:402.

40 Hidalgo, J. U., Spear, V. D., Garcia, M., Maduell, C. R., and Burke, R. The precision reconstruction of radium implants. *Am. J. Radiol.* 1967; **100**:852.

41 Holt, J. A nomographic wheel for three dimensional localization of radium sources and calculation of dose rate. *Am. J. Radiol.* 1956; **75**:476.

42 Johns, H., and Cunningham, J. *The Physics of Radiology*, 3rd edition. Springfield, IL, Charles C. Thomas, 1969.

43 Kligerman, M., Vreeland, H., and Havinga, J. A graphical method for the localization of radium sources for dosage calculation. *Am. J. Radiol.* 1956; **75**:484.

44 Mussel, L. E. The rapid reconstruction of radium implants: A new technique. *Br. J. Radiol.* 1956; **29**:402.

45 Nuttal, J. R., and Spiers, F. W. Dosage control in interstitial radium therapy. *Br. J. Radiol.* 1946; **19**:133.

46 Shalek, R. J., and Stovall, M. Dosimetry in implant therapy. In *Radiation Dosimetry*, Vol. III (31), F. H. Attix and W. C. Roesch (eds.). New York, Academic Press, 1969.

47 Smith, M. A graphic method of reconstructing radium needle implants for calculation purposes. *Am. J. Radiol.* 1958; **79**:42.

48 Terta, E. Methods of dosage calculation for linear radium sources. *Radiology* 1957; **69**:558.

49 Vaeth, J., and Meurk, J. Use of Rotterdam radium reconstruction device. *Am. J. Radiol.* 1963; **89**:87.

50 Schoeppel, S. L., LaVigne, M. L., Martel, M. K., McShan, D. L., Fraass, B. A., and Roberts, J. A. Three-dimensional treatment planning of intracavitary gynecologic implants: Analysis of ten cases and implications for dose specification. *Int. J. Radiat. Oncol. Biol. Phys.* 1991; **28**:277–283.

51 Nag, S., Beyer, D., Friedland, J., Grimm, P., and Nath, R. American Brachytherapy Society (ABS) recommendations for transperineal permanent brachytherapy of prostate cancer. *Int. J. Radiat. Oncol. Biol. Phys.* 1999; **44**(4):789–799.

52 Yu, Y., Anderson, L. L., Li, Z., Mellenberg, D. E., Nath, R., et al. Permanent prostate seed implant brachytherapy: Report of the American Association of Physicists in Medicine Task Group No. 64. *Med. Phys.* 1999; **26**(10):2054–2076.

53 Nag, S. Brachytherapy for prostate cancer: Summary of American Brachytherapy Society recommendations. *Semin. Urol. Oncol.* 2000; **18**(2):133–136.

54 Blasko, J. C., Mate, T., Sylvester, J. E., Grimm, P. D., and Cavanagh, W. Brachytherapy for carcinoma of the prostate: Techniques, patient selection, and clinical outcomes. *Semin. Radiat. Oncol.* 2002; **12**(1):81–94.

55 Butler, W. M., Merrick, G. S., Lief, J. H., and Dorsey, A. T. Comparison of seed loading approaches in prostate brachytherapy. *Med. Phys.* 2000; **27**(2):381–392.

56 Hendee, W. R. (Ed.): *Biomedical Uses of Radiation*, Vol. 1 and 2. New York: VCH Publishers, 1999.

57 Nag, S., Bice, W., DeWyngaert, K., Prestidge, B., Stock, R., and Yu, Y. The American Brachytherapy Society recommendations for permanent prostate brachytherapy postimplant dosimetric analysis. *Int. J. Radiat. Oncol. Biol. Phys.* 2000; **46**(1):221–230.

58 Demanes, D. J., Rodriguez, R. R., and Altieri, G. A. High dose rate prostate brachytherapy: The California Endocurietherapy (CET) method. *Radiother. Oncol.* 2000; **57**(3):289–296.

59 Tewari, K. S., Cappuccini, F., Puthawala, A. A., Kuo, J. V., Burger, R. A., et al. Primary invasive carcinoma of the vagina: Treatment with interstitial brachytherapy. *Cancer* 2001; **91**(4):758–770.

60 Edmundson, G. K., Weed, D., Vicini, F., Chen, P., and Martinez, A. Accelerated treatment of breast cancer: Dosimetric comparisons between interstitial HDR brachytherapy, mammosite balloon brachytherapy, and external beam quadrant radiation. *Int. J. Radiat. Oncol. Biol. Phys.* 2003; **57**:S307– 308.

61 Vicini, F., Baglan, K., Kestin, L., Chen, P., Edmundson, G., and Martinez, A. The emerging role of brachytherapy in the management of patients with breast cancer. *Semin. Radiat. Oncol.* 2002; **12**(1):31–39.

62 Keisch, M., Vicini, F., Kuske, R., Hebert, M., White, J., et al. Two-year outcome with the mammosite breast brachytherapy applicator: Factors associated with optimal cosmetic results when performing partial breast irradiation. *Int. J. Radiat. Oncol. Biol. Phys.* 2003; **57**:S315.

63 Keisch, M., Vicini, F., Kuske, R. R., Hebert, M., White, J., et al. Initial clinical experience with the MammoSite breast brachytherapy applicator in women with early-stage breast cancer treated with breast-conserving therapy. *Int. J. Radiat. Oncol. Biol. Phys.* 2003; **55**:289–293.

64 Spencer, R. P. (ed.). *Therapy in Nuclear Medicine*, New York, Grune & Stratton, 1978.

65 Sartor, O. Overview of Samarium Sm-153 Lexidronam in the treatment of painful metastatic bone disease. *Rev. Urol.* 2004; **6**:S3–S12

66 Apisarnthanarax, S., and Chougule, P. Intravascular brachytherapy: A review of the current vascular biology. *Am. J. Clin. Oncol.* 2003; **26**:E13–E21.

67 Nath, R., Amols, H., Coffey, C., Duggan, D., Jani, S., et al. Intravascular brachytherapy physics: Report of the AAPM Radiation Therapy Committee Task Group No. 60. American Association of Physicists in Medicine, *Med. Phys.* 1999; **26**(2):119–152.

68 Nguyen-Ho, P., Kaluza, G. L., Zymek, P. T., and Raizner, A. E. Intracoronary brachytherapy. *Catheter Cardiovasc. Interv.* 2002; **56**:281–288.

18

RADIATION PROTECTION

Objectives

After studying this chapter, the reader will:
- Explain the philosophy of risk underlying radiation protection, including the linear, non-threshold model of radiation injury.
- Differentiate stochastic and nonstochastic effects of radiation exposure.
- Identify the key issues in the history of radiation protection, including the evolution and definition of radiation units.
- Identify the current occupational and public radiation exposure limits.
- Compute shielding requirements for primary, secondary, and neutron radiation, identifying the variables that influence the computations.
- Identify radiation protection principles important to the safe use of sealed brachytherapy sources.
- Describe the uses and limitations of various devices for radiation surveys and personnel monitoring.

Introduction

Within a few months after the discovery of x rays in 1895, x rays were being used in hospitals and physicians' offices in developed countries. Soon several cases of radiation-induced dermatitis were observed. For several years after their discovery, x rays and radioactive materials were used with little knowledge of their biological effects. However, the consequences of excessive exposure to radiation soon became apparent, including skin burns (erythema), hair loss (epilation), and, later, skin cancer (squamous and basal cell carcinoma). Persons affected included several physicians, physicists, and technicians who pioneered the early applications of ionizing radiation in medicine.[1]

Initial concern about radiation exposure focused more on the operator than on the patient because (1) patient exposures are intermittent while operators are exposed continually and (2) the

Hendee's Radiation Therapy Physics, Fourth Edition. Todd Pawlicki, Daniel J. Scanderbeg and George Starkschall.
© 2016 John Wiley & Sons, Inc. Published 2016 by John Wiley & Sons, Inc.

patient benefits directly from the exposure. William Collins, a Boston dentist, was a major early influence on radiation protection practices. He was the first to propose a *tolerance dose* limit for occupational radiation exposure.

By this time, ionizing radiation was proving to be helpful in medical diagnosis and therapy. The issue facing radiation experts was whether radiation could be used to benefit patients and society without exposing radiation users to unacceptable hazards. This issue is phrased today as a question of risk versus benefit. To reduce the risk, advisory groups were formed to establish upper limits for the exposure of radiation users, with the recognition that the risk to individual patients must always be balanced against medical benefits. Advisory groups have reduced the upper limits many times since the first limits were promulgated, as discussed later in this chapter. These reductions reflect the use of radiation by greater numbers of persons, the implications of new data concerning the sensitivity of biological organisms to radiation, and improvements in the design of radiation devices and the architecture of facilities where radiation sources are used.

The strategy underlying the control of radiation hazards is described as a *philosophy of risk*. In this approach, advisory groups attempt to establish standards for radiation protection that maintain radiation risks at an acceptable level to individuals and society without unnecessarily impeding the useful applications of radiation.[2] The philosophy of risk is portrayed in Figure 18-1. The total biological damage (the *radiation detriment)* to a population is the sum of various effects, such as mortality, morbidity, genetic damage, shortened life span, and reduced vitality, that may result from receipt of a particular dose rate of radiation averaged over the lifetime of individuals in the population. The total damage is assumed to increase gradually as the average dose rate increases to a value of about 0.01 Sv per week. Above this dose rate, the biological damage is assumed

to increase more rapidly. The *area of uncertainty* shown in Figure 18-1 is the region of greatest concern in radiation protection because it encompasses the dose rates typically encountered by radiation users. It is also the region where data are most limited. As indicated by curve c, the damage may remain at zero for dose rates below some threshold level, suggesting that biological repair of radiation injury may occur, provided that the damage does not take place so rapidly that repair mechanisms are overwhelmed. Considerable evidence supports this *threshold model of radiation injury* for certain types of exposures, including the induction of osteogenic carcinoma in individuals with significant bone concentrations of radium.[3] Conceivably the curve for biological effects might follow path d, suggesting that low dose rates are beneficial, a hypothesis known as *radiation hormesis*. Although considerable experimental evidence supports this hypothesis,[4] it continues to generate considerable controversy among radiation experts. Some persons suggest that the curve for total biological damage follows curve a,[5] but this *superlinearity theory of radiation damage* is not strongly supported by experimental data. Curve b suggests that the total biological damage to a population is linearly proportional to the average dose rate to individuals in the population down to a dose rate approaching zero. This model, known as the *linear non-threshold model of radiation injury*, is the model usually employed to estimate radiation risks and establish standards for radiation protection.[6]

Data are inadequate to identify which of the models for predicting biological damage is most appropriate within the area of uncertainty depicted in Figure 18-1. Consequently the cost of radiation protection (e.g., for shielding, remote control techniques, monitoring procedures, and personnel restriction) must be balanced against uncertain biological effects that may result at any given level of protection. The cost increases from almost zero for no restrictions on radiation exposure to a high cost if attempts are made to reduce exposures to a level approaching zero. Somewhere within the area of uncertainty, an upper limit must be established for permissible radiation exposures. This limit should reflect a risk that is acceptable to the exposed individuals and to society in general, without depriving society of the benefits derived from the judicious use of ionizing radiation. In addition, it should be recognized that exposures should always be kept *as low as reasonably achievable* (ALARA) consistent with reasonable costs and convenience and without compromising the benefits of radiation to society. ALARA was preceded by the protection philosophy of *as low as possible* (ALAP). It was soon recognized, however, that exposures can always be reduced further if enough resources are dedicated to the task. The substitution of "reasonably achievable" for "possible" was intended to reflect the need for common sense in resource allocation to radiation protection.

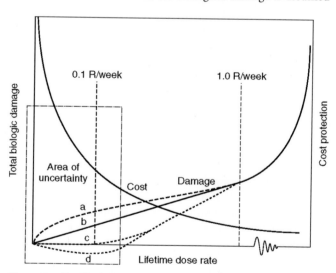

Figure 18-1 Total biological damage to a population expressed as a function of the average dose rate to individuals in the population. The cost of protection is reduced as greater biological damage is tolerated. *Source:* Claus 1958.[7]

Example 18-1

The lifetime risk of adverse biological effects from radiation exposure is approximately 5×10^{-2} Sv^{-1} for radiation workers.

Using the linear non-threshold model, estimate the lifetime risk for a whole-body x-ray dose equivalent of 0.01 Sv (1 rem):

$$\text{Lifetime risk} = (\text{Risk/Sv})[\text{Dose equivalent (Sv)}]$$
$$= (5 \times 10^{-2}\,\text{Sv}^{-1})(0.01\,\text{Sv})$$
$$= 5 \times 10^{-4}$$

That is, there is a risk of 5 chances in 10,000 that the radiation dose will cause an adverse biological effect over the lifetime of the exposed individual.

Effects of radiation exposure

Exposure to ionizing radiation can produce several effects in an individual, depending on (1) the type and amount of radiation producing the exposure, (2) the fraction of the body that is exposed, (3) the general health of the exposed individual, and (4) the quality of medical care available in the event of a relatively high exposure. If the exposure is relatively high, adverse effects may occur almost immediately or within several days or weeks. These effects are referred to as *immediate effects* of radiation exposure. At lower exposures, the effects, termed *delayed effects* of radiation exposure, may not appear for several years. Immediate effects of radiation exposure are also referred to as *early effects*, while delayed effects are frequently termed *late effects* of radiation exposure.

Stochastic radiation effects

It is well understood today that the incidence of leukemia and several forms of solid cancers began to increase in the atomic bomb survivors in Hiroshima and Nagasaki several years after the explosions occurred. This increase has been associated with exposure of the survivors to ionizing radiation released during the explosions. Increased likelihood of cancer *carcinogenesis* is the principal delayed (long-term) effect of exposure to radiation. Other delayed effects include *teratogenesis* (the induction of birth defects by irradiation of the fetus) and *mutagenesis* (the induction of genetic disorders in future generations by irradiation of germ cells).

Biological effects that appear several months or years after exposure to radiation have several characteristics in common: (1) the probability of occurrence of the effect (i.e., the number of persons in an exposed population who exhibit the effect) increases with dose; (2) the severity of the effect in a single individual is unrelated to the magnitude of the dose (i.e., the effect is an "all or none" response); and (3) no definitive threshold exists below which it can be said with certainty that the effect will not occur. These effects are probabilistic in nature and probably reflect the action of radiation to trigger mechanisms in the body that may lead ultimately to the appearance of an effect. Whether an effect actually does appear may depend on the presence of other *promoting* factors in the body. Such effects are known as

probabilistic or *stochastic effects*, in which the probability of occurrence but not the severity of the disorder is related to the dose of radiation received without a threshold dose.

Precise estimates of the role of an initiating agent such as radiation in producing stochastic effects are difficult to obtain because the effects also occur in the absence of radiation. That is, there is a *natural incidence* of the effects related to causes other than radiation exposure. Cancer, birth defects, and genetic mutations all occur naturally at relatively high rates in human populations, and identifying an increase in these rates caused by exposure to small amounts of ionizing radiation is subject to considerable uncertainty. The impact of stochastic radiation effects in a population depends on the dose and the number of persons exposed. These factors are combined in the concept of *collective dose*, sometimes called *population dose*, expressed in units of person-Sieverts.

Nonstochastic effects

Nonstochastic radiation effects, also known as *deterministic effects*, are those effects that exhibit a dose threshold. Deterministic effects of radiation are associated with levels of radiation far above those received by persons working in a modern radiation facility. These acute effects, known as *acute radiation syndromes*, are divided into three categories that differ in the relative radiation sensitivities of the involved organ systems and in the time required for the effects to occur. The three categories are the *hematopoietic syndrome*, *gastrointestinal syndrome*, and *cerebrovascular syndrome*. The stem cells of the hematopoietic system, residing primarily in the bone marrow as precursors of mature blood cells, can be inactivated in significant numbers at a dose level of a few Gray. Loss of stem cells may not become apparent until the time arrives for the precursor cells to reach maturity when the body may lose its ability to combat infection. This latency period of a few weeks provides an opportunity to reestablish the stem cell population by a bone marrow transplant.

Cells in the gastrointestinal tract, particularly epithelial cells that line the intestinal surface, are highly vulnerable to radiation injury. Following an absorbed dose of several Gray, diarrhea, hemorrhage, electrolyte imbalance, dehydration, and other gastrointestinal effects may appear within a few days as a consequence of cell damage.

At doses above about 50 Gy, cellular injury may be severe in the relatively radiation-insensitive neurological and cardiovascular compartments of the body. This effect may produce life-threatening changes almost immediately after exposure. Death in a few hours or days usually is caused by the destruction of blood vessels in the brain, fluid accumulation, and neuronal damage.

Fertility can also be impaired at relatively high doses of ionizing radiation. Temporary sterility occurs in the male at single doses above about 0.15 Gy to the testes, and permanent

Table 18-1 Differences between stochastic and deterministic effects of radiation.

	Dose-response relationship	Threshold
Stochastic effects	Severity independent of absorbed dose; probability of occurrence depends on dose	No dose threshold
Deterministic effects	Extent of damage depends on absorbed dose	Existence of dose threshold

sterility may occur at doses above about 3.5 Gy.[8] Single ovarian doses above about 0.65 Gy may cause temporary sterility in the female, and permanent sterility has been observed at doses above 2.5 Gy.[9] Doses required to produce temporary or permanent sterility are increased by orders of magnitude if delivered in fractions or continuously at low dose rates.[2] Table 18-1 summarizes the differences between stochastic and deterministic effects of radiation.

History of radiation protection standards

As appreciation of the adverse effects of radiation exposure grew in the early years of the century, advisory groups of radiation experts were established to develop upper limits of exposure for radiation users (referred to as *radiation workers* or *occupationally exposed individuals*). In 1921, the British X-ray and Radium Protection Committee developed the following recommendations for physicians and other radiation workers:[10]

- No more than 7 working hours/day; Sundays and two half-days off per week.
- As much leisure time as possible spent outdoors .
- Annual holiday of 1 month or two 2-week holidays annually.
- Personnel working full-time in x-ray and radium departments should not be expected to perform other hospital services.

Numerical limits for radiation exposure required a quantitative measure of radiation and were not proposed until the Röntgen (R) was defined in 1931. In 1934, the International Committee on X-ray and Radium Protection, later renamed the International Commission on Radiological Protection (ICRP), established a limit of 0.2 R/day for exposure of persons using radiation sources.[11] Two years later, the U.S. Advisory Committee for X-Ray and Radium Protection (now the National Council on Radiation Protection and Measurements, or NCRP) recommended a tolerance dose of 0.1 R/day. Both groups believed that the recommended limits were well below exposure levels at which immediate effects might occur. Initially the standards were intended only for x-ray exposure. However, the NCRP standard was later applied to γ rays from radium and served as a protection standard for workers on the atomic bomb (Manhattan) project during World War II.[12] Both the ICRP and NCRP are voluntary efforts, and their recommendations are purely advisory. In the United States, NCRP recommendations are frequently codified into radiation regulations by federal and state agencies, including the Nuclear Regulatory Commission and the Environmental Protection Agency.

In 1949, the NCRP substituted the concept of *maximum permissible dose* (MPD) for tolerance dose in response to the growing recognition of the leukogenic and mutagenic effects of ionizing radiation and the possibility that these effects might not exhibit a dose threshold. The assumption underlying the importance of cumulative dose is that at least some radiation-induced bioeffects are irreversible. The possibility of a dose threshold for radiation-induced cancer is an ongoing controversy which is ultimately impossible to resolve. An MPD of 0.3 R/week (15 R/year) was established for radiation workers, principally in response to concerns about the genetic effects of radiation, the dependence of the extent of occurrence of these effects on the number of individuals exposed, and the growing number of persons employed in the postwar nuclear industry.[13]

In 1956, the first of several reports on radiation effects was released by the Committee on the Biological Effects of Atomic Radiation (BEAR) of the U.S. National Academy of Sciences' National Research Council.[14] This report suggested that the total dose accumulated by an individual is more important than the dose received over any limited period in terms of effects on the health of the individual or the individual's progeny. A year later, the NCRP established a limit of $0.05(N - 18)$ Gy as the *maximum cumulative dose* for a radiation worker, with N equal to the age in years.[15] This limit implies that a person less than 18 years of age could not be considered a radiation worker. A person was permitted to receive up to 0.12 Gy/year, provided that the cumulative dose limit of $0.05(N - 18)$ was not exceeded. In 1959, the ICRP adopted the same limit,[16] and this protection standard remained in place for the next 18 years. Several later committees of the National Academy of Sciences have guided the estimation of radiation risk over the years. These committees are referred to as *BEIR* (Biological Effects of Ionizing Radiation) *committees*. Responses to concerns over radioactive fallout in the 1950s and early 1960s led to an effort to reduce the much greater exposures for medical radiation. One consequence of this effort was passage of the Radiation Control for Health and Safety Act of 1968. This act established manufacturing performance standards for radiation-emitting devices.

In 1977, the ICRP introduced a conceptual change in protection standards by restating radiation limits in terms of the *effective dose equivalent* (H_e).[17] The (H_e) was intended to permit summation of external and internal exposures in evaluating the overall risk to an exposed individual, and the unit Sievert (Sv) was used to express differences in the capacity of various types of radiation to affect the overall well-being of exposed individuals. A numerical limit of 0.05 Sv/year was recommended consistent with the cumulative dose limit of $0.05(N - 18)$, and radiation-induced cancer (carcinogenesis) replaced genetic effects (mutagenesis) as the principal health concern. This shift in concern reflected data from studies of the survivors of the atomic explosions at Hiroshima and Nagasaki revealing that the cancer risk of radiation exposure significantly exceeds the genetic risk. However, the use of Hiroshima and Nagasaki data for generalization of radiation-induced cancer risks has been criticized for the following reasons:

- Cancer incidence varies with population groups, and Japanese data may not describe other groups.
- Exposures at Hiroshima and Nagasaki were acute, not chronic, exposures.
- Social support and medical care were severely compromised in Hiroshima and Nagasaki, and they may have affected cancer incidence and mortality.

The ICRP also recommended that radiation protection standards be based on acceptable health risks rather than on arbitrary dose limits, and that these risks be determined by comparison with the health risks of individuals working in "safe" industries that do not employ radiation. The 1977 recommendations of the ICRP established a risk-oriented philosophy of radiation protection standards that continues to guide the work of both the ICRP and the NCRP.[18] In 1987, the NCRP recommended discontinuance of the 0.05(N – 18) cumulative dose limit, and its replacement by a cumulative limit of N/100 Sv, where N is the age of the exposed individual in years.[19]

In the early years of radiation protection, exposure standards were developed principally for the protection of radiation workers. With expansion of the nuclear weapons industry in the early 1950s and because of growing concern about exposure to fallout from atmospheric weapons tests, advisory groups began to consider *protection standards for the general public*. In 1955, the ICRP suggested that no member of the public (i.e., anyone other than a radiation worker) should be exposed to more than 1/10 of the MPD for an occupationally exposed person.[20] A lower limit was justified for members of the public because these individuals receive no direct benefits from radiation exposure (i.e., their jobs do not require radiation exposure), and they constitute a much greater population group compared with radiation workers. In 1957, the NCRP restated the ICRP recommendation as a dose limit of 0.005 Sv/year (5 mSv/year) for individual members of the public, consistent with its standard of 0.05 Sv/year for radiation workers.[15] The ICRP later added a population dose limit of 0.05 Sv over 30 years averaged over the entire population, principally in response to concern about the possible genetic consequences of radiation exposure of large populations.[16] In 1977, the ICRP reinforced the 5 mSv/year limit for members of the public but added that the cumulative dose to these individuals should not exceed 1 mSv/year averaged over a lifetime.[17] The NCRP officially adopted the ICRP recommendation in 1987.[19]

Current limits on radiation exposure

In Chapter 5, the *mean dose equivalent*, $\overline{H}$, (sometimes termed the *equivalent dose*) is defined as the average absorbed dose to a region of tissue multiplied by an effective quality factor, $\overline{Q}$, that depends on the *linear energy transfer* (LET) of the radiation

Table 18-2 Weighting factors (W_r) for different types of radiation.

Type and Energy	W_r
X and γ rays, electrons[a] positrons, muons	1
Neutrons, energy	
<10 keV	5
>10–100 keV	10
>100 keV–2 MeV	20
>2–20 MeV	10
>20 MeV	5
Protons other than recoil protons, energy >2 MeV	2[b]
Alpha particles, fission fragments, nonrelativistic heavy nuclei	20

Notes:
All values apply to radiation incident on the body or, if internal sources, emitted from the source.
[a]Excluding Auger electrons emitted from nuclei bound to DNA.
[b]For body irradiated by protons of > 100 MeV energy, W_r of unity applies.
Source: Adapted from National Council on Radiation Protection 1993.[21]

averaged over the region of exposed tissue. When the radiation dose is delivered by more than one type of radiation, the total $\overline{H}$ is the sum of the average absorbed dose, $\overline{D}_r$, times the effective quality factor, $\overline{Q}_r$, for each type of radiation ($\overline{H} = \sum \overline{D}_r \cdot \overline{Q}_r$), where Q is a function of the LET of the radiation. The mean dose equivalent is a measure of the biologically effective radiation dose averaged over a tissue region of interest. However, it does not address the need for a dose unit that considers the different sensitivities of specific tissues for the expression of radiation-induced biological effects. Hence, a unit is needed that accounts for nonuniform exposures of tissues and their significance in terms of the overall biological effect on the exposed organism. The effective dose equivalent has been created to address this need. Values of the radiation weighting factor for different types of radiation are displayed in Table 18-2.

The *effective dose equivalent*, H_e, (sometimes referred to as the *effective dose*, although the two quantities are not numerically identical) to an irradiated organism (i.e., an exposed person) is the sum over all exposed tissues of the mean dose equivalent, H, to each region multiplied by a *weighting factor* for the tissue, w_t, in the region. The effective dose equivalent is given by $H_e = \sum \overline{H} \cdot w_t$, where w_t accounts for influences such as the probability of cancer mortality and morbidity linked to irradiation of a specific tissue, the risk of hereditary effects related to irradiation of the tissue, and the relative length of life lost per unit dose caused by exposure of the specific tissue. The H_e is the sum of the absorbed doses to various regions multiplied by the weighting factors Q_r and w_t appropriate for each region:

$$H_e = \sum w_t \cdot \sum Q_r \cdot D_{t,r} = \sum Q_r \cdot \sum w_t \cdot D_{t,r}$$

As implied in this equation, the effective quality factor, Q_r, is independent of the tissue or organ, and the tissue weighting factor, w_t, is independent of the radiation type or energy. Weighting factors for different tissues and organs are shown in Table 18-3.

Table 18-3 Weighting factors (w_t) for different tissues.

0.01	0.05	0.12	0.20
Bone surface	Bladder	Bone marrow	Gonads
Skin	Breast	Colon	
	Liver	Lung	
	Esophagus	Stomach	
	Thyroid		
	Remainder[a,b]		

Notes:
[a]The remainder includes the following additional tissues and organs: adrenals, brain, small intestine, large intestine, kidney, muscle, pancreas, spleen, thymus, and uterus.
[b]In exceptional cases in which one of the remainder tissues or organs receives an equivalent dose in excess of the highest dose in any of the 12 organs for which a weighting factor is specified, a weighting factor of 0.025 should be applied to that tissue or organ and a weighting factor of 0.025 should be applied to the average dose in the other remainder tissues or organs.
Source: National Council on Radiation Protection and Measurements, 1993.[22]

The establishment of an *effective dose equivalent limit* on radiation exposures to workers and the general public is based on several assumptions. First, no exposure is justified unless there is a commensurate benefit to the exposed person, other individuals, or society at large. The benefit must always outweigh the risk, no matter how small the risk may be. Second, radiation exposures must be kept ALARA, consistent with sound economic and administrative practice. Third, no specific individual or group should be subjected to a risk greater than that judged acceptable. Fourth, a lower limit of radiation exposure also exists for individuals, below which the risk is negligible and does not warrant extensive administrative control. Although most radiation advisory groups subscribe philosophically to this last assumption, referred to as a *negligible individual dose* (NID), or *negligible individual level* (NIL), identification of a specific value for the lower level has not been possible to date. Efforts to establish an NIL of 0.01 mSv/year have been unsuccessful.[19] Although there is general agreement that the benefit of radiation exposure must outweigh the risk, considerable disagreement exists concerning the magnitude of benefit and risk. Furthermore, benefit and risk should be expressed in identical terms (e.g., the numbers of lives saved and lost per unit exposure) if a comparison of benefit and risk is to be meaningful.

Finally, upper limits of radiation exposure should be established to restrict the maximum risk to individuals in terms of both the immediate and the long-term effects of radiation exposure. An upper limit of radiation exposure should ensure that risks to which radiation workers are exposed are no greater than those encountered by workers in other "safe" industries. Radiation risks should be based on the *total biological detriment* resulting from radiation exposure, including the risk of fatal cancer, hereditary defects caused by genetic mutations, relative length of life lost, and the contribution of nonfatal cancer to compromised quality of life.

The current guidance of the NCRP concerning radiation limits for occupationally exposed persons can be summarized as:[19–21]

- The lifetime total effective dose equivalent in mSv should not exceed 10 times the individual's age in years. Note that recommendations of the ICRP are slightly different. Rather than 10 mSv × (age in years), the ICRP recommends a limit of 100 mSv over 5 years cumulative.
- Occupational exposure to radiation should not be permitted for persons below age 18.
- The annual total effective dose equivalent should be limited to 50 mSv, provided that the limit on lifetime total effective dose equivalent is not exceeded.
- Exposures should always be maintained at levels ALARA.

Expression of radiation protection standards in terms of effective dose equivalent reduces the need to identify dose limits for specific regions of the body. Use of such standards, however, could conceivably permit doses of several Sv/year to certain body regions that have relatively small values of w_t. To prevent excessive doses to these regions, the following additional dose limits have been established:

- 150 mSv to the crystalline lens of the eye.
- 500 mSv to all other tissues and organs, including the red bone marrow, breast, lung, gonads, extremities, and localized areas of the skin.

These limits on total effective dose equivalent are generally consistent with recommendations of the ICRP.[17,20,23]

Reports suggest that mental retardation may be the greatest risk of radiation exposure of the human fetus, especially if exposures are received 8–15 weeks following conception. The risk of radiation-induced mental retardation during this period is estimated as 0.4/Sv, which has also been expressed as a reduction in IQ of about 30%/Sv.[24] Some investigators have suggested that mental retardation may not occur for doses below about 0.4 Sv, although a mechanism has not been delineated to explain a dose threshold for this effect. Some evidence also exists that the risk of adult cancer may be significantly greater in persons exposed to radiation in utero compared with unexposed individuals.[25] The NCRP recommends that exposures to the embryo-fetus be limited to no more than 0.5 mSv/month once pregnancy is known.[19] The ICRP recommends a limit of 2 mSv to the woman's abdomen over the course of pregnancy once pregnancy is known. Both the NCRP and the ICRP suggest that restrictions beyond those appropriate for radiation workers in general should not be applied to workers who are fertile women but are not known to be pregnant.

Circumstances such as planned special exposures and emergency situations may arise occasionally during the course of a radiation worker's career. Specific guidelines for control of radiation exposures during these circumstances have been developed by the NCRP.[19] For planned special exposures, a few workers may be allowed to exceed 50 mSv for essential tasks planned well in advance. In emergency situations, no guidelines are intended to inhibit actions necessary to save lives in the event of a catastrophe. Exposures greater than 100 mSv, however, must be justified in any post-catastrophe review of actions of individuals confronted with a life-saving situation.

Radiation limits for members of the public are proposed as a maximum H_e of 5 mSv/year and an H_e of 1 mSv/year averaged over a lifetime. This average H_e is comparable to the average exposure to natural background radiation excluding exposure to radon. The NCRP has stated that a higher limit of 5 mSv/year is permissible for a small group within the general public, provided that it is not repeated in subsequent years for the same group. For the general public, the NCRP recommends an annual limit of 50 mSv to the lens of the eye, skin, and extremities. In 1992, the U.S. Nuclear Regulatory Commission adopted a revision of the Code of Federal Regulations (10CFR20) in which public exposure to reactor-produced radioactive sources is limited to 1 mSv/year (0.02 mSv/week). In 1994, the Conference of Radiation Control Program Directors recommended in its Suggested State Regulations for Control of Radiation that the same limit be applied for exposure of the public to all sources of radiation. Radiation limits are summarized in Table 18-4.

If an exposure exceeds the limit for an individual by a small amount, the expectation of harm to the individual is small. Nevertheless, this occurrence should be investigated to identify the reason for the excessive exposure. Questions such as whether there was a lapse in institutional safety procedures and what will be done to prevent a reoccurrence of the exposure should be answered. To permit identification of problems before a significant exposure occurs, institutions should set action levels based on review of personnel exposure records. These action levels (typically referred to as *ALARA limits*) are below effective dose equivalent limits but above exposures thought to be necessary to perform typical tasks requiring radiation exposure.[26] Many institutions set action levels at 1/10 of the limits on effective dose equivalent. If an individual's exposure falls between the action level and the effective dose equivalent limit, an investigation is conducted to determine the cause, while the individual continues to function as a radiation worker.

In addition to the risks discussed above, radiation oncologists and medical physicists need to be aware of radiation risks to therapy patients in order to evaluate and plan the safest and most effective treatments for an individual patient. As more and more

mature data become available, there are increasing numbers of reports of late effects and secondary malignancies that can help in the understanding of long-term radiation effects. Consideration of these long-term toxicities and secondary cancer risks needs to be included in the planning of curative courses of radiation therapy. A few examples include secondary cancers (general), cardiac toxicities and secondary lung cancers in patients treated for breast cancer, and growth issues in pediatric patients.

Two studies have been published linking computed tomography (CT) scans in pediatric patients and cancer induction. One study published in the *Lancet* in 2011 retrospectively analyzed over 170,000 patients and found a positive link between radiation dose from CT scans and leukemia and brain tumors.[27] A similar study was performed in Australia and published in the *BMJ* in 2013. It analyzed over 680,000 pediatric patients, along with over 10 million unexposed individuals in the same age bracket, and also showed cancer incidence was associated with radiation dose from CT scans.[28] The reader is also referred to review articles by Little[29] and Tubiana[30] concerning secondary cancers associated with radiotherapy procedures.

In regards to toxicities associated with breast cancer treatments, Darby et al.[31] used the SEER database (Surveillance Epidemiology and End Results) to investigate the mortality from heart disease and lung cancer after radiation therapy for breast cancer. It was concluded that radiation techniques from the 1970s and 1980s showed an increase in mortality; however, modern techniques should reduce those risks. Examples of modern techniques used to reduce toxicity by increasing distance between the irradiated tissue and heart in left-sided breast cancers are *deep inspiration breath hold* (DIBH) and *prone breast* treatments. Additionally, like DIBH treatment, respiratory-gated treatments have also been employed to decrease normal tissue dose in breast cancer patients.

Growth issues have also been associated with radiation treatment of pediatric patients. Sasso et al.[32] studied almost 100 patients treated for Wilms tumors and, of those, 34 had a minimum follow-up of at least 5 years allowing for reporting of late toxicities. Of those 34 patients, 23 (68%) presented with late toxicities such as scoliosis, muscular hypoplasia, length inequality, kyphosis, iliac wing hypoplasia, or intestinal occlusion.

The examples discussed above can all be related back to the principle of ALARA. Not only do physicians and physicists need to keep that in mind when designing and building new facilities and shielding current ones, but they need to keep that in mind in terms of patient care as well. Image acquisition parameters should be optimized to deliver a low dose while obtaining a high-quality image and treatment plans should deliver an effective treatment dose while keeping normal tissue dose ALARA.

Protective barriers for radiation sources

The walls, ceiling, and floor of a room containing an x-ray or radioactive source may be constructed to permit use of

Table 18-4 Annual radiation exposure limits.

Occupational Exposures	Dose in Sv
Whole body	0.05
Organ or tissue (not eye)	0.5
Lens of eye	0.15
Skin, Extremities	0.5
Embryo, Fetus during entire pregnancy	0.005
Public Exposure limit	0.001

adjacent rooms when the x-ray source is energized or the radioactive source is exposed. With an effective dose equivalent limit of 50 mSv/year for occupational exposure, the maximum permissible average dose equivalent equals 1 mSv/week. This dose rate is used in computations of the thickness of radiation barriers required for controlled areas. For uncontrolled areas (i.e., areas outside of direct supervision), a value of 0.1 mSv/week is usually used. Controlled areas are areas under the direct supervision of a *radiation safety officer* (RSO), sometimes called a *radiation protection officer* (RPO).

NCRP Report no. 116 recommends that a limit of 50 mSv/year [1 mSv/week] for controlled areas "should be utilized only to provide flexibility required for existing facilities and practices. The NCRP recommends that all new facilities and the introduction of all new practices be designed to limit annual exposures to individuals to a fraction of the 10 mSv/year limit implied by the cumulative dose limit by occupation."[21] Because $Q_r = 1$ for x rays and γ rays and because radiation around shielded facilities usually is assumed to produce whole-body exposures ($w_t = 1$), exposure limits for shielding purposes can be expressed as 1 mGy/week (0.1 rad/week) in controlled areas and 0.1 mGy/week (0.01 rad/week) in uncontrolled areas. Finally, the conversion from Röntgens to rads is nearly unity for x rays and γ rays. Hence, the exposure limits sometimes are still expressed as 0.1 R/week in controlled areas and 0.01 R/week in uncontrolled areas around rooms containing an x-ray or γ-ray source. In a shielded room, *primary barriers* are designed to attenuate the primary (useful) beam from a radiation source and *secondary barriers* are constructed to reduce scattered and leakage radiation from the source. Stated slightly differently, room surfaces (e.g., walls, floor, and ceiling) that are exposed to the primary beam are known as *primary barriers*. Other surfaces are termed *secondary barriers* because they are exposed only to secondary (scatter and leakage) radiation.

Protection from small sealed gamma-ray sources

The dose in Gy to an individual in the vicinity of a point source of radioactivity is given by:

$$D = \Gamma_\infty A t B / d^2$$

where Γ_∞ is the dose rate constant in units of (Gy-m²/hr-MBq) at 1 m, A is the activity of the source in MBq, t is the time in hours spent in the vicinity of the source, d is the distance from the source in meters, and B is the fraction of radiation transmitted by a protective barrier between the source and the individual. Dose rate constants for several γ-emitting sources are given in Table 18-5. The dose may be reduced by (1) decreasing the time, t, spent in the vicinity of the source, (2) increasing the distance, d, between the source and the individual, and (3) increasing the attenuation (reducing the transmission B) of the protective barrier. The thickness of lead required to provide a given transmission factor B can be determined from

Table 18-5 Dose rate constants, Γ_∞, for selected radionuclides.

Radionuclide	Exposure Rate Constant (R-m²/hr Ci)	Dose Rate Constant ($\times 10^7$) [Gy-m²/hr-MBq]
^{60}Co	1.31[a]	3.41
^{125}I	0.1.45[a]	0.378
^{137}Cs	0.328[a]	0.856
^{192}Ir	0.462[a]	1.21
^{198}Au	0.238[a]	0.619
^{222}Rn	1.02[a,b]	2.65
^{225}Ra	0.825[b,c]	2.15

Notes:
[a]Unfiltered.
[b]In equilibrium with progeny.
[c]Filtered by 0.5 mm Pt.
Six half-value layers (6 × 8 mm = 4.8 cm) of lead are required to reduce the dose rate to less than 1 mGy/hr.

Figure 18-2 for three radionuclide sources (^{182}Ta, ^{60}Co, and radium).

The three factors *(time, distance, and shielding)* are often referred to as the *three options for radiation protection*. The exposure to an individual varies directly with the activity of the source and the time spent in its vicinity, and inversely with the square of the distance between the source and the individual.

Example 18-2

What is the dose rate at a distance of 1 m from a 50 mCi (1.85 × 10⁵ MBq) point source of radium filtered by 0.5 mm Pt(lr) with a dose rate constant of 2.15 × 10⁻⁷ Gy-m²/hr-MBq? What

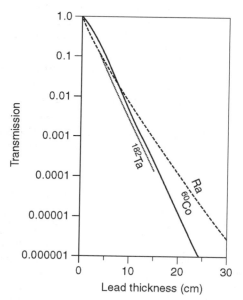

Figure 18-2 Transmission of γ radiation through lead for three radionuclides (^{182}Ta, ^{60}Co, ^{226}Ra).[33]

thickness of lead is required to reduce the dose rate to less than 1 mGy/hour if the HVL is 8 mm lead for radium?

$$D = \Gamma_\infty AtB/d^2$$
$$= (2.15 \times 10^{-7}\ \text{Gy-m/hr-MBq})(1.85 \times 10^5\ \text{MBq})(1\ \text{m})^2$$
$$= 39.8\ \text{mGy/hr}$$

Design of structural shielding

The design of shielding for radiation sources is discussed extensively in several reports of the NCRP.[21,33–35] The fundamental considerations of shielding design are presented in this section; published reports should be consulted for technical details important to the design of specific shielding configurations.

Several factors are important to the design of shielded facilities for x-ray sources used in radiation therapy. Among the factors to be considered are:

- The *workload*, W, describes the "output" of the x-ray unit. For units operating below 500 kVp, the workload is usually expressed as milliampere-minutes per week (0.01 mA-min/week), computed as 1/100 times the average mA per treatment multiplied by the approximate minutes/week of beam "on time." The factor of 1/100 reflects the observation that the dose rate is approximately 0.01 Gy/min (1 R/min) at a distance of 1 m from an x-ray tube. For units above 500 kVp, the workload is described as a weekly dose (Gy/week) delivered at 1 m from the source, estimated as the number of patient treatments per week multiplied by the dose in Gy delivered per treatment at 1 m.
- The *use factor*, U, is the fraction of the operating time during which the primary radiation beam is directed toward a particular protective barrier. Typical values of U are given in Table 18-6. The use factor is always unity for scattered and leakage radiation because these radiations impinge on the barrier for all orientations of the primary beam.
- The *occupancy factor*, T, is the fraction of the operating time of the x-ray unit that a particular area to be shielded is occupied. Representative values of T are given in Table 18-7. Note

Table 18-6 Typical use factors for a radiation therapy installation.

Full use (U = 1)	Floors of radiation rooms except dental installations, doors, walls, and ceilings of radiation rooms exposed routinely to the primary beam
Partial use (U = 1/4)	Doors and walls of radiation rooms not exposed routinely to the primary beam; also, floors of dental installations
Occasional use (U = 1/16)	Ceilings of radiation rooms not exposed routinely to the primary beam. Because of the low use factor, shielding requirements for a ceiling are usually determined by secondary rather than primary beam considerations

Source: International Commission on Radiological Protection 1960.[36] Copyright 1960, Elsevier.

Table 18-7 Typical occupancy factors for a radiation therapy installation.

Full occupancy (T = 1)	Control spaces, offices, corridors, and waiting spaces large enough to hold desks, darkrooms, workrooms and shops, nurse stations, rest and lounge rooms used routinely by occupationally exposed personnel, living quarters, children's play areas, and occupied space in adjoining buildings
Partial occupancy (T = 1/4)	Corridors too narrow for desks, utility rooms, rest and lounge rooms not used routinely by occupationally exposed personnel, wards and patients' rooms, elevators with operators, and unattended parking lots
Occasional occupancy (T = 1/16)	Closets too small for future occupancy, toilets not used routinely by occupationally exposed personnel, stairways, automatic elevators, pavements, and streets

Source: International Commission on Radiological Protection 1960.[36] Copyright 1960, Elsevier.

that the values of T in Table 18-7 are suggested values in areas where occupancy factors specific for the facility are not known. The occupancy factor is always unity for a controlled area.

- The distance, d, is the separation in meters between a source of radiation and a protective barrier. In calculating shielding requirements, the factor d asserts that the radiation intensity decreases as the square of the distance from a radiation source (inverse square falloff of intensity with distance).

Primary radiation barriers

For a maximum permissible dose, P, in a protected area (1 mGy/week in a controlled area, 0.1 mGy/week in an uncontrolled area), the required transmission, B, of a primary barrier is:

$$P = (WUTB)/d^2$$
$$B = Pd/(WUT)$$

By consulting broad-beam attenuation curves for the radiation energy of the primary beam, the required barrier thickness can be determined (Example 18-3). Typical broad-beam attenuation curves are shown in Figure 18-3 and Figure 18-4. A full range of attenuation curves is available in the literature.[33,34]

Example 18-3

A 6 MV linear accelerator delivers up to 300 treatments per week, with each treatment averaging 2 Gy tumor dose at a distance of 1 m from the target. The unit is pointed no more than 1/4 of the time toward a particular wall 4 m from the target. The laboratory on the other side of the wall is a controlled area. What thickness of concrete is required for the wall?

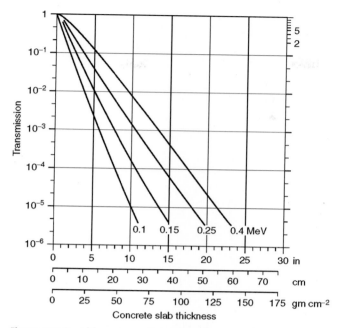

Figure 18-3 Broad-beam transmission through concrete (density 2.35 g/cm³) of x rays produced by 0.1 to 0.4 MeV electrons.[34]

With an estimated average tissue-air ratio of 0.7, the workload, W, of the therapy unit is:

(2 Gy/treatment)(300 treatments/week)/0.7

= 860 Gy/week at 1 m

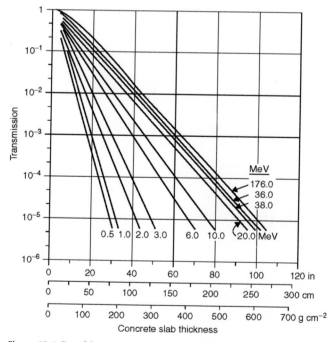

Figure 18-4 Broad-beam transmission of x rays through concrete, density 2.35 g/cm³. Energy designations refer to monoenergetic electrons incident on a thick x-ray target.[29]

For a controlled area, $P = 0.001$ Gy/week and $T = 1$. The distance $d = 4$ m and $U = 1/4$:

$$B = Pd^2/WUT$$
$$= [0.001][4^2]/[860][\tfrac{1}{4}][1]$$
$$= 7.4 \times 10^{-5}$$

From Figure 18-4, the required thickness is 140 cm concrete.

In Example 18-3 and in following examples, shielding computations are designed to limit occupational exposures to 50 mSv/year (1 mSv/week). To shield to lower limits, the value of P should be reduced (e.g., from 0.001 Gy/week to 0.0002 Gy/week to achieve a lower limit of 10 mSr/year).

The type of barrier material to be employed (e.g., concrete, lead, or steel) depends on several factors, including structural, space, and cost considerations, and the efficiency with which different materials attenuate radiation of a particular energy. For radiation therapy units, concrete is usually employed except in cases in which space is at a premium, in which case steel or lead may be preferred. For megavoltage x rays, the equivalent thickness of various materials can be estimated by comparing *tenth value layers* (TVL). The TVL is the thickness of a material required to reduce the beam intensity to 1/10 of its original value. TVL = 3.32 HVL. The number, N, of TVLs required to achieve a barrier transmission, B, is $N = \log(1/B)$. A coarse approximation can be obtained by comparing physical densities. Densities and TVLs for various materials and beam energies are given in Table 18-8.

Secondary barriers for scattered radiation

In radiation therapy, the patient is the principal source of scattered radiation. The amount of scattered radiation varies with the dose rate, beam energy, beam area incident on the patient, and the angle of scatter. The ratio of radiation scattered at various angles at 1 m from the patient to the amount of radiation incident on the patient is denoted as α. Values of α for different scattering angles and beam energies are given in Table 18-9 for an incident beam area of 400 cm². For megavoltage x-ray beams, α is usually taken as 0.1% for 90° scatter from a 400 cm² beam. The value of α increases with decreasing scattering angle. Values of α for incident beam areas other than 400 cm² can be estimated by multiplying α by area/400.

Scattered radiation is usually lower in energy than the primary beam. At relatively low energies (<500 kVp), however, the difference is not great, and the scattered energy is usually assumed to be equal to the energy of the primary beam. For higher-energy x-ray beams (>500 kVp), the energy of the x rays scattered at 90° cannot exceed 511 keV, and the required barrier thickness can be determined with the transmission curve for 500 kVp x rays. The energy of scattered radiation increases as the scattering angle decreases.

Table 18-8 Physical densities and tenth-value layers for various materials and beam energies.

Peak Voltage (kV)	Lead (mm) $\rho = 11.36$ g/cm³		Concrete (cm) $\rho = 2.35$ g/cm³		Iron (cm) $\rho = 7.8$ g/cm³	
	HVL	TVL	HVL	TVL	HVL	TVL
50	0.06	0.17	0.43	1.5	—	—
70	0.17	0.52	0.84	2.8	—	—
100	0.27	0.88	1.6	5.3	—	—
125	0.28	0.93	2.0	6.6	—	—
150	0.30	0.99	2.24	7.4	—	—
200	0.52	1.7	2.5	8.4	—	—
250	0.88	2.9	2.24	7.4	—	—
300	1.47	4.8	3.1	10.4	—	—
400	2.5	8.3	3.3	10.9	—	—
500	3.6	11.9	3.6	11.7	—	—
1000	7.9	26	4.4	14.7	—	—
2000	12.5	42	7.4	24.5	—	—
3000	14.5	48.5	7.4	24.5	—	—
4000	16	53	8.8	29.2	2.7	9.1
6000	16.9	56	10.4	34.5	3.0	9.9
8000	16.9	56	11.4	37.8	3.1	10.3
10,000	16.6	55	11.9	39.6	3.2	10.5
Cesium-137	6.5	21.6	4.8	15.7	1.6	5.3
Cobalt-60	12	40	6.2	20.6	2.1	6.9
Gold-198	3.3	11.0	4.1	13.5	—	—
Iridium-192	6.0	20	4.2	14.7	1.3	4.3
Radium-226	16.6	55	6.9	23.4	2.2	7.4

Table 18-9 Ratio α of scattered to incident radiation, with the scattered radiation measured 1 m from a phantom with a field area of 400 cm², and the incident radiation measured at the center of the field 1 m from the source in the absence of the phantom.

Source	Scattering Angle (from Central Ray)					
	30	45	60	90	120	135
X rays						
50 kV[a]	0.0005	0.0002	0.00025	0.00035	0.0008	0.0010
70 kV[a]	0.00065	0.00035	0.00035	0.0005	0.0010	0.0013
100 kV[a]	0.0015	0.0012	0.0012	0.0013	0.0020	0.0022
125 kV[a]	0.0018	0.0015	0.0015	0.0015	0.0023	0.0025
150 kV[a]	0.0020	0.0016	0.0016	0.0016	0.0024	0.0026
200 kV[a]	0.0024	0.0020	0.0019	0.0019	0.0027	0.0028
250 kV[a]	0.0025	0.0021	0.0019	0.0019	0.0027	0.0028
300 kV[a]	0.0026	0.0022	0.0020	0.0019	0.0026	0.0028
4 MV[b]	—	0.0027	—	—	—	—
6 MV	0.007	0.0018	0.0011	0.0006	—	0.0004
Gamma rays						
137Cs[d]	0.0065	0.0050	0.0041	0.0028	—	0.0019
60Co[e]	0.0060	0.0036	0.0023	0.0009	—	0.0006

Notes:

[a]Average scatter for beam centered and beam at edge of typical patient cross-section phantom. Peak pulsating x-ray tube potential. (Trout and Kelley 1972.)[37]

[b]Cylindrical phantom. (Greene and Massey 1961.)[38]

[c]Cylindrical phantom. (Karzmark and Capone 1968.)[39]

[d]These data were obtained from a slab placed obliquely to the central ray. A cylindrical phantom should give smaller values. (Interpolated from Frantz and Wyckoff, 1959.)[40]

[e]Modified for $f = 400$ cm². (Mooney and Braestrup 1967.)[41]

Source: National Council on Radiation Protection and Measurements 1976.[33]

For a maximum permissible dose rate, P, in Gy/week from radiation scattered from a patient, the required transmission, B, of a secondary barrier can be estimated as:

$$P = [(\alpha \cdot W \cdot U \cdot T)/d^2(d')^2] \cdot [F/400] \cdot B$$
$$B = [P/(\alpha \cdot U \cdot W \cdot T)] \cdot [400/F] \cdot d^2 \cdot (d')^2$$

where α is the fractional scatter at 1 m for a beam area of 400 cm^2, F is the actual beam area in cm^2, d is the source–patient distance in meters, and d' is the distance in meters from the patient to the barrier. For radiation scattered at 90°, U is usually assumed to be unity. The barrier thickness that provides the required transmission is determined from the appropriate attenuation curve in Figure 18-3 and Figure 18-4 (primary energy curve for beams <500 kVp and the 500 kVp curve for beams >500 kVp for scatter at 90 degrees; curves such as those in Figure 18-5 are used for radiation scattered at angles other than 90°).

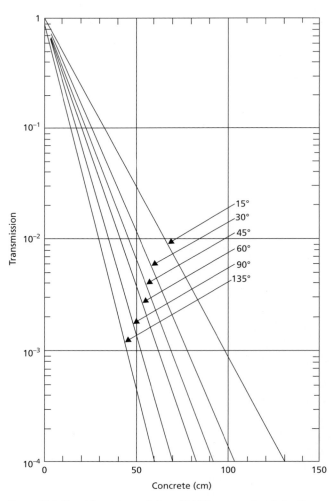

Figure 18-5 Broad-beam transmission of 6 MV x rays scattered at various angles.

Secondary barriers for leakage radiation

For therapy x-ray units operating below 500 kVp, the maximum leakage of radiation from the tube housing is 1 rad/hour (0.01 Gy/hour) at a distance of 1 m. For therapy units above 500 kVp (i.e., ^{60}Co γ-ray and megavoltage x-ray units), the maximum leakage radiation at 1 m in any direction from the source is confined by regulatory statute to 0.1% of the dose rate from the useful beam at 1 m from the source. The required secondary barrier, B, for leakage radiation to yield a permissible dose rate, P, (Gy/week) at 1 m from the source is determined as:

For therapy units operating at energies below 500 kVp, we obtain:

$$P = WTB/(d^2 \times 60I)$$
$$B = Pd^2 \cdot 60I/WT$$

where I is the maximum tube current for continuous operation of the x-ray source, W is the workload expressed as 0.01 mA-min/week, the number 60 converts minutes to hours, and d is the distance from the source to the barrier.

For therapy units operating at energies above 500 kVp, we obtain:

$$P = 0.001 WTB/d^2$$
$$B = Pd^2/(0.001 WT)$$

where 0.001 is the 0.1% leakage through the source housing measured at 1 m.

The energy of leakage radiation is approximately the same as the energy of the primary beam, and the transmission curve for primary radiation should be used to determine the barrier thickness for leakage radiation. Also, leakage radiation is assumed to be isotropic (equal intensity in all directions), so $U = 1$ in barrier computations for leakage radiation.

For therapy x-ray beams, a barrier thickness for primary radiation greatly exceeds that for secondary radiation. Hence, secondary radiation can be ignored when barrier thicknesses are determined for primary radiation because a primary barrier also reduces secondary radiation to a negligible level. For megavoltage x-ray beams, shielding requirements for leakage radiation usually significantly exceed those for scattered radiation because the leakage radiation is more energetic. Hence, requirements for secondary barriers are usually dominated by leakage radiation except in situations in which small scattering angles must be considered. For lower-energy beams, differences may be small between the requirements for scattered and leakage radiation. Shielding requirements for secondary barriers are computed separately for scattered and leakage radiation. If the difference in shielding requirements exceeds 3 HVLs (or 1 TVL) for the primary beam, the greater of the two thicknesses provides adequate shielding for both. If the difference is less than 3 HVLs, 1 HVL of shielding thickness should be added to the larger thickness to provide adequate shielding against both scattered and leakage radiation.

Door shielding

Unless the entrance to a room housing a radiation therapy unit is constructed as a maze, the room door must provide radiation shielding equivalent to the contiguous wall. For higher-energy therapy beams, the door contains massive quantities of lead or steel and requires a motor drive for opening and closing. A manual means of moving the door must be available in the event that electrical power fails. In most cases, a maze entranceway is preferable to a motorized door because it greatly reduces the shielding requirements for the door. The maze is designed so that radiation must be scattered at least once, and usually multiple times, before it reaches the door (Figure 18-6). With each scattering, the intensity and energy of the radiation is decreased, and the required door shielding is reduced. The shielding requirements of the door can be determined by using the equation given earlier for the intensity of scattered radiation for each scattering angle in the pathway from the radiation source to the door. In most cases, the use of an entrance maze can reduce the required door shielding to a few millimeters of lead. A few different examples of maze design are shown in Figure 18-7.

Example 18-4

The 6 MV linear accelerator described in Example 18-3 is equipped with a primary beam stopper that transmits less than 0.1% of the primary beam. Radiation scattered by the patient through angles of up to 30° is also intercepted by the beam stopper. Under these conditions and for use and occupancy factors of unity, what thickness of concrete is required for the wall described in Example 18-3?

From Table 18-9, the fraction of the incident radiation scattered at 1 m through a scattering angle of 30° is 0.007 for a 400 cm^2 field. With the patient 1 m from the target, the distance, d', from the patient to the wall is:

$$d' = (3\ \text{m})/(\cos 30°) = (3\ \text{m})/(0.866)$$
$$= 3.46\ \text{m}$$

If the average field size for patient treatment is 400 cm^2, the required attenuation factor, B, is:

$$B = [P/(aWUT)][400/F]d^2/d')^2$$
$$= [0.001/(0.007)(860)(1)(1)][400/400]](1)^2/(3.46)^2]$$
$$= 2.0 \times 10^{-3}$$

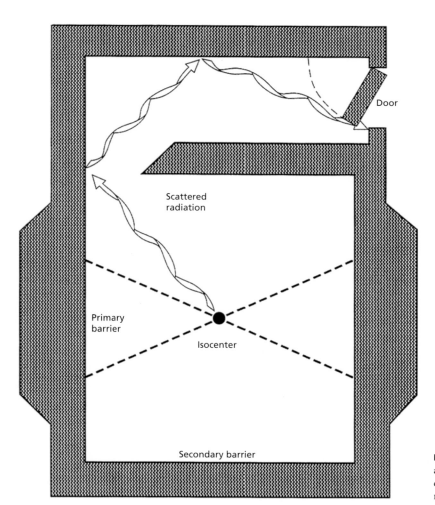

Figure 18-6 Entrance maze for a high-energy accelerator used in radiation therapy. The maze is designed so that only multiply scattered radiation can reach the door.

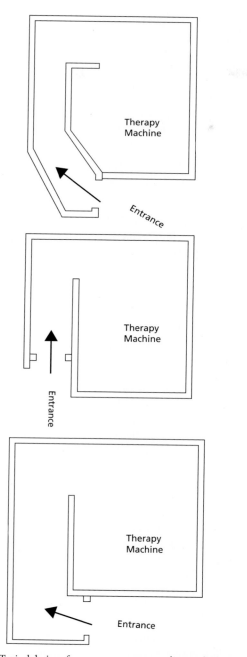

Therapy
Machine

Entrance

Therapy
Machine

Entrance

Therapy
Machine

Entrance

Figure 18-7 Typical designs for maze entrances to radiation therapy rooms. *Source:* Jayaraman and Lanzl 1996, with permission.[42]

From Figure 18-5, 70 cm of concrete is required to provide an attenuation factor of 2.0×10^{-3} for 6 MV x rays scattered through 30°. This thickness provides more than adequate protection against scattered radiation because scattered radiation skims past the beam stopper and strikes the wall only when the therapy unit is oriented toward the wall (i.e., $U = 1/4$ could have been used in this computation). The remainder of the time the unit is oriented in a different direction in which the scattering

angle is greater and both α and the average energy of scattered photons are reduced.

Example 18-5

For the 6 MV accelerator described in Example 18-3 a wall perpendicular to the axis of rotation of the unit is never exposed to the primary beam. The wall is 4 m from the patient and the average field size at the patient is 20×20 cm. What thickness of concrete is required to shield non-occupationally exposed individuals ($P = 0.0001$ Gy/week) in the adjoining room from scattered radiation if the occupancy factor for the room is 1/4?

$$B = [P/(\alpha W 400/F]d^2/d')^2$$
$$= \frac{(0.0001)(400/400)(1)^2/(4)^2}{0.0006)(860)(1/4)}$$
$$= 1.2 \times 10^{-2}$$

From the 500 kVp curve in Figure 18-4, 33 cm of concrete is required to reduce scattered radiation to an acceptable level.

Example 18-6

For the wall described in Example 18-5, determine the thickness of concrete required to protect the non-occupationally exposed individuals from leakage radiation:

$$B = \frac{Pd^2}{0.001 \, WT}$$
$$= \frac{(0.0001)(4)^2}{(0.001)(860)(1/4)}$$
$$= 7.4 \times 10^{-3}$$

Leakage radiation has essentially the same energy as primary radiation, so attenuation curves for the primary beam are consulted when leakage is considered. The required thickness of concrete is 70 cm.

Example 18-7

For the wall described in Examples 18-5 and 18-6, 33 cm of concrete is required to shield against scattered radiation, and 70 cm is needed to shield for leakage radiation. The difference of 37 cm in these thicknesses slightly exceeds the 35 cm of concrete described as 1 TVL, hence, the required barrier thickness is 70 cm of concrete. If the difference had been less than 35 cm, 1 HVL (11 cm of concrete) would have to be added to the 70 cm thickness of concrete.

Neutron shielding

Neutrons are released when electrons and x rays produced in a high-energy accelerator interact with the target, flattening filter, collimator, patient, and materials in the accelerator room. Hence, the x-ray beam from a high-energy (>10 MV) accelerator is contaminated with neutrons. The electron beam from a high-energy accelerator is contaminated with neutrons to a much smaller degree than the x-ray beam because electrons produce neutrons with a much lower efficiency compared with x rays. The neutron contamination increases rapidly with increasing x-ray energy from 10 to 20 MV and remains relatively constant above 20 MV.[43] For x rays between about 15 and 25 MV, the neutron dose equivalent rate along the central axis of the beam is about 0.5% of the x-ray dose-equivalent rate and falls to about 0.1% outside the primary beam.[44] The energy of the neutrons extends over a wide range with a maximum of about 1 MeV. The neutron energy is rapidly degraded by multiple scattering. Neutrons are attenuated efficiently in concrete, and concrete barriers for x-ray shielding almost always provide adequate shielding against neutrons.

The degradation (*moderation*) of neutron energy occurs most efficiently by elastic scattering with hydrogen nuclei (protons) and other light nuclei. Heavy nuclei such as lead are poor moderators because they deflect neutrons with little energy loss. The door to a treatment room for a high-energy accelerator often presents a special challenge with regard to neutron shielding.[33] A maze entranceway can be designed to reduce greatly the quantity and energy of neutrons reaching the door. In most cases, a few inches of a hydrogenous material such as polyethylene in the door are sufficient to reduce the neutron dose equivalent to an acceptable level outside the treatment room. Boron is a strong absorber (i.e., it has a high cross-section) for low-energy neutrons. Hence, polyethylene impregnated with boron is often used to shield the treatment-room door.[34] However, as the neutrons are absorbed by (n, γ) reactions in the door, γ rays (called *neutron-capture γ rays*) are released with energies in the range of a few MeV. These γ rays must be attenuated by lead in the door so that dose rates outside the room do not exceed acceptable levels.

The determination of shielding barriers for high-energy accelerators required to reduce x rays, neutron-capture γ rays, and neutrons to acceptable levels outside a treatment room is a complex process. NCRP Report no. 79 provides the following expressions for computation of TVLs for reduction of absorbed dose for neutrons of average energy, E, in MeV:

Concrete: $\text{TVL(cm)} = 15.5 + 5.6E$

Polyethylene: $\text{TVL(cm)} = 6.2 + 3.4E$

Several references are available to aid these computations.[34,35,42–46] However, the computations should be performed by persons who are expert in shielding design for high-energy accelerators and the computations can be checked by an on-site clinical physicist.

Protection for sealed radioactive sources

The safe handling, transport, and storage of sealed radioactive sources used for brachytherapy require supervision by an individual with extensive knowledge of radiation protocols and safety. A few principles are discussed in this section, but detailed safety procedures are required for the safe use of high-activity sealed sources of radioactivity in radiation therapy.[47–49]

Long-lived brachytherapy sources are stored in a lead-lined *safe* with lead-filled drawers designed to hold sources in the shape of needles, capsules, and other configurations. The safe should be designed to facilitate rapid removal and return of sources. A shielded area, often equipped with an *L-block* of lead with a lead-glass window, should always be used when sealed sources are handled. The shielded area may be equipped with mirrors to permit handling of the sources under conditions in which direct viewing of the sources is undesirable. Beta-emitting sources such as ^{90}Sr–^{90}Y ophthalmic applicators should be manipulated behind a low-Z shield such as acrylic. High-Z shielding materials such as lead are undesirable for β sources because they generate more Bremsstrahlung during absorption of β particles.

Sealed sources should always be handled with forceps and never with the hands. A sink trap should always be present in the sink used to clean brachytherapy applicators to prevent loss of a sealed source that has been left accidentally in the applicator. Brachytherapy sources should be sterilized only by chemical treatment. They should never be subjected to heat or steam sterilization methods. Afterloading procedures should be used whenever possible to reduce the exposure to personnel engaged in brachytherapy. The three principles of radiation protection (time, distance, and shielding) are particularly applicable in the handling and transport of sealed radioactive sources.

Brachytherapy sources should always be transported in a lead-shielded container, often a cart that can be rolled to the application site. The cart should be well balanced so that it cannot tip over and spill its contents. The container should display a radiation warning sign and should never be left unattended while radioactive sources are inside. The container should be used only to transport brachytherapy sources and should not be used for the permanent storage of sources.

An accurate inventory of long-lived brachytherapy sources must be maintained. An inventory is especially challenging when radioactive wires (e.g., ^{192}Ir, ^{182}Ta, or ^{198}Au) are present that can be cut into segments of variable length. Sealed radioactive sources must be *leak tested* at periodic intervals, not to exceed 6 months by regulation. Most sealed sources are tested by wiping the surface with a moistened cloth or cotton swab and determining whether any radioactivity has been transferred to the wiping material. A source is considered *leaky* if 0.005 μCi (185 Bq) or more activity is present on the material. A leaking source should be sealed in a container and returned to the supplier. Radium sources are particularly hazardous and subject to radon leakage. Although these sources are no longer recommended for brachytherapy, they are still occasionally found in storage receptacles in medical facilities.

Discharge instructions are also an important radiation safety consideration for patients who are sent home after a temporary, or permanent, seed implant. Typical discharge paperwork for a seed implant will include instructions on interactions with pregnant individuals and children as well as what to do if a seed is dislodged and found. For permanent prostate seed implant patients, it will usually include additional instructions regarding sexual intercourse (such as wearing a condom for 6 months post-procedure).

Radiation surveys

After installation or modification of radiation equipment, a radiation survey must be performed to verify that exposure levels in all occupied areas are within acceptable limits and that the integrity of the shielding material has not been compromised. The survey should also ensure that the equipment is functioning properly and that safety interlocks and emergency procedures are appropriate, functional, and well understood by all employees. Three instruments commonly employed in radiation protection surveys are the portable ionization survey meter, G-M counter, and neutron detector.

Ionization chambers

Exposure rates in the range of a few mR/hour can be measured with a portable survey meter such as that depicted in Figure 18-8. This instrument contains a pressurized ionization chamber as the radiation-sensitive component. The measured current is displayed directly on a meter scale denoting radiation units such as mR/hour. The response of the chamber must be calibrated periodically against a standard source, such as ^{137}Cs and an energy-dependence correction applied if the measured photons differ significantly in energy from those used for instrument calibration. A correction may also be required if the

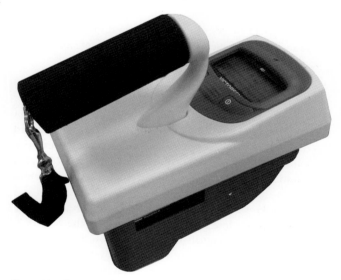

Figure 18-8 Pressurized ionization-chamber survey meter.

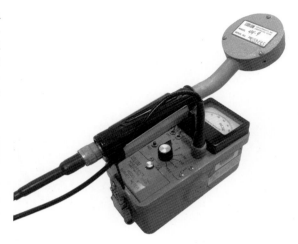

Figure 18-9 Geiger–Müller survey meter with pancake probe.

instrument varies in sensitivity with the direction of impinging radiation. Some ionization-chamber survey instruments are unsealed, and corrections may be necessary for the ambient temperature and pressure if the chamber is calibrated under conditions greatly different from those encountered during routine use.

Geiger–Müller counters

The *Geiger–Müller (G-M) counter* uses a sealed cylindrical detector filled with an inert gas containing small amounts of impurities (Figure 18-9). When radiation interacts with the gas, an avalanche of ionization is created as a result of the relatively high voltage (~1000 V) applied across the chamber. As this ionization is collected, a voltage pulse is produced across the detector electrodes that indicates that an ionization event has occurred inside the detector. This indication is displayed by a meter with units of counts/min. The G-M counter records individual interactions and is not useful for measurement of actual exposure or dose rates around a radiation unit. It is much more sensitive than a cutie pie, however, and is helpful in identifying the presence of small amounts of radioactivity or small voids in radiation shields. However, G-M counters have a relatively long resolving time (50–300 μsec). Hence, high activities can paralyze a G-M counter, resulting in suppression of the count rate.

Neutron detectors

Various types of instruments are available to detect and measure the presence of neutrons in occupied areas outside the treatment room. A common instrument is an ionization chamber or proportional counter filled with BF_3 gas or composed of walls coated with lithium, boron, or a hydrogenous material. A BF_3 proportional counter is shown in Figure 18-10 in which the detector is surrounded by a nine-inch cadmium-loaded polyethylene sphere to slow (*moderate*) the neutrons so

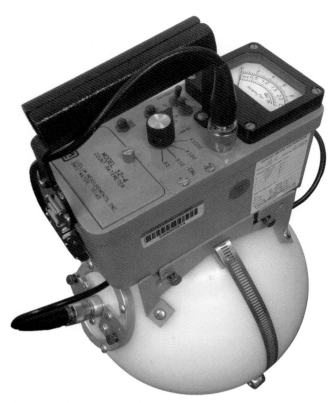

Figure 18-10 BF_3 proportional counter used for surveys of neutron levels.

that they interact efficiently with the detector. Measurements with the chamber are recorded in units of mSv/hour.

Personnel monitoring

Radiation exposures must be monitored for persons working with or near sources of ionizing radiation. Individuals who have a potential of receiving doses of one-tenth or more of the permissible limit must wear one or more radiation monitors that can be read out periodically (e.g., biweekly or monthly) to determine their actual exposure to radiation. Over the years, the monitor used most often has been the film badge containing two or more dental-size x-ray films in a sealed packet. The films differ in sensitivity to permit measurement over a wide range of exposures. A film badge is worn on the collar or trunk of the body, or sometimes in both locations during each workday. Periodically, the films are replaced, and the optical densities of the exposed films are measured as an index of the exposure received by the person wearing the badge. Radiations detectable with the film badge include x rays, γ rays, high-energy electrons, and neutrons. In many *film badges* in use today, optically stimulated luminescent dosimeters (OSLDs) have replaced x-ray film and thermoluminescent dosimeters (TLDs) as the sensitive element in the monitor. Modifications of the OSLD whole-body monitor

have yielded wrist and finger dosimeters to monitor the radiation exposure to the extremities. These monitors are especially useful in angiography and nuclear medicine.

Small ionization chambers about the size of a fountain pen can be worn in the pocket while an individual is engaged in a procedure involving exposure to ionizing radiation. Many of these pocket chambers can be read at any time by the individual and permit periodic assessment of exposure as the procedure progresses. Pocket chambers are sometimes used by persons engaged in brachytherapy procedures.

Summary

- Standards for radiation are based on estimates of risk derived from the linear non-threshold model of radiation injury.
- Stochastic effects of radiation exposure include carcinogenesis, teratogenesis, and mutagenesis.
- Nonstochastic effects of radiation exposure include the hematopoietic syndrome, gastrointestinal syndrome, and cerebrovascular syndrome.
- Organizations important to the evolution of radiation protection standards include the International Commission on Radiological Protection and the U.S. National Council on Radiation Protection and Measurements.
- Radiation limits expressed as effective dose equivalents are influenced by the average absorbed dose to tissue and weighted by factors that account for the linear energy transfer (LET) of the radiation and for mortality and morbidity linked to irradiation of specific tissues.
- Shielding barriers for x rays include (a) primary barriers to protect against the primary beam and (b) secondary barriers to protect against secondary radiation (scatter and leakage).
- Factors that influence the thickness of primary and secondary barriers include the workload W, use factor U, occupancy factor T, and distance from the radiation source to the barrier.
- Shielding against neutrons may be required for high-energy accelerators (>10 MV). Instruments used for radiation surveys include cutie pies, G-M counters, and, for high-energy accelerators, a neutron survey instrument.

Problems

18-1 The lifetime risk of a particular form of radiation-induced cancer is estimated as 10^{-3} Sv^{-1}. What is the lifetime risk for a whole-body dose equivalent of 0.05 Sv? Does your estimate assume that the dose response follows a linear, non-threshold model?

18-2 For a 45-year-old radiation worker, what is the maximum cumulative dose limit recommended by the NCRP? If the worker's cumulative dose were below this limit, what would be the dose limit for the next year? What would be the maximum cumulative dose limit if the individual were a member of the public?

18-3 What is the dose rate at a distance of 2 m from a 200 mCi (7.4×10^3 MBq) point source of $^{137}Cs(\Gamma_\infty = 8.5 \times 10^{-8} \frac{Gy-m^2}{hr-MBq})$? What thickness of lead (HVL 7 mm) is required to reduce the dose rate to less than 0.02 mGy/hr (2 mR/hr)? What additional thickness of lead would keep the dose rate at the same level if the source activity were increased to 800 mCi (29.6×10^4 MBq)?

18-4 A therapy facility is designed to treat as many as 60 patients per week with a 6 MV linear accelerator. Treatments will deliver a tumor dose of 2 Gy on the average with a tissue-air ratio of approximately 0.7. For an uncontrolled adjacent room at a distance of 6 m and full occupancy, what is the required thickness of concrete wall for a use factor of $^1/_4$? If four inches of lead (attenuation factor 10^{-2}) are placed along the wall, how much additional concrete would be needed?

18-5 Repeat the computation in Problem 18-4 for a wall 6 m away that never receives the primary beam ($P = 10^{-4}$ Gy/wk, $T = 1$).

18-6 For the wall described in Problem 18-3, what thickness of concrete is required to protect against leakage radiation? Is additional shielding required when scattered and leakage radiation are considered together?

18-7 If IMRT treatment volumes are expected to be 30% of the patient volume on a typical linear accelerator (e.g., 30 patients/day), and the number of monitor units triples for these patients to deliver step and shoot segmented MLC shapes, how will this affect shielding calculations regarding head leakage? If the original design had an additional tenth value layer of shielding built in as a safety margin and only 6 MV x rays are used for IMRT, do you think this will still be enough?

References

1 Stannard, J. N. *Radioactivity and Health: A history*. Springfield, VA, Department of Energy, National Science and Technology Information Service, (DOE/RL101830-759), 1988.

2 Moeller, D. History and perspective on the development of radiation protection standards. In *Radiation Protection Today: The NCRP at 60 Years*, W. K. Sinclair (ed.). *Proceedings of the 25th Annual Meeting*. Bethesda, MD, National Council on Radiation Protection and Measurements, 1990.

3 Stebbings, J. H., Lucas, H. F., and Stehney, A. F. Mortality from cancers of major sites in female radium dial workers. *Am. J. Ind. Med.* 1984; **5**:435–459.

4 Luckey, T. D. *Hormesis with Ionizing Radiation*. Boca Raton, FL, CRC Press, 1980.

5 Gofman, J. W. *Radiation and Human Health*. San Francisco, Sierra Club, 1981.

6 Edwards, F. M. Development of radiation protection standards. *Radiographics* 1991; **11**:699–712.

7 Claus, W. The concept and philosophy of permissible dose to radiation. In *Radiation Biology and Medicine*, W. Claus (ed.). Reading, MA, Addison-Wesley, 1958.

8 International Commission on Radiological Protection. *Nonstochastic Effects of Ionizing Radiation*, ICRP Publication No. 41. Oxford, Pergamon Press, 1984.

9 United Nations Scientific Committee on the Effects of Atomic Radiation. (UNSCEAR). *Ionizing Radiation: Sources and Biological Effects Report E.82.1X.8*. New York, United Nations, 1982.

10 British X-Ray and Radium Protection Committee. X-ray and radium protection. *J Roentgen Soc.* 1921; **17**:100.

11 International Commission on Radiological Protection (ICRP). International recommendations for x-ray and radium protection. *Radiology* 1934; **23**:682 and *Br. J. Radiol.* 1934; **7**:695.

12 Taylor, L. S. The development of radiation protection standards (1925–40). *Health Phys.* 1981; **41**:227–232.

13 Taylor L. S. Organization of radiation protection. *The Operations of the ICRP and NCRP—1928–1974*, DOE/TIC-10124. Washington, DC, U.S. Department of Energy, Office of Technical Information, 1979.

14 National Academy of Sciences, National Research Council. *The Biological Effects of Atomic Radiation: Summary Report*. Washington, DC, National Academy of Sciences Press, 1956.

15 National Council on Radiation Protection and Measurements (NCRP). Maximum permissible radiation exposure to man: A preliminary statement of the National Committee on Radiation Protection and Measurements. *Am. J. Roentgenol.* 1957; **68**:260–267.

16 International Commission on Radiological Protection. *Recommendations of the ICRP*, ICRP Publication No. 1. London, Pergamon Press, 1957.

17 International Commission on Radiological Protection: *Recommendations of the ICRP*, ICRP Publication No. 26. London, Pergamon Press, 1977.

18 Kocher, DC. Perspective on the historical development of radiation protection standards. *Health Phys.* 1991; **61**:519–527.

19 National Council on Radiation Protection and Measurements. *Recommendations on Limits for Exposure to Ionizing Radiation*. NCRP Report No. 91. Bethesda, MD, NCRP, 1987.

20 International Commission on Radiological Protection. *Statement and Recommendations of the 1980 Brighton Meeting of the ICRP*, ICRP Publication No. 30. Elmsford, NY, Pergamon Press, 1980.

21 National Council on Radiation Protection and Measurements: *Limitations of Exposure to Ionizing Radiation*, NCRP Report No. 116. Bethesda, MD, NCRP, 1993.

22 National Council on Radiation Protection and Measurements: *Limitation of Exposure to Ionizing Radiation*, NCRP Report no. 116. Bethesda, MD, NCRP, 1993.

23 International Commission on Radiological Protection. *Nonstochastic Effects of Ionizing Radiation*. ICRP Publication No. 41. Elmsford, NY, Pergamon Press, 1984.

24 Meinhold C. Past-President, National Council on Radiation Protection and Measurements: Personal communication, 1992.

25 United Nations Scientific Committee on the Effects of Atomic Radiation. *Genetic and Somatic Effects of Ionizing Radiation: UNSCEAR Report to the General Assembly with Annexes*. New York, United Nations, 1981.

26 National Council on Radiation Protection and Measurements. *Implementation of the Principle of as Low as Reasonably*

Achievable (ALARA) for Medical and Dental Personnel. NCRP Report No. 107. Bethesda, MD, NCRP, 1990.

27 Pearce, M. S., Salotti, J. A., Little, M. P., McHugh, K., Lee, C., et al. Radiation exposure from CT scans in childhood and subsequent risk of leukaemia and brain tumours: a retrospective cohort study. *Lancet* 2011; **380**: 499–505.

28 Mathews, J. D., Forsythe, A. V., Brady, Z., Butler, M. W., Goergen, S. K., et al. Cancer risk in 680,000 people exposed to computed tomography scans in childhood or adolescence: data linkage study of 11 million Australians. *BMJ* 2013; **346**: f2360.

29 Little, M. P. Cancer after exposure to radiation in the course of treatment for benign and malignant disease. *Lancet Oncol* 2001; **2**: 212–20.

30 Tubiana, M. Can we reduce the incidence of Secondary primary malignancies occurring after radiotherapy? A critical review. *Radiotherapy and Oncology* 2009; **91**: 4–15

31 Darby, S. C., McGale, P., Taylor, C. W., and Peto, R. Long-term mortality from heart disease and lung cancer after radiotherapy for early breast cancer: prospective cohort study of about 300000 women in US SEER cancer registries. *Lancet Oncol* 2005; **6**: 557–65.

32 Sasso, G., Greco, N., Murino, P., and Sasso, F. S. Late Toxicity in Wilms Tumor Patients Treated with Radiotherapy at 15 years of Median Follow-up. *J. Pediatr. Hematol. Oncol.* 2010; **32**: e264.

33 National Council on Radiation Protection and Measurements. *Structural Shielding Design and Evaluation for Medical Use of X Ray and Gamma Rays of Energies Up to 10 MeV*, NCRP Report No. 49. Bethesda, MD, NCRP, 1976.

34 National Council on Radiation Protection and Measurements. *Radiation Protection Design Guidelines for 0.1–100 MeV Particle Accelerator Facilities*, NCRP Report No. 51. Bethesda, MD, NCRP, 1977.

35 National Council on Radiation Protection and Measurements. *Medical X-ray, Electron Beam and Gamma-Ray Protection for Energies Up to 50 MeV (Equipment Design, Performance and Use).* NCRP Report No. 102, NCRP, Bethesda, MD, 1989.

36 International Commission on Radiological Protection. *Report of Committee III on Protection Against X Rays Up to Energies of 3 MeV and Beta and Gamma Rays from Sealed Sources*, ICRP Publication No. 3. New York, Pergamon Press, 1960.

37 Trout, D. and Kelley, J. P. Scattered radiation from a tissue-equivalent phantom for x rays from 50 to 300 kVp. *Radiology* 1972; **104**: 161.

38 Greene, D., and Massey, J. B. Some measurements on the absorption of 4 MV x rays in concrete. *Br. J. Radiol.* 1961; **34**:389–391.

39 Karzmark, C. J., and Capone, T. Measurements of 6 MV x-rays: I: Primary radiation absorption in lead, steel and concrete. *Br. J. Radiol.* 1968; **41**:33–39.

40 Frantz, F. S. Jr, and Wyckoff, H. O. Attenuation of scattered cesium-137 gamma rays. *Radiology* 1959; **73**:263–266.

41 Mooney, R. T., and Braestrup, C. B. *Attenuation of scattered cobalt-60 radiation in lead and building materials.* Atomic Energy Commission Report NYO 2165, 1957.

42 Jayaraman, S., and Lanzl, L. (eds.). *Clinical Radiotherapy Physics*, Vol II. Bethesda, MD, CRC Press, 1996, p. 171.

43 Sohrabi, M., and Morgan, K. Z. Neutron dosimetry in high-energy x-ray beams of medical accelerators. *Phys. Med. Biol.* 1979; **24**:756–766.

44 Axton, E., and Bardell, A. Neutron production from electron accelerators used for medical purposes. *Phys. Med. Biol.* 1972; **17**:293–298.

45 Kersey, R. Estimation of neutron and gamma radiation doses in the entrance mazes of SL 75-20 linear accelerator treatment rooms. *Medicamundi* 1979; **24**:151.

46 National Council on Radiation Protection and Measurements: *Neutron Contamination for Medical Linear Accelerators*, NCRP Report No. 79. Bethesda, MD, NCRP, 1984.

47 National Council on Radiation Protection and Measurements. *Protection Against Radiation from Brachytherapy Sources*, NCRP Report No. 40. Bethesda, MD, NCRP, 1972.

48 American Association of Physicists in Medicine. *Remote Afterloading Technology*, AAPM Report No. 41. New York, American Institute of Physics, 1993.

49 International Electrotechnical Commission. *Particular Requirements for the Safety of Remote Controlled Automatically Driven Gamma-Ray Afterloading Equipment*, International Standard IEC 601, Medical Electrical Equipment, Part 2. Geneva, Bureau de la Commission Electrotechnique Internationale, 1989.

CHAPTER

19

QUALITY ASSURANCE

Objectives

After studying this chapter, the reader should be able to:
- Describe the components of an effective quality assurance program in radiation therapy.
- Identify standard equipment for performing quality assurance measurements.
- List resources for recommended testing procedures and tolerances for relevant equipment.
- Differentiate between commissioning tests and patient-specific tests.
- Describe aspects of a quality assurance program for brachytherapy.

Hendee's Radiation Therapy Physics, Fourth Edition. Todd Pawlicki, Daniel J. Scanderbeg and George Starkschall.
© 2016 John Wiley & Sons, Inc. Published 2016 by John Wiley & Sons, Inc.

Introduction

A comprehensive quality assurance (QA) program should address all sources of variability in the treatment of patients in an effort to minimize the overall uncertainty of treatment. The ICRU has recommended that the uncertainty in dose delivery be maintained below approximately 5%.[1] Delivering a dose to a patient within a tolerance of 5% is no simple task.[2] It has been estimated that the equipment used by most medical physicists to calibrate therapeutic radiation beams is accurate to an overall uncertainty (expressed at the 95% confidence level) of approximately 1.5%.[3] However, one should remember that there are other sources of uncertainty related to treatment, such as patient thickness, transmission factors, and dose calculation, so that the overall uncertainty in dose delivered to the patient is about 5%.

A good QA program should be designed specifically for each facility. Differences in equipment design and reliability, staffing levels, patient mix, and other variables may justify a tightening, or possibly a relaxation, of the recommendations presented in this chapter. The development of a good QA program is an evolutionary process. QA programs must be balanced against the resources available to provide quality care. With rapidly advancing technologies, QA programs must be adaptable to new techniques and must permit obsolete processes to be abandoned. An efficient and adaptable framework for QA programs for new technologies and procedures should be based on established hazard analysis techniques (see Chapter 20).

Recommended quality assurance procedures

The recommendations summarized in this chapter have evolved over a number of years as a product of the authors' experiences in several institutions. Furthermore, this chapter focuses on conventional equipment as opposed to more recent delivery methods, such as robotic devices, tomotherapy, or proton delivery. Each unique delivery method will have its own set of special measurements, which can be found elsewhere.[4] In general, however, there are overarching components of a robust QA program regardless of the equipment. These include: safety, mechanical, software operation, radiation properties, and radiation/mechanical coincidence. Testing the integration and function of connected systems from different vendors is also very important.

As previously mentioned, the frequency of QA procedures should be determined individually, by each institution, for each piece of equipment. Equipment that demonstrates instability, or that has not yet demonstrated a record of stability, should be tested frequently. Once a piece of equipment has demonstrated stability, or aspects of its performance have been shown to be stable, consideration might be given to reducing the frequency of certain testing procedures. Any proposed reduction in test frequency must always be balanced against the risk of failure to detect poor performance and the potential adverse consequences of said failure. For example, the output of many linear accelerators has been shown to be very stable. However, the failure to detect an unexpected change in output could be catastrophic. Therefore, daily measurements of output constancy continue to be recommended.

The decision of what tests should be performed is determined by trying to minimize the risk of possible harm to the patient. Recommendations are made here for tests to be conducted biennially, annually, semiannually, quarterly, monthly, and daily. To reduce the time required to perform annual tests, some procedures may be distributed among the monthly or quarterly checks. If this approach is taken, the procedures should be designed carefully to ensure that none of the measurements is overlooked. Most daily QA procedures should always be performed at the beginning of the day, before patient treatments are delivered. This is because malfunctions sometimes occur as equipment is being turned off at the end of the day, or turned on at the beginning of the day, possibly due to a change in power status or to the time interval since last usage. Performing QA tests during the day or at the end of the treatment day carries an increased risk that patients might be treated with malfunctioning equipment.

When a measured parameter falls outside the action or tolerance limits, a decision should be made that is commensurate with the deviation from the stated tolerance and the severity of possible harm. Daily constancy measurements should indicate that beam symmetry is constant to within 3%. If beam symmetry on a particular day is outside baseline by, say, 15%, patient treatments should not start until the asymmetry is corrected. On the other hand, if the measured value is different from baseline by 4% (only 1% outside tolerance), one could argue that patient treatments should continue and that corrective actions could be postponed until the end of the treatment day. The decision depends on many factors, such as the types of treatments that day and the past history of symmetry deviations. Lastly, it is important that a comprehensive set of measurements be obtained before taking action on the basis of any single measurement.

QA should be reflected in the patient's chart through continuity of process. When auditing a chart, the person performing the audit should be able to trace the treatment delivered through all aspects of the QA program. For example, there should be continuity among the monitor units (MUs) delivered, the dose determined from the treatment plan, QA of the planning system, and QA of the treatment machine.

Physics instrumentation

Instruments used to perform QA procedures should be incorporated into a comprehensive QA program. Clearly, the reliability of major pieces of radiation therapy equipment cannot be demonstrated satisfactorily with instruments of questionable

Table 19-1 Quality assurance procedures for physics instrumentation.

Measurement Equipment	Procedure	Frequency	Comments
Calibration Equipment			
Ionization chamber and electrometer (local standard)	ADCL calibration	Biennially	Should include a measurement of linearity (within 0.5%) and venting
All ionization chambers and electrometers used clinically	Inter-comparison	Semiannually	With a radioactive source or another instrument
Scanning Equipment			
Detectors	Linearity	Annually	Document and apply correction
	Stem effect	Annually	Document and apply correction
	Leakage current	Initial use	Document and apply correction
	Short-term stability	Initial use	Document and apply correction
	Energy dependence	Initial use	For diode detectors only
Positioner	Accuracy and reproducibility	At each use	
Dosimetry Accessories			
Solid phantom materials	Inspect for damage	At each use	Pay particular attention to development of voids or cracks, or damage to recess for detector
Thermometer (mercury in glass)	Inter-comparison with calibrated standard	Initial use	Less than 0.1 °C error
Thermometer (electronic)	Inter-comparison with calibrated standard	Monthly	Less than 0.5 °C error
Barometer (aneroid or electronic)	Inter-comparison with calibrated standard	Monthly	Less than 2 mmHg error
Linear rule	Inter-comparison with calibrated standard	Initial use	0.3%
Miscellaneous Dosimetry Devices			
TLD system	Calibration	At each use	Document and apply correction
	Linearity	Initial use	Document and apply correction
Film	Dose response	Initial use	Test each box of film, for each modality and energy including the response of associated equipment

reliability. QA procedures should address not only ionization chambers used for calibrations but also instruments used for determining other beam characteristics, such as water phantom scanning systems, film scanners, diodes, and thermoluminescent dosimeters (TLDs). Ancillary devices such as thermometers and barometers should also be incorporated into the QA program. This section offers advice on procedures and frequencies for the QA of these devices. The recommendations are summarized in Table 19-1.

Ionization chambers and electrometers

Under normal conditions, the instruments used for calibration of therapy equipment are very stable.[5] Unless careful QA procedures are followed, a change in response might not be detected. The Nuclear Regulatory Commission (NRC) and several states require that instruments used to calibrate treatment units (i.e., ionization chamber and electrometer) must themselves be calibrated at intervals of no more than 2 years by a dosimetry laboratory that has been accredited by the American Association of Physicists in Medicine (AAPM). These *accredited dosimetry calibration laboratories* (ADCLs) have been established to transfer calibration factors from instruments calibrated by the National Institute for Standards and Technology (NIST) to a customer's instrument. The ADCLs are supervised by the AAPM,

to which they provide frequent reports of their workload and experiences, and by which they are inspected on a regular basis.[6,7] Through the use of carefully designed equipment and well-defined procedures, the ADCLs are able to assign a calibration factor to a customer's instrument with only a slight increase in the uncertainty associated with national standards maintained at NIST.[3] The calibration factor for an ionization chamber is determined by its geometry, collecting volume, and composition and is required for a chamber to be used for absolute calibration of a radiation beam (i.e., following AAPM Task Group 51 or equivalent calibration document).[8]

Biennial ADCL calibrations of ionization chambers and electrometers should not be substituted for regular QA procedures. An instrument submitted for calibration, called the *local standard*, cannot be assumed to maintain its calibration factor throughout the two-year interval. Instead, twice-yearly inter-comparisons with another instrument or an isotope source are recommended between ADCL calibrations. For the same measurement conditions, the signal detected in two similar chambers (i.e., same model number) should be equal to the ratio of their calibration values. Inter-comparisons also should be performed before and after an instrument is sent to an ADCL to reveal damage sustained during shipping. An ideal redundant system can be assembled from two ionization chamber/electrometer systems and an isotope source.[7] An institution should make available a second ionization chamber and electrometer, as well as some type of isotope source (either a ^{60}Co treatment unit or a ^{90}Sr source) to establish this redundant system. An ongoing record should be kept of inter-comparisons of the components of this redundant system so that the behavior of each component can be monitored over time.

Several other performance indicators for ionization chambers and electrometer systems should be evaluated. Before the initial use of each piece of equipment, the *stem effect* should be determined. The stem effect is a measurement of extracameral signal resulting from ionization events occurring in the chamber stem and cable.[9,10] Each ionization chamber should also be tested for losses due to ionic recombination. This measurement should be made for each beam modality and energy for which the ionization chamber is used.

Ideally, each time an ionization chamber and electrometer system is used, a simple capacitance test should be performed as a quick check of the constancy of response of the system. The capacitance check is made by measuring the charge integrated by the electrometer as the chamber bias is applied or removed. The quotient of measured charge over applied collecting potential indicates the capacitance of the chamber and electrometer system. This value should remain constant from one use to the next.

Beam scanning systems

Instruments used to characterize radiation beams are not generally used to calibrate these beams. Instead, they are used to make measurements of relative dose or ionization distributions, and the resulting data are sometimes used for treatment-planning calculations. The detectors associated with these systems need not be calibrated, but tests should be performed to evaluate their reliability and constancy of response over the time interval required to make a full set of measurements. Upon receipt, the detectors should be investigated to verify that, over the course of a day, their response is constant, they remain waterproof, and the leakage current does not change significantly or exceed acceptable values. Scanning mechanisms should be tested to ensure that they move smoothly and reliably and that the detector can be positioned reproducibly. The linearity of positioning and of readout devices should be ensured. Similar procedures should be applied to scanning film densitometers and flatbed scanners.

Beam scanning systems are expected to provide accurate distance measurements, and to respond appropriately in regions of high-dose rate (HDR), low-dose rate (LDR), and high-dose gradients. To remove the effects of linac dose-rate variations, a reference chamber is often used. A setup of a three-dimensional (3D) beam scanning system is shown in Figure 19-1. For the same linear accelerator, the dose profiles and depth dose curves should be the same when measured with two systems. It may be wise to spot-check measured profiles for accuracy using a system other than the primary system employed for collecting data

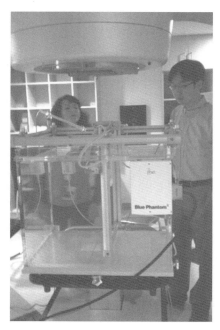

Figure 19-1 Representative beam scanning system. The system consists of a water tank, a computer-controlled positioning system, and radiation detectors. The software driving the computer also displays measurement results and can analyze data with a variety of protocols. Data can often be saved in a format for direct input into the treatment planning system. The water tank is positioned under the treatment beam.

(e.g., film, diode array, another scanner, or point measurements with ion chamber). A sample profile without the reference chamber may be noisy but it will indicate whether the ratio is correctly accounted for, particularly in low-dose regions outside of the field.

Ancillary equipment

Accurate calibration of a treatment unit depends as much on the careful placement of the detector and accurate measurements of environmental conditions as it does on the calibration of the ionization chamber. Devices used to position the calibration instrument in a phantom should be inspected for wear and damage on a regular basis. These devices include rulers, chamber positioning devices, and solid phantom materials. Positioning and scanning equipment should be reproducible to within 1 mm and should report the detector position to within 1 mm accuracy.

Devices for determining environmental conditions should be tested regularly. Thermometers, particularly electronic devices, should be compared with a reference instrument on a regular basis. The frequency of comparison depends on the type of instrument. Electronic devices should be inter-compared at weekly or monthly intervals. Mercury-in-glass thermometers should be inter-compared with a similar instrument before their initial use.

Relative dose measuring equipment

Dosimeters used for measurement of relative dose (e.g., diodes and TLDs) or dose distributions (e.g., film) do not require calibration. However, their performance should be monitored as part of the ongoing QA program. The response of devices such as TLDs and radiographic or radiochromic film should be measured frequently, even at each use, and appropriate corrections applied. Similarly, behavior that can affect the response of these devices, such as the linearity of response, should be evaluated before their initial use, and corrections (if necessary) should be applied when measurements are taken.

Survey meters

Devices used to measure dose levels around patients, such as Geiger–Müller (G-M) counters and survey meters, should be calibrated yearly. This is often a state or NRC requirement, and it is likely that the calibration status of these instruments will be verified during an inspection. If they are battery operated, the batteries must be operational and tested prior to use. A check source is a reliable method for verifying operation of these devices.

Conventional linear accelerators

Conventional linear accelerators are considerably more complex than earlier devices, and they rely increasingly on computer technology. The application of advanced technology may eliminate some sources of error but may introduce other sources, and the risk of injury to the patient must be guarded against.[11] A comprehensive QA program can help to reduce these risks. Recommended procedures and measurement frequencies are summarized in Table 19-2 and Table 19-3. The AAPM Task Group 40 provided early guidance for the necessary QA tests for linear accelerators, ^{60}Co units, and conventional simulators.[12] This Task Group also provided recommendations on overall quality management practices. For linear accelerator QA, the Task Group 40 report has been updated by the AAPM Task Group 142 report.[13] Task Group 142 has recommendations for the expanded functionality of modern linear accelerators, including multileaf collimators (MLCs), dynamic wedges, gating techniques, and imaging systems attached to the linear accelerator.

Safety procedures

At the time of installation of new megavoltage equipment, a complete radiation protection survey should be performed.[14] It is not necessary to repeat the survey unless changes in the equipment, treatment facility, workload, or use of the space surrounding the facility are made. On an annual basis, it is advisable to review the conditions under which the original protection survey was performed and to determine whether the conditions are still applicable. For example, it is not unusual for the workload of a megavoltage treatment unit to change with time. If the present workload exceeds that anticipated at the time of installation, the original protection survey and associated calculations may no longer be valid. At the same time, the use of space around the treatment facility should be reviewed and compared with the conditions at the time of installation. One should be alert not only for changes in construction but also for changes in the use and duration of occupancy of the space as the space adjacent to the therapy room might not be under the control of the therapy clinic. Finally, the review should include an inspection of the physical condition of the facility. Any indication of deterioration in the construction warrants a repeat protection survey. The physical condition of the treatment unit itself should not be overlooked, although a thorough inspection can rarely be accomplished without removing the covers of the equipment. In a few reported instances, sections of shielding in the treatment head of a megavoltage treatment unit that were inadvertently removed during service procedures were not replaced. Should one suspect an event of this type, a leakage survey of the accelerator head should be performed.[14,15] Regions exhibiting high radiation leakage can be identified by closing the collimator jaws and covering the head of the accelerator in radiographic or radiochromic film followed by a long beam-on time. Measurements of leakage from these areas may also be made with a large-volume ionization chamber instrument placed 1 m from the photon beam target in the head of the linear accelerator.

Modern computerized linear accelerators are equipped with software to test many of the interlocks. Simple interlocks that directly affect the safety of the patient or staff should be tested at least daily. An example of this is the door interlock. Other interlocks that are more difficult to test should be checked at longer intervals (e.g., the emergency beam-off linac shutdown and the auxiliary power to the couch should be tested annually). Other items such as the radiation "on" indicator lights should also be checked daily as operational.

It is good practice to have megavoltage treatment rooms equipped with closed-circuit television and audio monitoring systems. This allows the therapists to be in constant contact with the patient while the patient is in the treatment room. These devices should be checked every day for proper operation.

Mechanical alignment

At the time of acceptance testing, mechanical tests are conducted to ensure that the collimator axis of rotation is stable and deviates from intersection with the gantry axis of rotation by no more than a specified small amount. On an annual basis, the deviation of the collimator and gantry axes of rotation should be re-tested with a mechanical device. This is most conveniently done with the mechanical front pointer provided with most linear accelerators (Figure 19-2).

On a monthly basis, this test may be conducted using the crosshairs projected within the light field using graph paper. Again, the center of the crosshairs should not wander outside a

Table 19-2 Frequency of quality assurance procedures and recommended tolerances for megavoltage treatment units.

Procedure	Annually	Monthly	Daily
Safety Procedures			
Protection survey	Limited survey	Watch for signs of deterioration and use of adjacent space	—
Test of interlocks and patient audio/visual monitoring systems	Check for proper operation	Check for proper operation	Check for proper operation
Mechanical Alignment			
Collimator isocenter	1 mm radius circle–use mechanical pointer	1 mm radius circle–use light field/crosshairs	—
Jaws parallel and orthogonal, symmetrical about collimator axis	Parallel 0.5°, orthogonal 0.5°, symmetrical about collimator axis ±2 mm	—	—
Light field versus jaw position indicators	±2 mm each jaw, 2 mm overall for field sizes 5×5 to 20×20 and 1% overall for fields >20×20	Meet specifications of annual test at selected field sizes	±2 mm overall in a single field size. Central axis indicator ±2 mm from center of light field at one field size
Collimator angle indicator	±1° mechanical,±0.5 digital over full range of motion	±1° mechanical, ±0.5° digital at selected angles	—
Gantry isocenter	1 mm radius sphere	—	—
Gantry angle indicator	1°mechanical, ±0.5°digital over full range of motion	±1° mechanical, ±0.5° digital at selected angles	—
Couch isocenter	1 mm radius circle	—	—
Couch angle	±1° mechanical, ±0.5° digital over full range of motion	±1° mechanical, ±0.5° digital at selected angles	—
Couch position indicators	2 mm	±2 mm	Couch height 2 mm
Couch top sag	2 mm	—	—
Range light	±1 mm at isocenter, ±5 mm elsewhere	±1 mm at isocenter, ±5 mm elsewhere	±2 mm at isocenter
Localizing laser	±1 mm	±1 mm	±2 mm
Beam Alignment Tests			
Light versus radiation field congruence	±2 mm each jaw, ±2 mm overall for field sizes 5×5 to 20×20, ±1% overall for fields >20×20	Meet specifications of annual test at selected field sizes	—
Collimator rotation	1 mm radius circle	—	—
Gantry rotation	1 mm radius circle	—	—
Couch rotation	1 mm radius circle	—	—
Calibration			
Output calibration	±2% (dose to water)	±2% (constancy check)	±3% (constancy check)
Monitor chamber linearity	≤1%	—	—
Output variation with gantry angle	≤1% at selected angles	—	—
Photon Beam Characterization			
Field size dependence of output	±2% constancy over full range of field sizes	±2% constancy at selected field	—
Percent depth dose (or tissue-maximum ratio)	±2% constancy over full range of depths and field sizes	±2% constancy at selected depths and field sizes	—
Beam flatness	±3% over central 80% of fields up to 30×30 cm at 10 cm depth, for selected gantry angles	±2% constancy in selected field sizes	—
Beam symmetry	≤2% difference between points equidistant from the beam axis for selected gantry angles	±2% constancy in selected field sizes	±3% constancy in a single field size
Transmission factor of wedge filters and treatment accessories	2% constancy over applicable range of field sizes	2% constancy at a single field size, or check of alignment	—
Electron Beam Characterization			
Dependence of output on applicator size	±2% constancy over full range of applicator sizes	—	—
Percent depth dose	±2% constancy over full range of depths and applicator sizes (2 mm in region of steep dose gradient)	±2 mm constancy with selected applicator size in region of steep dose gradient	—
Beam flatness	±3% over central 80% of fields up to 30×30 cm at 10 cm depth, for selected gantry angles	±2% constancy in selected field sizes	—
Beam symmetry	±2% difference between points equidistant from the beam axis	±2% constancy in selected field sizes	±3% constancy in a single field size

Table 19-3 Multileaf collimator quality assurance.

Frequency	Test	Tolerance
Patient specific	Check of MLC-generated field versus simulator film or digitally reconstructed radiograph (DDR) before each field is treated	2 mm
	Double-check MLC field by therapists for each fraction	Expected field
	Online imaging verification for patient on each fraction	Physician discretion
	Port film approval before second fraction	Physician discretion
Weekly	Qualitative picket fence test	Visual inspection for any changes in transmission or misalignment of picket fence
Monthly	Setting versus light field versus radiation field for two designated patterns	2 mm
	Quantitative picket fence test (at cardinal gantry angles)	1 mm leaf positions in pickets
	Check of interlocks	All must be operational
Annually	Setting versus light versus radiation field for patterns over range of gantry and collimator angles	2 mm
	Leaf position repeatability	1 mm
	Film/EPID scans to evaluate interleaf leakage and abutted leaf transmission	50% radiation edge within 1 mm
	MLC spoke shot	Interleaf leakage <3%, abutted leakage <25%
	IMRT patterns (step-and-shoot, moving window)	1 mm radius
	Review of procedures and in-service with therapists	<0.35 cm max error RMS
		95% of error counts <0.35 cm
		All operators must fully understand operation and procedures

circle of 1 mm radius during rotation of the collimator. Similarly, the collimator jaws should be parallel, orthogonal, and symmetrical about the collimator axis, and this can be verified using graph paper.

With most conventional megavoltage therapy units, the dimensions of the radiation field are indicated by a light field projected through the collimator jaws by a light source mounted inside the collimator. The digital display of the field size should agree with the dimensions of the light field within 2 mm.

The accuracy of the angle indicator can easily be assessed by rotating the gantry of the accelerator to the horizontal position and positioning a digital level against either the collimator jaw or a machined surface that is parallel to one of the jaws. Once each year, the accuracy of the angle indicator should be tested over the full range of collimator rotational motion. Monthly tests of accuracy should be made at a few selected angles.

The gantry isocenter is the axis of rotation of the gantry. Ideally, this is a point, but due to limitations on mechanical precision it has a wobble and transcribes a small circle. Determining this circle to quantify the variation of the gantry axis of rotation is achieved using mechanical methods. The mechanical pointer can be used to demonstrate the isocenter variation. For reference, a metal pointer such as a small-diameter drill bit should be taped to the treatment couch and raised to the approximate location of the isocenter. The collimator pointer should be extended until it almost touches the couch pointer. The gantry should be rotated throughout its entire range of motion while observing the variation in position of the tip of the collimator pointer (see Figure 19-2). If necessary, the length of the collimator pointer should be adjusted to reduce the motion of the tip to a minimum. Variations both within and perpendicular to the gantry plane of rotation should be observed. The motion of the tip of the pointer should be confined within a sphere of 1 mm radius. The center of this sphere is considered the isocenter. This test should be repeated annually.

Digital angle indicators should be accurate to within 0.5°, while mechanical scales should be accurate to within 1°. The

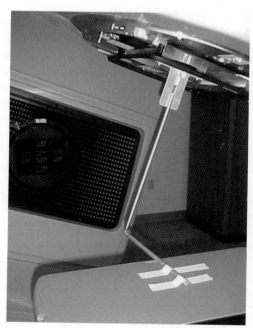

Figure 19-2 The use of mechanical pointers to measure the stability of rotation of the collimator, the gantry, and the patient treatment couch.

accuracy should be tested annually over the full range of motion, and monthly at selected angles.

The stability of the couch axis of rotation is most conveniently tested with the pointers previously positioned for the gantry and collimator isocenter tests. The collimator pointer should be adjusted so that it indicates the center of the sphere containing the gantry isocenter. The couch should be rotated through its complete range of motion while observing the movement of the pointer attached to the couch top (see Figure 19-2). The tip of the couch pointer should describe a circle of radius no more than 1 mm. This test should be performed annually.

Digital scales for the treatment couch should be accurate to within 0.5° and mechanical scales should be accurate to within 1°. The couch angle indicators should be tested over their full range once each year and at selected angles every month.

Almost all treatment couches for conventional linear accelerators are of a cantilevered design. Consequently, the extension of the couch top combined with the patient's weight causes the table top to sag slightly. Therapists often set patients up using the table top, for which the distance from the surface of the table to the laser line is measured using a ruler. If the table is not level, the table-top values will be different from one side to the other. A measurement of the couch top sag is made by extending the couch fully toward the gantry and by raising the couch top to the level of the isocenter. A small amount of weight, such as 10 kg (22 lb), should be placed at the gantry end of the couch top. The position of the couch top relative to a point of reference should be noted. The alignment lasers or the collimator front pointer can be used for this purpose. Additional weight should then be added to the couch top to simulate the distributed weight of a 75 kg (170 lb) patient. It is acceptable to add 25 kg (55 lb) to the gantry end of the couch for this purpose. The displacement of the couch top relative to the reference point should be noted. The displacement should not exceed 2 mm. This test should be performed once each year.

Longitudinal, vertical, and lateral couch position indicators should be accurate to within 2 mm. The accuracy of the indicators should be tested over their full range each year and at selected positions every month. A test of couch height indicator accuracy should be performed on a daily basis at one location.

The *optical distance indicator* (ODI) is one of several valuable aids for ensuring correct patient positioning. Its accuracy should be determined by comparison with a mechanical front pointer, or by measurements made from a reference point on the collimator. The design of most optical indicators permits the greatest accuracy at the position of the isocenter; at this location the optical distance indicator should be accurate to within 1 mm. At other distances, an error of ±3 mm is acceptable. Optical indicators may lose accuracy with time and should be tested over their full range on an annual as well as monthly basis. A daily test of accuracy at the level of the isocenter should be performed. The ODI should be most accurate over the range of common use. For most clinical situations with 100 cm source–axis distance (SAD) linear accelerators, this range is 80–120 cm.

The localizing laser lights indicate the isocenter of the linear accelerator and are used to position the patient under the treatment beam. Checking the localizing laser lights is done with the front pointer still in place from previous tests. The alignment of the localizing lasers with the isocenter can be observed to intersect with the front pointer. The position of the laser should be within 1 mm of the isocenter. The therapists often perform patient setup using the lasers at 30 cm or more from the isocenter. Thus, the accuracy of alignment lasers over the range of use must be verified. A detailed test of the lasers should be performed monthly. On a daily basis, a simpler test can be performed to confirm that the laser alignment is within 2 mm of the isocenter.

Beam alignment tests

On conventional linear accelerators, the dimensions of the radiation field are indicated by a light field projected through the collimator by a light source mounted inside the collimator. The light source may be positioned at the location of the x-ray target by a rotating carousel or a sliding drawer assembly, or it may be positioned to one side of the collimator axis of rotation, with the light reflected from a mirror. In either case, the location of the light source must agree with the actual or virtual location of the radiation source. The agreement of the light field with the radiation field can most easily be verified through the use of film or other device such as an electronic portal imaging device. The light field should agree with the radiation field to within 2 mm along each edge. In addition, the overall dimensions of the light field should agree with the dimensions of the radiation field to within 2 mm for field sizes up to 20 cm × 20 cm, and to within 1% of the field dimension for fields larger than 20 cm × 20 cm.

At the same time, the agreement between the radiation field and the collimator size indicators should be checked. The specifications indicated above should apply to the agreement between the field size indicators and the radiation field size. Otherwise, errors between the field size indicators, the light field size, and the radiation field size could accumulate to unacceptable levels. The test of light field and radiation field congruence should be performed annually over the full range of field sizes and monthly at selected field sizes. Projection of the light field is sensitive to the position of the transmission mirror within some linear accelerators. If the mirror is replaced or if it is moved while repairs take place, it is important to verify the light/radiation field alignment immediately.

The mechanical test described earlier ensures that the collimator axis of rotation is stable. However, it does not ensure that the radiation beam also rotates about the same axis. Failure of the radiation beam and mechanical axes of rotation to coincide may indicate that the radiation source is not positioned properly on the collimator axis of rotation. A test of collimator rotation stability is easily performed by positioning the treatment couch top at the isocenter and taping a film to the couch top. One pair of collimator jaws should be opened to a moderate size (say,

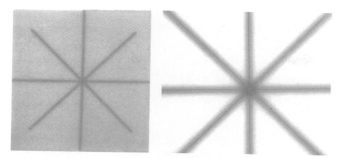

Figure 19-3 A spoke film indicating good stability of collimator rotation. The image on the right is zoomed in on the center of the image on the left. *Source:* Courtesy of Rich Goodman, Waukesha Memorial Hospital.

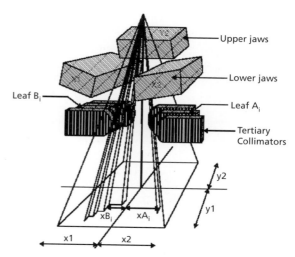

Figure 19-4 Generic configuration for multileaf tertiary collimators. This figure shows double-focused leaves in addition to primary collimation jaws X and Y. Note jaw Y2 is not shown, for clarity. *Source:* AAPM Report No. 72, 2001.[16]

15 cm), while the other pair should be closed to the minimum achievable symmetrical position. Several exposures should then be made on a single film, with the collimator rotated between exposures. The collimator angle should be chosen so that exposures do not overlap one another. Exposures should be made throughout the entire range of collimator motion; making five or six exposures usually yields an adequate test. After processing, the film should exhibit a pattern reminiscent of the spokes of a wheel (Figure 19-3). If the spokes are more than 1–2 mm wide, a pencil line should be drawn carefully down the center of each spoke. Ideally, the spokes should all intersect at a single point. In most circumstances, the spokes will pass within a short distance of a point representing the collimator axis of rotation. The spokes should all fall within 1 mm of the collimator axis of rotation, indicating a circle of radius of no more than 1 mm. The test should then be repeated with the jaw positions reversed. This test should be repeated annually. A similar test is done for the treatment couch where the collimator position is fixed, and the couch is rotated between exposures. Variation in the position of the spokes on the developed film indicates the variation in rotation of the couch axis.

A spoke image of gantry rotation can be generated by positioning a film upright on the table top so that it is perpendicular to the gantry axis of rotation. The collimator jaws whose edges are parallel to the gantry axis of rotation are closed to their minimum symmetrical setting, while the opposite jaws are opened to an intermediate size. Exposures are made with the gantry at several different angles, with care taken to avoid overlapping exposures. For this test, it is important that the film be located exactly in the plane described by the beam central axis as the gantry is rotated. In addition, it is important that the collimator be rotated so that the edges of the jaws closed to minimum setting be exactly parallel to the gantry axis of rotation. The film is evaluated as before. The spokes should all pass within 1 mm of the gantry axis of rotation. This test should be repeated annually.

Multileaf collimator quality assurance

Most modern linear accelerators incorporate tertiary field-shaping in the form of MLCs in their design. In many treatment applications, MLCs eliminate the need for customized blocking and are able to conform to relatively complex shapes. Several configurations are available, depending on the manufacturer, as either intrinsic to the treatment device or as an add-on accessory. A sample configuration is shown in Figure 19-4 to illustrate a possible mechanical arrangement. As mechanical devices, the radiation properties of MLCs in treatment delivery are largely dependent on their physical design.

The original intent of the MLC was to provide an outer field boundary to eliminate the hazards and tedious work of creating custom blocks. With the delivery of intensity modulated radiation therapy (IMRT) using MLCs, their physical characteristics are now integral to therapeutic dose delivery. Now a more thorough understanding of the design of MLCs is required for treatment planning and QA. For example, whether the path of the radiation follows beam divergence or is linear creates differing penumbra effects.

Some basic properties of MLCs are presented in this text. For more information, one may refer to the manufacturer's documentation. Developing a QA program for MLCs should be consistent with the institution's program for treatment delivery.[16] Initial tests should characterize the mechanical and radiation properties, whereas components for daily, monthly, and annual tests generally involve ensuring proper operation and monitoring for any changes. Some of the important tests and characteristics of MLCs include leaf calibration, leaf transmission, inter-leaf leakage, light field versus radiation field congruence, the tongue-and-groove effect, and stability with gantry and collimator rotation. The components of leaf transmission, inter-leaf leakage, and the tongue-and-groove effect are shown in Figure 19-5.

The effects of gravity on leaf operation should be investigated by testing patterns over a variety of gantry and collimator angles. This is typically done using a *picket fence test*. This test

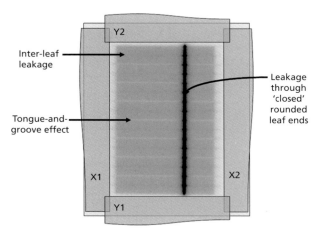

Figure 19-5 Effect of different components of multileaf collimators, including inter-leaf leakage, tongue-and-groove effect, and leakage.

consist of several (5–10) MLC leaf movements so that all the leaves move together in a straight line with a small opening of 1–2 cm between the leaf banks. Film or an electronic portal imaging device (EPID) is irradiated, and the resulting image resembles a picket fence. This test is useful to identify any leaves that are not moving together with the others. A summary of recommended tests and frequency adapted from the AAPM Task Groups 50 and 142 reports is shown in Table 19-3.

Beam calibration

The AAPM Task Group 51 document recommends that the monitor chamber indicate dose to water at the depth of maximum dose in a 10 cm × 10 cm field, with the phantom surface positioned at the normal treatment distance (usually 100 cm).[8] However, the measurement used to determine dose is obtained at another depth, such as 10 cm. Once each year, the accuracy of the output monitoring system should be determined from fundamental measurements. Accuracy to within 2% is required. On a monthly basis, a constancy check of output should be performed using the local standard measurement equipment rather than the ADCL-calibrated equipment. This check may be performed using a solid phantom for ease of setup. The measurement should be constant to within 2% from one month to the next. A daily measurement of output constancy should be also made. Commercial devices are available for such tests and these are designed to facilitate the measurement, as well as to perform several other routine QA measurements such as beam flatness and symmetry (Figure 19-6). The daily constancy check should be reproducible to within 3%. Lastly, the output should be verified annually by an independent measurement from outside the institution. This is typically done using TLDs or optically stimulated luminescent dosimeters that are mailed to the institution and then mailed back to determine the absolute dose.

Monitor output calibration is generally performed at a single representative MU setting, such as 100 MU. Because patient

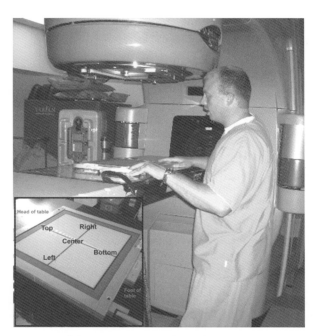

Figure 19-6 Daily beam measurements that readily measure beam output, flatness, and symmetry. The inset shows a beam's-eye-view and orientation of the device.

treatments may involve the delivery of MU settings over a wide range, the linearity of the monitor system must be verified. Readings with an ionization chamber may be made at a number of different MU settings, and the output is graphed as a function of MU setting. A straight line fit to the data should fall within 1% of all the data points and pass within 1% of the origin.

Output calibration measurements are most often made with the beam oriented in the vertical-downward position. Many treatments, however, are delivered with the gantry at other angles, and it is essential that the output not vary significantly as the gantry is rotated. The output calibration test is not easily performed with a water phantom at other gantry angles, but a solid phantom or even a suitable buildup cap may be used to measure the radiation output for other gantry angles. It is important only to ensure that the ionization chamber is located at the same distance from the source for each measurement. The variation with gantry angle should not exceed 1%. The variation should be measured once each year.

Photon beam characterization

Measurements at representative field sizes should be made annually to confirm that output dependence has not changed by more than 2% from original measurements. Changes of more than 2% indicate that data used for treatment planning calculations may require revision. The constancy of the beam energy should be checked, to ensure both consistent operation of the treatment unit and that the data in use for treatment planning calculations remain valid. Percent depth dose should be checked annually at a large number of depths and field sizes to verify that the data remain within 2% of the original measurements. Once a month, a limited set of such measurements should be made.

Beam flatness as measured in water phantom should be repeated annually, again not only to ensure proper operation of the treatment unit but also to verify that the data in use for treatment planning remain valid. Beam flatness is specified at 10 cm depth in water or water equivalent material, at field sizes up to at least 30 cm × 30 cm. Over the central 80% of the field width along the major axis of the field, the maximum and minimum dose values should be determined. The difference between these values divided by their sum should not be more than ±3% of the mean. At monthly intervals, measurements should be made to ensure constancy of beam flatness. These measurements may be made in one or a few field sizes and should demonstrate that the flatness remains constant to within 2%. Beam flatness is largely a physical parameter determined by the flattening filter used and not readily adjustable. Symmetry, on the other hand, can be controlled by beam steering and needs to be monitored to make sure the beam has not drifted from baseline.

Acceptance and commissioning testing procedures generally include measurements of beam symmetry at which time baseline values are acquired. An accepted procedure for measuring and describing beam symmetry consists of measuring the beam profile at the depth of maximum dose and examining the dose at points equidistant from the central axis. Corresponding points on each side of the central axis should not vary by more than 2% of the central axis value.

Beam symmetry can be altered by a change in the position of the flattening filter as well as by electrical changes in the operation of the treatment unit. Such asymmetries can introduce distortions into the dose distribution throughout a patient's target volume.

Monthly spot checks of beam symmetry constancy should be made to verify continued agreement with initial commissioning measurements. Daily or weekly measurements of beam symmetry should also be made. Several commercially available devices that permit making such measurements with minimal effort are available (e.g., Figure 19-6). Daily QA should indicate constancy of the beam symmetry to within 3% of baseline. Measurements should be made in large, medium, and small field sizes, as well as at representative gantry angles on an annual basis.

Treatment accessories such as blocking trays and wedge filters are unlikely to change in ways that would affect the transmission of radiation through them. A transmission factor is measured using an ionization chamber by taking the ratio of the device in place and a reading for the corresponding open field. However, periodic measurements of the transmission factors of these devices are important because they can expose two important sources of error. First, devices such as blocking trays are subject to wear and breakage, and they must periodically be replaced. Blocking trays have on occasion unintentionally been replaced with trays having a different thickness or having been made from different material, so that the transmission factor in

use is no longer applicable. Second, removable "hard" wedge filters are mounted on trays that can occasionally become damaged; this necessitates their replacement, possibly with a tray having different transmission characteristics. In addition, damage to the wedge tray can result in a misalignment of the wedge. A measurement of the wedge transmission factor is often the most straightforward way to uncover such misalignment. Annually, measurements should be made of wedge and tray transmission factors in selected field sizes covering the applicable range. Constancy to within 2% of measurements made at the time of commissioning should be demonstrated. Measurements of hard wedge factors are done by averaging the readings at two opposing wedge orientations. This approach is used to account for any perceptibly small misalignment of the wedge about the central axis of the radiation beam. Wedges and other devices should be inspected monthly to ensure their proper alignment. As indicated previously, a transmission measurement indicating constancy within 2% may be the best way to demonstrate continued alignment.

Unflattened treatment beams are used for patient treatments.[17] These types of beams are created by removing the flattening filter. One benefit of an unflattened beam is that very high output can be achieved without the flattening filter thus speeding up beam delivery during treatment. There are also indications that doses outside the treatment room and doses due to activation of the accelerator are reduced with a flattening-filter-free accelerator.[18] It should be noted that shielding requirements should not be modified based on this without analyzing other radiation shielding aspects such as workload and use factors. The trade-off with these benefits is that one has an unconventional dose distribution for open beams. Figure 19-7 shows the difference of unflattened and conventional flat beams. Unflattened beams should always be used with CT-based treatment planning dose calculations to ensure that appropriate coverage of the target volume and normal tissue sparing is achieved at points away from the central axis of the fields. Dosimetric

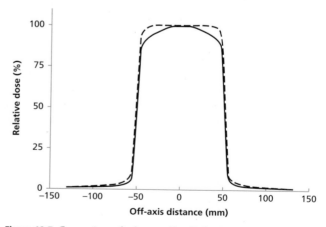

Figure 19-7 Comparison of a dose profile of a flattened and unflattened beam for a 6 MV 10 cm × 10 cm at the depth of maximum dose.

analysis of unflattened beams indicates that such beams have reduced head scatter and lower out-of-field doses compared to flattened beams.[19,20] When measuring dose with open-air ion chambers for unflattened (high-output) beams, the ion collection efficiency can be reduced by about 1% compared to conventional output beams.[21] The usual care must be taken when commissioning and performing QA of unflattened beams.[22] For unflattened beams, all the same QA tests and frequencies apply, with the exception of beam flatness requirements.

Electron beam characterization

As is the case with photon beams, electron beams should be thoroughly characterized at the time of treatment unit commissioning. Electron beam output varies with field size; depending on the design of the collimation system; however, the variation may not be straightforward. Linear accelerators that employ electron applicators, or *cones*, can use different collimator jaw settings to create a useful clinical electron beam for different applicators sizes. Small variations in the setting of the collimator jaws, or minor damage to the electron applicators, might result in a change in the electron beam output. It is recommended that periodic measurements be made of electron beam output as a function of applicator size. The agreement between annual measurements and the original commissioning data should be within 2%.

Percent depth dose is generally the means by which electron beam energy is characterized. It is important that the electron beam characteristics do not vary from the data used in the treatment planning system by more than a small amount. Measurements should be made annually of percent depth dose at a variety of depths and applicator sizes. Agreement with original measurements should be within 2% in regions of low-dose gradient and within 2 mm in regions of high-dose gradient as a method to check electron beam energy constancy. Recall that dose is a derived quantity related to the energy of electrons crossing the cavity of an ionization chamber. Dose is not simply equal to a reading of charge for a given irradiation. For electron beams, the electron energy changes significantly with depth in the phantom, and different factors (e.g., stopping power ratios) must be applied for different depths to convert a charge reading to dose. However, relative charge readings may be used for constancy checks. Monthly relative ionization measurements should be acquired at a point corresponding to the depth of maximum dose, as well as at a second point located in the region of steep dose gradient. The relative reading at the deeper point should be compared with the original depth-ionization data to ensure that the curve has not shifted by more than 2 mm. This test is easily conducted by use of a parallel plate ionization chamber in a solid phantom, but other techniques are acceptable. Electron beam energy checks should be combined with the monthly checks of output calibration.

Electron beam flatness should meet the same specification as does photon beam flatness, with the exception that

measurements are made at the depth of maximum dose. Annual measurements should be made to ensure that the beam flatness continues to meet the original specifications, in a range of field sizes and throughout the range of gantry angles. Monthly, the constancy of beam flatness should be tested in selected field sizes. This measurement might easily be made by exposing a film at the depth of maximum dose in a solid phantom, or by moving an ionization chamber off the central axis of the beam to representative locations. Commercially available devices discussed earlier may also be used. Constancy within 2% of the original measurements should be demonstrated.

As with photon beams, several procedures for determining electron beam symmetry have been suggested, including the procedure described above for photon beams. The ionization at representative points equidistant from the beam's central axis can be used. The difference in readings at these points should be less than 2% of the average reading. Complete measurements of beam symmetry for a variety of field sizes and gantry angles should be done annually. The constancy of beam symmetry should be checked monthly to ensure less than 2% variation from measurements obtained at the time of commissioning. This test can easily be combined with the previous measurement of beam flatness. A verification of the constancy of beam symmetry should also be made on a daily or weekly basis, with an instrument sufficiently reliable to indicate constancy to within 3% of the original commissioning measurements. These tests should be designed to ensure that the measurements are made at or near the depth of maximum dose.

In-room image-guidance quality assurance

Safety procedures

The x-ray tube used with a linear accelerator is regarded as a diagnostic x-ray device; therefore it must meet the same standards as those of conventional diagnostic x-ray equipment. A measurement of tube leakage radiation should be made annually to ensure that the ICRP recommendation of 0.1 R/hr at 1 m is not exceeded. The measurement is to be made at the highest-rated kVp setting for the x-ray tube, as well as with the largest mA permitted for continuous operation. Because the x-ray tube is used in a room for megavoltage x-rays, the shielding is always acceptable if deemed acceptable for the therapy x-ray beam. Interlocks intended to halt the motion of the equipment if a collision is detected should also be tested at regular intervals.

X-ray beam performance

Specific recommendations for imaging systems on linear accelerators can be found in table 6 of the AAPM Task Group 142 document.[13] Measurements should be made of several parameters that indicate x-ray beam performance.

Half-value layer (HVL; i.e., beam energy) measurements should be performed at least annually. The measurement of the

HVL is straightforward; it can be made with the equipment frequently found in a radiation oncology department. An ionization chamber with a flat energy response in the diagnostic range should be used. Exposure measurements should be made under easily reproduced conditions, with all removable graticules and trays removed from the beam. Aluminum filters are added until the exposure is reduced to half the original value. From a graph on semi-logarithmic paper, the beam HVL can be determined. Reproducible measurements of HVL ensure that both the x-ray beam and the x-ray generator are stable.

While not specifically included in the AAPM Task Group 142 document, several other parameters are worth checking.[13] These include kVp accuracy, in which a noninvasive test device can be used to determine the effective kVp of the x-ray beam. This value should be compared with the kVp selected at the operator's control panel and the measured kVp should not disagree with the selected kVp by more than 5 kVp. The mA linearity should be checked so that as the x-ray tube current increases the exposure rate should increase proportionally. Measurements should be made periodically of the exposure for several different mA settings. During these measurements, the kVp and timer settings should be kept constant. When plotted on graph paper, the radiation exposure as a function of mA setting should fall on a straight line that passes through the origin. The mA's linearity also needs to be checked. Measurements of radiation exposure should be made as the mA's is changed, for constant settings of kVp. Checking the automatic exposure control (a *phototimer* that can turn off the x-ray beam when a predetermined radiation exposure has been reached) is appropriate and can be done using Lucite phantoms of several different thicknesses with a different-size phantom for each exposure. Exposures should be made at kVp settings that span the range commonly used in clinical practice. Films or an EPID device (see next section) should all indicate approximately the same optical density. Significant variations among the films indicate that the phototimer is not properly terminating the beam.

The *spatial resolution* can be evaluated with a line pair test tool. Several types of test tools are available; any tool that provides a high-contrast pattern with variable spacing can be used. A measurement of *contrast resolution* should also be made.[23] In addition, tests related to sensitivity, modulation transfer function (MTF), noise power spectra (NPS), and detective quantum efficiency (DQE) have been performed.[24] With the adoption of new digital imaging techniques, concepts familiar to diagnostic radiological physicists become integral to QA in radiation therapy. The tests of imaging characteristics should ensure that the equipment performs its intended function (i.e., the equipment produces comparable or better portal images). The AAPM Task Group 142 table 6 gives the specific recommendations of these systems.[13]

Modulation transfer function (MTF) is a measure of how well information presented to the imaging system in the form of a sine wave is represented in the image. As the frequency of the sine wave increases, the ability of the system to represent the information in the image decreases. *Detective quantum efficiency* (DQE) is a measure of the detection efficiency that includes the effects of noise. It may be defined as the ratio of the signal-to-noise at the output of the system to the signal-to-noise at the input of the system.

Quality assurance procedures for conventional simulators

With the widespread use of CT scanners in radiation oncology departments and virtual simulation software, conventional simulators are becoming less common. Their mechanical specifications are similar, if not identical, to those of megavoltage units. Consequently, they are subject to comparable QA procedures. Advice regarding simulator QA procedures is available from several sources.[12,24,25]

CT simulator quality assurance

Simulation of patients using computed tomography is commonplace in many centers. Features of these systems, such as moving lasers (either wall-mounted or internal CT lasers), must be evaluated with a quality assurance program to ensure accuracy in patient alignment. In addition, differences in geometry between the CT scanner and the treatment unit must be correctly accounted for. For example, in cases where the patient is scanned feet first but treated head first, the transformation of patient data in treatment planning is critical. For centers that have a dedicated CT simulator in radiation oncology, routine image quality evaluation will likely be the responsibility of the radiation oncology physicist. Changes in Hounsfield units (CT numbers) may affect image quality slightly, but could affect dose calculation accuracy. CT simulator QA not only includes the scanner but also the virtual simulation software and procedures. The QA for CT Simulator systems is specified in AAPM Task Group 66.[26] An example list of CT simulator tests is provided in Table 19-4.

Lasers

To identify the reference point on the CT images, small fiducials (bb's) are often used. This approach eliminates reliance on the laser localizing lights of the CT scanner, other than perhaps to level the patient. When CT simulation is performed, an accurate laser marking system is required. One complicating factor is any physical shift between the wall laser isocenter and the isocenter of the CT gantry. In addition, the CT scanner internal laser localizers need to be accurate if used, and the wall lasers may in fact be "movable" to assist in marking the patient. To verify that the laser isocenter matches the CT isocenter, a phantom is used that is first aligned to the lasers using crosshairs with corresponding fiducials, then the phantom is shifted to the gantry isocenter using the couch and a known shift increment (Figure 19-8). A

Table 19-4 CT simulator daily, monthly, and annual QA tests.

	Item Tested	Description
Daily	Lasers	Verify isocenter location on wall lasers and correct transformation to CT coordinates
	Tube warmup	CT simulator in radiation oncology often not used continually as in radiology. May require warmup prior to patient scanning
	Water phantom	Verify CT number of water
	Interlocks	Test scanner interrupt button
	Patient viewing and intercom	Test functionality
Weekly	Detector calibration	Run calibration routine for CT detector ring
	Isocenter shift	For movable lasers, correct translation to new isocenter coordinates
	Couch	Accuracy of travel
Monthly	Lasers	Verify isocenter and transformation of coordinates from CT simulation software
	Density check	Verify density of water, low-density object, and high-density object
	Interlocks	Test safety interlocks and interrupt
	Slice thickness	Verify slice thickness using phantom
	Table increment	Verify table increment by scanning object of known length
Annual	Resolution	Check high- and low-contrast resolution. Check spatial resolution
	Tube parameters	Measure kVp and mAs
	CT density table	Verify computed tomography to density table or graph over full range of densities encountered
	Exposure rate	Check exposure rates for commonly used scanning configurations

single scan at this point should have the fiducial markers intersecting the gantry isocenter. For movable lasers, positioning should be accurate to within ±2 mm. This can be verified using a ruler or graph paper positioned on the treatment couch.

CT couch

Key parameters in CT imaging studies include slice thickness and table increment. For diagnostic studies, slight inaccuracies in table increment may not affect diagnosis. For radiation therapy, however, an inaccurate table increment will produce a false data set, notably in the superior/inferior direction. The result is incorrect tumor volumes, beam blocking, jaw positions, and DDRs. Patient anatomy on portal films will not match, even though the isocenter may be exact. Accurate couch positioning and calibration is important and must be verified for axial and helical modes. Since the flat couch top is often removable to allow conventional CT scanning using a rounded table top, a check is required to ensure that the flat couch top is level when

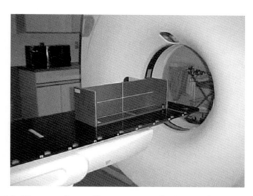

Figure 19-8 Phantom for quality assurance of a CT simulator.

reinstalled. Finally, couch sag should be evaluated, particularly when the couch is extended far into the gantry (e.g., scanning a prostate patient head first). Progressive couch sag on the images will appear as a slight table angle when viewed in a sagittal plane.

Image orientation

The correct translation of imaging coordinates to treatment coordinates is critical. Since axial images are often symmetric, an incorrect transformation of coordinates may not be apparent. One simple solution to this problem is to create a known asymmetric geometry by placing a wire on one side of the treatment couch. This marker should always be on the same side of the image set, regardless of patient position. To evaluate correct transformation of patient position, a cube with imageable markers (A, anterior; P, posterior; L, left; R, right; S, superior; I, inferior) can be scanned in various treatment positions (Figure 19-9).

Image quality

Any deterioration in the images will adversely affect the ability to delineate the structures in the process of contouring tissues for treatment planning. Use of a standard CT phantom to test variables such as spatial resolution, low contrast resolution, slice positioning, and spatial accuracy can accomplish this task.

Computed tomography to density table

Correct mapping of Hounsfield numbers to electron densities (relative to that of water) contributes to accurate treatment planning calculations. By scanning a phantom of known densities, a table or graph can be generated for the treatment planning computer (Figure 19-10). Care must be taken to scan objects that

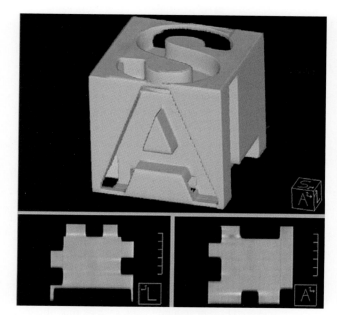

Figure 19-9 Reconstruction of an orientation phantom to verify proper patient position in the treatment planning system.

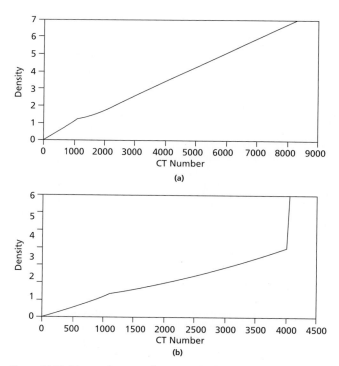

Figure 19-10 Measured computed tomography to density graphs for a treatment planning system. For this system, the pixel values became saturated at a value of 4096 and data were extrapolated to a density of 7. In part (b), it is assumed that any pixel values that are saturated most likely reflect the presence of a metal prosthesis, and a density of 6 is used as an estimation of the object's density.

adequately represent the range of densities encountered within the body, including high-density objects such as dense bone or a hip prosthesis. One should avoid objects that have an unnaturally high atomic number since the photoelectric effect in these objects will inflate the observed CT number. A standard commercial phantom can be used for this analysis.

Care must be taken when phantom materials in radiation oncology, namely those phantoms intended for megavoltage dose measurement, are imaged on a CT scanner. One must be careful that the phantom properties are correctly accounted for in treatment planning. For example, the physical density and chemical makeup of some phantoms are designed so they are water-equivalent at megavoltage energies. Atomic number and density effects may yield higher or lower CT numbers for these phantoms, and the planning system may interpret these numbers as representing materials different from water for the purpose of dose calculation. One simple solution is to use only phantoms that are truly water-equivalent at megavoltage energies.

Treatment planning computers

Treatment planning computers are widely used in radiation therapy departments. Modern treatment planning systems can generate isodose distributions for multiple rectangular beams, calculate the dose at selected points in irregular fields, and calculate the dose throughout a complete 3D volume, making corrections for the patient contour as well as for the presence of inhomogeneities. Fully 3D treatment planning programs consider the effects of tissue densities throughout the irradiated volume and thus permit the entry of beams whose central axes do not lie in the same plane (*noncoplanar* beams). The MU setting (or treatment time) required to deliver the prescribed dose according to the treatment plan is also determined by these systems.

Because of the complexity of the software, it is virtually impossible to test every conceivable computational situation. Therefore, a QA program for treatment planning computers can only address a finite range of treatment situations, computational requirements, and specific calculations (Table 19-5). It is possible, however, to design a QA program that gives the user confidence that the treatment planning system provides acceptable accuracy over a clinically useful range of situations.[27–29]

Most treatment planning computer systems require the entry of measured beam data. The computer calculates dose distributions for a wide variety of treatment conditions. In this case, it is up to the user to confirm that the computer is able to successfully mimic these situations from the small amount of data provided. The commissioning of a treatment planning system therefore requires the following steps:

1 Understanding, in a broad sense, the treatment planning software algorithms and their dependence on measured data.
2 Collection of appropriate data required by the treatment planning system, and entry of these data.

Table 19-5 QA for treatment planning systems and monitor unit calculations.

Frequency	Test	Tolerance[a]
Commissioning and following software update	Understand algorithm	Functional
	Single field or source isodose distribution	2%[a] or 2 mm[b]
	MU calculations	2%
	Test cases	2% or 2 mm
	I/Q system	1 mm
Daily	I/O devices	1 mm
Monthly	Checksum	No change
	Subset of reference QA test set (when checksums not available)	2% or 2 mm[c]
	I/Q	1 mm
	DRR display	Spatial linearity
	DVH calculation	Accurate volume calculation
Annual	MU calculations	2%
	Reference QA test set	2% or 2 mm[d]
	I/O system	1 mm

[a]Percent difference between calculation of the computer treatment planning system and measurement (or independent calculation).
[b]In the region of high-dose gradients, the distance between isodose lines is more appropriate than percent difference. In addition, less accuracy may be obtained near the end of single sources.
[c]These limits refer to the comparison of dose calculations at commissioning to the same calculations subsequently.
[d]These limits refer to comparison of calculations with measurement in a water tank.
Source: Kutcher et al. AAPM Radiation Therapy Committee Task Group 40, 1994.[12] Reproduced with permission from American Association of Physicists in Medicine.

3 Collection of additional data (a) fully characterizing the beams for which treatment planning will be done and (b) representing a range of clinical situations.
4 Calculation of dose distributions, point doses, and MU or treatment time settings, along with comparison of these calculations with the measured data.

The steps described above are complex and may be quite time-consuming. The collection and analysis of large amounts of data cannot be avoided if a treatment planning system is to be thoroughly evaluated. Even if a treatment planning system operates on a limited set of measured data, the user must still make extensive measurements to fully evaluate the system. A complete set of measured data and test cases has been prepared to assist in the commissioning of treatment planning systems.[30] A summary of acceptability agreement for different parameters of the treatment planning system is shown in Table 19-6.

Once the initial commissioning and evaluation of a treatment planning system has been completed, an ongoing program of QA is required to ensure the continued reliable operation of the system. Computer systems have been characterized as being both unlikely to fail at all and unlikely to fail in any but obvious and catastrophic ways. This statement is probably true for most computer hardware, such as the central processing unit

(CPU), memory, and disk-storage devices. Failures are rare, and when they do occur they are generally obvious. This rule does not always hold, however. A highly publicized failure of the Intel Pentium processor chip resulted in frequent incorrect calculations.[31–33] The magnitude of the error was so small as to be negligible except when iterative calculations were performed.

A QA program for treatment planning computer systems must address several major sources of uncertainty (the operator as a source of inaccuracy is not considered here but in the next chapter).[34]

Measured data fall into two categories: (a) measurements of beam data and (b) measurements of patient-specific data. Inaccuracies in measured beam data may be caused by incorrect or inappropriate measurements, or by changes in the treatment beam or beam parameters that have occurred since the original measurements were made. There have been documented cases of many patients having been harmed because of improperly measured beam data being entered into the treatment planning system.[35] Uncertainties in patient-specific data may include the incorrect interpretation of imaging data, such as that obtained from CT scans. This last category would include an incorrect relationship between CT information and electron densities.

Under certain conditions, beam data stored in a computer can be changed unintentionally by the user. To guard against the risk of undetected changes in stored data, careful records should be kept of data entry sessions and software upgrades. A checksum is another tool to validate the integrity of stored data. A checksum is a unique identifier that is related to the data in the file and to the software using the data. When the data are changed outside the software, the system will generate an incorrect checksum, which will flag the data as invalid. Only if the data are changed within the system will the checksum correctly reflect the changes. In addition, calculations should be repeated on a regular basis to test the veracity of stored data. A subset of the dose calculations performed during commissioning of the planning system would ensure consistency and accuracy.

Many beam scanning systems provide software for the direct electronic transfer of data from the scanning system to the treatment planning computer. Such systems are generally reliable. Without such software, it is necessary to plot the data obtained by the scanning system and then digitize them manually into the treatment planning system. Opportunities for error exist in the digitizing and storing of these data as does data transfer from one computer system to another.[36]

The output of a treatment planning system may be in the form of graphic isodose plots and DRRs. Either type of output may be produced on a video monitor or other digital format such as portable document format (PDF). Graphic output data must be accurate, regardless of their means of production, because they are used frequently to position the patient relative to the treatment beam. Alphanumeric data must likewise be accurate because this information is often used to program the treatment unit. Tests for evaluating the accuracy of data output devices may

Table 19-6 Criteria of acceptability for photon and electron beam dose calculations.

Descriptor	Criterion
I Photon beams	
A Homogeneous calculation (no shields)	
1 Central ray data (except in buildup region)	2%
2 High dose region-low dose gradient	3%
3 Large dose gradients (>30%/cm)	4 mm
4 Small dose gradients in low dose region (ie., <7% of normalization dose)	3%
B Inhomogeneity corrections	
1 Central ray (slab geometry, in regions of electron equilibrium)	3%
C Composite uncertainty, anthropomorphic phantom	
Off axis	
Contour corrections	
Inhomogeneities	
Shields	
Irregular fields	
In regions of electronic equilibrium	
Attenuators	
1 High dose region–low dose gradient	40%
2 Large dose gradient (>30%/cm)	4 mm
3 Small dose gradients in low dose region(i.e., <7% of normalization dose)	3%
II Electron beams	
A Homogeneous calculation (no shields)	
1 Central ray data (except in buildup region)	2%
2 High dose region-low dose gradient	4%
3 Large dose gradients (>30%/cm)	4 mm
4 Small dose gradients in low dose region i.e., <7% of normalization dose)	4%
B Inhomogeneity corrections	
1 Central ray (slab geometry, in regions of electron equilibrium)	5%
C Composite uncertainty, anthropomorphic phantom	
Contour correction	
Inhomogeneities	
Shields	
Irregular fields	
Off axis	
1 High dose region-low dose gradient	7%
2 Large does gradient (>30%/cm)	5 mm
3 Small dose gradients in low dose region (i.e., <7% of central ray dose)	5%

Note: Percentages are quoted as a percent of the central ray normalization dose.
Source: Van Dyk 1993 [28]. Reproduced with permission of Elsevier

be conducted simultaneously with the tests of input devices. In addition, it is advisable to retain a standard test case on the computer's hard disk; this case should be output on occasion to test the device independently of the source of input data.

Inaccuracies in the computational algorithm are not easily detected or controlled by the operator of the system. Radiation therapy treatment planning presents complicated situations that can only be approximated by computational techniques. Although these techniques may prove sufficiently accurate over a range of frequently encountered treatment techniques, they may not always perform satisfactorily as the limits to these approximations are approached. Evaluation of the software should therefore cover the full range of complexity encountered in the clinic. Inaccuracies may also result from decisions made in implementing the software. For example, selection of a large grid spacing for the computational algorithm may yield increased computational speed but also isodose lines that show

a scalloped appearance, and rounding or truncation errors when multiple beams are used.

Two types of computational accuracy tests should be performed. A test of reproducibility involves repeating a standard treatment plan on a regular basis. All input information should be identical, so that the output is expected to be identical from one test to the next. Several simple tests should be devised to test calculations using single beams, multiple fields, wedges, and the presence of inhomogeneities. Comparable tests should be devised for verifying the repeatability of calculations using implanted sources, both singly and in arrays.

The second type of test should evaluate the accuracy of calculations. To provide a valid test, the data used for comparison should have been measured at the same time as the data used in the computations. Similar tests can be conducted to compare measured data with calculated doses at points irradiated by multifield and intensity-modulated treatment plans. Note that if isodose curves are generated it may be adequate to determine the dose at only a small number of points and then to examine the calculated isodose curves for consistency with these few values. Tests of computational reproducibility should be performed frequently, and monthly intervals are suggested. Tests of computational accuracy need to be performed less frequently but should be performed at no less than yearly intervals, or whenever changes are made to the stored data or software.

Quality assurance for intensity-modulated radiation therapy

As with other specialty procedures, IMRT has its own specific QA procedures. By *intensity modulated*, we are referring to either fixed-field IMRT or volumetric modulated arc therapy (VMAT). The procedures encompass radiation safety, treatment planning calculations, machine characteristics, and patient-specific dosimetric verification. The primary goals of QA are to identify safe parameters for treatment and to verify that the dose intended is the dose delivered.

Radiation safety

Generally speaking, a given treatment field using IMRT will have more MUs than a comparable conformally shaped field. Depending on the amount of modulation (roughly corresponding to the complexity of the fluence map or the number of segments), it is common to use three to four times the number of MUs to deliver an IMRT field. Since there are often more beam directions with IMRT, the effect on primary barriers is not a major concern. However, the ability of secondary barriers to handle leakage radiation becomes an issue, particularly if higher energies are used.[37] The calculations used in evaluating secondary barriers for the original vault design should be re-visited using the increased workload for an IMRT patient volume. Also, increased neutron dose to the patient should be considered when x rays above 10 MV are used.

Treatment planning

The planning system should be commissioned for IMRT by verifying that the dose predicted by the planning system is accurate to within acceptable limits. Since actual patient plans are quite complex, it may be best to start with geometric test patterns with a predictable or known dose. For example, computing the expected dose on a segment as shown in Figure 19-11 and then measuring the delivered dose in a phantom will illustrate the ability of the planning system to predict dose in a simple geometry. Then, by combining several segments, one can determine whether the cumulative dose for multiple segments is correctly computed, accounting for such parameters as MLC transmission within the field. Finally, a complex dose distribution using multiple segments from several beam directions can simulate an actual patient treatment.

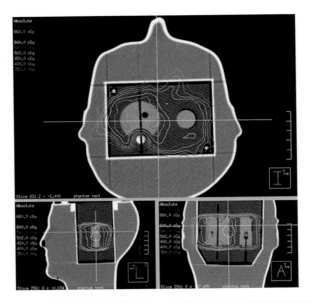

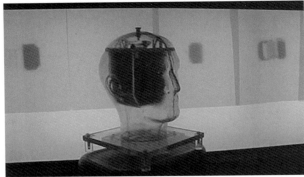

Figure 19-11 IMRT head and neck phantom from the Imaging and Radiation Oncology Center – Houston at MD Anderson. This phantom is designed to independently test the ability of the institution to deliver IMRT treatments for participation in the RTOG IMRT head and neck protocol. The top figure shows the planned dose distribution, and the bottom figure shows the phantom and delivered fluence maps.

Machine characteristics

Two general classifications of machine characteristics must be investigated to provide QA for IMRT: (a) MLC performance and (b) dose delivery. Parameters to be tested for MLC characteristics are detailed earlier in this chapter in the section for MLC QA; they refer to the mechanical properties of MLC leaf design, and monitoring them for any aberrant behavior. With heavily blocked segments, in which the jaws remain fixed for each segment, the jaws move with each segment, or the MLCs replace one set of jaws, leaf and jaw transmission contribute to the therapeutic dose delivery. This must be correctly calculated in the planning system. With the potential for segments with small numbers of MUs, the ability of the treatment unit to deliver the correct dose must be investigated.

Patient-specific dose verification

The ASTRO/ACR guidelines (American Society for Radiation Oncology, www.astro.org, and American College of Radiology, www.acr.org) for IMRT treatment delivery indicate that the dose delivery must be documented for each course of treatment by irradiating a phantom that contains either calibrated film to sample the dose distribution or an equivalent measurement system to verify that the dose delivered is the dose planned. This guideline implies that each and every IMRT plan must be verified by measuring the dose delivered. Several techniques are available to accomplish this task, including point dose or planar dose measurements for individual fields and for all fields.[38–40]

- Point Dose Measurements for a Single Field. This can be measured using film or ion chamber. Film measurements may involve sampling locations specified on the planar dose map. Ion chamber measurements in a phantom are generally acquired at a single specified point such as the isocenter.
- Point Dose Measurements for All Fields. A composite film can be used to sample the dose at a specified point (or points), or an ion chamber may be used.
- Planar Dose Measurements for a Single Field. Dose is computed at a specified depth in the phantom, perpendicular to the central axis of the beam. It may be measured using film or an array of diodes (e.g., MapCheck from Sun Nuclear Corporation; Figure 19-12) or the electronic portal imaging device. Dose profiles or isodose lines may be compared quantitatively using specialized software to scan and analyze the film (e.g., RIT, Radiological Imaging Technologies, Inc.; Figure 19-13).

- Planar Dose Measurements for Multiple Fields. These are typically measured using film. Dose profiles or isodose lines may be compared to the treatment plan.

The approach implemented in a clinic is largely a matter of personal preference, and it may change over time as a comfort level with IMRT treatment is established. It is important to mention that expertise with one type of intensity-modulated treatment (e.g., static field IMRT) does not imply expertise with a different intensity-modulated modality such as VMAT or IMRT using physical compensators. When setting acceptable tolerances for dosimetric measurements, limits should be set for individual fields as well as for overall delivery. These limits may be expressed in terms of absolute error or percentage error. For example, individual field tolerances could be set at 5% or 3 cGy, whichever is less, and the tolerance for overall dose delivery could be set at 3%. Several commercial software systems are also available that can perform an independent MU check for IMRT fields, as well as predicted fluence maps. Tools available for IMRT analysis are also quite useful for QA of other delivery techniques, such as stereotactic radiosurgery (SRS) and dynamic wedges. They may also be used to compare a typical 3D treatment with an IMRT treatment to evaluate the differences between these two techniques.

Stereotactic radiosurgery and radiotherapy

SRS is utilized for small lesions requiring precision localization and highly conformal dose distributions. It has been used most often for the treatment of brain tumors because the patient

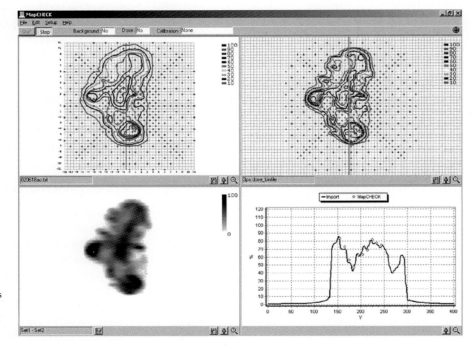

Figure 19-12 Quality assurance tool consisting of 400 diodes to generate a two-dimensional map of delivered dose. This tool allows instantaneous evaluation of IMRT fields without processing film. *Source:* Courtesy of Sun Nuclear.

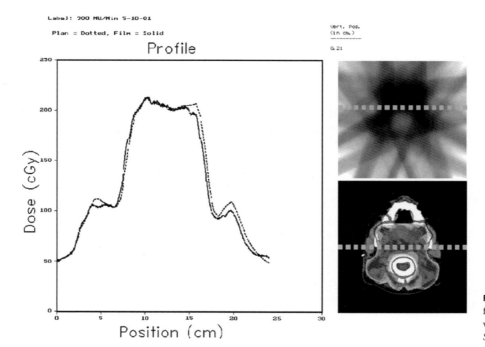

Figure 19-13 Composite dose verification for multiple fields. Profiles through the target volume and parotids are compared.
Source: Courtesy of Chester Ramsey, Ph.D.

can be easily immobilized. Advances in internal localization techniques, however, have prompted the use of the procedure for extracranial treatment sites. With stringent requirements for precise localization and accurate dosimetry, QA for cranial stereotactic treatment is quite involved.[41]

The first aspect of QA is the immobilization of the target during treatment. In the case of SRS of brain tumors, immobilization is often accomplished by a rigid frame attached to the skull. For stereotactic radiotherapy, in which the patient will return for several fractions, a re-locatable frame or mask approach may be used.[42] Care must be taken to ensure that the immobilization system provides reproducible setups for fractionated treatments. Newer methods are less reliant on immobilization but use surface imaging to locate and track the patient during treatment and to stop the beam if the patient moves out of position.[43,44] For non-frame-based SRS programs, additional QA is required for the additional tertiary systems used in the procedure.[45]

The second aspect of QA is localization, accomplished using either an external coordinate system referenced to the immobilization device or fiducials. In both cases, the location of the target relative to the localization system is known, and it must be accurately positioned on the treatment unit.

Brachytherapy quality assurance procedures

As is true of all radiation oncology equipment, brachytherapy equipment and sources should be subjected to routine QA procedures to ensure the safety of patients and staff, as well as to improve the quality of patient treatments.[46,47] In addition, the NRC and many states require that certain QA procedures be performed routinely. Failure to adhere to regulations can subject an institution to a notice of violation and a monetary fine.

Applicators

Applicators for brachytherapy procedures should be inspected and radiographed before their initial use. Frequently, these devices are made from several pieces of metal that have been welded together, and there is a risk that flaws can develop and pieces of the applicator can separate. In the case of remote afterloading systems, using radio-opaque dummy markers in conjunction with an autoradiograph of the source in corresponding dwell positions will verify the positional accuracy of the applicator as well as an understanding of the geometry of the applicator for treatment planning purposes. Documentation of this initial inspection and storage of the original films may be valuable for later comparison. After each use, the applicator should be cleaned and then examined for flaws. This inspection can take place before the equipment is sterilized for the next use.

Radioactive sources

The sources used for radioactive implants should be inspected periodically. Inspection is done most conveniently at the time an inventory is conducted. In most localities, an inventory of radioactive sources is required annually. A systematic program of recordkeeping is an essential part of a brachytherapy program.[48] It is also convenient to perform a brief inspection of sources at the time of each use. Tube sources of ^{137}Cs should be inspected for curvature, because these sources can become caught between the drawers of a safe and bent to the point at which they either begin to leak radioactive material or become

Table 19-7 Brachytherapy QA procedures and frequencies.

Procedure	At Source Change	Monthly	Daily
Safety Procedures			
Protection survey	Limited survey	—	Watch for signs of deterioration. Be aware of changes in design/use of adjacent space
Test of interlocks	Test safety interlocks	Test safety interlocks	Test safety interlocks
Applicator integrity	—	Inspect for damage or deterioration	—
Patient monitoring device operation	—	—	Check for proper operation
Dose Delivery			
Source activity	Measure source activity	Perform check of activity and verify agreement with calculated value	—
Stored and computed value	Enter measured source activity	Check calculated activity for agreement with measured activity	Verify displays of time, date, and current source activity
Dwell time accuracy	Performed as part of source calibration	Performed as part of activity check	Verify with QA device
Mechanical Alignment			
Programmed dwell position alignment	Verify with radiograph	Verify with radiograph	Verify with QA device

difficult to remove from an implant applicator. Leak testing of radioactive sources is required before their initial use and on a regular basis thereafter. Generally, leak testing is required semi-annually, but some cesium sources are certified for leak testing only every 3 years.

Remote afterloading equipment

As is the case with treatments using any radioactive material, treatments with remote afterloading devices require safety procedures to avoid the unintended exposure of the patient or personnel, or the loss of radioactive material. The high activity of sources provided with HDR remote afterloading equipment demands that close attention be paid to the whereabouts of the source at all times. QA procedures must be designed to ensure that the equipment functions as intended. Safety procedures must also be designed, and attending personnel must be trained in these procedures to ensure that the treatments are delivered safely and that employees respond appropriately in emergencies.

The NRC has published regulations requiring that a physician and a physicist be nearby whenever HDR treatments are performed. The term *nearby* is vague and it is generally considered to be equivalent to *within speaking distance*. Radiation monitors must be available in the room and accessible to personnel entering the room. Immediately following treatment, a survey of the patient is required to ensure that the source has been removed properly from the patient.

Careful documentation of the treatment is required. If multiple applicators are used and are left in place, they must be clearly identified to facilitate connecting the device for subsequent treatment. Finally, all personnel must be adequately trained in emergency procedures. Only properly trained individuals should be permitted to respond in the case of emergencies, and departmental operating procedures should ensure that those trained individuals are available at the time of treatment.

Safety procedures

Whenever brachytherapy is performed, attention must be paid to the use of occupiable space surrounding the treatment room. HDR brachytherapy generally is performed in a dedicated room, and shielding is designed and installed at the time of equipment installation. However, LDR brachytherapy treatments are typically given in hospital patient rooms, and it is not always possible or practical to provide radiation shielding. The rooms in which remote afterloading devices are installed must be equipped with a door interlock, to ensure that the source is retracted when the door is opened. The room must be equipped with a functioning radiation area monitor. Staff must be trained in appropriate emergency procedures and must practice these procedures on a regular basis. Recommendations for emergency procedures have been published.[49,50]

The following QA procedures apply equally well to HDR units. A complete QA program should address not only the treatment unit but also the treatment planning system and treatment procedures. A QA program for a remote afterloading system can be divided into three phases: (1) procedures associated with a source change, (2) procedures to be performed on a daily basis prior to patient treatments, and (3) procedures to be performed monthly.[49] A summary of the procedures appears in Table 19-7.

Source-change quality assurance

A radiation safety survey should be conducted to ensure adequate shielding of the radioactive source when it is housed in the head of the treatment unit. Areas adjacent to the treatment room should be surveyed with the source exposed. In areas where a

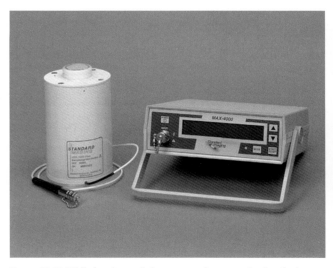

Figure 19-14 Well chamber and electrometer for measuring brachytherapy source strength.
Source: Courtesy of Standard Imaging, Middleton Wisconsin.

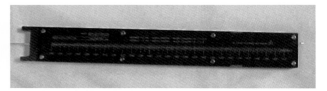

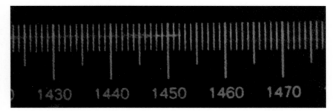

Figure 19-15 Source position check ruler. The source is programmed to a given position (1450 mm in this case) and the center of the source as remotely observed should be within 1 mm of the programmed position.
Source: Courtesy of Richard Goodman, Waukesha Memorial Hospital, Wisconsin.

reading above background is detected, the area should be surveyed with the source retracted as well.

A measurement of the source activity must be made before the source is used for patient treatment. Although no national calibration standard for ^{192}Ir exists, a technique that can be followed by hospital physicists has been developed by the AAPM ADCLs. In addition, the ADCLs calibrate well-type re-entrant chambers designed specifically for use with high-activity iridium sources (Figure 19-14).[51,52]

Date	
Time	
Operator	
Accuracy of source positioning to within ±1 mm of the programmed position Programmed position Actual position If > ±1 mm, notify authorized physicist and the authorized users	_____ _____
Timer linearity 1. T1 sec reading (nC) 2. Calculated current reading (nA) 3. T2 sec reading (nC) 4. Calculated current reading (nA) 5. Current reading (nA) Ratio 2:4 Ratio average (2,4):5	
Timer accuracy (set 10 sec)	
Measurement of the source guide tubes and connectors (±1 mm)	Pass/Fail
Backup battery test to verify emergency source retraction upon power failure	Pass/Fail
Source strength verification Manufacturer Treatment unit model number and serial number Radioactive source serial number Well chamber Manufacturer Model serial number Measured source strength	
Source homogeneity (autoradiograph, at source change only)	Pass/Fail
Comments	

Note: T1 and T2 readings have the charge collected during source transit subtracted. The transit charge is determined using a dwell position of zero seconds.

Figure 19-16 Sample monthly quality assurance form.

Daily quality assurance

Daily QA procedures are to be performed every day of patient treatment, and they should be performed prior to initiating a patient treatment (for the same reason that daily QA for external beam treatment is done prior to the first patient, as mentioned earlier in this chapter).

1 All monitors and interlocks should be checked, including the door interlocks, emergency off buttons, treatment interrupt buttons, audiovisual monitors, and room radiation monitors. The interlocks that detect missing or misconnected applicators or transfer tubes should be tested.
2 The treatment unit displays of time, date, and current source strength should be verified for accuracy.
3 A test of source-position accuracy, dwell-time accuracy, and normal termination of treatment should be performed. Most HDR and PDR manufacturers provide a test jig to assist in performing this procedure (Figure 19-15).
4 The mechanical integrity of applicator connections to the treatment unit should be verified. The availability and integrity of emergency response equipment should be verified daily.

Monthly quality assurance procedures

Monthly QA procedures should be performed at the time of source exchange, and at monthly intervals between source changes. A monthly HDR QA form is shown in Figure 19-16.

Source positioning accuracy can be checked by verifying the alignment of radiographic markers with the programmed source position. This may be accomplished by attaching treatment catheters to radiochromic film, inserting radiographic markers into each catheter, and making an exposure with an x-ray unit. The radiographic markers are removed and the remote afterloading source is programmed to (a) enter each catheter and (b) stop briefly at each of the positions identified by the radiographic markers. Afterwards, the film is processed to verify that the source positions correspond with the location of the radiographic markers (Figure 19-17). Alternatively, one can check that the programmed position matches the actual dwell position using the room camera or built-in treatment unit camera.

The integrity of the applicators used most often should be checked for mechanical damage, ease of coupling, kinks, and mechanical deformation. Transfer tubes should be inspected and measured to verify that they are in proper working condition. A power failure test should be performed where the power to the system should be interrupted to verify that the source retracts. Lastly, the activity and timer should be checked. The source activity should be checked to verify agreement with the calculated activity. The timer should be checked to verify accuracy and linearity.

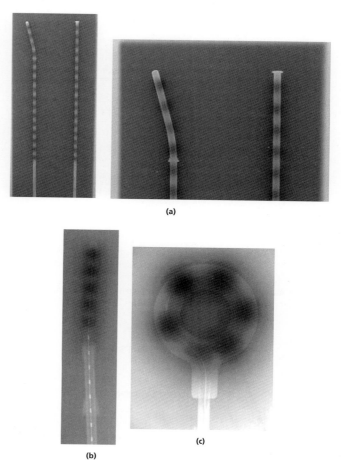

(a)

(b)

(c)

Figure 19-17 The positioning of an HDR source can be checked using an autoradiograph of source positions. (a): Dwell positions relative to the applicator are shown to aid in treatment planning; (b), (c): dummy markers are also visible indicating correlation between expected (light-colored dummy markers) and actual (darkened areas) dwell positions. Note that in (c) a slight discrepancy is observed due to the difference in the path of travel between the dummy markers and source cable for a circular path (the dummy markers are 20 and 15 mm apart starting at the tip, while the dwell positions are every 10 mm).

Patient-specific brachytherapy treatment plan quality assurance

The outline below includes some of the important checks to include in a patient-specific QA program.

1 Target Coverage. Does the isodose surface selected for the prescription cover the target volume adequately?
2 Homogeneity. Does the maximum significant dose remain below the predefined range acceptable at the institution?
3 Dose Prescription. Does the prescribed dose correspond to a protocol for the disease, and does it account for contributions from external beam treatments?
4 Normal Structure Doses. Do the doses to normal structures remain within their tolerances?

TANDEM AND OVOIDS

FOR POSITION 5:

$$\frac{(\text{Dwell Time For Position 5}) \times (\text{Source Activity})}{\text{Dose To Point M}}$$

Accepted Range: 34 to 44

FOR TOTAL TREATMENT:

$$\frac{(\text{Total Dwell Time}) \times (\text{Source Activity})}{(\text{Dose To Point M}) \times (\text{Number of Dwell Positions})}$$

Accepted Range: 24 to 30 (2.0 cm ovoids, 31 to 36 corpus)
28 to 36 (2.5 cm ovoids)

Figure 19-18 Sample dosimetry index for tandem and ovoid treatment. Note that Point M in this case is based on the University of Wisconsin system for HDR brachytherapy of the cervix.[53,54]
Source: Courtesy of Bruce Thomadsen, University of Wisconsin.

VOLUME IMPLANTS
(e.g. Prostate)

FOR TOTAL TREATMENT:

$$\left[\frac{\dfrac{\text{Activity(Ci)} \times \text{Time(s)}}{\text{Dose(Gy)}}}{\text{Volume(cc)}} - 64.3 \right] \quad \text{for volume} < 40\text{cc}$$

Accepted Range: 5.44 to 6.64

$$\left[\frac{\dfrac{\text{Activity(Ci)} \times \text{Time(s)}}{\text{Dose(Gy)}}}{\text{Volume(cc)}} - 172.7 \right] \quad \text{for volume} > 40\text{cc}$$

Accepted Range: 3.03 to 3.70

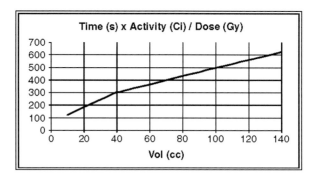

Figure 19-19 Sample dosimetry index for volume implant. Note that the volume is the volume treated to full dose, obtainable from the dose volume histogram.
Source: Adapted from information provided by California Endoenric Institute.

5 Consistency. Does the total strength used in the application correspond to that normal for the dose specified to the isodose surface?

6 Duration. Has the total duration of the application been calculated correctly?

7 Independent Dose Check. For a particular type of treatment, it is possible for an institution to develop a set of indices to check that the activity (and time for temporary implants) is appropriate. The units for these tests could be in mCi/Gy for permanent implants, mCi-hr/Gy for LDR temporary implants, or Ci-s/Gy for HDR implants. Sample indices for common treatment sites are included below.

Several patient-specific QA forms are shown in Figures 19-18 to 19-21. A sample for tandem and ovoid treatment is shown in Figure 19-18. Figure 19-19 provides a form for volume implants. A single-dwell implant patient-specific QA form is shown in

SINGLE DWELL POSITION

$$\frac{(\text{Dwell Time}) \times (\text{Source Activity})}{\text{Dose} \times r^2} \times g(r)$$

Note: time in seconds, activity in Ci, distance 'r' in cm, dose in Gy

Accepted Range: 75 to 90 (average anisotropy constant of 0.963)

72 to 87 (anisotropy constant of 1.0, e.g. mammosite)

Radius	g(r)
10	1.000
15	1.003
20	1.007
25	1.008
30	1.008
35	1.007
40	1.004
45	1.000
50	.995
55	.988
60	.981
65	.973
70	.964
75	.953
80	.940
85	.927
90	.913
95	.898
100	.882
105	.864
110	.844
115	.822
120	.799
125	.774
130	.747
135	.716
140	.681

Figure 19-20 Sample dosimetry index for single dwell position. For complex geometries that do not fit into any other index, this can be used as a point source approximation so long as the calculation point is relatively distant from the implant.
Source: Courtesy of Waukesha Memorial Hospital, Wisconsin.

HDR Handcalc v1.02 secondary calculation detailed results							
Patient name:	BRACHY PHANTOM						
Patient ID:	7112012						
Date:	2/26/2014						
Source strength:	12902.33	mCi					
Exposure constant:	4.69	R-cm^2 / mCi-hr					
fmed:	0.971						
Calculation point information							
X (cm)	Y (cm)	Z (cm)			Dose (cGy)		
-4	0	0			200		
Dwell position information							
X (cm)	Y (cm)	Z (cm)	Dist (cm)	H2O/air	Dwell (s)	Dose (cGy)	
0.01	0	0.04	4	1.014	198.2	203.96	
				Totals:	198.2	204	
				Percent difference:		1.98%	

Figure 19-21 Sample treatment plan quality assurance form.

Figure 19-20 and a general patient-specific QA form is provided in Figure 19-21.

Summary

- The ICRU has recommended that the uncertainty in dose delivery should be no greater than 5%.
- QA needs to be performed for physics instrumentation including radiation measuring devices and equipment for evaluating mechanical performance.
- Devices used in the calibration of radiation-producing equipment should be calibrated by a method traceable to national standards.
- The goal of a QA program in radiation therapy is accurate and safe treatment delivery.
- The QA program should be based on current recommendations such as those provided by Task Group reports from the American Association of Physicists in Medicine (AAPM).
- Daily checks for linear accelerators emphasize operational safety checks and output constancy. Monthly checks include output and mechanical checks. Yearly checks include output calibration and evaluation of treatment planning parameters.
- Diagnostic x-ray tube performance should be included in the QA tests for simulators (conventional and CT).
- The accuracy of dose calculation in the treatment planning system is evaluated prior to use and anytime there may be a change in software performance, such as during a software version upgrade or change in hardware.
- Provisions should always be in place for QA in intensity-modulated radiation therapy (IMRT) to verify that the dose delivered is the dose intended.

- For precision localization systems, such as external coordinate systems used in stereotactic radiosurgery (SRS), stringent QA is required to ensure accurate patient positioning.
- Brachytherapy QA includes source strength verification, treatment plan accuracy, and patient safety. Institutions must abide by state and/or federal regulations for brachytherapy.

Problems

19-1 Calculate the effect of a systematic error in patient source-to-skin distance (SSD). Assume that the actual treatment distance is 2 cm greater than the indicated distance and that the patient is being treated with a 6 MV linear accelerator (see data in Table 7-3 and Table 7-8). The patient's area of exposure is 20 cm in diameter and is being treated with opposing anterior and posterior 10 × 10 cm fields. Calculate the effect for both (a) 100 cm SSD setup and (b) 100 cm SAD setup.

19-2 It is discovered that a tray factor of 0.95 was not considered in a patient's treatment for the first 15 fractions. If 135 MU were given for each of these fractions, and there are 25 fractions remaining, how many MUs should be used for the remaining fractions?

19-3 The source in an HDR remote afterloader contains 10 Ci of ^{192}Ir. If, during a patient treatment, the source retraction mechanism were to jam, causing the source to remain in the patient for 60 seconds longer than intended, what additional dose would the patient receive at 1 cm from the source? Assume that the exposure to dose conversion factor for iridium is 0.96.

19-4 During the event described in problem 19-3 above, a staff member manually retracts the iridium source from the patient into the remote afterloader. This process takes approximately 15 sec, during which time the staff member is at an average distance of 0.6 m from the source. What is the exposure to the staff member?

19-5 The following measurements are made at 10 cm depth in a water phantom from a 20 ×20 cm field provided by a 6 MV linear accelerator. The maximum reading, found at a point 5 cm to the left of the central axis, is 101.3. The minimum reading, found at a point 8 cm to the right of the central axis, is 94.9. Calculate the beam flatness. Is this flatness acceptable?

19-6 List four parameters of simulator operation that should be checked before a service person is called to address poor fluoroscopic image quality.

19-7 Several afterloading devices are designed as a *closed system*. Why is it important to try to maintain a closed system when dealing with an emergency situation?

19-8 What effect results in lines of lower dose parallel to the direction of leaf motion?

19-9 Point dose measurements are performed on an IMRT patient. The calibration field reading of 0.333 nC corresponds to 175.5 cGy. The readings and expected doses for the seven IMRT fields are:

Field 1:	0.040 nC	20.2 cGy
Field 2:	0.031	15.9
Field 3:	0.042	23.4
Field 4:	0.102	53.1
Field 5:	0.044	23.4
Field 6:	0.044	23.5
Field 7:	0.058	31.6

What is the overall error in the delivered dose? Are any fields more than 3 cGy off from their expected value?

References

1 International Commission on Radiation Units and Measurements. Determination of absorbed dose in a patient irradiated by beams of x or gamma rays in radiotherapy procedures. ICRU Report No. 24, Washington, DC, 1976.

2 Leunens, G., et al. Assessment of dose inhomogeneity at target level by in vivo dosimetry: Can the recommended 5% accuracy in the dose delivered to the target volume be fulfilled in daily practice? *Radiother. Oncol.* 1992; **25**:245–250.

3 Ibbott, G. S., et al. Uncertainty of calibrations at the accredited dosimetry calibration laboratories. *Med. Phys.* 1997; **24**(8):1249–1254.

4 Pawlicki, T, Dunscombe, P., Mundt, A. J., Scalliet, P. (eds.). 2011. *Quality and Safety in Radiotherapy.* Boca Raton, FL: Taylor & Francis.

5 Hanson, W. F., Grant, W. 3rd., Kennedy, P., Cundiff, J. H., Gagnon, W. F., et al. A review of the reliability of chamber factors used clinically in the United States (1968–1976). *Med. Phys.* 1978; **5**:552– 554.

6 Lanzl, L. H., Rozenfeld, M., and Wootton, P. The radiation therapy dosimetry network in the United States. *Med. Phys.* 1981; **8**:49–53.

7 Rozenfeld, M., and Jette, D. Quality assurance of radiation dosage: Usefulness of redundancy. *Radiology* 1984; **150**(l):241–244.

8 Almond, P. R., Biggs, P. J., Coursey, B. M., Hanson, W. F., Huq, M. S., et al. AAPM's TG-51 protocol for clinical reference dosimetry of high-energy photon and electron beams. *Med. Phys.* 1999; **26**(9):1847–70.

9 Campos, L. L., and Caldas, L. V. Induced effects in ionization chamber cables by photon and electron irradiation. *Med. Phys.* 1991; **18**(3):522–526.

10 Ibbott, G. S., et al. Stem corrections for ionization chambers. *Med. Phys.* 1975; **2**(6):328–330.

11 Karzmark, C. J. Procedural and operator error aspects of radiation accidents in radiotherapy. *Int. J. Radiat. Oncol. Biol. Phys.* 1987; **13**:1599–1602.

12 Kutcher, G. J., Coia, L., Gillin, M., Hanson, W. F., Leibel, S., et al. Comprehensive QA for radiation oncology: Report of AAPM Radiation Therapy Committee Task Group 40. *Med. Phys.* 1994; **21**(4):581–618.

13 Klein, E. C., Hanley, J., Bayouth, J., Yin, F. F., Simon, W., et al. Task Group 142 report: Quality assurance of medical accelerators. *Med. Phys.* 2009; **36**(9):4197–4212.

14 National Council on Radiation Protection and Measurements, Medical x-ray, electron beam and gamma ray protection for energies up to 50 MeV (Equipment design, performance and use), NCRP Report No. 102: Bethesda, MD, 1989.

15 Bureau Central de la Commission Electrotechnique Internationale. Radiotherapy simulators: Particular requirements for the safety of electron accelerators in the range of 1 MeV to 50 MeV, International Electrotechnical Commission Standard No. 601-2-1, Geneva, Switzerland, 1993.

16 Radiation Therapy Committee, Basic Applications of Multileaf Collimators, Report of Task Group No. 50 AAPM Report No. 72, Medical Physics Publishing, 2001.

17 Georg, D., Knöös, T., and McClean, B. Current status and future perspective of flattening filter free photon beams. *Phys. Med. Biol.* 2011; **38**(3):1280–1293.

18 Vassiliev, O. N., Titt, U., Kry, S. F., Mohan, R., and Gillin, M. T. Radiation safety survey on a flattening filter-free medical accelerator. *Radiat. Protect. Dosim.* 2007; **124**(2):187–190.

19 Vassiliev, O. N., Titt, U., Pönisch, F. Kry, S. F., Mohan, R., and Gillin, M. T. Dosimetric properties of photon beams from a flattening filter free clinical accelerator. *Phys. Med. Biol.* 2006; **51**:1907–1917.

20 Cashmore, J. The characterization of unflattened photon beams from a 6 MV linear accelerator. *Phys. Med. Biol.* 2008; **53**:1933–1946.

21 Lang, S., Hrbacek, J., Leong, A., and Klöck, S. Ion-recombination correction for different ionization chambers in high dose rate flattening-filter-free photon beams. *Phys. Med. Biol.* 2012; **57**:2819–2827.

22 Hrbacek, J., Lang, S., and Klöck, S. Commissioning of photon beams of a flattening filter-free linear accelerator and the accuracy of beam modeling using an anisotropic analytical algorithm. *Int. J. Radiat. Oncol. Biol. Phys.* 2011; **80**(4):1228–1237.

23 Samei, E., et al. Performance evaluation of computed radiography systems. *Med. Phys.* 2001; **28**(3):361–371.

24 Perez, C. A. The critical need for accurate treatment planning and quality control in radiation therapy. *Int. J. Radiat. Oncol. Biol. Phys.* 1977; **2**:815–818.

25 McCullough, E. C., and Earle, J. D. The selection, acceptance testing, and quality control of radiotherapy treatment simulators. *Radiology* 1979; **131**:221–230.

26 Mutic S., Palta, J. R., Butker, E. K., Das, I. J., Huq, M. S., et al. Quality assurance for computed-tomography simulators and the computed tomography-simulation process: Report of the AAPM Radiation Therapy Committee Task Group No. 66. *Med. Phys.* 2003; **30**(10):2762–2792.

27 Jacky, J., and White, C. P., Testing a 3-D radiation therapy planning program. *Int. J. Radiat. Oncol. Biol. Phys.* 1989; **18**:253–261.

28 Van Dyk, J., Barnett, R. B., Cygler, J. E., and Shragge, P. C. Commissioning and quality assurance of treatment planning computers. *Int. J. Radiat. Oncol. Biol. Phys.* 1993; **26**(2):261–273.

29 Fraass, B., Doppke, K., Hunt, M., Kutcher, G., Starkschall, G., et al. American Association of Physicists in Medicine Radiation Therapy Committee Task Group 53: Quality assurance for clinical radiotherapy treatment planning. *Med. Phys.* 1998; **25**(10):1773–1829.

30 American Association of Physicists in Medicine. Radiation treatment planning dosimetry verification. AAPM Task Group 23 Test Package, 1987. AAPM Report No. 55, 1995.

31 Cipra, B. How number theory got the best of the Pentium chip. *Science* 1995; **267**:175.

32 Coe, T., Mathisen, T., Moler, C., and Pratt, V. Computational aspects of the Pentium affair. IEEE Comp. Sci. Eng. 1995; (Spring):18–30.

33 Fisher, L. M. Flaw reported in new Intel chip. New York Times 1997 (May 5). Available at http://www.nytimes.com/library/cyber/week/050697intel-chip-flaw.html, accessed September 15, 2015.

34 McCullough, E. C., and Krueger, A. M. Performance evaluation of computerized treatment planning systems for radiotherapy: External photon beams. *Int. J. Radiat. Oncol. Biol. Phys.* 1980; **6**:1599–1605.

35 Bogdanich, W., and Ruiz, R.R. Radiation errors reported in Missouri. New York Times 2010 (February 24), http://www.nytimes.com/2010/02/25/us/25radiation.html?˙r=0, accessed September 15, 2015.

36 Leunens, G., Verstraete, J., Van den Bogaert, W., Van Dam, J., Dutreix, A., and van der Schueren, E. Human errors in data transfer during the preparation and delivery of radiation treatment affecting the final result: "Garbage in, garbage out." *Radiother. Oncol.* 1992; **23**:217–222.

37 Intensity Modulated Radiation Therapy Collaborative Working Group. Intensity-modulated radiotherapy: Current status and issues of interest. *Int. J. Radiat. Oncol. Biol. Phys.* 2001; **51**(4):880–914.

38 Dong, L., Antolak, J., Salehpour, M., Forster, K., O'Neill, L., et al. Patient-specific point dose measurement for IMRT monitor unit verification. *Int. J. Radiat. Oncol. Biol. Phys.* 2003; **56**(3):867–877.

39 Jursinic, P., and Nelms, B. A 2-D diode array and analysis software for verification of intensity modulated radiation therapy delivery. *Med. Phys.* 2003; **30**(5):870–879.

40 Vieira, S. C., Dirkx, M. L., Heijmen, B. J., and de Boer, H. C. SIFT: a method to verify the IMRT fluence delivered during patient treatment using an electronic portal imaging device. *Int. J. Radiat. Oncol. Biol. Phys.* 2004;**60**(3):981–93.

41 Report of Task Group 42. Stereotactic Radiosurgery, AAPM Report No. 54, 1995.

42 Bova, F. J., Buatti, J. M., Friedman, W. A., Mendenhall, W. M., Yang, C. C., and Liu, C. The University of Florida frameless high-precision stereotactic radiotherapy system. *Int. J. Radiat. Oncol. Biol. Phys.* 1997; **38**(4):875–82.

43 Cerviño, L. I., Detorie, N., Taylor, M., Lawson, J. D., Harry, T., et al. Initial clinical experience with a frameless and maskless stereotactic radiosurgery treatment. *Pract. Radiat. Oncol.* 2012;**2**(1):54–62.

44 Pan, H., Cerviño, L. I., Pawlicki, T., Jiang, S. B., Alksne, J., et al. Frameless, real-time, surface imaging-guided radiosurgery: clinical outcomes for brain metastases. *Neurosurgery.* 2012; **71**(4):844–51.

45 Wooten, H. O., Klein, E. E., Gokhroo, G., and Santanam, L. A monthly quality assurance procedure for 3D surface imaging. *J. Appl. Clin. Med. Phys.* 2010; **12**(1):234–238.

46 Nath, R., Anderson, L. L., Meli, J. A., Olch, A. J., Stitt, J. A., and Williamson, J. F. Code of practice for brachytherapy physics: Report of the AAPM Radiation Therapy Committee Task Group No. 56 *Med. Phys.* 1997; **24**(10):1557–1598.

47 Kubo, H. D., Glasgow, G. P., and Pethel, T. D., Thomadsen, B. R., Williamson, J. F. High dose-rate brachytherapy treatment delivery: Report of the AAPM Radiation Therapy Committee Task Group No. 59. *Med. Phys.* 1998; **25**(4):375–403.

48 Slessinger, E., Grigsby, P., and Williams, J. Improvements in brachytherapy quality assurance. *Int. J. Radiat. Oncol. Biol. Phys.* 1988; **16**:497–500.

49 Hicks, J., and Ezzell, G. A. Calibration and quality assurance. In Activity, Special Report No. 7. Veenendaal, The Netherlands, Nucletron-Oldelft, 1995.

50 Spicer, B. L., and Hicks, J. A. Safety programs for remote afterloading brachytherapy: High dose rate and pulsed low dose rate. In Activity, International Nucletron-Oldelft Radiotherapy Journal, Quality Assurance, Special Report No. 7, Veenendaal, The Netherlands, Nucletron-Oldelft, 1995.

51 Goetsch, S. J., Attix, F. H., DeWerd, L. A., Thomadsen, B. R. A new re-entrant ionisation chamber for the calibration of iridium-192 high dose rate sources. *Int. J. Radiat. Oncol. Biol. Phys.* 1992; **24**:167–170.

52 Goetsch, S. J., et al. Calibration of iridium-192 high dose rate afterloading systems. *Med. Phys.* 1991; **18**:462–467.

53 Stitt, J., et al. High dose rate intracavitary brachytherapy for carcinoma of the cervix: The Madison system: I. Clinical and radiobiological considerations. *Int. J. Radiat. Oncol. Biol. Phys.* 1992; **24**(2):335–348.

54 Thomadsen, B. R., Shahabi, S., Stitt, J. A., Buchler, D. A., Fowler, J. F. et al. High dose rate intracavitary brachytherapy for carcinoma of the cervix: The Madison system: II. Procedural and physical considerations. *Int. J. Radiat. Oncol. Biol. Phys.* 1992; **24**(2):349–357.

20

PATIENT SAFETY AND QUALITY IMPROVEMENT

Objectives

After studying this chapter, the reader should be able to:
- Describe how human biases affect patient safety.
  Understand and use aids to mitigate the effects of human biases.
- Perform a failure modes and effects analysis.
- Perform a root cause analysis.
- List the components of an incident learning system.
- Outline the plan–do–study–act paradigm.
- Describe aspects of lean/six-sigma.
- Understand process variation and process control.
- Construct and use an individual's control chart for process analysis.

Introduction

"It is not enough to do your best; you must know what to do, and then do your best."

–W. Edwards Deming, Ph.D.
(Quality pioneer)

Compassion and the desire to do a good job alone are not sufficient to produce the safest and highest quality care for patients. One must first learn new tools and techniques and then apply them in clinical practice to achieve higher levels of quality and safety. In this chapter, quality and safety techniques are presented that are not routinely taught in medical or graduate school. Many of these concepts will be new to the reader, so the goal of this chapter is to provide the reader with an overview and basic working knowledge of the information herein.

With the exception of peer review (e.g., chart rounds), quality assurance (QA) has typically been the responsibility of the medical physicist. New quality and safety techniques are evolving in radiation oncology. To be most effective, all leaders of a department should be fluent with the techniques of quality and safety. In this chapter, several aspects of quality and safety that have recently entered the domain of radiation oncology practice are introduced. Effects of cognitive biases on safety are discussed, together with simple mitigation strategies. Both prospective and retrospective risk assessment techniques are described.

Hendee's Radiation Therapy Physics, Fourth Edition. Todd Pawlicki, Daniel J. Scanderbeg and George Starkschall.
© 2016 John Wiley & Sons, Inc. Published 2016 by John Wiley & Sons, Inc.

The structure and formation of incident learning systems (ILSs) are explained. Lastly, the quality improvement paradigms of six-sigma and plan–do–study–act (PDSA) are described, including process control and the construction and use of control charts. Additional information related to radiation therapy quality and safety can be found in a designated textbook on the topic.[1]

Human factors

Humans have an impact on quality and safety. One of the goals of a quality and safety management program is to mitigate the effects of human factors. Generally, the term *human factors* refers to the effects of environment, culture, organization, and equipment on job performance.[2–4] *Human-factors engineering* relates to the functional design that incorporates comfort and the ability to do one's job effectively and without error. These can be applied to both hardware scenarios (e.g., the type of chair you sit on) and to software (e.g., an electronic medical record user interface). When applied to patient safety, appropriately addressing human factors requires a broader view to include cognitive biases and human error. This broader view will be the focus of this section. Many types of human factors play important roles in treating patients with radiation.

Human performance can be divided into the following categories: skill-based, rule-based, and knowledge-based performance.[5] Any activity can encompass more than one level of performance. The reason for making the distinction among human performance categories is that all areas of human performance are susceptible to errors. Making this distinction can help to understand contributing factors to an error and how one might prevent future errors. *Skill-based performance* refers to routine tasks. These tasks are usually repetitive activities in which skill is obtained and increased through repetition. Rarely is any documentation referred to for skill-based activities. Examples of skill-based performance include performing morning warm-up of a machine, acquiring patient-specific intensity-modulated radiation therapy (IMRT) QA measurements, or performing a patient's history and physical exam. *Rule-based performance* refers to complex or critical tasks that are occasionally performed. In these situations, documentation needs to be readily accessible to follow the rules. Examples of rule-based performance include adjusting patient-setup lasers, calculating appropriate amounts of radiation shielding, or contouring a target for a patient under a specific protocol. *Knowledge-based performance* refers to unfamiliar tasks for which prior specific documentation is not available or applicable. This type of performance relies heavily on education rather than training. Examples of knowledge-based performance include deciding what to do if a patient is setting up differently in the treatment room from the setup in CT simulation, commissioning a novel treatment technique, or contouring and re-planning a shrinking target in the middle of a course of therapy.

Example 20-1

Assign the following tasks to the most appropriate human performance category:
1 Determining the appropriate prescription dose for a cranial radiosurgery retreatment.
2 Reviewing orthogonal setup images for a prostate case with fiducials.
3 Contouring the target and normal tissues for a patient in a clinical trial.

A knowledge-based
B skill-based
C rule-based (although one could also argue that there is a component of knowledge-based activity in this example as well).

The traditional view of safety is that a chain of failure events leads to a loss. A loss can include a patient being harmed, an error or mistake that does not reach the patient (usually called a *near-miss*, although calling it a *near hit* may be more appropriate), or even a delay in a patient's treatment. This approach is not sufficient to address complex systems. In complex systems, many factors from different components of a process can fail, leading to an error. Eliminating one component does not imply that an error will be prevented.

The lack of serious events or near-misses does not imply a safe department. Safety does not equal reliability. It is well known that accidents happen even when equipment and processes are working as designed. Conversely, equipment and processes may not be working properly but accidents do not always happen. Therefore, mitigating errors requires a different focus from that of simply checking the performance of equipment as described in Chapter 19.

Understanding accidents

Radiotherapy equipment is fairly robust against software or hardware failures, but catastrophic equipment failures can still occur.[6,7] The traditional QA programs described in Chapter 19 are designed, in part, to identify equipment failures before they arise in clinical practice. However, even when equipment fails, mitigating human circumstances can contribute to failures that reach the patient. Current safety thinking is that errors are not a simple sequential chain of events in which one event fails and an error results. There are always several contributing factors to an error, with the human playing a prominent role. The human condition leading to errors is addressed in this section. It should be recognized that the human can also play an important role in preventing errors and recovery from them.[8]

Humans have many biases; some that people are consciously aware of and many that they are not aware of. Human biases can arise from information-processing shortcuts (heuristics), motivational factors, social influence, and a host of other sources. Therefore, it is prudent to understand some of the human biases and how they can affect human performance. Additionally, understanding human biases will be helpful to performing an effective causal analysis after an error has occurred.

The notion of human biases related to behavioral economics was first introduced in the 1970s by Tversky and Kahneman.[9] There is a connection between behavioral economics and patient safety.[10] Behavioral economists and safety researchers identify replicable ways in which human judgment and decisions differ from rational choice theory. The biases described below, as well as information about many other human biases, can be found in popular books by Ariely[11] and Kahneman[12].

Current research suggests that the far majority of our human operations are performed in an automatic fashion (i.e., skill-based performance) without much consideration as to what is actually happening.[12,13] The automatic mode (unconscious) control is primarily influenced by past experience, which can lead to a "strong but wrong" reaction to a set of environmental circumstances. Similarly, the unconscious can present information even when it is not requested. Because the methods of human cognition are fixed, one can change the work environment (context) to decrease the likelihood of errors or, when an error does occur, increase the likelihood of detection and correction in the future. These are used during *root cause analysis* (RCA), which is discussed later in this chapter.

Examples of human biases that have an impact on patient safety are self-herding and choice blindness. The first of these, *self-herding*, refers to the tendency to repeat decisions that have been made in the past. This tendency is commonplace in healthcare. Once a person acts on something (makes a decision), that person tends to repeat that behavior without questioning it. Therefore, initial decisions can have a disproportional effect on future decisions.[14] A related bias is *anchoring* or *early information bias*, which is the overemphasis on early information (often the first piece received) when making decisions. When a medical error occurs, causal analysis techniques usually uncover multiple contributing factors at the operator level. Therefore, understanding the situational factors leading up to the error can provide new insights to address all the contributing factors.

Choice blindness is the bias in which people produce confabulatory explanations when asked to describe the reasons behind the choices they make.[15] Choice blindness can occur during a causal analysis procedure in which those involved in a medical error are interviewed to understand what they were thinking just before the error occurred. Even for an optimal interview of a healthcare professional involved in a medical error, the interviewer can still be inadvertently misled by the interviewee when explaining their decisions leading up to the error. Thus, any error-mitigation strategy based on confabulatory explanations may not necessarily prevent the error from happening in the future. At the same time, *hindsight bias* may come into play, which occurs when people perceive events as more predictable than they really are.[16,17]

The tendency to favor information or categorize new evidence as confirming one's existing beliefs is referred to as *confirmation bias*.[18] Operationally, confirmation bias manifests itself by jumping to a conclusion as to the cause of an error (usually only one cause) and then looking for or interpreting new information as confirming the initial conclusion. Confirmation bias is typically found in causal analysis when determining the reasons that an error has occurred and is an artifact of how information is stored in long-term memory. Information is not stored as raw data, for example, like that stored on a computer's hard disk. Rather, information is stored as *mini-theories* that also contain a schematic of how the world works. Therefore, even the most experienced people can make significant errors if the situation they are presented with is not described by the mini-theory retrieved from long-term memory.[8] Biases and workload are major factors affecting job performance.

Workload can be assessed by a tool called the *Task Load Index*, which was developed in part by the United States National Aeronautics and Space Administration and is called *NASA-TLX*. The NASA-TLX is a multi-dimensional rating scale that quantifies the magnitude and sources of six workload-related factors.[19] The factors assessed in the NASA-TLX are mental demands, physical demands, temporal demands, frustration, effort, and performance. These are combined to derive a sensitive and reliable estimate of workload. This type of quantitative objective analysis has been used to identify that workload levels for some radiation oncology workers might exceed what is considered safe in other industries.[20] The NASA-TLX tool was also used to quantify and compare physician workload for several common treatment planning tasks and to relate workload levels to errors for routine clinical tasks to determine situations in which performance is expected to decline.[21,22] As the NASA-TLX scores increased, the physician was less comfortable with approving the treatment plan. The NASA-TLX can be used as a way to identify tasks at risk of reduced human performance where scores greater than about 50 indicate an amount of workload that needs to be addressed. In general, the results of this type of research indicate that there is much work to be done toward improving safety in radiation therapy.

Mitigating errors

A safe department cannot be assured solely by checks that were described in the previous chapter, such as chart checks, machine performance checks, and the like. Safety must be designed into departmental processes. Not only must the technical components be considered but perhaps more importantly must the human, managerial, and organizational components be considered. In response to an error, human or system causes need to be mitigated. While training on job function is not a particularly powerful tool to use in response to an error, learning about errors has been suggested as a strategy to help prevent them.[23] There are many types of aids that facilitate human performance. Both general and specific aids can help mitigate human biases toward the reduction of errors and safety improvement.

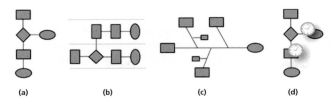

Figure 20-1 Representation of different types of process maps: (a) flowchart, (b) swim lanes, (c) fishbone, Ishikawa, or cause-and-effect diagram, and (d) value-stream map.

In this section, five tools for mitigating errors are reviewed. These tools are process maps, checklists, time-outs, no-interruption zones, and peer review. Using these aids adds extra time to normal departmental workflow and can be difficult to use during times of busy clinical activities. However, it is at these times that these aids can be most effective. Time and space should be provided to make use of these tools. At the same time, the use of an aid can have unintended negative consequences. Therefore, the introduction of an aid should be monitored carefully using an ILS. ILSs will be described later in this chapter.

A process map is a pictorial representation of the sequence of steps that comprise a process and a general-purpose tool to facilitate effective communication. It is generally recognized that "a picture is worth a 1000 words," and therein lies the value of process maps. Representations of process maps include flowcharts, swim-lane diagrams, cause-and-effect diagrams, and value stream maps. A flowchart shows a serial sequence of events, and a swim-lane diagram shows a parallel sequence of events. A cause-and-effect diagram represents a start and end with various branches and sub-branches that contribute to the main trunk. The cause-and-effect diagram is typically used when investigating an accident, but can also be used as part of prospective process analysis. Lastly, the value stream map is similar to a flowchart, but includes a duration or capacity component for the different steps in the flowchart. The various process maps are shown in Figure 20-1. This classification is an oversimplification of these different types of process maps, but it does provide a high-level overview. Some types of process maps are more appropriate than others in different situations. When starting out, any type of process map can be used and will be better than not using any process map at all.

The different symbols have different meanings, particularly when working with flowcharts. A rectangle denotes a process (action) step, a diamond denotes a binary (yes/no) decision, and an oval denotes a point where inputs enter or the process ends or begins. Sometimes arrows are used to connect the boxes to indicate the direction of the process if it is not immediately obvious from the process map. A value-stream map is similar to a flowchart except that a duration is associated with the transition from one box to the next. A very high-level process map for radiation therapy is shown in Figure 20-2.

One approach to creating effective process maps has four steps:

1 Decide what process will be mapped, focusing on the start and end points. It is best not to try to cover too large a process, so a helpful strategy is to ensure the process map is of a manageable size. For example, the process in Example 20-2 can be reduced in scope by considering only the treatment-planning component for prostate IMRT cases.
2 Form a group and identify someone to lead the process-mapping exercise to ensure it is completed. Although it could be helpful for the entire group to meet to discuss the process map, early on it is sufficient to know who is expected to participate.
3 Create an initial process map by starting with a draft that captures the workflow. It may be sufficient for the group leader or one to two other members to create the process map. The initial version should be verified with others in the designated group as to its appropriateness.
4 Use an iterative strategy in which the process map is refined with the input from the group. The main point is that the people directly involved in the process being mapped need to have input into creating the final version of the process map. If the group is able to meet together to complete the map, it is useful to plan a fixed amount of time (e.g., 1–2 hours) and the leader makes sure the map is completed within that timeframe.

There is value in the exercise of creating the process map. At the end of the process-mapping procedure, everyone should have the same understanding of the process steps and functions.

Example 20-2

Create a process map (flowchart) that describes an image-guided treatment fraction. Make it six symbols that include one decision symbol (diamond).

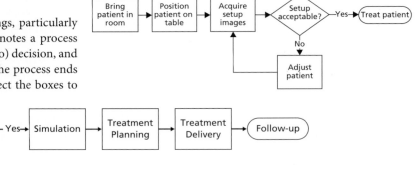

Figure 20-2 Example of a high-level process map for radiation therapy.

Note, one possible answer is shown below and other answers may be equally acceptable depending on the processes in your department and your understanding of the image-guidance procedure.

The second tool that can be used to mitigate errors is a checklist. A checklist is simply a document containing a list of items of actions to be performed and is used as a reminder of these actions. It serves as a memory aid to successfully complete a task by making the optimal set of steps explicit. The use and value of checklists is described by Gawande.[24] Checklists can be introduced to reduce variability in decision making, particularly under stressful situations, and to ensure compliance with standards.[25]

Generally, there are two different types of checklists: do–confirm checklists and read–do checklists.[24] The intent of a do–confirm checklist is that the user does the job from memory and experience and then stops to confirm that everything which was supposed to be done was actually done. Conversely, in using a read–do checklist, the user performs the tasks and checks them off as they are completed. The read–do checklist facilitates rule-based performance, whereas the do–confirm checklist works in the skill-based domain. Creating an effective checklist requires a domain expert (i.e., someone actually doing the work) to identify the most critical steps that even a highly skilled professional could miss.

In either checklist type, the checklist should consist of five to nine items which, without special training, is the number of steps most people can keep in working memory.[26] A checklist does not spell everything out as would be found in a standard operating procedure. The checklist should be designed to be completed by the user in less than two minutes depending on the context of the process. For example, a dosimetrist preparing a treatment plan, which can take several hours, can benefit from spending a few minutes to review a checklist. On the other hand, a few extra minutes in the treatment room can be a significant burden, as each patient is treated within 10–15 minutes. If the checklist is too long for a given process, people will start to cut corners and avoid using the checklist altogether. To achieve the two-minute requirement, an effective checklist should contain wording that is simple and exact using familiar language. The checklist should be streamlined to fit on one page, be free from clutter and unnecessary colors, and be easy to read whether the checklist is printed on paper or on a computer (e.g., Web or mobile-device-based).

To implement a checklist effectively, clear pause points in the workflow must be identified or created. The use of an automated checklist has also been shown to be effective.[27] The items on the checklist must be interpreted in the same way by multiple people. Therefore, a new checklist will likely need a few revisions before it is perfected. Once implemented, the issues identified by a checklist should be tracked and analyzed on a routine basis. The analysis should include a determination as to the effectiveness of the implemented checklist. Checklists are living documents and will need to be altered or discontinued in the face of changing clinical processes and technology. It is recommended to review checklists at least annually. The AAPM has also provided guidance on using checklists in clinical practice.[28]

The third error-mitigation tool, the time-out, is closely related to the checklist. In fact, the checklist can be considered as a type of time-out. Therefore, checklists and time-outs are frequently used together. A time-out is a pause immediately prior to the initiation of patient treatment or other procedure that improves communication.[29] It can also be used in an ad hoc fashion any time that a question or potential discrepancy is noted. A time-out generally consists of verification of the patient, the verification of the correct treatment site or process, and verification of the procedure. Additional items that can be verified for radiotherapy treatments are the treatment parameters (e.g., number of monitor units, dose, site, and energy), patient positioning, patient name, date of birth, and medical record number. While a time-out can be an effective error-mitigation strategy, implementation requires diligence, and methods to ensure compliance should be considered.[30]

The fourth tool for mitigating errors is the no-interruption zone. In many clinics, it is accepted practice to interrupt a therapist about to turn the beam on, a physicist checking a plan, or a radiation oncologist contouring a target volume. Self-interruptions are also routinely used. Interruptions need to be recognized as safety hazards that need to be actively minimized. Limiting interruptions is a straightforward and inexpensive error-mitigation strategy. A no-interruption zone is a designated protected area in space or time for someone to get work done without interruptions. It allows concentration on the task in hand without distractions. In 1981, the United States' Federal Aviation Authority adopted a policy that prohibits non-essential tasks and communication in the cockpit during flight operations below 10,000 ft (sterile cockpit rule). No-interruption zones are recognized as being useful safety tools in health care as well.[31]

The fifth error mitigation strategy is that of peer review. Quality and safety improvement has two broad areas: execution-based aspects and decision-based aspects. Execution-based aspects have a clear right or wrong outcome. Conversely, decision-based aspects have no clear right or wrong outcome. An example is drawing a gross target volume on a CT scan. There is a range of justifiable outcomes (i.e., target volumes). It is in the cases of decision-based aspects that peer review can be an effective quality and safety improvement strategy.

Peer review is the evaluation of one's work by an equivalently trained professional, and includes feedback to the person being reviewed. Previous studies have noted that about 5–10% of cases undergo modification as a result of peer review.[32,33] An appropriate organizational culture must exist for effective peer review. Namely, an open and collaborative environment will facilitate the learning cycle of peer review. Feedback should be given respectfully and received with the collaborative intent upon which it was delivered.

Targets for peer review can be separated into three levels.[34] Level 1 is the highest priority of items needing peer review, and includes target definition and first day of treatment delivery. Level 2 is for items for which there are guidelines or potential ambiguities such as the decision to treat with radiation, the planning directive, and technical plan quality. Level 3 is the lowest level of items that could benefit from peer review. These include the general radiation treatment approach and normal tissue segmentation. While peer review is primarily thought of as a physician-oriented activity, medical physicists can also benefit from peer-review activities.[35] Radiation therapy peer-review activities and requirements are still evolving. Studies suggest the existence of a large variation in the implementation of peer review that still results in both minor and major changes in patient management.[36,37] Peer review for all members of a department should be a standard of practice.

A final issue that needs to be addressed in mitigating errors is the use of workarounds. A workaround is a way to bypass the workflow as designed. This can be for vendor hardware or software but can also apply to standard operating procedures in a department. Workarounds are pervasive in healthcare. However, relying too much on workarounds is a safety hazard.[38,39] The stress created by consistent reliance on workarounds can manifest errors in other parts of the system even if problems are not observed at the point of the workaround. The accepted practice of workarounds can lead to doing too much with too little and losing the heightened awareness of the possibility of errors. Active efforts to identify and remove workarounds should be an integral part of any safety management program.

Error-mitigation strategies are essential to maintaining a quality and safety program. Process maps are an excellent tool to ensure everyone has the same understanding of the process. Checklists and time-outs can serve as effective safety barriers at critical steps in a process. A safety barrier is something (hard constraint, process change, etc.) that reduces the chance that an error will occur. Being aware of the deleterious effects of interruptions and workarounds is important. A designated no-interruption zone can be used as an area in time or space for concentrated slow-thinking work and a notification to others to not interrupt the work being done. Lastly, peer review is an excellent tool to evaluate clinical decision where there is no absolute right or wrong answer. All of these tools are simple but helpful to include in error-mitigation strategies.

Hazard analysis

Errors can be categorized as sporadic or systematic. A sporadic error is one that happens once and is not likely to occur at the same place in the process again. The term *sporadic* is used to distinguish it from *random*, which has a statistical meaning. Sporadic errors have causes related to equipment failures or human biases. Categorizing an error as systematic indicates that the same error will occur repeatedly under the same set of circumstances. Systematic errors can affect multiple patients. Systematic errors have causes related to improper procedures or workarounds and can be addressed by adjusting the standard operating procedures to accommodate the circumstances.

Prospective analysis

Failure modes and effects analysis (FMEA) is the systematic evaluation of the components of a piece of equipment or a process for the purpose of mitigating risk.[40] FMEA is an inductive (bottom-up) method and is known as a *component-based probabilistic hazard model*. One begins with a postulated fault and then attempts to figure out what the effect of the fault might be.

Many approaches for performing an FMEA have been developed. One such method has the following steps:

1 Define the equipment or process to be analyzed.
2 Identify all potential failure modes and define their effects on the system.
3 Estimate the severity (S) of each failure mode.
4 Estimate the probability of detecting (D) each failure mode.
5 Estimate the probability of occurrence (O) of each failure mode.
6 Calculate the risk priority number (RPN) as the product of the severity (Step 3), probability of detection (Step 4), and probability of occurrence (Step 5) for each failure mode (i.e. $RPN = O \cdot S \cdot D$).
7 Rank the RPNs and take action to mitigate the highest risk failure modes.

The relative risk of the failure modes is determined by the RPN values and is used to guide risk-mitigation efforts. Many different scales for severity, probability of detection, and probability of occurrence have been proposed. The scales proposed by the AAPM are shown in Table 20-1a, b, and c.[41] RPN values range from 1 to 1000. For example, using Table 20-1, a failure mode that has a 1% chance of occurrence, a 1% chance of being detected, and a minor dosimetric error will have an RPN of about 96 to 112.

When choosing a process or piece of equipment to analyze, a process map can be used to understand the process or equipment. Then, all possible failure modes are imagined together with the occurrence, severity, and detection values. It is important to check the assumptions with others such as other physicists, therapists, physicians, dosimetrists, and nurses. The last step is to multiply values together for each failure mode and rank the RPN numbers. From there, one would address the failure modes by changing (re-engineering) the process or equipment and creating safety barriers. After implementing changes or adding safety barriers, a new FMEA can be performed and the RPN numbers can be correspondingly decreased.

FMEA is relatively straightforward to understand and implement. The O, S, and D values are not scientific, meaning that FMEA is not an exact science with an exact answer. One should not worry about getting it correct. The important thing is to complete the project and start with something simple and small. It is also important to take action on the results and revisit the analysis after subsequent events.

Example 20-3

Perform an FMEA on the process of HDR brachytherapy.
1 Begin by creating a process map of some form. We have used the cause and effects diagram type of process map.

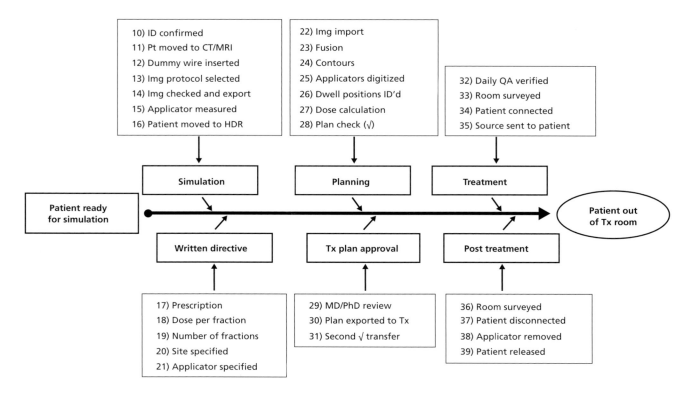

2 Define the failure modes and the effects of the failure modes.
3 Establish the O, S, and D values.
4 Calculate the RPNs.

Table 20-2 illustrates RPNs for some of the steps on the process of high-dose rate (HDR) brachytherapy.

FMEA has been successfully applied to radiotherapy in a number of areas.[42–47] However, even though FMEA is straightforward to understand and use, it does have some shortcomings. It relies somewhat on the assumption that the likelihood of errors is linearly proportional to the RPN value, namely, that if one decreases the RPN value for a failure mode, the system is proportionally safer. Therefore, uncertainty in the probabilities can limit the effectiveness of an FMEA. Traditional hazard models do not consider issues for which the probability of failure is difficult to estimate reliably. This includes effects of organizational culture, effects of process changes over time, and computer software failures. Hazard models based on systems theory have been developed as a more robust hazard analysis to get around the shortcomings of the probabilistic chain of event hazard models.[48] One such method is known as *systems theoretic process analysis* (STPA) and is a deductive method based on systems theory. In this method, safety is posed as a system control problem rather than a component failure problem.[49]

Retrospective analysis

Chance plays a part in accident causation. The apparent sporadic nature of errors is largely a matter of perspective; from a far

(e.g., an administrator's view), errors seem to arise sporadically. But from a close-up view of a department's operations, errors are actually predictable. RCA is used to understand and mitigate the predictable aspects of an error after an error or near-miss has occurred. The goal of an RCA is to explain the event, predict how it could happen in the future, and then propose and implement mitigation strategies to prevent it from happening again.

An RCA consists of four simple steps:

1 Collect information: identify what happened.
2 Identify causes: postulate why it happened.
3 Propose recommendations for remediation: ensure it does not happen again.
4 Implement the solution and monitor for effectiveness.

Collecting relevant information is critical to performing an effective RCA. Besides process maps, which were previously discussed, the tools of brainstorming and 5-whys are useful when performing an RCA. Brainstorming is a method for a group of people to generate a large number of ideas in a short period of time. In a typical brainstorming session, a group of people gather in a room. The brainstorming session starts with a statement of the topic or problem being discussed then the discussion ensues. A designated note taker and moderator are identified. The basic rules of a brainstorming session are to capture ideas without criticism or discussion about the significance of the idea. All ideas are recorded, typically on a whiteboard or easel pad, and there are no bad ideas in a brainstorming session. Expanding, combining, or modifying any ideas brought forward is allowed. The technique of 5-whys is the simple procedure of asking why four or five times as to the cause of an error or near-miss to force an

Table 20-1 The FMEA scales for the probability of occurrence (a), probability of detection (b), and severity (c).

(a)

Frequency	Qualitative	Occurrence Value (O)
1/10,000	Failure unlikely	1
2/10,000		2
5/10,000	Relatively few failures	3
1/10,000		4
<0.2%		5
<0.5%	Occasional failures	6
<1%		7
<2%	Repeated failures	8
<5%		9
>5%	Failure inevitable	10

(b)

Estimated probability of going undetected (%)	Detection Value (D)
0.01	1
0.2	2
0.5	3
1.0	4
2.0	5
5.0	6
10	7
15	8
20	9
>20	10

(c)

Qualitative	Categorization	Severity Value (S)
No effect		1
Inconvenience	Inconvenience	2
		3
Minor dosimetric error	Suboptimal plan or treatment	4
Limited toxicity or under-dose	Wrong dose, dose distribution, location or volume	5
		6
Potentially serious toxicity or under-dose		7
		8
Possible very serious toxicity	Very wrong dose, dose distribution, location or volume	9
Catastrophic		10

in-depth analysis. At each successive question, the group probes either deeper or laterally as to possible reasons why an event has occurred. The answers are recorded, analyzed, and categorized as part of the RCA.

There are characteristics of recurrent accidents. For example, consider an error of patient setup for a treatment in the thorax (e.g., treatment for spinal cord compression). Environment-specific characteristics must be considered, such as the fact that the error happened at the treatment machine, and characteristics of the task or work area must be considered. In this example, characteristics of the task would be treatment around the thoracic spine and the software that is used to review the images and setup. In addition, broader issues related to organizational issues must be considered, such as the culture of operations and whether physicians or other support staff are required to review the images in a timely manner. All characteristics need to be considered in an effective RCA.

Initially, it is important to focus on Step 1, identifying what happened rather than why it happened. A narrative can be helpful. Brainstorming can generate a large number of ideas in a short time at this step. Process maps can provide a description of the separate steps in the process. In Step 2, one should identify causes; focusing on the why. Tools to help are brainstorming and 5-whys. Next, one should provide recommendations to mitigate future events of the same type (Step 3). Coming up with optimal solutions requires domain experts. One should focus on low-cost, high-impact solutions that are within the domain experts' sphere of influence.[50] The last step of an RCA is to implement and monitor the solution(s). RCA is best used in conjunction with an ILS (see next section) to determine and monitor the effectiveness of the solutions. As previously discussed, issues to be aware of are confirmation bias and hindsight bias when performing an RCA. The point is to keep an open mind so that several possible causes of an error or near-miss are uncovered. Once a possible mitigation strategy has been identified and implemented, it is important to remember that the mitigation strategy might not get it right, so any solution should be monitored with an ILS and one should be prepared to try another solution if the one implemented is not working.

Table 20-2 RPN values for some of the steps in the process of HDR brachytherapy.

Process Step	Potential Failure Mode	Effect of Failure Mode	O	S	D	RPN
34) Patient connected	Wrong channels connected	Wrong dose delivered	10	9	10	900
27) Dose calculated	Wrong Rx entered in TPS	Wrong dose delivered	7	10	8	560
9) Applicator inserted	Wrong applicator documented	Wrong dose delivered	7	7	8	392
25) Applicators digitized	Wrong channel, wrong length	Geographical miss	9	8	5	360
27) Dose calculated	Wrong reference point	Wrong dose delivered	9	9	4	324
35) Source sent to patient	Patient dislodges applicator	Geographical miss	2	10	9	180
23) Fusion	Incorrect fusion	Wrong dose delivered	4	6	6	144
35) Source sent to patient	Patient kinks guide tubes	Source gets stuck—Overdose	5	9	2	90
37) Patient disconnected	Device forcibly removed	Patient trauma	7	7	1	49
22) Image import	Wrong data set	Geographical miss	1	6	5	30

Incident learning

Over the course of this chapter, it should be clear that accidents happen in the context of a complex, dynamic process and are not simply a sequence of chain of failure events. Interactions among humans, machines, and the environment constitute a complex, dynamic environment. The purpose of an ILS is to capture, categorize, and troubleshoot errors and near-misses, leading to overall quality improvement and a positive worker experience. An optimally run ILS can also provide insight into processes and guide resource and effort allocation as well as whether quality and safety interventions are working.

Incident learning systems

An ILS is any methodology to capture information about errors and near-misses for the purpose of analyzing data and developing mitigation strategies to prevent future occurrences. An ILS works by people entering information pertaining to an error or near-miss shortly after it has occurred. A department structure needs to be in place to effectively deal with the data coming into an ILS. A taxonomy, which is simply a standardized terminology to facilitate communication, needs to be established in order to properly handle and categorize the data that is entered.[51] For example, the classification of causal factors is part of a safety taxonomy. The taxonomy also needs to include a severity scoring scale so events can be classified consistently as to the severity of an incident. Several reports of ILSs from around the world have appeared for radiotherapy.[52–57]

In the development of an optimal ILS, it is important that all levels of department leadership support a reporting culture (to be discussed in the next section) and actively promote and support incident learning. Reporting of errors and near-misses should be an integral component of the departmental operations and safety improvement efforts. The actual reporting process should require minimal time and effort for initial reporters and should be designed to be used within the busy clinical environment. Feedback to the department on disposition of their reports and corrective actions should be provided routinely. The ILS should be used to proactively monitor effectiveness of corrective actions. Lastly, to be most effective, all faculty and staff in the department need to participate in reporting errors and near-misses. It has been reported that physician and physician-trainees are significantly less likely to report errors than others in the department.[58]

Learning from errors and near-misses requires explicit support from department leadership. The learning process must include a system for reporting, as well as guidelines for sharing data and providing feedback. Those assigned to review and resolve errors should have the competence to interpret reported data, the ability to make process changes, and the ability to reinforce the appropriate organizational culture.[59]

To summarize, benefits of using an ILS include learning to focus safety efforts in the department, understand which mitigation strategies are working, and disseminate information about errors and near-misses to raise awareness that errors are always possible no matter how well defended a department is and how robust a safety culture is about errors. Longer-term benefits afforded by the consistent use of an ILS are to understand how seemingly small issues can lead to larger problems and also to reveal patterns of cause and effect around errors.

Organizational culture

Organizational culture refers to the shared values and shared beliefs to produce behavioral norms. *Shared values* indicate what is important and *shared beliefs* refer to how things work. There is no single measure of a department's safety health. However, continued efforts toward defining measures for safety assessment are on-going.[60]

The different components of organizational culture are a safety culture, a reporting culture, and a just culture. All cultures are built from the top down and must be driven by department leadership. A safety culture is the explicit declaration from leadership that safety is a priority for the department. The caveat is that the decisions of leadership should reinforce the commitment to safety rather than subvert it. For example, urgently starting cases without proper support goes against an optimal safety culture. A simple start to building a safety culture is to create a declaration from leadership about how the department values safety.

Example 20-4

Create a four-point safety declaration for your department.
   A simple four-point safety declaration is:
1 All injuries and accidents are preventable.
2 We will not compromise safety to achieve any other objective.
3 Every member of the department has a responsibility for patient safety.
4 Department members will be empowered to stop and report any unsafe conditions.

A reporting culture requires an efficient method to submit all event types and an indemnity against retribution for reporting. There are ways this can be facilitated, for example, by separating the data collection from those with authority to discipline. An effective reporting culture also includes feedback to the radiation oncology department in order to keep everyone engaged in the system and realizing its benefits. A just culture is different from a safety or reporting culture. In a just culture, it is recognized that not all errors result from acceptable actions and that blanket immunity sends the wrong message to staff. Performance standards and expectations of behavior need to be established and department members should be expected to perform to those standards. Disciplinary action is still warranted if department members do not perform to those standards.

In the 1960s and 1970s, the human resources department of IBM's European headquarters investigated the ways in which cultures differ from one another. One of the cultural aspects investigated was to determine the extent that less powerful members of organizations and institutions accept and expect that power is distributed unequally. One result of this work was to find that the social norms in which people are raised play a significant role in how they think and work even if they do not explicitly realize it.[61] This is known as the *power distance index* (PDI). High-PDI cultures have poor communication between those in authority and the regular workers compared to low-PDI cultures. The PDI can have a negative impact on safety by limiting communications.

Low-PDI cultures are more *transmitter oriented*, in which it is considered the responsibility of the speaker to communicate ideas clearly and unambiguously. High-PDI cultures are more *receiver oriented*, which means that it is up to the listener to make sense of what is being said. High-PDI communication can be effective when the listener is capable of paying close attention, and if the two parties in a conversation have time to decipher the correspondence. In 1994, Boeing first published safety data showing a clear correlation between a country's plane crashes and its ranking on cultural dimensions including PDI.[62] A version of transmitter/receiver-orientated communications can exist in micro-environments of a department or even person-to-person exchanges (e.g., physicians to therapists).

A department's commitment is not enough to make a successful safety program. The department should include competence and cognizance related to safety, that is, education on safety and awareness that errors are always possible. From a leadership perspective, targets cannot be set on the number of errors or near-misses since the stochastic nature of errors (as seen at the level of department leadership) means that errors are not controllable. Therefore, the optimal organizational strategy is to consistently focus on the department's long-term safety fitness program. Effective safety management requires the use of both reactive and proactive measures. In combination, they provide information about the state of the defenses and about the systemic and workplace factors known to contribute to bad outcomes.

Quality improvement

To assess and improve quality in health care, it has been found helpful to consider health care in the three broad areas of structure, process, and outcome.[63] The structure aspect encompasses the adequacy of facilities, the credentials of staff, and the administrative organization. The process aspect entails the appropriateness of care, including issues such as the thoroughness of physical exams and diagnostic tests, the technical competence with which procedures are performed, and the medical justification for tests and therapies administered. The outcome aspect is gauged in terms of recovery, restoration of function, and survival. The problem with outcome-based metrics is that poor quality can be camouflaged as complications in radiotherapy. The issue is how to make operational aspects of quality related to structure, process, and outcome.

To ensure quality improvement, a broader approach must be taken than just verifying the technical aspects.[64] An accessible structured approach to data-based quality improvement using a wide variety of tools and techniques tied to the goals of department leadership including overall time and/or cost savings for the department needs to be implemented. Different paradigms of quality improvement have been developed for this purpose. Simple strategies exist to engage all levels of department leadership. This approach is known generally as *total quality management* (TQM), which was developed by the U.S. Navy to improve quality and productivity performance.[65] The TQM system includes four critical concepts: (1) quality is defined by customers' requirements, (2) top management has direct responsibility for quality improvement, (3) increased quality comes from systematic analysis and improvement of work processes, and (4) quality improvement is a continuous effort and conducted throughout the organization. The TQM strategy developed by the U.S. Navy relied in part on the *plan–do–study–act* (PDSA) quality improvement cycle. The first development of the PDSA appeared as the Shewhart cycle.[66] The PDSA as it is known today was described by W. Edwards Deming in 1993.[67] This is sometimes called *plan–do–check–act* (PDCA), but these are essentially the same. A newer paradigm, known as *six-sigma*, was developed in 1986[40] and is sometimes combined with a related methodology called *lean*, resulting in *lean/six-sigma*. All of these methodologies are meant to apply the scientific method to quality improvement. The keys to success are protected time for participants and to make use of guided problem solving. The most difficult parts of any quality improvement strategy are data collection and analysis.

Plan–do–study–act

The PDSA methodology is meant to describe a continuous improvement cycle, as shown in Figure 20-3. PDSA is a simple, perhaps obvious, methodology for quality improvement. The PDSA cycle originates from statistical process control work in the 1920s by Walter Shewhart.[66] It was then introduced to Japan after World War II by W. Edwards Deming.[67] The main idea of PDSA is to create structured quality improvement.

Act   Plan

Study   Do

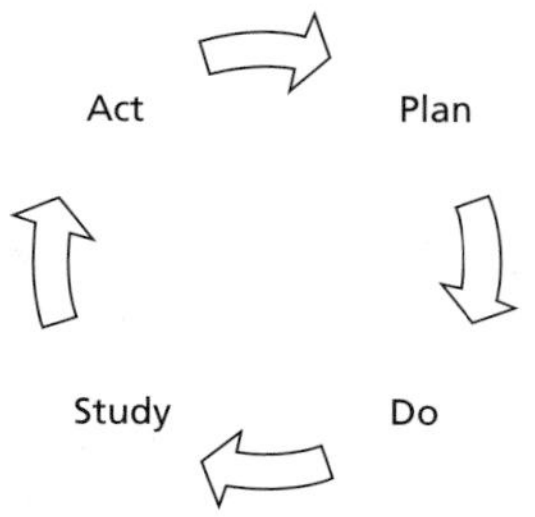

Figure 20-3 Plan–do–study–act cycle for quality improvement.

The first step in the cycle is to create the *plan*, which involves identifying the goal or purpose of the quality improvement initiative, defining metrics, and proposing a method to carry out the quality improvement initiative. This is followed by the *do* step, which is the implementation of the plan. The third step of the PDSA cycle is *study*. In this step, data from the metrics are evaluated to see whether the plan is having the intended outcome. The fourth and last step is *act*, which is either to implement the plan and make it part of routine processes or to modify the plan if it was found that it was not having the intended effect. The four steps of the PDSA cycle are repeated as part of a continuous cycle of quality improvement.

Six-sigma and lean

Bill Smith, an engineer at Motorola, created six-sigma in the 1980s as a TQM spinoff and a better way to achieve continuous quality improvement. Similar to the PDSA cycle, six-sigma is a data-based approach to quality improvement. Six-sigma has its own mnemonic: DMAIC, which stands for *define, measure, analyze, improve, control*. A host of tools can be systematically applied at each step. Six-sigma explicitly ties quality improvement initiatives to financial accountability and department leadership.

Six-sigma originally referred to a manufacturing process that produced no more than 3.4 defects per million parts. The number comes from assuming a normal distribution to describe process variability and a process drift of ± 1.5 standard deviations. A one-sided integration under the normal curve beyond 4.5 standard deviations results in an area of about 3.4/1,000,000. Although defective parts per million does not have a direct application in radiation therapy, the six-sigma methodology can be very effective for quality improvement since it provides the tools to improve to perform quality improvement initiatives.

The six-sigma approach has been developed and implemented in radiotherapy[68] and in particular as a "no-fly" policy[69]. In this implementation, a checklist-based approach to stopping the work if it is not completed before going to the next step was developed and implemented. This resulted in demonstrable improvements in workflow standardization where slip days (defined as delays in task completion) were reduced from 4.6 days to 1.0 days. More importantly is that the standard deviation of the slip-day metric decreased from 16.2 days to 4.7 days, which indicates a significant improvement in standardized practice. The DMAIC is a useful way to apply the scientific method to quality improvement.

Lean was developed from the Toyota production system around the 1950s. Lean, frequently used together with six-sigma, is a methodology focused on eliminating waste in a process. The lean methodology includes the specification of the value desired by the customer. Then the value stream for the process is identified, which is the interrogation of the process for wasted steps. In this effort, the process should flow continuously (e.g., no workarounds) and, if possible, each successive step should create pull from one step to the next. Lean is focused on eliminating waste and creating naturally occurring efficiencies, while six-sigma is focused on ensuring that quality is maintained in the process. Lean techniques have been used to streamline the treatment of patients referred for radiation treatment of bone and brain metastasis.[70] Initially, a current state value stream map is created of the process of radiation treatment of bone and brain metastasis. The second step is to create a future state value stream map that contains a very different series of process steps that allows the treatments to happen sooner, using fewer resources and without additional errors. The final step is to create a detailed work plan for implementing future state map to make that proposed process a reality. The result is a much more efficient process of getting patients treated. Before the lean event, 27 steps were required to get a patient treated in the same day as the referral, and after the lean event, 16 steps were required. Lean must be used properly to have the most beneficial effects. After all, it is easy to make a process so lean and efficient that it becomes unstable and prone to error.

Process control

As discussed in the previous section, quality and quality improvement initiatives need to be data-driven to be effective. However, QA tests must allow for reasonable judgment of next actions based on the results as there can be adverse effects when strict QA guidelines interrupt patient treatment. A quality-improvement program must be able to allow normal fluctuations in measured values to detect problematic errors, but not to shut down treatment due to a statistical fluctuation that may require monitoring. For example, daily linear accelerator output checks have limits of acceptability within which patients can continue to be treated. How to address the issue of random process fluctuations is the domain of process control. Furthermore, a defense in depth error mitigation strategy works only for stable and predictable processes. It is the goal of process control (also known as *statistical process control*, or SPC) to provide the tools to create and maintain stable and predictable processes using data acquired from the process as would be obtained in the "do" and "measure" steps of the PDSA and DMAIC methodologies, respectively.

Quality and process variation

It is most desirable for process variation to remain within acceptable levels, that is, to not cross beyond defined action limits. A long-held tenet in industrial and systems engineering is that optimal quality is defined as process performance being on-target with minimum variance. Control charts were created specifically to provide workers with a tool to achieve optimal quality.[71] The goal of quality improvement is to reduce process variation to be within the action limits. Action limits in healthcare are set by clinical experience so that variation of a specified parameter outside the action limits is likely to cause harm to a patient. Once process variation is well within action limits, it is difficult to achieve further quality improvement for that process without redesigning how the work is done. Continued effort to reduce process variation toward zero has an opportunity cost of not allowing focusing on other areas for improvement. After process variation is well within action limits, it is advisable for one to monitor the process to ensure that the process remains stable. One aspect of quality management is to specify which processes are undergoing active improvement efforts and which processes require only monitoring.

Use and interpretation of control charts

When analyzing data from a process, it is important to determine whether each data point is outside the limits of normal random variation in the process. Control charts were invented for this purpose.[71] In process control methodology, two charts are defined to achieve this purpose. One chart provides a measure of location for the data and one provides a measure of dispersion for the data. Each chart has statistically determined upper and lower limits that define random versus non-random process behavior. If the data acquired over a period of time are within the limits, then the process that created the data is considered stable, that is, in control. Otherwise, the process is considered out of control and needs to be stabilized.

Several applications of control charts have been used in radiotherapy.[72-79] These have mostly been related to the QA of technical parameters, but the charts can be equally applied to process-oriented quality improvement projects. In this section, the concept of control chart is explained. For simplicity, only the development of the chart for individual values (I-Chart) is covered. The I-Chart can be used for all continuous data and is simple to understand and implement. The limits are insensitive to the distribution of data being analyzed.

A control chart is a longitudinal plot of data with an upper control limit (UCL), lower control limit (LCL), and centerline (CL). For a quality indicator, the charts are calculated for $\mu \pm \sigma$. The process mean, μ, is estimated by the average and this becomes the CL. The sample standard deviation, s, is a biased estimator of σ so that $\sigma = mR/d_2$ is used where d_2 is a bias correction factor.[80] The quantity $2.660 \cdot \overline{mR}$ is an estimator of s and $d_2 = 1.128$ for the case when $n = 1$. The control limits are calculated using the following recipe:

1 Calculate the CL using as the average of a portion of the data:

$$CL = \bar{x} = \frac{1}{n}\sum_{j=1}^{n} x$$

2 Calculate the moving range, mR, and then the average moving range, $\overline{mR}$, over the data used to calculate the CL:

$$\overline{mR} = \frac{1}{n-1}\sum mR = \frac{1}{n-1}\sum_{j=2}^{n}\left|x_j - x_{j-1}\right|$$

3 Calculate the UCL:

$$UCL = CL + 2.660 \cdot \overline{mR}$$

4 Calculate the LCL:

$$LCL = CL - 2.660 \cdot \overline{mR}$$

5 Plot the data, CL, UCL, and LCL on the I-Chart.

The control limits and CL are point binominal estimates and therefore have a statistical uncertainty associated with them. However, this uncertainty is not typically incorporated in the use of the charts for process analysis and quality improvement.

A step-by-step example of how to create an I-Chart is described below (courtesy of TreatSafety, LLC). The process of treatment planning throughput is investigated. In the example, each of two physicians is asked to approve a treatment plan after the plan has been completed by a dosimetrist. The data gathered are the interval from the time the plan is completed by the dosimetrist to the time the physician approves the plan for treatment. The requirements (clinical action limits) for this process is for plan approval to be completed within 25 hours from the time the dosimetrist completes the plan. The data for two physicians are shown in Table 20-3.

The I-Charts for physicians #1 and #2 are shown in Figure 20-4 and Figure 20-5. The LCLs are both set to zero since that

Table 20-3 Data for the duration of time it takes two physicians (Physician #1 and Physician #2) to approve a treatment plan after it is completed by the dosimetrist. The duration, x, is measured in hours and the moving range, mR, is calculated from the duration.

Case Number	Physician #1		Physician #2	
	x (hrs)	mR (hrs)	x (hrs)	mR (hrs)
1	24.48	—	8.47	—
2	1.75	22.73	10.02	1.55
3	4.88	3.13	35.22	25.20
4	9.18	4.30	0.97	34.25
5	9.78	0.60	2.60	1.63
6	8.58	1.20	5.42	2.82
7	0.00	8.58	2.58	2.84
8	0.07	0.07	0.48	2.10
9	8.85	8.78	0.92	0.44
10	12.35	3.50	5.30	4.38
11	22.23	9.88	9.15	3.85
12	20.60	1.63	14.78	5.63
13	13.62	6.98	0.93	13.85
14	2.40	11.22	29.55	28.62
15	3.75	1.35	1.43	28.12
16	1.53	2.22	2.95	1.52
17	0.20	1.33	6.68	3.73
18	7.20	7.00	14.05	7.37
19	11.70	4.50	25.48	11.43
20	4.85	6.85	5.53	19.95
21	7.18	2.33	11.62	6.09
22	2.83	4.35	22.48	10.86
23	0.00	2.83	10.73	11.75
24	21.70	21.7	35.45	24.72
25	11.67	10.03	11.70	23.75
26	2.90	8.77	11.40	0.30

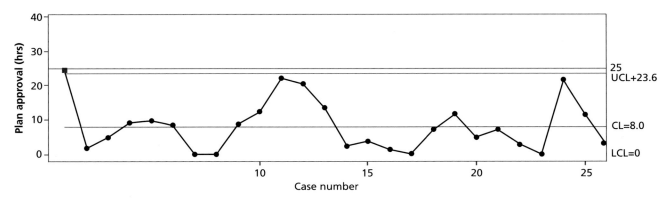

Figure 20-4 I-Chart for Physician #1.

is a limit of the process (i.e., there cannot be a negative plan turnaround time). The first 10 cases are used to calculate the CL and UCL. The process requirement of 25 hours is also shown in the figures.

The charts are used in the following way to understand process performance for the two physicians. The performance of Physician #1 lies within the process requirements because the UCL is equal to 23.6 hours, which is less than 25 hours. The process of Physician #1 is said to be in control. Physician #2 is performing outside the process requirements (UCL > 25 hours) and the process of Physician #2 is said to be an out-of-control process. In practice, after the first 10 data points and the control limits were calculated, each case would be plotted and monitored for out-of-control behavior (i.e., point outside the control limits). Therefore, cases 14 and 24 for Physician #2 would be investigated for opportunities to identify and fix any causes for the out-of-control behavior. Conversely, case 19 is outside the 25-hour process requirement but inside the control limits and is within the noise of the system so it is not likely to find a cause for this case to be outside the process requirements.

Cases would continue to be plotted on the charts. The CL and UCL would only be recalculated if there was a process change (either by removing a systematic cause or by re-engineering the process). When comparing the control limits to the process

requirements, four states and related actions should be taken from a quality perspective. The four states are:[81]

1 Process is in control and control limits are within process requirements. Action: Continue monitoring process indefinitely.

2 Process is in control and control limits are outside of process requirements. Action: Re-engineer process or widen process requirements.

3 Process is out of control and control limits are within action limits. Action: Analyze process and remove systematic causes of variation.

4 Process is out of control and control limits are outside of process requirements. Action: Analyze process and re-commission and/or re-engineer process.

Other quality tools can be helpful, for example, when a point is out of control, one may perform an RCA to find out why. Process mapping and value stream mapping can also be useful. When the process is out of control and the control limits are outside of process requirements, one should better understand the process and any reasons that the process is changing; FMEA and a review of incident learning error logs may be helpful. The conclusions derived from the use of control charts should confirm subject matter knowledge and experience. Several other types of control charts for specific processes or specific data types can

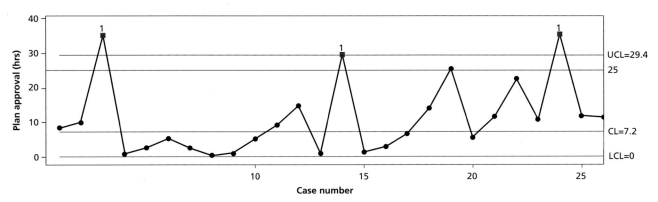

Figure 20-5 I-Chart for Physician #2.

be used and are mentioned below.[81] For processes that create a large amount of data in a short period of time (e.g., from real-time linear accelerator beam steering data), subgroup average and standard deviation charts are appropriate, whereas number or fraction non-conforming parts are better addressed by p-, np-, c-, or u-charts. The charts mentioned thus far are good for detecting large changes in process performance. To detect slow drifts of a process, either *exponentially weighted moving average* (EWMA) or *cumulative sum* (CUSUM) charts are appropriate. Once statistical control is achieved then process improvement can take place, defined as either minimizing variation or moving the average closer to the optimum value or both.

Summary

- Human biases related to patient safety have been presented, such as confirmation bias and hindsight bias.
- There are many different aids to mitigate human biases that can lead to errors. Aids presented are process maps, checklists, and no-interruption zones.
- Failure modes and effects analysis (FMEA) is a prospective risk assessment tool.
- Root cause analysis (RCA) is a retrospective risk assessment tool.
- The components of an incident learning system (ILS) include a reporting culture, a method for filing reports, knowledgeable people to review data, and feedback to the reporters.
- The plan–do–study–act quality improvement paradigm is known as *PDSA* and used for quality-improvement efforts.
- Six-sigma is another quality improvement methodology that uses the *define, measure, analyze, improve, control* mnemonic (DMAIC). It is also data-based and requires the direct input from department leadership as well as financial accountability for the quality improvement project.
- Process variation should be controlled to create a predictable process.
- Process control is the procedure of using control charts for process data analysis.
- Individual control charts (I-Charts) are one type of control chart that can be used to analyze any type of continuous data.

Problems

20-1 Explain confirmation bias and hindsight bias. Where or when might these human biases be relevant?

20-2 If you were using the process map in Example 20-2 to troubleshoot patient setup problems, what other steps might you include in the process map that would need to be investigated? You can add boxes or steps in addition to the process steps shown in the example.

20-3 Create a process map for a clinical process. Ask a colleague to create a process map for the same clinical process but on their own. Compare the two maps. What can you conclude?

20-4 What does FMEA and RPN stand for? Describe FMEA in your own words.

20-5 On your own, perform an FMEA on the patient setup in the treatment room using the process map of Example 20-2. In particular, assume the treatment is a conventionally fractionated VMAT prostate, the setup image is a CBCT, which is compared to the treatment planning CT. Focus on the step "Setup acceptable?" What is your highest RPN value? What might you do to reduce the RPN value?

20-6 List the steps of a root cause analysis (RCA).

20-7 What does *PDSA* and *DMAIC* stand for? What do these represent? How do PDSA and DMAIC differ?

20-8 Create an I-Chart for the following two data sets. Use the first five data points to calculate *CL*. What can you conclude about the processes that created these data, including a comparison to clinical limits of ± 5.0?

Case Number	Data Set 1	Data Set 2
1	0.00	1.39
2	0.50	−1.14
3	−0.25	−0.50
4	4.40	0.77
5	0.35	0.04
6	2.44	3.14
7	−0.86	1.93
8	3.52	4.23
9	−1.01	2.68
10	0.65	2.03

20-9 Choose a radiotherapy accident from the IAEA analyses found at https://rpop.iaea.org/RPOP/RPoP/Content/AdditionalResources/Publications/5_RadiologicalAccidents/index.htm. Then perform your own RCA on the accident.

References

1 Pawlicki, T., Dunscombe, P. B., Mundt, A. J., and Scalliet, P. *Quality and Safety in Radiotherapy*. Boca Raton, FL, CRC Press, 2011.

2 Munoz, M. I., Bouldi, N., Barcellini, F., and Nascimento, A. Designing the safety of healthcare: Participation of ergonomic to the design of cooperative systems in radiotherapy. *Work*. 2012; **41**(Suppl 1):790–796.

3 Chan, A. J., Islam, M. K., Rosewall, T., Jaffray, D. A., Easty, A. C., and Cafazzo, J. A. The use of human factors methods to identify and mitigate safety issues in radiation therapy. *Radiother. Oncol.* 2010; **97**(3):596–600.

4 Chan, A. J., Islam, M. K., Rosewall, T., Jaffray, D. A., Easty, A. C., Cafazzo, J. A. Applying usability heuristics to radiotherapy systems. *Radiother. Oncol.* 2012; **102**(1):142–147.

5 Rasmussen, J. Skills, rules, and knowledge: Signals, signs, and symbols, and other distinctions in human performance models. *IEEE Trans. Cybern.* 1983; **13**(3):257–266.

6 Leveson, N. G., and Turner, C. S. An investigation of the Therac-25 accidents. *IEEE Computer.* 1993; **26**(7):18–41.

7 Bogdanich, W. Radiation offers new cures, and ways to do harm. *New York Times*, 2010 (January 23), http://www.nytimes.com/2010/01/24/health/24radiation.html?pagewanted=all&_r=0, accessed September 15, 2015.

8 Reason, J. *The Human Contribution: Unsafe acts, accidents, and heroic recoveries.* Farnham, U. K., Ashgate Publishing, 2008.

9 Tversky, A., and Kahneman, D. Judgment under uncertainty: Heuristics and biases. *Science.* 1974; **185**(4157):1124–1131.

10 Battmann, W., and Klumb, P. Behavioural economics and compliance with safety regulations. *Safety Science.* 1993; **6**:35–46.

11 Ariely, D. *Predictably Irrational.* New York, HarperCollins, 2008.

12 Kahneman, D. *Thinking, Fast and Slow.* London, Macmillan, 2011.

13 Evans, J.S. Dual-processing accounts of reasoning, judgment, and social cognition. *Annu. Rev. Psychol.* 2008; **59**:255–278.

14 Ariely, D., and Norton, M. I. How actions create: Not just reveal: Preferences. *Trends Cogn. Sci.* 2008; **12**(1):13–16.

15 Johansson, P., Hall, L., Sikström, S., and Olsson, A. Failure to detect mismatches between intention and outcome in a simple decision task. *Science.* **310**(5745):116–119.

16 Fischhoff, B., and Beyth, R. I knew it would happen: Remembered probabilities of once-future things. *Organ. Behav. Hum. Perform.* 1975; **13**(1):1–16.

17 Henriksen, K., and Kaplan, H. Hindsight bias, outcome knowledge and adaptive learning. *Qual. Saf. Health Care.* 2003; **12**(Suppl II):ii46–ii50.

18 Koehler, J. J. The influence of prior beliefs on scientific judgments of evidence quality. *Organ. Behav. Hum. Decis. Process.* 1993; **56**:28–55.

19 Hart, S. G., and Staveland, L. E. Development of NASA-TLX (Task Load Index): Results of empirical and theoretical research. *Advances in Psychology.* 1988; **52**:139–183.

20 Mazur, L. M., Mosaly, P., Jackson, M., et al. Quantitative assessment of workload and stressors in clinical radiation oncology. *Int. J. Radiat. Oncol. Biol. Phys.* 2012; **83**(5):e571–e576.

21 Mazur, L. M., Mosaly, P. R., Hoyle, L. M., Jones, E. L., and Marks, L. B. Subjective and objective quantification of physician's workload and performance during radiation therapy planning tasks. *Pract. Radiat. Oncol.* 2013; **3**(4):e171–e177.

22 Mazur, L. M., Mosaly, P. R., Hoyle, L. M., Jones, E. L., Chera, B. S., and Marks, L. B. Relating physician's workload with errors during radiation therapy planning. *Pract. Radiat. Oncol.* 2014; **4**(2):71–75.

23 Reason, J. Beyond the organisational accident: The need for "error wisdom" on the frontline. *Qual. Saf. Health Care.* 2004; **13**(Suppl II):ii28–ii33.

24 Gawande, A. *The Checklist Manifesto: How to get things right.* New York, Metropolitan Books, 2010.

25 Levin, D. C. A surgical safety checklist to reduce morbidity and mortality in a global population (Letter to the Editor). *N. Engl. J. Med.* 2009; **360**(5):2374.

26 Miller, G. A. The magical number seven, plus or minus two: Some limits to our capacity for processing information. *Psychological Review.* 1956; **63**(2):84–97.

27 Breen, S. L., and Zhang, B. Audit of an automated checklist for quality control of radiotherapy treatment plans. *Radiother. Oncol.* 2010; **97**:579–584.

28 Fong de los Santos, L., Evans, S., Ford, E. C., et al. Medical physics practice guideline Task Group 4a: Development, implementation, use and maintenance of safety checklists. *J. Clin. Appl. Med. Phys.* 2015; **16**(3).

29 Meginniss, A., Damian, F., and Falvo, F. Time out for patient safety. *J. Emerg. Nurs.* 2012; **38**:51–53.

30 Gillespie, B. M., Chaboyer, W., Wallis, M., and Fenwick, C. Why isn't "time out" implemented? An exploratory study. *Qual. Saf. Health Care.* 2010; **19**:103–106.

31 Trbovich, P. L., Griffin, M. C., White, R. E., Bourrier, V., Dhaliwal, D., and Easty, A. C. The effects of interruptions on oncologists' patient assessment and medication ordering practices. *J. Healthc. Eng.* 2013; **4**(1):127–144.

32 Brundage, M. D., Dixon, P. F., Mackillop, W. J. *et al.* A real-time audit of radiation therapy in a regional cancer center. *Int. J. Radiat. Oncol. Biol. Phys.* 1999; **43**:115–124.

33 Boxer, M., Forstner, D., Kneebone, A. *et al.* Impact of a real-time peer-review audit on patient management in radiation oncology. *J. Med. Imaging Radiat. Oncol.* 2009; **53**:405–411.

34 Marks, L. B., Adams, R. D., Pawlicki, T., et al. Enhancing the role of case-oriented peer review to improve quality and safety in radiation oncology: Executive summary. *Pract. Radiat. Oncol.* 2013; **3**:149–156.

35 Halvorsen, P. H., Das, I. J., Fraser, M., et al. AAPM Task Group 103 report on peer review in clinical radiation oncology physics. *J. Clin. Appl. Med. Phys.* 2005; **6**(4):50–64.

36 Lawrence, Y. R., Whiton, M. A., Symon, Z., et al. Quality Assurance Peer Review Charts Rounds in 2011: A survey of academic institutions in the United States. *Int. J. Radiat. Oncol. Biol. Phys.* 2012; **84**(3):590–595.

37 Hoopes, D. J., Johnstone, P. A., Chapin, P. S., et al. Practice patterns for peer review in radiation oncology. *Pract. Radiat. Oncol.* 2015; **5**:32–38.

38 Tucker, A. L., and Edmondson, A. C. Why hospitals don't learn from errors: Organizational and psychological dynamics that inhibit system change. *Calif. Manage. Rev.* 2003; **45**:55–72.

39 Banja, J. The normalization of deviance in healthcare delivery. *Bus. Horiz.* 2010; **53**(2):139–152.

40 Tague, N. R. *The Quality Toolbox.* Milwaukee, WI, ASQ Quality Press, 2005.

41 Thomadsen, B., Brown, D., Ford, E., Huq, M. S., and Rath, F. Risk assessment using the TG-100 methodology. In B. Thomadsen, P. Dunscombe, E. Ford, S. Huq, T. Pawlicki, and S. Sutlief (eds.). *Quality and safety in radiotherapy: Learning the new approaches in task group 100 and beyond. Med. Phys. Monograph.* 2013; **36**:95–112.

42 Ford, E. C., Gaudette, R., Myers, L., et al. Evaluation of safety in a radiation oncology setting using failure mode and effects analysis. *Int. J. Radiat. Oncol. Biol. Phys.* 2009; **74**(3):852–858.

43 Ciocca, M., Cantone, M. C., Veronese, I., et al. Application of failure mode and effects analysis to intraoperative radiation therapy using mobile electron linear accelerators. *Int. J. Radiat. Oncol. Biol. Phys.* 2012; **82**(2):e305–e311.

44 Perks, J. R., Stanic, S., Stern, R. L., et al. Failure mode and effect analysis for delivery of lung stereotactic body radiation therapy. *Int. J. Radiat. Oncol. Biol. Phys.* 2012; **83**(4):1324–1329.

45 Denny, D. S., Allen, D. K., Worthington, N., and Gupta, D. The use of failure mode and effect analysis in a radiation oncology setting: The Cancer Treatment Centers of America experience. *J. Healthc. Qual.* 2014; **36**(1):18–28.

46 Ford, E. C., Smith, K., Terezakis, S., et al. A streamlined failure mode and effects analysis. *Med. Phys.* 2014; **41**(6):061709.

47 Masini, L., Donis, L., Loi, G., et al. Application of failure mode and effects analysis to intracranial stereotactic radiation surgery by linear accelerator. *Pract. Radiat. Oncol.* 2014; **4**(6):392–397.

48 Leveson, N. A new accident model for engineering safer systems. *Safety Science.* 2004; **42**:237–270.

49 Leveson, N. *Engineering a Safer World: Systems thinking applied to safety.* Cambridge, MA, MIT Press, 2012.

50 Jing, G. G. Flip the switch: Root cause analysis can shine the spotlight on the origin of a problem. *Quality Progress.* 2008; **October**:50–55.

51 Ford, E. C., Fong de Los Santos, L., Pawlicki, T., Sutlief, S., and Dunscombe, P. Consensus recommendations for incident learning database structures in radiation oncology. *Med. Phys.* 2012; **39**(12):7272–7290.

52 Ford, E. C., Smith, K., Harris, K., and Terezakis, S. Prevention of a wrong-location misadministration through the use of an intradepartmental incident learning system. *Med. Phys.* 2012; **39**(11):6968–6971.

53 Terezakis, S. A., Harris, K. M., Ford, E., et al. An evaluation of departmental radiation oncology incident reports: Anticipating a national reporting system. *Int. J. Radiat. Oncol. Biol. Phys.* 2013; **85**(4):919–923.

54 Clark, B. G., Brown, R. J., Ploquin, J., and Dunscombe. P. Patient safety improvements in radiation treatment through 5 years of incident learning. *Pract. Radiat. Oncol.* 2013; **3**(3):157–163.

55 Yang, R., Wang, J., Zhang, X., et al. Implementation of incident learning in the safety and quality management of radiotherapy: The primary experience in a new established program with advanced technology. *Biomed. Res. Int.* 2014; 392596.

56 Kusano, A. S., Nyflot, M. J., Zeng, J., et al. Measurable improvement in patient safety culture: A departmental experience with incident learning. *Pract. Radiat. Oncol.* 2014; **5**(3):e229–e237.

57 Rahn, D. A. 3rd, Kim, G. Y., Mundt, A. J., and Pawlicki, T. A real-time safety and quality reporting system: Assessment of clinical data and staff participation. *Int. J. Radiat. Oncol. Biol. Phys.* 2014; **90**(5):1202–1207.

58 Smith, K. S., Harris, K. M., Potters, L., et al. Physician attitudes and practices related to voluntary error and near-miss reporting. *J. Oncol. Pract.* 2014; **10**(5):e350–e3577.

59 Frankel, A. S., Leonard, M. W., and Denham, C. R. Fair and just culture, team behavior, and leadership engagement: The tools to achieve high reliability. *Health. Serv. Res.* 2006; **41**(4 Pt 2):1690–1708.

60 Austin, J. M., D'Andrea, G., Birkmeyer, J. D., et al. Safety in numbers: The development of leapfrog's composite patient safety score for U.S. hospitals. *J. Patient Saf.* 2014; **10**:64–71.

61 Hofstede, G. *Culture's Consequences: International differences in work-related values.* New York, Sage Publications, 1980.

62 Gladwell, M. *Outliers.* New York, Little, Brown and Company, 2008.

63 Donabedian, A. Evaluating the quality of medical care. *Milbank Memorial Fund Q.* 1966; **44**:166–206.

64 Kehoe, T., and Rugg, L.-J. From technical quality assurance of radiotherapy to a comprehensive quality of service management system. *Radiother. Oncol.* 1999; **51**:281–290.

65 Houston, A. *A Total Quality Management Process Improvement Model.* San Diego, California: Navy Personnel Research and Development Center, pp. vii–viii, OCLC 21243646, AD-A202 154, 1988.

66 Shewhart, W. A. *Statistical Method from the Viewpoint of Quality Control.* Washington, D. C., Dover Publications, 1939.

67 Deming, W. E. *The New Economics.* Cambridge, MA, MIT Press, 1993.

68 Kapur, A., and Potters, L. Six sigma tools for a patient safety-oriented, quality-checklist driven radiation medicine department. *Pract. Radiat. Oncol.* 2012; **2**(2):86–96.

69 Potters, L., and Kapur, A. Implementation of a "no fly" safety culture in a multicenter radiation medicine department. *Pract. Radiat. Oncol.* 2012; **2**:18–26.

70 Kim, C. S., Hayman, J. A., Billi, J. E., Lash, K., and Lawrence, T. S. The application of lean thinking to the care of patients with bone and brain metastasis with radiation therapy. *J. Oncol. Practice.* 2007; **3**(4):189–193.

71 Shewhart, W. A. *Statistical Methods from the Viewpoint of Quality Control.* New York, Dover Publications, 1986.

72 Pawlicki, T., Whitaker, M., and Boyer, A. L. Statistical process control for radiotherapy quality assurance. *Med. Phys.* 2005; **32**(9):2777–2786.

73 Breen, S. L., Moseley, D. J., Zhang, B., and Sharpe, M. B. Statistical process control for IMRT dosimetric verification. *Med. Phys.* 2008; **35**(10):4417–4425.

74 Gérard, K., Grandhaye, J. P., Marchesi, V., Kafrouni, H., Husson, F., and Aletti P. A comprehensive analysis of the IMRT dose delivery process using statistical process control (SPC). *Med. Phys.* 2009; **36**(4):1275–1285.

75 Ung, N. M., and Wee, L. Fiducial registration error as a statistical process control metric in image-guidance radiotherapy with fiducial markers. *Phys. Med. Biol.* 2011; **56**(23):7473–7485.

76 Nordström, F., af Wetterstedt, S., Johnsson, S., Ceberg, C., and Bäck, S. J. Control chart analysis of data from a multicenter monitor unit verification study. *Radiother. Oncol.* 2012; **102**(3):364–370.

77 Sanghangthum, T., Suriyapee, S., Srisatit, S., and Pawlicki, T. Retrospective analysis of linear accelerator output constancy checks using process control techniques. *J. Appl. Clin. Med. Phys.* 2013; **14**(1):4032.

78 Sanghangthum, T., Suriyapee, S., Kim, G. Y., and Pawlicki, T. A method of setting limits for the purpose of quality assurance. *Phys. Med. Biol.* 2013; **58**(19):7025–7037.

79 Gagneur, J. D., and Ezzell, G. A. An improvement in IMRT QA results and beam matching in linacs using statistical process control. *J. Appl. Clin. Med. Phys.* 2014; **15**(5):4927.

80 Keen, J., and Page, D. J. Variability from the differences between successive readings. *J. R. Stat. Soc. Ser. C Appl. Stat.* 1953; **2**(1):13–23.

81 Wheeler, D. J., and Chambers, D. S. *Understanding Statistical Process Control.* Knoxville, TN, SPC Press, 1992.

82 Pawlicki, T., Yoo, S., Court, L. E., et al. Moving from IMRT QA measurements toward independent computer calculations using control charts. *Radiother. Oncol.* 2008; **89**(3):330–337.

APPENDIX: ANSWERS TO SELECTED PROBLEMS

Chapter 1: Atomic structure and radioactive decay

1.1 $Z = 8$; $A = 17$; mass defect = 0.141367 amu; E_b = 131.6 MeV; $(E_b)_{\text{avg/nucleon}} = 7.74$ MeV

1.2 15.999 amu

1.3 W: 58.2 keV; H 10.1 eV

1.4 e: 0.51 MeV; p: 937.7 MeV

1.5 2.37×10^{24} fissions; 0.85 g

1.6 isotopes : $^{14}_{6}C$, $^{15}_{6}C$; $^{14}_{7}N$, $^{15}_{7}N$, $^{16}_{8}O$, $^{17}_{8}O$

isotones : $^{14}_{6}C$, $^{15}_{7}N$, $^{16}_{8}O$, $^{15}_{6}C$, $^{16}_{7}N$, $^{17}_{8}O$

isobars : $^{14}_{6}C$, $^{14}_{7}N$; $^{15}_{6}C$ $^{15}_{7}N$; $^{16}_{7}N$, $^{16}_{8}O$

1.7 28.6 days; 42.9 days

1.8 1600 years

1.9 essentially 100%

1.10 9.5 ng; N = 17.8×10^{13} atoms; 49.0 ng

1.11 37%

1.12 1 MeV; $\lambda = 1.24 \times 10^{-3}$ nm; $\nu = 2.4 \times 10^{20}$ s^{-1}

15 MeV; $\lambda = 0.08 \times 10^{-3}$ nm; $\nu = 36.3 \times 10^{20}$ s^{-1}

1.13 $^{126}_{53}I \rightarrow {}^{126}_{54}Xe + {}^{0}_{-1}\beta + \ddot{\upsilon}$

$^{126}_{53}I \rightarrow {}^{126}_{54}Te + {}^{0}_{1}\beta + \upsilon$

$^{126}_{53}I + {}^{0}_{-1}e \rightarrow {}^{126}_{54}Te + \upsilon$

1.14 6.15×10^{14} atoms; 9.2×10^{-8} g

1.15 691×10^{3} MBq

1.16 ^{131}I negatron decay; ^{125}I electron capture and possibly positron decay

1.17 160

1.18 0.018 MeV; 0.018 MeV

1.19 1.98 MeV; 0.96 MeV

Chapter 2: Interactions of x rays and gamma rays

2.1 $I = (1/10)I_0 \, I_{O_e}^{-\mu(\text{TVL})}$

$\ln(l/10) = 2.30 \log(l/10) = -\mu(\text{TVL})$

$-2.30 = -\mu \, (\text{TVL})$

$\text{TVL} = 2.30/\mu$

2.2 —

2.3 0.59

2.4 2.5 cm

2.5 2 keV; 25 keV

2.6 138 keV; 12 keV; decreased

2.7 86.5 keV

2.8 $\Delta\lambda = 0.00243(1 - \cos\emptyset)$

for $\emptyset \geq 60°$, $\cos\emptyset \leq 0.5$

$\Delta\lambda \geq 0.00124$ nm

For high-energy photons, $\lambda \ll \Delta\lambda$

and can be ignored

$\lambda' = \lambda + \Delta\lambda \approx \Delta\lambda$

$h\nu \leq 1.24/0.00124$ nm

≤ 1000 keV, which is below threshold for pair production

2.9 13.2 cm

2.10 0.9 cm^2/g

2.11 1000 cm of absorber will not attenuate all the photons in the beam. The interpretation of the linear attenuation coefficient as the fraction of photons attenuated per unit thickness of absorber is only valid for a thin absorber. An absorber thickness of 1000 cm in this case would be considered a thick absorber.

2.12 A homogeneity coefficient greater than unity would be possible if the beam were to soften passing through an absorber. This could be possible if the higher-energy components of the beam were selectively attenuated more than the lower-energy components. This would occur for very high-energy photon beams, where pair production was the primary interaction, and the attenuation coefficient increased with increasing energy.

2.13 The scattered dose would be more dependent on field size for 6 MV photons.

Hendee's Radiation Therapy Physics, Fourth Edition. Todd Pawlicki, Daniel J. Scanderbeg and George Starkschall.
© 2016 John Wiley & Sons, Inc. Published 2016 by John Wiley & Sons, Inc.

Chapter 3: Interactions of particulate radiation with matter

3.1 3.3
3.2 2.04 keV/cm
3.3 5150 IP/cm
3.4 3 cm; 10 cm
3.5 0.054; 0.180
3.6 The collision stopping power is the rate of energy loss resulting from the sum of the soft and hard collisions. The energy spent in collision interactions produces ionization and excitation contributing to the dose near the particle's track.

Chapter 4: Machines for producing radiation

4.1 1.25×10^{18}; 20 kW (20,000 J/sec)
4.2 11.3 degrees
4.3 250 keV; 0.023; 0.005 nm
4.4 0.58 cm; 10.6 cm
4.5 a) 0.98 cm
        b) 34% smaller (0.53 cm)
4.6 1137 Ci/g
4.7 See Problem 1-12; $\lambda = 0.21 \times 10^{-3}$ nm
4.8 1.005; 1.15; 7.09
4.9 7.4 cm; 14.22 – 15.78 MeV ($\pm 5.2\%$)
4.10 A magnetron transforms DC power to radiofrequency power. The central cylindrical cathode is surrounded by an anode block made of copper that has resonant cavities with a circular layout. The magnetron is placed in a homogeneous magnetic field. Electrons emitted from the central cathode follow a complex cycloidal path to the anode because of the effect of DC pulses and the magnetic field. The radiofrequency energy induced in the magnetic field by this process is trapped in the resonant cavities. A loop antenna inserted in one of the cavities taps the radiofrequency energy in the cavities and transfers it to a waveguide for transmission to the accelerator waveguide. The klystron, on the other hand, is not a high-frequency generator but a microwave amplifier. The tube requires a low-power radiofrequency oscillator (driver) to supply RF power to the first cavity (buncher). As electron bunches arrive at the second cavity (catcher cavity), they are decelerated and their energy is transformed into a pulse of microwave power.
4.11 In a standing wave linear accelerator, microwaves are reflected from the ends of the accelerator waveguide. The backward traveling wave interferes with the forward traveling wave. The resulting standing wave has a magnitude of approximately double that of the traveling wave. In alternate spaces between discs, the magnitude of the wave is always at, or near, zero.

Chapter 5: Measurement of ionizing radiation

5.1 69×10^{15} IP; 1.11×10^{-2} Coulombs; 48.4×10^{-2} J/m^3; 37.4×10^{-2} J/kg; 37.4×10^{-2} Gy
5.2 65.7 R/min
5.3 7.8×10^{10} MeV/m^2 – sec; 15.6×10^{11} MeV/m^2
5.4 2.28×10^{15} photons/m^2; 2.28×10^{15} MeV/m^2
5.5 7.4
5.6 0.28 nA
5.7 47 pFd
5.8 300 R or 7.7×10^{-2} Coulombs/kg
5.9 10 J/kg; 8 J
5.10 0.85
5.11 2.5 cSv
5.12 0.014°C
5.13 9.6×10^{17}
5.14 1.5 mm A1; 2.25 mm A1; 0.7

Chapter 6: Calibration of megavoltage beams of x rays and electrons

6.1 75.2 R/min; 0.95 Gy/min
6.2 2.04; 4.37; 0.963
6.3 0.12%
6.4 0.996
6.5 1.009
6.6 80.7%; 0.972

Chapter 7: Central-axis point dose calculations

7.1 28.2%; 129 cGy
7.2 1.272
7.3 353.6 cGy
7.4 268 cGy; 102 cGy
7.5 89% primary; 11% scatter
7.6 10.1×10.1 cm^2; 274 cGy; 95 cGy
7.7 increase by a factor of 2.12
7.8 0.763 cGy/MU; 262 MU
7.9 5.28 min; 0.76 rev/min
7.10 0.54
7.11 61.0

Chapter 8: External beam dose calculations

8.1 $\frac{(20 \times 20 \times 15)}{(10 \times 10 \times 15)} \times \frac{5^3}{4^3} = 4 \times 1.95 = 7.8$, or almost a factor of 8
8.2 Primary dose, Direct beam phantom scatter dose, Head scatter dose, and Contaminant charged particle dose. Dose calculation uncertainty plays a role in modeling the

patient surface dose and at tissue interface boundaries between high- and low-density tissue (or materials such as metal implants).

8.3   **a)** $Dose_{point} = Dose_{primary} + Dose_{scatter}$
   b) $Dose_{point} = 70\ cGy + 30\ cGy = 100\ cGy$

8.4 $Dose_Q = 0.03 \times Dose_P + Dose_{scatter} = 0.03 \times 200\ cGy + 2\ cGy = 8\ cGy$; A block in radiation therapy is about 5 HVLs resulting in about 3% transmission of the primary beam. The dose falls off rapidly outside the open field and it was estimated that only 1% of the direct beam contributed to the scatter dose ($0.01 \times Dose_p$).

8.5   Monte Carlo calculated dose distributions have an associated statistical uncertainty due to the random sampling of the transport parameters from the probability density functions. Other dose calculation methods have associated systematic uncertainty.

8.6   The calculation speed for Monte Carlo electron beam dose calculations is faster than Monte Carlo photon beam dose calculations because electrons deposit dose directly and fewer histories are needed to achieve a statistically reliable result.

Chapter 9: External beam treatment planning and delivery

9.1   —

9.2   In forward planning, the treatment planner must choose the beam weighting (how much dose per beam) for each beam, whereas in inverse planning, a computer algorithm (optimization algorithm) chooses the beam weighting. In current practice, the treatment planner must also choose the beam angles (or arcs in VMAT) for both forward and inverse treatment planning.

9.3   DRR stands for *digitally reconstructed radiograph*. The DRR is a computer-generated x-ray image that is used to compare to a planar image captured on the treatment machine of the patient in the treatment position. The DRR is created by ray-tracing from a virtual x-ray source through the patient's CT scan and calculating the attenuation of rays. The slice thickness of the CT scan plays a role in the quality of the DRR image so that ray tracing through a thin slice CT data (e.g., 0.25 cm slice thickness) set will produce a clearer DRR than ray-tracing through a thick slide CT data set (e.g., 1.0 cm slice thickness).

9.4   Beam's eye view (BEV) represents the vantage point of looking *from* the radiation machine (as if you were the radiation source) *toward* the patient (through the beam collimating devices) so that you see what the radiation beam sees.

9.5   GTV = gross tumor volume, which represents demonstrable disease by physical exam or imaging.

CTV = clinical tumor volume, which is the region of the patient that includes microscopic disease based on knowledge of tumor spread.

PTV = planning target volume, which is a not a physical concept but represents any additional margin needed to ensure GTV and CTV dose coverage during a course of radiotherapy. It includes patient setup inaccuracies.

ITV = internal tumor volume, which includes the CTV and accounts for intrafractional tumor motion and interfractional anatomic variation. For targets in the thorax, for example, the ITV can be determined in part by using a 4D-CT scan.

PRV = planning organ at risk volume, which is the normal tissue organ to be spared during radiotherapy including a margin for patient setup uncertainty and motion.

9.6   Cumulative dose matrix:

0	0	0	0	0	20	20	0	0	0
0	0	0	0	0	45	45	0	0	0
0	0	0	0	0	90	90	0	0	0
35	65	120	160	175	330	315	120	85	40
35	65	120	160	175	365	350	120	85	40
35	65	120	160	175	330	315	120	85	40
0	0	0	0	0	90	90	0	0	0
0	0	0	0	0	45	45	0	0	0
0	0	0	0	0	15	15	0	0	0

Normalized dose matrix: The skin is everything inside the matrix; the thick dashed line is the OAR and the thick solid line is the PTV.

0	0	0	0	0	5	5	0	0	0
0	0	0	0	0	12	12	0	0	0
0	0	0	0	0	25	25	0	0	0
10	18	33	44	48	90	86	60	23	11
10	18	33	44	48	100	96	60	23	11
10	18	33	44	48	90	86	60	23	11
0	0	0	0	0	25	25	0	0	0
0	0	0	0	0	12	12	0	0	0
0	0	0	0	0	4	4	0	0	0

DVH

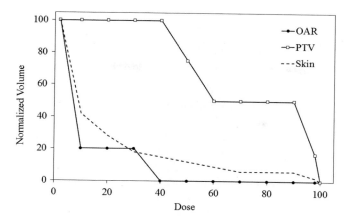

9.7 An objective or cost function is a mathematical expression that quantifies the difference between a target value and the actual value of some parameter. It is used in an optimization algorithm. For radiotherapy, the objective or cost function is typically the difference between the prescribed dose and the dose as calculated in the treatment planning. The two categories of optimization algorithms are deterministic (e.g., gradient decent) and stochastic (e.g., simulated annealing).

9.8 $(15 \times 2) \times (15 \times 2) \times 9 = 8100$, or over eight thousand adjustable parameters.

9.9 brain < 6000 cGy (< 3% symptomatic necrosis), spinal cord < 5000 cGy (< 0.2% myelopathy), cochlea mean < 4500 cGy (< 30% sensory-neural hearing loss), larynx < 6600 cGy (< 20% vocal dysfunction), and parotids < 2500 cGy (< 20% long-term salivary function < 25%)

For SRS Tx, brain = V12 < 5–10 cc (< 20% symptomatic necrosis), spinal cord < 1300 cGy (1% myelopathy), cochlea < 1400 cGy (< 25% sensory-neural hearing loss).

Chapter 10: The basics of medical imaging

10.1 From the Hubbell and Seltzer tables (see reference 1 in Chapter 10), the mass attenuation coefficients of relevance are:

	Density	(μ/ρ) 20 keV	(μ/ρ) 40 keV
Breast tissue	0.9 g/cm³	6.89×10^{-1} cm²/g	2.53×10^{-1} cm²/g
Calcification	1.5 g/cm³	1.31×10^{1} cm²/g	1.83×10^{0} cm²/g

At 20 keV:
- Breast tissue:
$$\frac{I}{I_0} = exp\left(-0.9 \times 6.89 \times 5\right) = 0.0450$$

- With calcification:
$$\frac{I}{I_0} = exp(-0.9 \times 6.89 \times 10^{-1} \times 4.9 - 1.5 \times 1.31$$
$$\times 10^{-1} \times 0.1) = 0.0067$$

In the presence of the calcification, the 20 keV beam intensity is reduced to 0.0067/0.0450, or a factor of 0.149 of its value in the absence of the calcification.

At 40 keV:
- Breast tissue:
$$\frac{I}{I_0} = exp\left(-0.9 \times 2.53 \times 10^{-1} \times 5\right) = 0.3202$$

- With calcification:
$$\frac{I}{I_0} = exp(-0.9 \times 2.53 \times 10^{-1} \times 4.9 - 1.5 \times 1.83$$
$$\times 10^{0} \times 0.1) = 0.2490$$

In the presence of the calcification, the 40 keV beam intensity is reduced to 0.2490/0.3202, or a factor of 0.778 of its value in the absence of the calcification.

10.2 In Example 10-3, we found that the precision of a digital thermometer in which temperatures were represented by 16 bits is the dynamic range (140°) divided by 216, or 0.002°. If we reduce the bit representation to 8 bits, we have 28 = 256 levels, so the precision is 0.5°.

10.3 A typical CT image data set is $512 \times 512 \times 12$ bits = 3×106 bits. If we represent the images as 2 byte images, we have $512 \times 512 \times 2 = 500$ kB = 0.5 MB. That is a good number to remember.

10.4 If the field of view is 50 cm, each pixel is approximately 1 mm × 1 mm. A typical dose matrix in a radiation treatment planning system is in the range 2 mm × 2 mm to 5 mm × 5 mm.

Chapter 11: Diagnostic imaging and applications to radiation therapy

11.1 4.2 MB

11.2 2.5 lp/mm

11.3 air – 1000; bone + 1000

11.4 0.23%

11.5 160 μsec

11.6 63.9 MHz

Chapter 12: Tumor targeting: Image-guided and adaptive radiation therapy

12.1 If too great a pitch were used, part of the CT image would be undersampled. In some of the older implementations of 4D image acquisition, blank spaces could be seen in coronal and sagittal reconstructions, where incomplete information in a transverse plane was acquired.

12.2 An MIP image encompasses the envelope of the GTV motion during respiration. Adding a CTV margin to the MIP does not take account of regions where microscopic spread is unlikely, such as spread into the chest wall or across lobar boundaries, which would not be included in a CTV based on the GTV at each phase. Hence an ITV generated from an MIP image is an upper limit to the true ITV.

12.3 Suppose the ITV was spherical with a radius of 1 cm. With a total margin of 0.86 cm, the radius of the PTV would be 1.86 cm, giving a volume of 27.0 cm^3. Removing the systematic uncertainty gives a PTV radius of 1.33 cm and a volume of 9.85 cm^3.

12.4 Because of the shielding required in the head of a linear accelerator, it would take an inordinately large force to stop a fast gantry rotation in the event of an emergency. Consequently, limitations are placed on the speed of gantry rotation.

12.5 A typical 4D-CT data set consists of 10 3D CT data sets. Each data set corresponds to a different phase of the respiratory cycle. Therefore, a 30 cm scan length at 2.5 mm slice thickness will have 120 CT scan slices. For 10 data sets, a 4D-CT scan would have 1200 individual CT slices. Note that larger regions of the patient will result in a correspondingly greater number of scan slices. For the above example, including the diaphragm as a surrogate for tumor motion could result in 2000 CT scan slices.

Chapter 13: Computer systems

13.1 **a)** ROM
13.2 **c)** input, processing, output, storage
13.3 **d)** Secure Socket Layer
13.4 **a)** 100 TB; kilo (K) is 10^3, mega (M) is 10^6, giga (G) is 10^9, and tera (T) is 10^{12}
Bytes (B) is a unit of storage.
13.5 **b)** pixels, width by height or 1280 columns by 800 rows of pixels
13.6 Decimal: 59037
13.7 Binary: 111 1100 1011
13.8

	1	0	0	1	1		19
		1	0	1			×5
	1	0	0	1	1		
	0	0	0	0	0		
1	0	0	1	1	0	0	
1	0	1	1	1	1	1	95

13.9 2.36 minutes for a 1 Mb per second network
0.14 seconds for a 1 Gb per second network

13.10 3,616 CT data sets for a 64 GB storage device
56,514 CT data sets for a 1 TB storage device

Chapter 14: Radiation oncology informatics

14.1 A representation of information and knowledge within a specific area of interest (domain knowledge)

14.2 Concepts can be well defined as well as the relationship among concepts so that information, research, and clinical findings can be collected, organized and characterized.

14.3 DICOM-RT contains several extensions to DICOM version 3 standard, including: RT Image, RT Plan, RT Dose, RT Structure Set, and RT Treatment Record.

14.4 Examples are quantities related to 4D-CT and treatment planning, such as phase-tagged CT images and dose distributions and respiratory traces. These might eventually be incorporated into the DICOM-RT standard at some later date, however.

14.5 A major advantage of structured database is ease of performing longitudinal studies among many patients. Freeform text is probably much easier for the user to enter information.

14.6 Obstacles can be: unwillingness of the user to adapt to the change, difficulty using software, and undefined or unclear new procedures for the user.

14.7 Software as a Service, Infrastructure as a Service, and Platform as a Service.

Chapter 15: Physics of proton radiation therapy

15.1 The relativistic mass is given by:

$$m = \frac{E_{tot}}{c^2}$$

where:

$$E_{tot} = KE + m_0 c^2$$

The kinetic energy of the proton is 250 MeV, and the rest energy is 931 MeV, so the total energy is 1181 MeV. The relativistic mass is then 1181/931 = 1.27 times the rest mass of the proton.

15.2 From Table 15-2, we see that a 140 MeV proton beam has a range of 10.2 cm in a 10 cm × 10 cm field. The next lower energy of 120 MeV would have a range of 6.9 cm, which would not be sufficient to cover the target.

15.3 From Figure 15-2, it appears that approximate weights of 40% of the weight of the highest energy component are necessary to yield the SOBP in the figure.

15.4 The smearing radius is an amount added to the thickness of a compensating filter to account for setup uncertainties, motion, and multiple scattering of the protons. Using the formula:

$$SR = \sqrt{(IM + SM)^2 + (0.03 \times \text{range})^2}$$

we find the smearing radius to be given by:

$$SR = \sqrt{(1.0 + 0.5)^2 + (0.03 \times 8.0)^2}$$
$$= 1.5 \text{ cm}$$

15.5 Conversion of CT number to stopping power contributes a range uncertainty of 2–3%; uncertainties in proton scattering affect range compensation to 3% of the range of the protons.

15.6 The factors that go into the dose rate are the relative output factor (change in dose per MU for a different beam energy with a designated RMW and a second scatterer for the deepest range with no range shifter in the beam), the SOBP factor (change in dose per MU with the change in the SOBP width), the range shifter factor (change in dose per MU with the thickness of the range shifter), the SOPB off-center factor (change in dose per MU with the location of the measurement point in the direction of beam away from the center of the SOBP), the off-center ratio, the field size factor (change in the dose per MU with a change of open field size), the inverse square factor (correction from distance of reference measurement to actual distance of dose calculation), the compensator and patient scatter factor (accounts for the presence of the compensator as well as scatter from inhomogeneities in patient anatomy).

Chapter 16: Sources for implant therapy and dose calculation

16.1 —
16.2 **a)** Once the daughters are in secular equilibrium, their activities equal that of the parent (10 mCi).
 b) 6.5×10^{-8} g (0.65 ng)
16.3 2.6×10^{-4} cm^3. No, an inert "filler" material is mixed with the RaSO$_4$.
16.4 1.76 mCi; 0.63 mCi
16.5 1.27 cGy · cm^2/hr
16.6 1.61 mCi
16.7 0.19 R/hr
16.8 **a)** 1.98 cGy/hr; 0.32 cGy/hr
 b) 1.85 cGy/hr; 0.30 cGy/hr

Chapter 17: Brachytherapy treatment planning

17.1 2.1 cm

17.2 33,303 cGy (using the air kerma strength calculation method)
17.3 24.4 hr; 483 cGy
17.4 1.1 mR/hr
17.5 5.26 cGy/hr; 197 days

Chapter 18: Radiation protection

18.1 5×10^{-5}; yes
18.2 0.45 Sv (45 rem); 0.05 Sv (5 rem); 0.045 Sv (4.5 rem)
18.3 0.16 mGy/hr; 2.1 cm; 1.4 cm
18.4 165 cm concrete; 90 cm
18.5 35 cm
18.6 80 cm; no
18.7 If about a third of the patients have three times the number of monitor units, this will effectively double the workload of the linear accelerator. A safety factor of 10 should still be able to accommodate this, but this type of analysis should be part of implementing an IMRT program in existing vaults.

Chapter 19: Quality assurance

19.1 **a)** 4% reduction in dose
 b) 0.1% reduction in dose
19.2 146 monitor units
19.3 739 cGy
19.4 71 milliröntgens
19.5 ±3.3%. No, it exceeds the specification of ±3%.
19.6 —
19.7 to reduce the risk of spreading radioactive contamination
19.8 tongue-and-groove effect
19.9 0.4% or 0.8 cGy; no

Chapter 20: Patient safety and quality improvement

20.1 Confirmation bias is the tendency to favor information as confirming one's existing beliefs. Hindsight bias is the perception that events that occurred in the past are more predictable than they really are. These biases are relevant to performing a root cause analysis.
20.2 Adding a CT simulation box to the process map could be helpful. The setup and creation of immobilization devices during the CT simulation process can lead to problems of patient setup at the time of treatment.
20.3 You will most likely find that people have different understandings of how clinical processes work. Therefore, it is important to use a multidisciplinary team when creating process maps as well as people who are directly involved in the process.

20.4 FMEA = failure modes and effects analysis; RPN = risk priority number

20.5 20-5. There is no single correct answer to this question. One possible answer is given here.

Potential failure mode	Effect of failure mode	O	S	D	RPN
The CBCT is poor quality and is incorrectly matched to the CT (i.e., anatomical structures are misidentified by the user)	The patient shifts are wrong or not optimal	2	9	3	54
The CBCT is good quality but is incorrectly matched to the CT (i.e., anatomical structures are misidentified by the user)	The patient shifts are wrong or not optimal	3	9	7	189
The CBCT is good quality and is matched correctly but the comparison software computes the shift incorrectly	The patient shifts are wrong or not optimal	1	9	10	90

The highest RPN value is for the failure mode of the CBCT being incorrectly matched to the CT (RPN = 189). The Detectability can be reduced by ensuring that the match of the CBCT to the CT is independently reviewed by a second qualified person before the shift is applied. The Occurrence can be reduced by ensuring that an adequate training and competency assessment program exists in the department. With these two mitigation strategies implemented, it can be estimated that O becomes 2 and D becomes 3, bringing the new RPN to 54. Note that these mitigation strategies do not help the failure mode, "The CBCT is good quality and is matched correctly but the comparison software computes the shift incorrectly." To mitigate this failure mode, other machine- and software-specific quality assurance checks would need to be implemented.

20.6 (1) collect information, (2) identify causes, (3) propose recommendations for remediation, and (4) implement the remediation and monitor for effectiveness

20.7 PDSA = plan–do–study–act; DMAIC = define, measure, analyze, improve, control. Both of these are quality improvement methodologies that utilize data-driven techniques and the scientific process. DMAIC is at the core of six-sigma and is a more structured approach to quality improvement than PDSA. Six-sigma also includes specific ties to senior management and financial gains of quality improvement efforts.

20.8 We can conclude that the Data Set 1 (see diagram) process is in-control and performing consistently but it is not able to meet the clinical requirements of ±5.0. The Data Set 2 (see diagram)process is performing within ±5.0 but the process is unstable. Specifically, case number 8 is out of control.

20.9 —

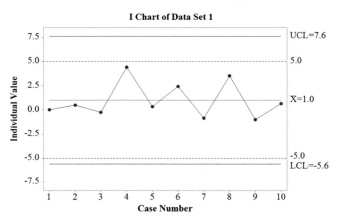

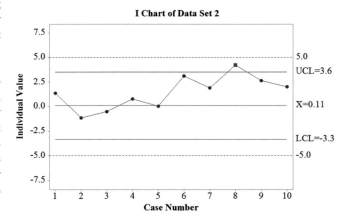

INDEX

Hendee's Radiation Therapy Physics, Fourth Edition. Todd Pawlicki, Daniel J. Scanderbeg and George Starkschall.
© 2016 John Wiley & Sons, Inc. Published 2016 by John Wiley & Sons, Inc.